PRIMARY CARE SECRETS

Second Edition

Publisher: HANLEY & BELFUS, INC.
                    Medical Publishers
                    210 South 13th Street
                    Philadelphia, PA 19107
                    (215) 546-7293; 800-962-1892
                    FAX (215) 790-9330
                    Web site: http://www.hanleyandbelfus.com

Note to the reader: Although the information in this book has been carefully reviewed for correctness of dosage and indications, neither the authors nor the editor nor the publisher can accept any legal responsibility for any errors or omissions that may be made. Neither the publisher nor the editor makes any warranty, expressed or implied, with respect to the material contained herein. Before prescribing any drug, the reader must review the manufacturer's current product information (package inserts) for accepted indications, absolute dosage recommendations, and other information pertinent to the safe and effective use of the product described.

Library of Congress Cataloging-in-Publication Data

Primary care secrets : questions you will be asked on rounds, in the clinic,
    on oral exams / edited by Jeanette Mladenovic. — 2nd ed.
        p.   cm. — (The Secrets Series®)
    Includes bibliographical references and index.
    ISBN 1-56053-305-6 (alk. paper)
    1. Internal medicine—Miscellanea.   2. Primary care (Medicine)—
Miscellanea.   I. Mladenovic, Jeanette., 1949–   . II. Series.
    [DNLM: 1. Primary Health Care examination questions.   2. Internal
Medicine examination questions.   W 18.2 P951 1999]
RC48.P736   1999
616'.0076—dc21
DNLM/DLC
for Library of Congress   98-42098
                                                           CIP

PRIMARY CARE SECRETS, 2nd edition   ISBN 1-56053-305-6

Last digit is the print number: 9   8   7   6   5   4   3   2   1

DEDICATION

To my total support system,

Steve

and

Ben, Jessica, Amy, Jeffrey

CONTENTS

CONTRIBUTORS

Irene Aguilar, M.D.
Instructor, Community Health, Denver Health Medical Center, Denver, Colorado

Stephen F. Albert, D.P.M.
Associate Professor, Department of Surgery, and Chief, Podiatric Section, Department of Surgery, University of Colorado Health Sciences Center, Denver; Chief, Podiatric Section, Surgery Service, VA Medical Center, Denver, Colorado

Catherine Amlie-Lefond, M.D.
Assistant Professor of Neurology and Pediatrics, State University of New York at Syracuse, Syracuse, New York

C. Alan Anderson, M.D.
Assistant Professor of Neurology and Emergency Medicine, Department of Neurology, University of Colorado School of Medicine, Denver, Colorado

Joseph Anderson, M.D.
Assistant Professor of Clinical Medicine, Departments of Gastroenterology and General Medicine, State University of New York at Stony Brook, Stony Brook, New York

Elizabeth L. Aronsen, M.D.
Clinical Assistant Professor, Department of Medicine, Pulmonary Division, University of Colorado Health Sciences Center, Denver; Vice-Chairman, Department of Medicine, Rose Medical Center, Denver, Colorado

Roberta K. Beach, M.D., M.P.H.
Associate Professor of Pediatrics and Adolescent Medicine, Department of Pediatrics, University of Colorado School of Medicine, Denver; Assistant Director, Community Health Services, Denver Health Authority, Denver, Colorado

Daniel H. Bessesen, M.D.
Assistant Professor of Medicine, Department of Medicine, Denver Health Medical Center and the University of Colorado Health Sciences Center, Denver, Colorado

Bahri Bilir, M.D.
Assistant Professor of Medicine, Department of Medicine, Division of Gastroenterology, University of Colorado School of Medicine, Denver, Colorado

Jon M. Braverman, M.D.
Director, Division of Ophthalmology, Denver Health Medical Center; Assistant Clinical Professor of Ophthalmology, University of Colorado Health Sciences Center, Denver, Colorado

John F. Bridges, M.D.
Assistant Professor, Department of Psychiatry, Denver Health Medical Center and University of Colorado School of Medicine, Denver, Colorado

Edmund Casper, M.D.
Associate Professor, Departments of Psychiatry and Behavioral Health, University of Colorado School of Medicine, Denver; Director, Behavioral Health, Denver Health, Denver, Colorado

Gayle S. Cekada, M.D.
Internal Medicine Physician, Department of Internal Medicine, University of Colorado School of Medicine, Denver, Colorado

Arlene B. Chapman, M.D.
Associate Professor of Medicine, Division of Renal Diseases and Hypertension, University of Colorado Health Sciences Center, Denver Health and Hospitals, Denver, Colorado

David H. Collier, M.D.
Associate Professor of Medicine, Department of Medicine, Division of Rheumatology, University of Colorado Health Sciences Center, Denver; Chief, Department of Rheumatology, Denver Health Medical Center, Denver, Colorado

Alan B. Cooper, M.D.
Formerly Fellow in Nephrology, Department of Medicine, University of Colorado Health Sciences Center, Denver, Colorado; currently in Private Practice

Mary Ann De Groote, M.D.
Instructor, Department of Medicine, University of Colorado Health Sciences Center, Denver, Colorado

Susan J. Diem, M.D., M.P.H.
Assistant Professor of Medicine, Department of Medicine, University of Minnesota Medical School, Minneapolis, Minnesota

B. Jane Disrud, M.D.
Formerly Resident, Department of Neurology, University of Colorado School of Medicine, Denver, Colorado

Robert H. Eckel, M.D.
Professor of Medicine, Department of Medicine, Endocrinology Division, University of Colorado Health Sciences Center, Denver, Colorado

Raymond Estacio, M.D.
Assistant Professor of Medicine, Department of General Internal Medicine, University of Colorado Health Sciences Center, Denver, Colorado

Michele A. Ferguson, M.D.
Assistant Professor, Department of Neurology, University of Colorado School of Medicine, Denver, Colorado

Richard C. Fisher, M.D.
Associate Professor, Department of Orthopaedics, University of Colorado Health Sciences Center, Denver, Colorado

Katherine M. Fitting, M.D.
Medical Director, Renal Transplant Program, Presbyterian–St. Luke's, Denver, Colorado

Mark E. Fogarty, M.D.
Assistant Clinical Professor, Department of Internal Medicine, St. Louis University Health Sciences Center, St. Louis, Missouri

Carlos E. Girod, M.D.
Assistant Professor, Department of Medicine, Division of Pulmonary and Critical Care Medicine, University of Texas Southwestern Medical School, Dallas, Texas

James Goff, M.D.
Formerly Fellow in Gastroenterology, Department of Medicine, University of Colorado Health Sciences Center, Denver, Colorado

Loren E. Golitz, M.D.
Clinical Professor, Departments of Pathology and Dermatology, University of Colorado School of Medicine, Denver, Colorado

Mary Chri Gray, M.D.
Assistant Professor of Medicine, Department of Medicine, University of Colorado Health Sciences Center, Denver, Colorado

Michael E. Hanley, M.D.
Associate Professor of Medicine, Division of Pulmonary Sciences and Critical Care Medicine, University of Colorado School of Medicine, Denver, Colorado

Donald B. Hansen, B.S. (Pharm), Pharm D.
Formerly Pharmacy Clinical Coordinator, Denver General Hospital, Denver, Colorado

Fred D. Hofeldt, M.D.
Professor of Medicine, Department of Medicine, University of Colorado Health Sciences Center, Denver Health Medical Center, Denver, Colorado

Richard Hughes, M.D.
Associate Professor of Neurology, Department of Neurology, University of Colorado School of Medicine, Denver, Colorado

Evelyn Hutt, M.D.
Assistant Professor, Department of Medicine, University of Colorado School of Medicine, Denver, Colorado

Joyce Seiko Kobayashi, M.D.
Associate Professor, Department of Psychiatry, University of Colorado Health Sciences Center, Denver, Colorado

Laura M. Lasater, M.D.
Assistant Professor of Medicine, Department of Medicine, Denver Health Medical Center and the University of Colorado Health Sciences Center, Denver, Colorado

David W. Lehman, M.D., Ph.D.
Assistant Professor of Medicine, Division of General Internal Medicine, University of Colorado School of Medicine, Denver; Clinical Advisor, HIV Early Intervention Services, Denver Health Medical Center, Denver, Colorado

Meg A. Lemon, M.D.
Clinical Assistant Professor, Department of Dermatology, University of Colorado Health Sciences Center, Denver, Colorado

Michael L. Lepore, M.D., FACS
Professor, Vice-Chairman of Academic Affairs, and Program Director, Department of Otolaryngology—Head and Neck Surgery, University of Colorado School of Medicine, Denver; Medical/Surgical Director, Division of Otolaryngology, Denver Health Medical Center, Denver, Colorado

Allan Liebgott, M.D.
Associate Clinical Professor of Medicine, University of Colorado Health Sciences Center, Denver; Director of Correctional Telemetry, Denver Health Medical Center, Denver, Colorado

Stuart L. Linas, M.D.
Chief of Nephrology, Department of Medicine, Denver Health Medical Center; Professor of Medicine, University of Colorado Health Sciences Center, Denver, Colorado

Terry Linn, D.O.
Formerly Fellow in Gastroenterology, Department of Medicine, University of Colorado Health Sciences Center, Denver, Colorado

Richard P. Lofgren, M.D., M.P.H.
Professor and Chief, Department of General Internal Medicine, Medical College of Wisconsin, Milwaukee, Wisconsin

Thomas D. MacKenzie, M.D., M.S.P.H.
Assistant Professor of Medicine, Division of General Internal Medicine, University of Colorado Health Sciences Center, Denver, Colorado

Eric T. McFarling, M.D.
Formerly Instructor of Medicine, University of Colorado School of Medicine, Denver, Colorado

Philip S. Mehler, M.D.
Chief, General Internal Medicine, Denver Health Medical Center, Denver; Associate Professor of Medicine, Department of Medicine, University of Colorado Health Sciences Center, Denver, Colorado

Lawrence A. Meredith, M.D.
Assistant Clinical Professor of Neurology, Department of Neurology, University of Colorado School of Medicine, Denver, Colorado

Jeanette Mladenovic, M.D.
Professor and Vice-Chair, Department of Medicine, University of Colorado Health Sciences Center, Denver; Chief of Medicine, HealthONE Affiliated Hospitals, Denver, Colorado

Kavita Nanda, M.D., M.H.S.
Fellow, Division of Health Services Research, Department of General Medicine, Duke University Medical Center, Durham; Gynecologist, Durham VA Medical Center, Durham, North Carolina

Kristin L. Nichol, M.D., M.P.H.
Chief of Medicine, Minneapolis VA Medical Center; Professor, Department of Medicine, University of Minnesota School of Medicine, Minneapolis, Minnesota

Jerry A. Nick, M.D.
Assistant Professor of Medicine, Division of Pulmonary and Critical Care Medicine, University of Colorado School of Medicine, Denver, Colorado

Kathleen Ogle, M.D.
Medical Oncologist, Methodist Hospital, St. Louis Park, Minnesota

Norman E. Peterson, M.D.
Professor, Department of Surgery/Urology, University of Colorado Health Sciences Center, Denver; Associate Director, Divisions of Surgery and Urology, Denver Health Medical Center, Denver, Colorado

Jeffrey Pickard, M.D.
Assistant Professor of Medicine, Department of Internal Medicine, University of Colorado Health Sciences Center, Denver, Colorado

Randall R. Reves, M.D., MSc
Associate Professor of Medicine, Department of Medicine, Division of Infectious Diseases, University of Colorado Health Sciences Center, Denver, Colorado

Terri L. Richardson, M.D.
Assistant Professor, Department of General Internal Medicine, University of Colorado Health Sciences Center, Denver, Colorado

Julie Rifkin, M.D.
Assistant Professor of Medicine, Department of General Internal Medicine, HealthONE and University of Colorado Health Sciences Center, Denver, Colorado

Andrew R. Robinson, M.D.
Assistant Professor, Department of Internal Medicine, University of Colorado Health Sciences Center, Denver, Colorado

Hanna Bloomfield Rubins, M.D., M.P.H.
Chief of General Internal Medicine and Primary Care, Minneapolis VA Medical Center; Associate Professor of Medicine, University of Minnesota School of Medicine, Minneapolis, Minnesota

Iqbal S. Sandhu, M.D.
Senior Fellow, Department of Gastroenterology, University of Colorado Health Sciences Center, Denver, Colorado

Archana Shrestha, M.D.
Chief Resident and Research Fellow in Neurophysiology, Department of Neurology, University of Colorado Health Sciences Center, Denver, Colorado

Jeffrey M. Sippel, M.D.
Fellow, Pulmonary and Critical Care Medicine, Oregon Health Sciences University, Portland, Oregon

Lawrence G. Smith, M.D.
Professor, Department of Medicine, Mount Sinai School of Medicine, New York, New York

Andrew W. Steele, M.D., M.P.H.
Assistant Professor, Division of General Internal Medicine, University of Colorado School of Medicine, Denver, Colorado

Stephen E. Steinberg, M.D.
Professor of Medicine and Surgery, University of Colorado School of Medicine, Denver, Colorado

Benjamin T. Suratt, M.D.
Fellow, Department of Pulmonary and Critical Care Medicine, University of Colorado Health Sciences Center, Denver, Colorado

Thomas E. Trouillot, M.D.
Formerly Fellow in Gastroenterology, Department of Medicine, University of Colorado Health Sciences Center, Denver, Colorado

Valerie K. Ulstad, M.D., M.P.A., M.P.H.
Clinical Assistant Professor, Department of Internal Medicine, University of Minnesota Medical School, Minneapolis, Minnesota

Robert J. Valuck, Ph.D., R.Ph.
Assistant Professor, Department of Pharmacy Practice, University of Colorado School of Pharmacy, Denver, Colorado

Thomas R. Vendegna, M.D.
Formerly Pulmonary and Critical Care Physician, Department of Pulmonary and Critical Care Medicine, University of Colorado Health Sciences Center, Denver, Colorado; currently Staff Physician, French and Sierra Vista Hospital, San Obispo, California

Danny C. Williams, M.D., FRCPC, FACP, FACR
Assistant Professor of Medicine, Division of Rheumatology, University of Colorado Health Sciences Center, Denver, Colorado

Timothy J. Wilt, M.D., M.P.H.
Associate Professor, Department of Medicine, University of Minnesota School of Medicine, Minneapolis, Minnesota

Lisa Corbin Winslow, M.D.
Assistant Professor, Department of Medicine, HealthONE and University of Colorado Health Sciences Center, Denver, Colorado

PREFACE

Primary Care Secrets, 2nd edition is designed for physicians, residents, students, and other health care providers who must develop and maintain a practical and scholarly breadth of knowledge to deliver the necessary daily care to their patients. As the first professional contact for both preventive and therapeutic needs, primary care providers are often faced with problems much different from those intensive experiences that led to educational opportunities on the classic inpatient service. For this reason, the abbreviated topics selected from this overwhelmingly broad subject matter were organized (where possible) according to problems commonly facing the health care professional in the outpatient setting. Answers to the questions posed are not meant to be proscriptive in nature, but rather to address approaches, rationales, and often cost-effectiveness. In the second edition, expanded and updated chapters have new questions that specifically address clinical practice from the standpoint of evidence-based medicine. Additionally, new chapters about the physical examination, smoking cessation, and alternative medicine are included. The contributors include medical and surgical specialists and subspecialists, in addition to generalists. They have frequently provided opinions about which patients should be referred for the next level of care or admitted to the hospital. While the subject matter does not specifically address the primary care of newborns and children, issues unique to the pediatric patient are discussed in several, especially nonmedical, chapters.

Primary Care Secrets, 2nd edition is another text in the popular and unique Secrets Series® originated by the late Dr. Charles Abernathy, who cleverly acknowledged the time-honored Socratic educational approach in written format. Dr. Abernathy was a practicing academic surgeon whose energy and passion for life and medicine were infectious and apparent to all who were fortunate enough to cross his path. His intense commitment to the art of medicine, the fun of learning, and the fundamentals of teaching are embodied in *Secrets*. These should serve as his reminder to us that the practice of medicine is based upon "secrets" divulged within a relationship between physician and patient, and interpreted in the light of sound clinical evidence.

I would like to express my appreciation to all the contributors for their time and efforts, and to Vicky Kalasountas, once again, for her exceptional organizational skills in preparation of manuscripts and coordination of this project.

Jeanette Mladenovic, MD

I. Health Maintenance

1. PRINCIPLES OF PREVENTIVE MAINTENANCE AND TEST SELECTION

Richard P. Lofgren, M.D., M.P.H.

1. Why buy a test?
   There are three reasons to obtain a laboratory or diagnostic test.
   1. **Screening or case finding.** The purpose is to detect a condition before symptoms occur in the hope of altering the natural history of the disease.
   2. **Diagnosis of disease.** The purpose is to refine the diagnostic hypothesis either to "rule in" a disease if the likelihood of disease is high or to "rule out" a disease if the likelihood is low.
   3. **Patient management.** Tests can aid patient management by (a) monitoring the status of diseases, (b) identifying complications, (c) providing prognostic information, and (d) ensuring therapeutic levels.

2. What is the most important characteristic of a test used to monitor the status of a patient?
   The reproducibility of the test.

3. How is an "abnormal" test result defined?
   Differentiating normal from abnormal is often more difficult than it seems. A test may be abnormal based on three different definitions:
   1. **Normal distribution**. For most analytic tests, normal limits are determined by measurements done in a large number of subjects and are arbitrarily defined as the range encompassed by 2 standard deviations from the mean. With a normal curve distribution, 95% of observations are within 2 standard deviations from the mean.
   2. **Biologically normal**. The results of tests that are statistically normal may not be biologically normal. The classic example is cholesterol. There is a three-fold increase in the risk of cardiovascular disease with a high-normal cholesterol versus a low-normal cholesterol level.
   3. **Abnormal as treatable**. Abnormal not only refers to a value that increases the risk of bad outcome, but also to a result that, if treated, results in improved outcome. Initially hypertension was defined as a diastolic blood pressure above 105 mmHg, since studies had shown that treatment at that level was beneficial. With further studies the definition of "normal" has steadily decreased and may vary for different populations such as diabetic versus nondiabetic patients.

4. What are the limitations inherent in using the normal distribution as a definition of normal?
   • **Chance phenomenon**. By definition, 5% of subjects will have results that lie at the extremes and will be labeled abnormal. With any given test, a normal individual has a 1 in 20 chance of having an "abnormal" result. The likelihood of having an abnormal result increases in proportion to the number of independent tests performed. Sixty-four percent of normal individuals will have at least one abnormal result on a chemistry panel of 20 tests. Therefore, it is distinctly abnormal for a normal person to have a normal screening "chem 20" panel.

- **Physiologic variable**. Some physiologic variables, such as the alkaline phosphatase, have a skewed distribution.
- **Reference group**. Often the normal range is determined in young healthy volunteers (such as medical students). For many tests the distribution will vary by age, gender, or other important parameters.

5. What are the sensitivity and specificity of a test?

Although the terms are often defined mathematically, it is helpful to remember what they mean in simple language.

Sensitivity is the probability that a test will be positive if the disease is present.

Specificity is the probability that a test will be negative if the disease is absent. The terms can also be defined using a 2×2 table:

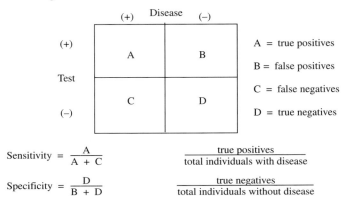

$$\text{Sensitivity} = \frac{A}{A + C} \qquad \frac{\text{true positives}}{\text{total individuals with disease}}$$

$$\text{Specificity} = \frac{D}{B + D} \qquad \frac{\text{true negatives}}{\text{total individuals without disease}}$$

6. If a test to detect a disease whose prevalence is 1/1000 has a 95% sensitivity and 95% specificity, what is the chance that a person found to have a positive result actually has the disease?

The answer is $< 2\%$. There is a 95% chance that the test will detect the one individual out of 1000 with the disease. However, with a 95% specificity or a 5% false-positive rate, 50 normal individuals will have an abnormal result. Therefore, only 1 of the 51 individuals with a "positive" result will actually have the disease.

This question was asked of 20 students, 20 residents, and 20 attending physicians, and only 18% gave the correct answer. The most common answer given was "95%," a gross overestimation of the likelihood of disease! Appropriately interpreting test results is not intuitively obvious. In order to interpret test results properly, it is essential the clinician make a "guesstimate" of the likelihood (or prevalence) of disease prior to obtaining the test. The most common mistake made in interpreting test results is failing to consider the probability of disease before the results are known. Once the results are in hand, clinicians tend to be swayed by the findings and inflate the accuracy of the test.

7. What is predictive value?

Sensitivity and specificity are characteristics of a test. They tell you the likelihood a test will be positive or negative if you already know if the disease is present or absent. Knowledge of test characteristics does not, per se, permit the accurate interpretation of the test result. In practice, the clinician needs to know the likelihood that the disease is absent or present when the result is positive or negative. This is the **predictive value** of a test. It is determined by the sensitivity and specificity of the test and the prevalence of the disease in the population. **Positive predictive value** is the probability that the disease is present given a positive test result. **Negative predictive value** is the probability that the disease is absent given a negative test result.

In order to accurately interpret the test results (i.e., the positive and negative predictive value), one has to know (or make an a priori educated guess) about the prevalence of the disease before obtaining the test. The predictive value can be calculated using Bayes' theorem or a 2×2 table if prevalence is known.

$$\text{Positive predictive value} = \frac{A}{A + B} \qquad \frac{\text{true positives}}{\text{total individuals with positive result}}$$

$$= \frac{(Se)(P)}{(Se)(P) + (1 - Sp)(1 - P)} \qquad \begin{array}{l} Se = \text{sensitivity} \\ Sp = \text{specificity} \\ P = \text{prevalence of disease} \end{array}$$

$$\text{Negative predictive value} = \frac{D}{C + D} \qquad \frac{\text{true negatives}}{\text{total individuals with negative result}}$$

$$= \frac{(1 - P)(Sp)}{(1 - P)(Sp) + (P)(1 - Se)}$$

8. When ruling out a disease, what kind of test is needed?

When ruling out a disease, the clinician suspects that the probability of disease is low (i.e., "it is possible but I doubt it"). In these situations, you must select a test that is almost always positive when the disease is present (a sensitive test). If such a test is negative, then the clinician can be confident that the likelihood of disease is remote. However, sensitive tests are not as specific and are subject to many false-positive results. If the pretest likelihood of disease is low and the test is positive, then it is likely a false-positive result. When the probability of disease is low, a negative result using a sensitive test yields a very high negative predictive value.

Conversely when ruling in disease, the clinician strongly suspects the disease is present. In these situations, the clinician wants a test that is rarely positive in people without the disease (a specific test). A positive result confirms the diagnosis, whereas a negative result is likely a false negative. When the probability of disease is high, a positive result using a specific test yields a very high positive predictive value.

In summary, there are two important rules to remember when interpreting laboratory results. When "ruling out" a disease, you should select a very sensitive test and you want the result to be negative. If it is positive, it is most likely a false-positive result and is not helpful (try to ignore the results). When "ruling in" disease, you should select a very specific test. If the result is positive, the diagnosis is confirmed. However, if the result is negative it is likely a false-negative result and not useful. Armed with these two simple rules, the clinician can correctly interpret test results without necessarily calculating the exact predictive value. Clinicians must resist being unduly influenced if the "unexpected" result is obtained.

9. How can you increase the sensitivity and specificity of your diagnostic strategy?

Often there is no single test that is sufficiently sensitive to rule out a disease (or sufficiently specific to rule in a disease). The clinician can improve the sensitivity or specificity of the diagnostic approach by using multiple tests. Using several tests in combination, or in parallel, will significantly increase the sensitivity (while decreasing the specificity) and thus the negative predictive value of the diagnostic strategy. If all of the tests used in combination are negative, then it is unlikely the disease is present. Conversely, using multiple tests in sequence, or series, significantly increases the specificity (while decreasing the sensitivity). If you do test A and if positive, do test B and if positive test C, then the clinician can be fairly certain the disease is present if all three tests are positive (a strong positive predictive value).

10. When should you screen for a disease?

There are important factors to consider before screening for a disease.

1. **Common disease**. The disease must be relatively common for a screening program to be cost-effective. If the disease is rare, a significant number of normal individuals will have a false-positive result and the predictive value will be poor. Individuals with a false-positive result may be subject to further expensive and perhaps invasive procedures.

2. **Cause significant morbidity**. The disease must result in significant suffering. For example, tinea pedis may be common but does not cause sufficient problems to warrant a screening program.

3. **An effective screening test must exist**. A screening program needs to have a test with reasonable test characteristics (sensitivity and specificity) and be practical, convenient, and inexpensive with few side effects. Because the majority of individuals will not have the disease, the screening process has to be acceptable to the patient. Although the complications of a cerebral aneurysm may be preventable, a screening program using cerebral angiograms is not practical or acceptable. However, screening for hypertension is simple and effective.

4. **Therapy must alter the natural history of disease**. Treatment early in the asymptomatic period should be superior to therapy started once symptoms develop. Data strongly suggest that removal of adenomatous colonic polyps decreases the incidence of colon cancer. Similarly, therapy of stage I breast cancer is superior to treatment of stage III disease. On the other hand, it is not clear that early treatment of asymptomatic hyperglycemia improves patient outcomes. Since early therapy is not clearly beneficial, screening for this important disease is questionable.

11. What is the difference between primary, secondary, and tertiary preventive care?

Primary prevention is an intervention designed to prevent a pathologic condition or disease from occurring. Examples include immunizations to prevent specific infectious diseases or wearing a seat belt to prevent bodily injury during an accident.

Secondary prevention is an intervention designed to prevent future morbidity and/or mortality by treating a condition during the asymptomatic period. Often early intervention is relatively simple and more effective therapy. Screening and treating malignancies such as cervical cancer, colon cancer, and breast cancer are examples of secondary prevention.

Tertiary prevention is an intervention designed to prevent complications in patients with an established disease. For example, treating an elevated cholesterol to prevent the progression of atherosclerosis in a patient with coronary artery disease is a tertiary preventive measure. Primary care physicians often spend considerable time delivering tertiary preventive services.

The distinction between the various types of preventive care can be blurred. For example, the treatment of hypertension could be primary intervention to prevent heart disease or tertiary intervention to prevent the progression of renal disease in a diabetic patient.

12. What is the purpose of the periodic health examination (PHE)?

1. **Preventing disease** (primary prevention), such as providing immunization
2. **Identifying risk factors** for common chronic disease, such as hyperlipidemia and obesity
3. **Case finding** (secondary prevention) to detect asymptomatic disease, such as screening for cervical or colorectal cancer, hypertension, and glaucoma
4. **Counseling and educating patients to promote health behavior such as diet, exercise, and smoking cessation**
5. **Updating the patient's clinical data**, including any new medical conditions, such as surgeries or allergies
6. **Enhancing patient/physician communication**. It is important that the patient knows and trusts the physician and becomes an active partner in his or her own health. Periodic examinations can help nurture this relationship.

The PHE is a time-honored but often maligned practice. Few preventive medicine procedures have been demonstrated to reduce mortality and morbidity by randomized trials. Discussions about the value of the PHE often fail to recognize the importance of points 5 and 6.

13. How well do physicians do in providing preventive service?

Unfortunately, not well. Studies from a variety of clinical settings report compliance rates from 75–99% for blood pressure determination, 40–80% for breast examination, 20–80% for Pap smears, 20–65% for hemoccult tests, 10–54% for mammograms, 8–20% for pneumococcal vaccines, and 5–40% for yearly influenza vaccines. Physicians fail to recognize more than 50% of patients with alcoholism and substance abuse. Physicians are knowledgeable, generally recognize the importance of preventive services, and typically overrate their own success. Providing preventive services often is not the top priority during an office visit.

14. How can physicians improve their success in providing preventive care?

To effectively implement a preventive medicine program into a busy practice setting, physicians need to develop a specific plan. Important elements include:

1. **Use of PHE**. Performance of the PHE improves provision of preventive measures. However, attendance rates are lower for purely preventive visits. It is often necessary to incorporate the services into regular office visits.

2. **Guidelines**. There are a number of competing and conflicting guidelines. The practice should adopt a set of guidelines that is acceptable and post it throughout the clinic setting.

3. **Flow sheet**. The use of a preventive medicine flow sheet in a prominent part of the medical records may help.

4. **Reminders**. A number of different strategies have been used to remind busy physicians to perform preventive service. In large clinics, automatic computer reminders, customized to individual patients, are effective.

5. **Allied health personnel**. Involving nursing and other professionals in the practice to initiate and implement preventive services can be effective.

15. Why and how do the recommended guidelines for preventive services vary?

Many professional organizations and societies, advisory panels, and federal organizations have issued guidelines. The content and frequency of the recommended preventive services are controversial and may vary significantly among published guidelines. In general, guidelines from specific professional societies, such as the American Cancer Society or the American Diabetes Association, are the most aggressive in recommending specific screening procedures.

On the other hand, the Canadian and U.S. Task Forces are more conservative in their recommendations. These task forces use explicit rules of evidence and criteria to generate recommendations. Recommendations to perform or not to perform a preventive service are based on the quality of the evidence that its performance would be beneficial. The strongest recommendations are reserved for interventions proved to be effective in well-designed studies. Measures are described as "clinically prudent" only if there is compelling *indirect* evidence. Many procedures receive no recommendations because the evidence of efficacy is lacking.

16. What is the difference between efficacy and effectiveness of preventive service?

Efficacy refers to the ability of an intervention to produce the desired outcome under optimal circumstances. Effectiveness is the performance of an intervention in a practice setting (i.e., does it still work in the heterogeneous environment of clinical practice?). Clinical studies usually involve highly motivated, selected patients with equally motivated health professionals. Oftentimes preventive services are not nearly as effective when applied in "real world" conditions. Unfortunately, the effectiveness of an intervention is rarely studied.

BIBLIOGRAPHY

1. Canadian Task Force on the Periodic Health Examination: Periodic health examination, 2: 1989 update. Can Med Assoc J 141:1136–1140, 1989.
2. Fletcher RH, Fletcher SW, Wagner EH: Clinical Epidemiology: The Essentials. Baltimore, Williams & Wilkins, 1982, pp 18–74.
3. Hayward RS, Steinberg EP, Ford DE, et al: Preventive care guidelines—1991. Ann Intern Med 114:758–783, 1991.
4. Holbrook JH: Periodic health examination for adults. In Stults BM, Dere W (eds): Practical Care of the Ambulatory Patient. Philadelphia, W.B. Saunders, 1989, pp 415–422.
5. Kern DE: Preventive medicine in ambulatory practice. In Barker LR, Burton JR, Zieve PD (eds): Principles of Ambulatory Medicine. Baltimore, Williams & Wilkins, 1991, pp 13–25.

6. US Preventive Services Task Force: Guide to Clinical Preventive Services. Baltimore, Williams & Wilkins, 1989.

7. Woolf SH: Analytic principles in assessing the effectiveness of clinical preventive services. In Goldbloom RB, Lawrence RS (eds): Preventing Disease Beyond the Rhetoric. New York, Springer-Verlag, 1990, pp 5–11.

2. EARLY CANCER DETECTION

Timothy J. Wilt, M.D., M.P.H.

1. Describe the four major biases that may result in invalid conclusions about the effectiveness of cancer screening methods.

1. **Lead time** is the length of time between detection of cancer with a screening test and the time at which the disease, by the presence of signs and symptoms, would have been detected in the absence of screening. Lead-time bias occurs when survival appears to be lengthened because screening simply advances the time of diagnosis, lengthening the period between diagnosis and death without altering the natural history of the disease.

2. **Length bias** also may overestimate the benefits of cancer screening. Less aggressive (slower-growing) tumors with relatively good prognoses are detected by screening programs more frequently because of their longer detectable preclinical phase compared with their more aggressive counterparts. Therefore, aggressive tumors are underrepresented in screening programs, resulting in apparent improved survival of screen-detected malignancies.

3. **Overdiagnosis bias** results when screening detects lesions that may not be clinically significant. Very early "cancers" detected during screening may never have caused symptomatic disease if they had been left undetected. Screening programs may overreport the number of malignancies that would have caused problems if not found by early detection.

4. **Selection bias** occurs because participants in screening programs are often different from the general population. They may participate because they are at higher risk for the disease, are more likely to comply with screening and treatment programs, and frequently have other health care practices that result in improved health outcome independently of the screening program.

2. The cancer detection and prevention guidelines of the United States Preventive Services Task Force (USPSTF) are based on a hierarchy of evidence in which greater importance is given to study designs that are less subjective to bias and misinterpretations. What study design provides the best evidence for effectiveness?

Randomized controlled trials. Participants are assigned in a randomized fashion to a group receiving the intervention or a control group. Randomization results in unbiased allocation of treatments and creation of comparable controls. Generalizability and representativeness of patients and results, however, may still be problematic.

3. Many cancers are rare. What type of study design is useful in investigating risk factors that may play a role in these diseases?

Case-control studies. Selection of study and control groups is based on whether participants have the disease rather than whether they have been exposed to a risk factor or intervention. By comparing people with and without the disease, investigators assess both groups for differences in risk factors preceding the onset of disease. Although useful for the study of rare diseases, this approach does not provide an estimate of incidence. In addition, representativeness of people with and without disease may be an issue.

4. Current evidence supports the practice of screening chest roentgenograms and/or sputum cytology to reduce lung cancer mortality. True or false?

False. The USPSTF has concluded that no good evidence supports screening for lung cancer, even in high-risk smokers. Chest roentgenograms and sputum cytology have been proposed as tests for early detection of lung cancer. However, several randomized controlled trials, a nonrandomized controlled trial, and two case-control studies have failed to demonstrate a reduction in lung cancer mortality from frequent screening with chest roentgenograms and sputum cytology. Currently, the National Cancer Institute is conducting the Prostate, Lung, Colorectal, and Ovarian Cancers (PLCO) Screening Trial to determine whether annual chest radiographic testing reduces lung cancer mortality compared with usual care.

5. What is the best method for preventing lung cancer?

Counseling patients against tobacco use is the best method of preventing lung cancer. Lung cancer is the leading cause of cancer-related mortality in both men and women. In 1997 there were an estimated 178,000 new cases of lung cancer and 160,000 lung cancer-related deaths. The 5-year survival rate of patients with lung cancer is less than 13%. Almost 90% of lung cancers are related to cigarette smoking and therefore should be preventable. Because smoking rates have increased in teenagers and women, efforts aimed at reducing smoking in these groups are particularly important. Passive or second-hand smoke also has been demonstrated to be associated with an increased risk of chronic lung and cardiac disease. Therefore, efforts have focused on developing smoke-free environments in public areas such as workplaces, airports, and restaurants.

6. Does screening for colon cancer with annual fecal occult blood tests reduce colon cancer mortality?

Yes. The results of three randomized controlled trials demonstrated that screening with fecal occult-blood testing (FOBT) reduces mortality from colorectal cancer by 15–33% compared with an unscreened control group. The reduction in colorectal cancer mortality was accompanied by a shift to detection at an earlier stage of cancer and improved survival in patients in whom cancer developed as compared with the control group. Screening annually with FOBTs and subsequent full colonoscopic evaluation for a positive FOBT reduce colon cancer deaths by about 3 per 1000 persons. The number of people who need to be screened to prevent 1 colon cancer death over 13 years is about 300. Colorectal cancer is one of the most common malignancies and the second leading cause of cancer-related death in the United States with approximately 130,000 new cases and 60,000 deaths annually.

7. What technical issues should be considered in conducting and interpreting the FOBT?

Screening with FOBTs involves many decisions, including identifying persons who should not be screened, type of test chosen, frequency of screening, restriction of diet and medication during screening, number of specimens collected, whether to rehydrate samples, and management of persons with a positive test.

FOBT should not be done in persons who are likely to have misleading results (e.g., active hemmorhoidal bleeding or symptoms and signs suggestive of colorectal cancer). Screening also should not be performed in people in whom additional evaluation and treatment are unlikely to be beneficial (life expectancy less than 10 years due to advanced age and/or comorbid conditions). The patient should prepare two slides from each of three consecutive bowel movements and should abstain from substantial doses of nonsteroidal antiinflammatory drugs, red meat, poultry, fish, some raw vegetables, and vitamin C. The slides should not be rehydrated and should be developed within 7 days. The optimal frequency (annual vs. biennial) for FOBT is not clear, but in general annual FOBT is recommended. If a patient has a positive test (one or more slide windows), the best approach for evaluation is to proceed directly to complete colorectal evaluation, preferably by colonoscopy. Because the sensitivity of the FOBT is limited for neoplasms (30–50%), a negative FOBT cannot rule out colorectal cancer. If signs or symptoms of colorectal cancer develop, the patient should undergo full colonoscopic evaluation.

8. Should flexible sigmoidoscopy or colonscopy be used for colon cancer screening?

In addition to FOBT, evidence from case-control studies suggests that screening with a 65-cm flexible sigmoidoscopy every 3–5 years (and possibly as infrequently as every 10 years) detects additional lesions in the distal colon. It is associated with reduced colon cancer deaths and should be performed for average-risk men and women between 50 and 75 years of age. There is no consensus about routinely screening with total colonic evaluation (e.g., colonoscopy or FOBT + air contrast barium enema). The American Cancer Society recommends that total evaluation with colonoscopy can be used instead of FOBT and flexible sigmoidoscopy. If such a strategy is followed, colonoscopy should be repeated every 10 years. High-risk people (i.e., previous history of colon cancer, large adenomatous polyps, polyposis syndromes, ulcerative colitis, family history of colon cancer) should undergo a full colonic evaluation.

9. Does digital rectal examination and/or prostate-specific antigen (PSA) reduce prostate cancer-specific mortality?

No. Despite widespread screening with PSA testing, neither early detection nor early treatment of prostate cancer has been demonstrated to reduce disease-specific morbidity or mortality. This has led to considerable controversy and confusion about the risks and benefits of early detection and treatment of prostate cancer.

The American Cancer Society and American Urological Association recommend that men at average risk for prostate cancer should have annual digital rectal examination and PSA test beginning at age 50; men at high risk (African-American men and men with a family history of prostate cancer) should begin at age 40. Evidence-based guidelines from the USPSTF, National Cancer Institute and American College of Physicians either recommend against early detection of prostate cancer or state that men should be counseled about the unproved benefits and known harms of screening and treatment. All groups state that the efficacy of early detection and treatment in reducing morbidity and mortality has not been demonstrated. The National Cancer Institute is conducting a large randomized trial to determine whether prostate cancer screening with annual digital rectal examination and PSA testing will reduce prostate cancer mortality.

Prostate cancer is the most frequently diagnosed cancer and second leading cause of cancer-related mortality in men. In 1997 it is estimated that 334,000 men will be diagnosed and that 41,000 men will die from prostate cancer. From 1990–1997 the incidence of prostate cancer rose 200% and the number of related deaths increased 39%. The marked increase in prostate cancer is most likely due to the greater frequency of PSA tests and subsequent prostate biopsy procedures that detect a large number of asymptomatic cancers.

10. Is PSA specific for prostate cancer?

No. Although the PSA blood test is specific for the prostate, it is not specific for prostate cancer. In addition to prostate cancer, other factors that commonly result in increased PSA levels include age, acute urinary retention, benign prostatic hypertrophy (BPH), infection, and biopsy or surgery of the prostate. Digital rectal examination does not produce clinically important elevations in PSA levels. The positive predictive value for prostate cancer in men over age 50 with PSA levels between 4 and 10 ng/ml is about 20%. This value does not vary substantially with age, suggesting that increased disease prevalence is balanced by decreased test specificity in older men. Use of PSA alone results in a cancer detection rate of about 3%. Elevations in PSA level of 4 and 10 ng/ml increase the odds of clinically significant intracapsular prostate cancer about 1.5–3-fold. Although PSA levels greater than 10 ng/ml may still reflect BPH, the odds of extracapsular cancer are increased by greater than 20-fold.

11. If a man is found to have prostate cancer believed to be confined to the prostate gland, of what treatment options should he be informed?

There are at least three standard treatment options for early stage or clinically localized prostate cancer: surgery to remove the entire prostate and surrounding tissue (radical prostatectomy), radiation to destroy the tumor (external beam or interstitial implants), and careful monitoring with palliative hormonal therapy or smaller surgical interventions for evidence of disease progression (watchful waiting). Results from a small clinical trial; case series of treatment with surgery, radiation, or watchful waiting; several structured literature reviews; and decision analysis modeling indicate that all three treatment approaches appear to provide similar survival rates. The American Urological Association recently concluded that all three treatments be considered options because the available evidence does not support the superiority of any one treatment in reducing disease-specific morbidity and mortality. The Department of Veterans Affairs, National Cancer Institute, and Agency for Health Care Policy and Research are currently conducting a randomized trial to determine whether radical prostatectomy or watchful waiting provides improved length and quality of life in men with clinically localized prostate cancer.

12. Why is the Pap smear a good screening test?

The Papanicolau smear, developed by George Papanicolau in the 1930s, is the recommended screening test for cervical cancer. The incidence and mortality rate of cervical cancer are relatively low compared with lung, breast, and colon cancer. However, the natural history with a long preinvasive stage and the availability of the Pap smear make screening for cervical cancer practical. Since the widespread practice of performing Pap smears, mortality has decreased from about 15/100,000 in the 1960s to approximately 8/100,000.

13. How often should Pap smears be performed?

Pap smears should be performed at least every 3 years in sexually active women who have a cervix. Screening should begin at the age of sexual intercourse. Screening can probably be discontinued at the age of 65 if multiple smears have been normal. The frequency of examinations depends on the presence of risk factors, including early onset of sexual intercourse, multiple sexual partners, and low socioeconomic status.

14. What should be done if the results are "atypical"?

The principal goal of cervical smears is not to diagnose overt clinical cancer but to detect occult carcinomas and precancerous abnormalities that may lead to invasive cancer. Therefore, clinicians should conduct further evaluation with colposcopy rather than repeat a Pap smear in women who have "atypical" or "precancerous" lesions on Pap smear.

15. Should CA-125 be used to screen women for ovarian cancer?

No. Although ovarian cancer is the fifth leading cause of cancer-related deaths in women (27,000 new cases and 14,000 deaths in 1995), routine screening with pelvic examination, Pap smears, transvaginal ultrasound (TVUS), or CA-125 blood testing is not generally recommended. The incidence of ovarian cancer increases with age, ranging from 14 per 100,000 at age 50 to 35 per 100,000 at age 70. Additional risk factors include low parity and family history of ovarian cancer. Although hereditary cancer syndromes account for less than 0.1% of women with ovarian cancer, the lifetime risk of developing ovarian cancer in women with a positive family history is up to 40%. Because the ovaries have a deep anatomic location, pelvic examination and Pap smear have poor sensitivity and specificity for detecting early-stage disease. The sensitivity and specificity of TVUS in the evaluation of a palpable ovarian mass are approximately 90% and 98% respectively; but because of the low prevalence of the disease, TVUS is not practical for routine screening (positive predictive value = 3%).

The sensitivity of CA-125 for ovarian cancer increases with clinical stage but is only 50% for clinically localized stage I and II neoplasms. In addition, CA-125 is elevated in 1% of healthy women, up to 40% of women with benign cysts, and 30% of women with nongynecologic tumors. It may be possible to improve the accuracy by combining ultrasound measurements with CA-125. However, the low prevalence of the disease will result in a large proportion of false-positive tests that require diagnostic laparotomy or laparoscopy. Recommendations for women at increased risk (presumed hereditary cancer syndromes) have included annual pelvic exams or prophylactic oophorectomy. The effectiveness of any of these strategies has not been determined.

An ongoing randomized trial is examining the effectiveness of multimodality screening (TVUS, CA-125, and pelvic exam) in reducing ovarian cancer mortality in 75,000 women aged 60–74.

16. What factors should physicians consider in screening patients for melanoma?

Physicians should recognize people with risk factors for melanoma; including moles, previously diagnosed basal or squamous carcinoma of the skin; fair complexion or poor tolerance to sunlight, and a family history of melanoma. One-third of newly diagnosed melanomas occur on non–sun-exposed areas that may not be routinely seen. Therefore, a complete skin examination is important at least once. People with multiple large moles or dysplastic moles should probably receive annual skin evaluations and education about worrisome changes that require a return visit. In African-American, Hispanic, and Asian patients, attention to palmar, plantar, and subungual areas is important because of a greater incidence of acral lentiginous melanomas.

17. What techniques are available to screen for breast cancer?

1. **Self breast examination** (SBE). Women who are trained to perform self breast examination can detect approximately 50% of lumps ranging in size from 0.25–3.0 cm in diameter. However, SBE also increases the false detection rate. No study has yet demonstrated the additional benefit of including SBE with clinical breast examination and mammography. The USPSTF states that there is insufficient evidence to recommend for or against SBE. SBE probably should be recommended on an individual basis that incorporates the women's desire to be trained in SBE.

2. **Physician-performed clinical breast examination**. Clinical breast examination (CBE) in combination with mammography has been shown to be effective in detecting early breast cancer and reducing mortality in women over the age of 50. However, CBE alone or the independent effect of CBE in women undergoing mammography has not been evaluated in randomized trials. CBE is probably not sufficiently sensitive to be used as a primary screening modality but is complementary to mammography. The USPSTF currently recommends annual CBE for women at average risk over the age of 40 years.

3. **Mammography**. Results from clinical trials, cohort studies, and uncontrolled projects demonstrate the effectiveness of annual screening mammography in women over the age of 50, either alone or with CBE, in reducing breast cancer mortality. Reduction in breast cancer mortality in the group receiving CBE and mammography ranged between 4% and 50%. Mammography with CBE is recommended in all women beginning at age 50.

The effectiveness of mammography in women under the age of 50 has been the subject of considerable debate. A recent consensus panel sponsored by the National Cancer Institute and American Cancer Society concluded that the data from 8 randomized clinical trials of mammography screening were insufficient to make a clear recommendation for or against mammography in women between the ages of 40–49. However, a reconvened panel decided that the evidence supported the recommendation that annual mammography should be performed for women beginning at age 40. The most recent meta-analysis suggested that annual screening reduces mortality by 18% among the group aged 40–49 and that its cost-effectiveness is within the range of other accepted screening procedures. Critics have suggested that the benefits of screening are small at best and are not actually obtained until women are aged 50 years and over and that the resource utilization and risk of mammography (radiation exposure, false-positive tests resulting in unnecessary biopsies, and increased detection and treatment of cancers that have a low risk of progressing to invasive breast cancer [ductal carcinoma in situ]) outweigh any potential benefit. An ongoing British trial is evaluating the effectiveness of annual screening in women 40–41 years old.

18. Can a positive FOBT be interpreted if the patient is on a daily aspirin?

Evidence suggests that a daily aspirin (and even warfarin) does not produce false-positive results in clinical practice. Patients should restrict higher doses of aspirin, nonsteroidal antiinflammatory agents, iron, vitamin C, and high peroxidase-containing foods (beets) for 3 days before ordering FOBT. A high-residue, meat-free diet during testing also may be beneficial to reduce the number of false-positive tests.

19. Is routine screening for testicular cancer likely to improve overall mortality?

It is unlikely that screening for testicular cancer would substantially improve the already favorable outcome of this uncommon disease. For example, the overall cure rate in the absence of systemic screening is 92%. Testicular cancer is a relatively uncommon disease (annual incidence of 8–14/100,000 men aged 20–35 years). Therefore, a primary care physician who has 1500 males in his or her practice can expect to detect one testicular cancer every 15–20 years. The vast majority of examinations would be normal or falsely abnormal. Screening and evaluation would result in considerable costs and possible morbidity with at best minimal benefit. Although men with a history of undescended testes or testicular atrophy are at increased risk for testicular cancer, the value of early detection has not yet been demonstrated.

20. What should primary care physicians do to reduce morbidity from oral cancer?

Identification and counseling of high-risk people against the use of tobacco or abuse of alcohol is probably the best strategy for reducing oral cancer complications. Because many patients have limited contact with dentists, the role of the primary care provider in identifying and counseling the high-risk individuals is critical. Over 90% of deaths due to oropharyngeal cancer are associated with smoking and alcohol. The use of snuff and chewing tobacco is also associated with oral cancer. The available screening tests are limited to oral examination of the mouth. Primary treatment of oral leukoplakia to prevent the development of oral cancer has not been widely accepted.

BIBLIOGRAPHY

1. American College of Physicians: Screening for prostate cancer. Ann Intern Med 126:480–484, 1997.
2. American College of Physicians: Suggested technique for fecal occult blood testing and interpretation in colorectal cancer screening. Ann Intern Med 126:808–811, 1997.
3. Bailar JC III, Gornick HL: Cancer undefeated. N Engl J Med 336:1569–1574, 1997.
4. Ernster VK, Barclay J, Kerlikowske K, et al: Incidence of and treatment for ductal carcinoma in situ of the breast. JAMA 275:913–918, 1996.
5. Fleming C, Wasson JH, Albertsen PC, et al for the Prostate Patient Outcomes Research Team: A decision analysis of alternative treatment strategies for clinically localized prostate cancer. JAMA 269:2650–2659, 1993.
6. Friedman GD: Primer of Epidemiology, 3rd ed. New York, McGraw-Hill, 1987.
7. Kerlikowske K, Grady D, Rubin SM, et al: Efficacy of screening mammography: A meta-analysis. JAMA 273:149–154, 1995.
8. Lederle FA, Niewoehner DE: Lung cancer surgery: A critical review of the evidence. Arch Intern Med 154:2397–2400, 1994.
9. Leitch AM, Dodd GD, Costanza M, et al: American Cancer Society Guidelines for the Early Detection of Breast Cancer: Update 1997. CA Cancer J Clin 47:150–153, 1997.
10. Mandel JS, Bond JH, Church TR, et al: Reducing mortality from colorectal cancer by screening for fecal occult blood. N Engl J Med 328:1365–1371, 1993.
11. Oboler SK, LaForce FM: The periodic physical examination in asymptomatic adults. Ann Intern Med 110:214–226, 1989.
12. Ransofhoff DF, Lang CA: Screening for colorectal cancer with the fecal occult blood test: A background paper. Ann Intern Med 126:811–822, 1997.
13. Richert-Boe KE, Humphrey LL: Screening for cancers of the lung and colon. Arch Intern Med 152:2398–2404, 1992.
14. Richert-Boe KE, Humphrey LL: Screening for cancers of the cervix and breast. Arch Intern Med 152:2405–2411, 1992.
15. Schapira MM, Matchar DB, Young MJ: The effectiveness of ovarian cancer screening: A decision analysis model. Ann Intern Med 118:838–843, 1993.
16. United States Preventive Services Task Force: Guide to Clinical Preventive Services, 2nd ed. Baltimore, Williams & Wilkins, 1996.
17. Wilt TJ, Brawer MK: The prostate cancer intervention versus observation trial: A randomized trial comparing radical prostatectomy versus expectant management for the treatment of clinically localized prostate cancer. J Urol 15:1910–1914, 1994.

3. CARDIOVASCULAR DISEASE PREVENTION

Hanna Bloomfield Rubins, M.D., M.P.H.

Cardiovascular disease is the leading cause of death for both women and men in the United States, claiming nearly one million lives a year. It is estimated that 70 million Americans have one or more manifestations of cardiovascular disease, including high blood pressure, stroke, and coronary heart disease (CHD). CHD alone affects over 13 million Americans, and every year half a million people suffer an acute stroke. This chapter focuses on the actions that primary care physicians can take to reduce the risk of cardiovascular disease (specifically CHD, cerebrovascular disease, and peripheral vascular disease) in their patients. Treatment of hypertension and certain other cardiovascular risk factors (e.g., obesity and dyslipidemia) is covered in detail in other chapters.

1. Is there a simple way to assess a patient's overall risk for atherosclerotic cardiovascular disease?

The major risk factors for atherosclerotic cardiovascular disease are listed below.

Major Risk Factors for Atherosclerotic Cardiovascular Disease

FIXED	MODIFIABLE
Advanced age	Cigarette smoking
Male gender or	Dyslipidemia (high LDL and/or low HDL cholesterol)
postmenopausal female	Hypertension
Family history of premature	Sedentary lifestyle
coronary heart disease	Diabetes
	Obesity

Multivariate risk functions that use a patient's risk factor profile to quantitate cardiac risk are available in either handbook or pocket calculator form. However, it is generally sufficient to assess a patient's risk status less quantitatively. High-risk patients have two or more major risk factors or a strong family history of premature CHD (even without other evident risk factors). Patients with one risk factor are considered to be at moderate risk, and patients with no risk factors are at low risk. Although some risk factors appear to be more important than others for specific manifestations of atherosclerotic disease (e.g., hypertension is a strong determinant of stroke), this is of little practical importance because the goal is to prevent all cardiovascular disease. A thorough assessment of all risk factors should be made at the initial visit and shared with the patient. A plan of action for modifiable risk factors should be initiated and close follow-up provided.

2. Should asymptomatic patients be screened for occult cardiovascular disease?

Screening for modifiable risk factors (e.g., hypertension, dyslipidemia, smoking) is strongly recommended, but screening asymptomatic people to detect occult atherosclerotic disease with modalities such as resting electrocardiography, exercise electrocardiography, or noninvasive carotid and peripheral vascular evaluation is not. Such tests have poor predictive value in asymptomatic populations; furthermore, the benefit of treating uncovered disease in asymptomatic patients is not established. In certain asymptomatic people, however, cardiac screening may be appropriate, including persons at very high risk for CHD (e.g., men over age 40 with several cardiac risk factors); persons in whom a catastrophic cardiac event would endanger public safety (e.g., airline pilots); and persons at moderate or high risk for CHD who wish to initiate a vigorous exercise program.

3. What can the physician do during a routine office visit to help patients quit smoking?

The National Cancer Institute recommends the following approach for physicians:

1. **Ask** about smoking at every visit, and assess the person's current motivation to quit.

2. **Advise** all smokers to stop with a clear, unequivocal statement. Personalize the message, if possible, with reference to the patient's particular social or health concerns.

3. **Assist** the patient in stopping. Methods include setting a quit date, providing self-help materials, and possibly prescribing nicotine replacement therapy for highly addicted patients. Patients who are currently unmotivated to stop smoking should be given motivational literature, and the issue should be raised again at the next visit.

4. **Arrange** follow-up visits. Patients should be reminded of the quit date by letter and contacted soon after the quit date to provide support and help prevent relapse. (These tasks can be delegated to office staff).

4. What is the role of nicotine replacement therapy for smoking cessation?

There is strong evidence that nicotine replacement therapy, either in gum or patch form, is highly efficacious for smoking cessation among heavy smokers (more than 10–15 cigarettes/day). Both therapies appear to work better if accompanied by psychosocial intervention. Gum tends to be less acceptable to patients because of unpleasant taste and texture and requires more clinician time and effort to train patients; the patch, therefore, is generally considered first-line therapy. Patch therapy is prescribed as 8 weeks of a tapering dose (see package insert for individual product prescribing information). Before starting nicotine replacement therapy, patients must stop smoking. To avoid skin irritation, which is common but rarely requires discontinuation of patch, the location of the patch should be rotated. Risks and benefits should be carefully considered before beginning therapy in pregnant or lactating women and in patients with unstable heart disease.

5. What useful diet advice can be given in 5 minutes or less?

The American Heart Association Step I diet, outlined in the table below, is recommended for all individuals over the age of two.

Recommended Diet for the General Population

1. Achieve ideal body weight.
2. Limit fat intake to 30% of calories: • Saturated fatty acids: 8–10%   • Polyunsaturated fatty acids: 10%   • Monounsaturated fatty acids: 10–15%
3. Limit cholesterol to 300 mg/day.
4. 50–60% of calories from carbohydrate.

The following recommendations are intended to translate this formal dietary plan into easily digestible nuggets for patients. It is helpful to acknowledge to the patient that lifetime habits are hard to change and to introduce only two or three of these suggestions at any one visit.

• For packaged foods, choose those with fewer than 3 gm of fat (and no more than 1 gm of saturated fat) per 100 calorie serving. Do not be fooled by foods advertised as "cholesterol-free" or "low cholesterol" because these may contain a lot of saturated fat.

• Use only low or nonfat dairy products.

• Use only lean beef.

• Avoid processed meats (bologna, salami, hot dogs, sausages) and organ meats.

• Increase intake of fruits, vegetables, legumes (beans, peas), grains, and fish.

• Eat no more than 4 egg yolks/week.

• Use spray or liquid fats for cooking (good choices: canola oil, olive oil).

It is extremely helpful to suggest specific alternatives for foods that your patient likes (e.g., pretzels instead of potato chips, no-fat frozen yogurt instead of ice cream, turkey breast instead of bologna, mustard instead of mayonnaise, jam instead of butter). The emphasis should be on substitution, not denial.

6. What advice should a physician give about alcohol?

Light-to-moderate alcohol consumption (< 3 drinks/day) has been linked with decreased risk of myocardial infarction and death due to CHD. This association may be explained at least partially by alcohol's propensity to raise high-density lipoprotein cholesterol (HDL-C). The relation between moderate alcohol intake and ischemic stroke is not clear; some data suggest that alcohol may increase the risk of both ischemic and hemorrhagic stroke. It is generally agreed that physicians should not actively recommend that nondrinkers start drinking alcohol. However, patients who drink fewer than 3 alcoholic beverages a day and have no associated social or medical problems may be reassured that this level of drinking is acceptable and may even be cardioprotective.

7. What are the benefits of exercise?

Numerous observational studies indicate that physical activity is associated with a reduced risk of CHD and total mortality independently of its beneficial effect on other risk factors such as serum lipids, obesity, diabetes, and hypertension. Physical activity also protects against osteoporosis and promotes mental well-being. In the past it was thought that only vigorous exercise would produce the desired health benefits; it is now believed that even a modest exercise program can have substantial positive effects.

8. When is it safe to start an exercise program?

The safety of starting an exercise program in an individual patient can be assessed with the Physical Activity Readiness questionnaire:

Physical Activity Readiness Questions

1. Have you ever been told that you have heart trouble?
2. Do you frequently get pain in your chest?
3. Do you often feel faint or have severe dizzy spells?
4. Have you ever been told that you have high blood pressure?
5. Have you ever been told that you have problems with bones or joints (such as arthritis) that may be made worse by exercise?
6. Do you have any other physical problem that may prevent you from exercising?
7. Are you older than 65 years and not used to regular, vigorous exercise?

Adapted from Harris SS, Caspersen CJ, DeFriese GH, Estes EH Jr: Physical activity counseling for healthy adults as a primary preventive intervention in the clinical setting. Report for the U.S. Preventive Services Task Force. JAMA 261:3588–3598, 1989.

A patient who answers "no" to all questions can safely undertake an exercise program without further testing or medical supervision. Patients who answer "yes" to any of the questions should be evaluated further. Exercise electrocardiography should be considered for older patients and patients with cardiac disease or risk factors who wish to undertake a vigorous exercise program. Screening exercise electrocardiography for young, asymptomatic patients with no cardiac risk factors is not recommended.

9. What should an exercise prescription include?

Prescriptions for exercise should specify intensity, duration, and frequency. Recommended intensity of exercise is in the range of 50–85% of maximal oxygen uptake (VO_2 max), which corresponds to 65–90% of the maximal heart rate. (The maximal heart rate is approximately equal to 220 minus the person's age). Patients should be told their target heart rate and shown how to take their pulse; for example, for a sedentary 60-year-old it may be 104 (220 – 60) × 0.65. The general recommendation for duration and frequency is 15–45 minutes 3–5 times/week. Patients should be told to work toward their exercise goal gradually. Brisk walking is in many ways the ideal exercise. It is easy, convenient, and free and has minimal risk of adverse effects (such as sudden death or musculoskeletal injury).

Patients should be told that increasing physical activity, even without embarking on a formal exercise program, has documented health benefits. A reasonable goal is to do 30 minutes/day of moderate-intensity activity, such as walking briskly, climbing stairs, mowing the lawn with a power mower, or general house cleaning. The 30 minutes can be accumulated through multiple shorter bouts of activity.

10. Who should be treated for high cholesterol?
Evidence from randomized, controlled outcome trials strongly favors treatment of high cholesterol in patients with established cardiovascular disease and patients at high risk of cardiovascular disease. The evidence indicates that patients with CHD and an LDL-cholesterol over 130 mg/dl should be treated with medication if diet fails to lower the level below 130 mg/dl (attempting to lower the LDL-cholesterol below 100 mg/dl has been advocated by some, but the evidence is not conclusive). For patients without CHD but at high risk (see question 1), an LDL-cholesterol greater than 160 mg/dl should be treated with medication if diet fails.

11. What should be done about low levels of HDL-C or high levels of triglycerides?
Although both low levels of HDL-C and high levels of triglycerides have been linked epidemiologically to increased risk of CHD, no clinical trials provide data on which to base firm treatment recommendations. Patients with HDL-C less than 35 mg/dl should be advised to achieve ideal body weight, discontinue smoking, and exercise regularly. Drug therapy is not recommended. Patients with triglycerides greater than 200 mg/dl should be advised to achieve ideal body weight, limit alcohol intake, and control diabetes (if present). Drug therapy is not recommended for the prevention of CHD. Patients with persistent elevations of fasting triglycerides above 750–1000 mg/dl should be considered for drug therapy (niacin or gemfibrozil) to reduce the risk of acute pancreatitis. For patients requiring drug treatment for high levels of LDL-C (see chapter 32), the level of HDL-C and triglycerides should be considered in choosing the most appropriate regimen.

12. Is hormone replacement therapy indicated for postmenopausal women to prevent CHD?
In the absence of definitive data from randomized, controlled clinical trials, the decision to initiate hormone replacement therapy must be individualized. The physician should discuss the pros and cons with each patient to help her make an informed decision based on her medical history and personal values. The following information may be useful for this discussion:

1. **CHD**. Observational data strongly suggest that unopposed estrogen reduces a woman's risk of CHD by about 35%; however, no randomized clinical trial data are yet available to confirm this observation.

2. **Hip and vertebral fractures**. Observational data suggest that unopposed estrogen reduces risk for hip and vertebral fractures by 25% and 50%, respectively. Addition of progestin probably does not attenuate this benefit.

3. **Endometrial cancer**. The risk of endometrial cancer is increased about 8-fold with prolonged use of unopposed estrogens. Addition of cyclic progestins for 12 days/month eliminates this increased risk.

4. **Breast cancer**. Observational data suggest that long-term (over 10 years) use increases the risk of breast cancer risk by 25–30% (i.e., from a 10% to a 13% lifetime risk in an average-risk 50-year-old woman). Use for less than 5 years does not seem to be associated with an increased risk of breast cancer.

5. **Side effects** may include vaginal bleeding, headaches, bloating, breast tenderness, irritability, and depression.

Recent guidelines recommend (1) unopposed estrogens for women who have had a hysterectomy and are not at increased risk for breast cancer; (2) combination therapy for women with a uterus who are at high risk or already have established CHD or osteoporosis; (3) no hormone replacement therapy in women at high risk for breast cancer; and (4) individualized decisions for all other women.

13. Which patients should take aspirin? What is the best dose?

Recent American Heart Association guidelines recommend aspirin therapy in the following situations (assuming no contraindications):

- For all patients with known CHD (dose: 75–325 mg/day)
- For men over 40 years old without CHD but with one or more risk factors for cardiovascular disease (dose: 75–325 mg/day).
- For all patients with a history of noncardiogenic stroke or transient ischemic attack (dose may need to be as high as 975–1500 mg/day, although lower doses may be equally effective).

14. Are vitamins indicated for the prevention of CHD?

In the past several years there has been tremendous interest in the potential of antioxidant vitamins, such as C, E, and beta-carotene to prevent atherosclerotic disease. It has been hypothesized that these vitamins may prevent the oxidation of LDL-cholesterol, a key step in the initiation of atherosclerotic lesions. Recent epidemiologic and clinical trial data, however, have not confirmed benefits from either vitamin C or beta-carotene. One study suggested that beta-carotene supplementation in fact may have increased the risk of cancer. The usefulness of vitamin E remains unclear. Large observational studies suggest that it is protective, and one randomized trial in patients with CHD demonstrated a reduction in nonfatal myocardial infarction in treated patients. From a practical standpoint, I encourage patients to eat a diet rich in fruits and vegetables (e.g., citrus fruits, carrots, spinach). I discourage them from wasting their money on beta-carotene or vitamin C supplements, and I let them know that the vitamin E question is still a toss-up.

15. What are the most important steps a physician can take to prevent stroke?

The most important risk factors for stroke are age, hypertension, atrial fibrillation, and history of transient ischemic attack. Other cardiac risk factors, such as smoking, dyslipidemia, and diabetes, also may play a role. To prevent stroke the following steps are recommended:

1. **Control of both systolic and diastolic hypertension** (see chapter 14)
2. **Anticoagulation of patients with atrial fibrillation**. Several well-designed, randomized, controlled clinical trials have established that low-intensity anticoagulation (international normalized ratio: 2–3) with warfarin reduces the risk of stroke in patients with atrial fibrillation by 50–80%.
3. **Antiplatelet treatment in patients with a history of transient ischemic attack**, either with aspirin (see question 13) or ticlopidine (for patients who cannot tolerate aspirin).
4. **Smoking cessation**

16. What is the role of carotid endarterectomy for stroke prevention?

One large, well-designed, randomized, controlled clinical trial has shown that carotid endarterectomy reduces stroke and total mortality in patients who have had a recent (within 4 months) transient ischemic attack or nondisabling stroke and who have high-grade (70–99%) ipsilateral carotid stenosis. The procedure should be recommended to eligible patients if the surgical mortality rate locally is comparable to the rate in the study (< 3% major stroke; < 1% mortality). The role of carotid endarterectomy for asymptomatic patients with high-grade stenoses remains controversial despite a recent trial suggesting that such patients do better with surgery than with aspirin. Because of this controversy, the U.S. Preventive Services Task Force does not recommend routine screening of patients for asymptomatic carotid disease.

17. Is aggressive treatment of risk factors appropriate in elderly patients?

Elderly patients are at very high risk for CHD, stroke, and peripheral vascular disease. Treating hypertension with medication and anticoagulating elderly patients in atrial fibrillation to prevent stroke have been proved beneficial in clinical trials. Smoking cessation, a reasonable exercise regimen, and weight control should be encouraged in patients of all ages. Most of the controversy revolves around drug treatment of dyslipidemia in elderly patients without evident CHD.

Patients over the age of 55 have not been included in clinical trials demonstrating that treatment of hypercholesterolemia decreases CHD-related morbidity and mortality. Furthermore, in several epidemiologic studies serum cholesterol levels were not as strongly associated with CHD risk in elderly as in middle-aged people. However, because the elderly are at such high baseline risk for CHD and stroke, dyslipidemia leads to a high number of cardiovascular events. Therefore, although decisions must be individualized, drug treatment of dyslipidemia should be considered in otherwise healthy, high-risk elderly people.

18. Which preventive measures are indicated in people who already have had a myocardial infarction (MI)?

Many modifiable risk factors, including cigarette smoking, dyslipidemia, physical inactivity, obesity, and hypertension, are important predictors of recurrent cardiac events among patients with a history of MI or other manifestations of CHD. Treating risk factors in patients with established heart disease (secondary prevention) may have a more substantial impact on CHD incidence than treating people without known disease (primary prevention) because the absolute risk of MI- and CHD-related death is so much higher in people with known disease. Clinical trials demonstrating beneficial effects of secondary prevention have been reported for hypercholesterolemia, hypertension, and exercise programs. In addition, aspirin (see question 13) and beta blockers are recommended.

CONTROVERSY

19. At what age should routine cholesterol screening be initiated? With what tests?

It is generally agreed that men and women of any age with a history of CHD should be screened and treated for high levels of cholesterol. The value of screening and treatment for persons without known CHD is highly controversial. The National Cholesterol Education Program recommends screening total cholesterol and HDL-cholesterol for all adults over the age of 20. The American College of Physicians and the U.S. Preventive Services Task Force, on the other hand, recommend screening for men aged 35–65 and women aged 45–65 with total cholesterol only. Proponents of screening at younger ages point to the fact that atherosclerosis starts decades before it becomes manifest and that intervention at younger ages has the potential to decrease future cardiac events. Those who advocate waiting until middle age to screen argue that younger people are at very low risk of cardiac events in the near future and that no clinical trial data in this population provide information about the risks and benefits of long-term treatment.

The controversy over whether to include HDL-cholesterol for general screening also revolves around lack of clinical trial data. The National Cholesterol Education Program, relying on the strong epidemiologic data linking low levels of HDL-cholesterol to CHD, believes that this is an important risk factor and should be measured to give a more accurate overall risk assessment for individual patients. Others argue that, because we do not know whether raising HDL-cholesterol will be of any benefit, there is no reason to measure it. Furthermore, general lifestyle and diet advice recommended for low HDL-cholesterol should be part of the counseling given to all patients.

Because neither of these controversies is likely to be resolved in the near future, when to start screening and with what tests must be determined by the provider-patient team.

BIBLIOGRAPHY

1. Albers GW, Atwood JE, Hirsh J, et al: Stroke prevention in nonvalvular atrial fibrillation. Ann Intern Med 115:727–736, 1991.
2. Agency for Health Care Policy and Research: Smoking cessation clinical guidelines. Washington, DC, U.S. Department of Health and Human Services. AHCPR Publ No. 96-0692, 1996.
3. American College of Physicians: Guidelines for counseling postmenopausal women about preventive hormone therapy. Ann Intern Med 117:1038–1041, 1992.

4. American College of Physicians: Guidelines for using serum cholesterol, high-density lipoprotein cholesterol, and triglyceride levels as screening tests for preventing coronary heart disease in adults. Ann Intern Med 124:515–517, 1996.
5. Andersen RE, Blair SN, Cheskin LJ, Bartlett SJ: Encouraging patients to become more physically active: The physician's role. Ann Intern Med 127:395–400, 1997.
6. Bucher HC, Griffith LE, Guyatt GH: Effect of HMGCoA reductase inhibitors on stroke: A meta-analysis of randomized, controlled trials. Ann Intern Med 128:89–95, 1998.
7. Diaz MN, Frei B, Vita JA, Keaney JF: Antioxidants and atherosclerotic heart disease. N Engl J Med 337:408–516, 1997.
8. Executive Committee for the Asymptomatic Carotid Atherosclerosis Study: Endarterectomy for asymptomatic carotid artery stenosis. JAMA 273:1421–1428, 1995.
9. Expert Panel on Detection, Evaluation, and Treatment of High Blood Cholesterol in Adults: Summary of the second report of the National Cholesterol Education Program (NCEP) Expert Panel on detection, evaluation, and treatment of high blood cholesterol in adults (Adult Treatment Panel II). JAMA 269:3015–3023, 1993.
10. Fuster V, Dyken ML, Vokonas PS, Hennekens C: Aspirin as a therapeutic agent in cardiovascular disease. Circulation 87:659–675, 1993.
11. Glynn TJ, Manley MW: How to help your patients stop smoking. Washington, DC, National Cancer Institute, NIH Publ No. 90-3064, 1990.
12. U.S. Preventive Services Task Force: Guide to Clinical Preventive Services, 2nd ed. Baltimore, Williams & Wilkins, 1996.

4. IMMUNIZATIONS AND SCREENING FOR INFECTIOUS DISEASES

Kristin L. Nichol, M.D., M.P.H.

1. Which vaccines are recommended for children?

Current recommendations are for all children to receive the following vaccines:

VACCINE	REGIMEN
Diphtheria/tetanus/pertussis	5 doses
Polio	4 doses
Measles/mumps/rubella (MMR)	2 doses
Hemophilus influenzae B (Hib—conjugate vaccine)	3–4 doses
Hepatitis B	3 doses
Varicella	1–2 doses

These vaccines are administered at various intervals from birth to age 12 years; 80% of injections are scheduled during the first 15–18 months of life. Several of these recommendations are new or have been modified within the past few years:

1. In 1996 routine varicella vaccination was recommended for all susceptible children.

2. In 1997 acellular pertussis (DTaP) vaccine became the preferred vaccine for protection against diphtheria, tetanus, and pertussis in infants and young children because of the reduced frequency of adverse reactions and equal or increased efficacy.

3. In 1997 two doses of inactivated poliovirus vaccine, followed by two doses of oral poliovirus vaccine, was recommended because of the slightly lower risk of vaccine-associated paralytic polio.

2. Which vaccinations are recommended for adults?

Vaccinations for adults, in contrast to those for children, are largely recommended only for persons in specific risk groups. The vaccines most often administered to adults include:

VACCINE	DOSE/TARGET GROUP
Influenza vaccine	Yearly for people who are elderly, at high risk of influenza-associated complications, or likely to transmit disease to high-risk persons
Pneumococcal vaccine	Once for elderly and people at high risk; revaccinate certain groups at highest risk
Tetanus/diphtheria	Booster every 10 years after primary series has been completed
Hepatitis B	3 doses for people at high risk, including international travelers and health care providers
Hepatitis A	2 doses for people at high risk, including international travelers
MMR	2 doses or other evidence of immunity (prior physician diagnosis of measles, laboratory evidence of immunity, or birth before 1957) for people at high risk, including health care providers

People aged 65 and older and people with chronic medical conditions (especially chronic heart and lung disease) are at particularly increased risk for complications from influenza and pneumococcal disease and should be offered both vaccines. Tetanus/diphtheria boosters are recommended routinely for all adults who have previously completed the primary series of three doses. Hepatitis B vaccine is recommended for people with high-risk life-styles (e.g., intravenous drug users, bisexual or homosexual men, people with other sexually transmitted diseases) or high-risk occupations (e.g., health care providers) and people who live or work in high-risk environments (e.g., prison inmates). Hepatitis B vaccination is also recommended for international travelers whose itineraries include much of eastern Europe, Asia, Africa, and Middle and South America. Hepatitis A vaccination is recommended for people at increased risk for infection as well as for food handlers. People at increased risk for infection include international travelers whose itineraries include countries with moderate or high rates of hepatitis A, such as eastern Europe, Asia, Africa, and Middle and South America, homosexual or bisexual men, users of street drugs, and people with chronic liver disease or clotting factor disorders. MMR is recommended for health care providers and students at colleges or other educational institutions after high school who have not previously received two doses of the vaccine and who lack evidence of adequate immunity (prior physician diagnosis of measles disease, laboratory evidence of immunity, birth since 1957).

In addition to routine immunizations, for travelers outside the United States the need for any other vaccines should be assessed. Special immunization requirements are geographically defined and may include immunizations for yellow fever, cholera, typhoid fever, hepatitis B, hepatitis A, and other diseases. Local and state health departments and the Centers for Disease Control and Prevention may be consulted for up to date information on immunization recommendations for international travelers.

3. Why do vaccine-preventable diseases continue to be major causes of illness and mortality?

The past several decades have seen dramatic decreases in the numbers of reported cases of vaccine-preventable diseases in the United States. Nevertheless, vaccine-preventable diseases continue to be major causes of illness and death each year in all age groups. Recent outbreaks of measles, congenital rubella syndrome, pertussis, and mumps underscore the continuing importance of these diseases among children. In addition, influenza and pneumonia continue to rank as the sixth leading cause of death in the United States, killing up to 60 times more people (85% or more of whom are elderly) than all other vaccine-preventable diseases in all age groups combined.

The major reason is that vaccination rates often fall far short of national goals. Among children aged 19–35 months, immunization rates have increased, with 90% coverage levels for diphtheria/pertussis/tetanus, polio, hemophilus B, and measles-containing viruses. Nevertheless, even among such children, 24% or more are not up to date for all of the recommended antigens. The lowest vaccination rates may be seen especially in certain difficult-to-reach groups including the urban poor and racial and ethnic minorities. Only 30% of targeted adults have received pneumococcal vaccine; only about 50–60% have received influenza vaccine; and up to 66% of adults may lack adequate immunity to tetanus.

Vaccine-preventable Diseases in the U.S.: Maximal Number of Cases Reported for a Calendar Year vs. Number of Cases Reported in 1995

DISEASE	MAXIMAL NO. OF CASES REPORTED DURING PREVACCINE ERA	YEAR(S) MAXIMAL NO. OF CASES REPORTED	NO. OF CASES REPORTED 1995	DECREASE IN MORBIDITY
Congenital rubella	20,000	1964–65	7	99.96%
Diphtheria	206,939	1921	0	99.99%
Invasive *Hemophilus influenzae*	20,000	1984	1164	94.18%
Measles	894,134	1941	309	99.97%
Mumps	152,209	1968	840	99.45%
Pertussis	265,269	1934	4315	98.37%
Polio (wild)	21,269	1952	0	99.99%
Rubella	57,686	1969	146	99.75%
Tetanus	601	1948	34	94.34%

Adapted from Centers for Disease Control and Prevention. Update: Vaccine side effects, adverse reactions, contraindications, and precautions. MMWR 45(RR-12), 1996.

Occurrences of Vaccine-preventable Diseases by Age Group, 1995

VACCINE-PREVENTABLE DISEASE	TOTAL REPORTED CASES (1995)	CASES BY AGE GROUP		
		< 25	25–64	65+
Pertussis	5137	4384	676	41
Tetanus	41	5	26	10
Measles	309	200	90	—
Mumps	906	700	179	6
Rubella	128	45	80	—
Polio	2	2	—	—
H. Influenzae	1180	397	338	427
Hepatitis B	10,805	2353	7725	441
Hepatitis A	31,582	15,101	14,961	1042

Adapted from Centers for Disease Control: Summary of Notifiable Diseases, United States, 1995. MMWR 44 (53), 1996.

Deaths Due to Vaccine-preventable Diseases, United States, 1989–1993

DISEASE	CASES	DEATHS
Influenza	(millions)	50,000–200,000*
Pneumococcal disease	(millions)	200,000*
Hepatitis A	138,990	412
Hepatitis B	92,011	4383
Measles	58,171	127
Mumps	19,532	5
Rubella	3274	14
Pertussis	22,115	36
Tetanus	267	49

* 85% of deaths are among the elderly.
Adapted from Centers for Disease Control and Prevention: Summary of Notifiable Diseases, U.S., 1995. MMWR 44 (No. 53), 1996.

4. How can vaccination rates be improved?

Although many opportunities have been missed to ensure adequate immunity to vaccine-preventable diseases among targeted persons in the U.S., many opportunities also exist for improving levels of immunity by increasing vaccination rates. Strategies to improve vaccination rates should address barriers to and facilitators of successful vaccination efforts, including:

Patient issues
- Physician's recommendation
- Access and convenience
- Cost
- Awareness of importance of vaccines, vaccine efficacy, and vaccine safety

Provider issues
- Up-to-date knowledge about vaccine recommendations, efficacy, and side effects
- Reimbursement
- Effective organizational structures in practice settings to ensure that vaccine is systematically offered and administered (including patient identification, tracking, and recall systems)
- Feedback using objective measures of performance

Public policy issues
- Public and provider education
- Reimbursement
- Vaccine purchase and distribution
- Regulations requiring evidence of immunity in specific situations (e.g., school enrollment, college matriculation)

Studies have shown that a physician's recommendation for immunization is among the most potent predictors of patient behavior. For providers, strategies aimed at improving organizational structures within their practice seem to be most effective in improving vaccination rates. Age-based strategies for assessing vaccination needs also may be effective. Recently recommendations have been made for assessment of immunization during a routine health visit for adolescents aged 11–12 years. It also has been recommended that all adults at age 50 should be assessed for immunization as well as other preventive health services. By age 50, 12% of adults have chronic lung disease and over one-third have chronic heart disease, placing them in target groups for influenza and pneumococcal vaccinations.

5. What are special considerations with regard to vaccinations and immunocompromised hosts?

Immunocompromised people may be at increased risk for vaccine-preventable diseases. This risk is determined by the nature and severity of the underlying process. Such people also may be at increased risk for adverse reactions to live-virus vaccines because viral replication after administration of live-virus vaccines may be enhanced in severely immunocompromised persons. Killed or inactivated vaccines, however, do not represent a danger to immunocompromised people and generally should be administered as recommended for otherwise healthy people.

Live vs. Killed or Inactivated Vaccines

LIVE (ATTENUATED) VACCINES*	KILLED/INACTIVATED VACCINES[†]	
Measles[‡]	Diphtheria	Influenza
Mumps[‡]	Pertussis	Pneumococcal
Rubella[‡]	Tetanus (toxoid)	*H. Influenzae*
Oral polio vaccine	Hepatitis B	Enhanced inactivated
Varicella	Hepatitis A	polio vaccine

* May be contraindicated for certain immunocompromised persons.
[†] Generally considered safe for administration to immunocompromised people.
[‡] Including MMR

6. Which three groups of immunocompromised patients should be specifically considered in choosing vaccine type?

1. People who are severely immunocompromised as a result of non-HIV diseases (e.g., congenital immunodeficiency, leukemia, lymphoma, generalized malignancy, therapy with alkylating agents, antimetabolites, radiation, or large amounts of corticosteroids)

2. People with HIV infection

3. Persons with conditions that cause limited immune deficits (e.g., asplenia, renal failure) that may require the use of special vaccines or higher doses but do not contraindicate use of any particular vaccine, including live-virus vaccines.

Live-virus vaccines are contraindicated for persons in group 1. In addition, oral polio vaccine should not be given to any household contact or nursing personnel in close contact with a severely immunocompromised person because of shedding of vaccine virus by the vaccine recipient. For persons in group 2, oral polio vaccine also should be avoided; if there is need for administration of polio vaccine, the enhanced inactivated form of the vaccine should be used (eIPV). MMR vaccination of people in group 2 should be considered. Vaccination early in the course of HIV disease is desirable because the immunologic response may decrease as HIV disease progresses. Furthermore, routine MMR vaccination of people in group 2 who have severe immunosuppression may result in an increased risk for adverse events associated with replication of vaccine viruses. Accordingly, recommendations for use of live-virus vaccines in people in group 2 are being reevaluated. For persons in group 3, live-virus vaccines may be administered according to the usual schedules.

People with certain medical conditions that impair immune responses, such as renal failure, asplenia, and diabetes, may be at increased risk for specific diseases. Bacterial polysaccharide (especially pneumococcal vaccine) and influenza vaccines are often recommended.

7. Can pregnant women be vaccinated?

All considerations about the use of vaccines during pregnancy should weigh the benefits to the mother and fetus against the possible risks; current immunization recommendations should be consulted before administering vaccines. There are, however, several general precautions for the use of vaccines during pregnancy. Because of potential risk to the developing fetus, live-virus vaccines (particularly MMR and varicella) usually should be avoided altogether for both pregnant women and women who are likely to become pregnant within 3 months. In addition, although no convincing evidence indicates an increased risk to the fetus from inactivated virus or bacteria vaccines or toxoids, it is a reasonable precaution to delay, if possible, administration of any necessary vaccine or toxoid until the second or third trimester to minimize any possible or theoretical risk of teratogenicity for the fetus. Tetanus/diphtheria toxoid, for example, may be administered to pregnant women in this fashion if indicated. Limited data from case reports and other studies suggest that pregnancy may increase the risk for hospitalization for serious complications of influenza as a result of increases in heart rate, stroke volume, and oxygen consumption as well as decreases in lung capacity and changes in immunologic function. Accordingly, routine influenza vaccination is recommended for all women who will be in the second or third trimester of pregnancy during the influenza season.

8. Which vaccines are recommended for health care providers?

Health care providers, including medical students, residents, and practicing physicians, are at increased risk for contracting and transmitting vaccine-preventable diseases, including influenza, MMR, hepatitis B, and varicella. Accordingly, health care professionals should have adequate immunity against these diseases. Often this means annual influenza immunization, two doses of MMR (unless they were born before 1957 or have other evidence of immunity as described above), and hepatitis B vaccine. Serologic screening before possible varicella immunization of health care workers with negative or uncertain histories may be cost-effective. In addition, it is prudent for health care professionals to receive tetanus/diphtheria boosters every 10 years.

9. What adverse events may occur after immunizations?

Modern vaccines are remarkably safe and effective. Although adverse events have been reported after the administration of all vaccines, the most frequent events are minor, local reactions. Hypersensitivity reactions are uncommon and are almost always caused by hypersensitivity to one or more vaccine components: (1) animal protein (e.g., residual egg protein from egg-grown virus vaccines such as measles, mumps, and influenza vaccines); (2) antibiotics (e.g., trace neomycin found in MMR); (3) preservatives (e.g., thimerosal in influenza vaccine); and (4) stabilizers. Other severe, systemic effects are rare; often a cause-and-effect relationship between symptom and vaccine is difficult or impossible to establish.

Although serious side effects are uncommon, health care providers may encounter patients who have temporally associated events serious enough to require medical attention. Since 1988, health care providers and vaccine manufacturers have been required by law to report adverse events associated with certain vaccines, including MMR or its component vaccines, DTP/DTaP or its component vaccines, and polio vaccines. Adverse events requiring medical attention after administration of any vaccine should be reported to the Vaccine Adverse Event Reporting Service (VAERS) of the U.S. Department of Health and Human Services.

10. Identify common contraindications to administration of vaccines.

Contraindications to administration of vaccines include certain disease states (e.g., live-virus vaccines are contraindicated for severely immunocompromised people); other medical conditions (e.g., live-virus vaccines are generally contraindicated during pregnancy); and known hypersensitivity to previous doses of vaccine or vaccine components (e.g., persons with a history of anaphylactic reactions to eggs or egg products should not receive egg-grown virus vaccines such as mumps, measles, and influenza vaccines). In addition, severe reactions to previous doses may preclude subsequent doses of certain immunizations (e.g., anaphylactic reaction or encephalopathy within 7 days of DTP/DTaP vaccination not attributable to another identifiable cause).

Certain conditions are commonly misunderstood to be contraindications to administration of vaccines. Physicians and other health care providers should maintain up-to-date knowledge about vaccine components and the indications and contraindications for vaccine administration to ensure appropriate immunization activities. Sources for this information include current vaccine package inserts and vaccination recommendations from expert groups such as the Advisory Committee on Immunization Practices (ACIP) of the Public Health Service.

Situations that Do Not Represent Contraindications to Vaccination

---

Reactions to a previous dose of DTP or other vaccine that involved only a mild-to-moderate local
   reaction or fever less than 40.5°C
Mild acute upper respiratory or gastrointestinal illness with fever less than 38°C
Current antimicrobial therapy or convalescent phase of illnesses
Premature infant
Pregnancy of household contact
Recent exposure to infectious disease
Breastfeeding
Personal history of nonspecific allergies
Family history of allergies or seizures

---

11. Describe some of the new developments in vaccine research.

Vaccine research currently focuses on a number of areas, including the development of new vaccines (e.g., for AIDS), improvement of existing vaccines to enhance immunogenicity (e.g., adjuvant vaccines to enhance the antigenic response to pneumococcal vaccine), and improvement of existing vaccines to decrease associated side effects (e.g., the recent release of acellular pertussis vaccine). In addition, researchers are working on new ways to combine multiple antigens into a single vaccine to decrease the numbers of injections required for the adequate immunization of children.

12. How should screening tests for infectious diseases be interpreted?

Screening tests are used to identify persons with disease before they become symptomatic and should be distinguished from diagnostic tests in symptomatic persons. In screening for any disease, two critical questions should be addressed: (1) Is the screening test accurate and reliable? and (2) Does early intervention improve the patient's outcome or benefit other persons? For all of the infectious diseases discussed below, earlier intervention is clearly of benefit.

13. Who should be screened for HIV?

In 1996 HIV infection was the second leading cause of death for persons aged 24–44 years and the eighth leading cause of death in all age groups. People at increased risk for HIV for whom screening may be indicated include persons receiving treatment for sexually transmitted diseases, homosexual or bisexual men, injection drug users, people with a history of multiple sexual partners or prostitution, residence or birth in an area with high prevalence of HIV infection, people undergoing treatment for tuberculosis or drug abuse, and history of a blood transfusion between 1978 and 1985. Recent data also confirm an increasing epidemic of HIV infection among pregnant women and their infants. Because treatment of HIV-infected pregnant women with antiretroviral agents reduces perinatal transmission, routine HIV counseling and voluntary HIV screening are now recommended for all pregnant women.

Screening is usually performed initially with an FDA-approved enzyme-linked assay (ELA) that detects antibodies to HIV. Even though this test reportedly has a sensitivity and specificity of about 99%, because of the implications of false-positive results, the ELA test should be repeated before being reported as positive. Positive ELA results should then be confirmed by an FDA-approved supplemental test (e.g., the Western blot test or immunofluorescence assay [IFA]) before a diagnosis of HIV infection is made. If the true prevalence of HIV positivity in a population is 0.5%, even with 99% sensitivity and specificity, the positive predictive value of a single ELA would be only 33%. In addition, because it may take up to 6–12 weeks after exposure for a person to develop detectable antibodies to HIV, people with a history of a recent, significant exposure and an initial negative ELA test should be considered for retesting. All screening should be accompanied by appropriate counseling and informed consent; people with positive tests should receive additional information, counseling, and follow-up as appropriate and should be informed of the need to notify sexual partners, people with whom intravenous needles have been shared, and others at risk of exposure. All seropositive cases also should be reported to local public health officials according to state guidelines.

14. Describe current recommendations for tuberculosis screening.

In contrast to the steady decline in incidence of tuberculosis (TB) from 1953–1984, over the 9 years from 1985–1992 there was a 20% increase. Over 28,000 more cases than expected were reported from 1985–1990 alone. Since 1992, there has again been a substantial decline in reported TB cases among U.S.-born persons and a slight increase among foreign-born persons. Adverse social and economic factors, the HIV epidemic, and immigration of persons with tuberculous infection are important risk factors. Screening programs represent a critical component of TB control and should focus on high-risk populations, including:

1. Household members and close contacts of persons with known or suspected TB, including health care workers with significant exposures (contact investigation)

2. People with HIV infection

3. People with medical risk factors known to increase the risk of disease, including diabetes mellitus, conditions requiring prolonged high-dose corticosteroid therapy, gastrectomy, and chronic renal failure

4. Foreign-born people recently arrived (within 5 years) from countries with high TB prevalence, including migrant and seasonal farm workers

5. Medically underserved, low-income populations

6. High-risk racial or ethnic minority populations, as defined locally

7. Persons who inject illicit drugs or other locally defined high-risk substance users (e.g., crack cocaine users)

8. Residents and employees of congregate settings (e.g., long-term-care facilities, correctional institutions, mental institutions, nursing homes/facilities, and homeless shelters)

9. Health care workers who care for high-risk patients

10. Infants, children, and adolescents exposed to adults in high-risk categories

Flexibility is important in defining and refining definitions of high-risk, high-priority groups for screening. The changing epidemiology of TB indicates that the risk for TB among groups currently identified as high-risk may change over time, whereas groups currently not identified as high-risk may become high-priority groups for screening in the future.

15. What are the screening methods for TB?

The tuberculin skin test is the standard method for demonstrating tuberculous infection. The most commonly used formulation of tuberculin is purified protein derivative (PPD); the usual dose is 5 tuberculin units (TU) (0.1 mm of PPD). The tuberculin may be administered intracutaneously (Mantoux test) or with the multiple-puncture technique and should be read at 48 and 72 hours after injection. The Mantoux test best detects infection and is the preferred test for screening. The tuberculin skin tests are interpreted according to the amount of induration at the injection site. Persons are considered to have positive reactions with the Mantoux test in the following situations:

Induration ≥ 5 mm: people with HIV infection, close contacts of infectious cases, and people with fibrotic lesions on chest radiographs

Induration ≥ 10 mm: all other persons with risk factors for TB

Induration ≥ 15 mm: all other persons (i.e., low-risk persons for whom screening is not recommended).

For the multiple puncture test, any vesicular reaction is considered positive. All papular reactions from the multiple puncture test should be followed by a Mantoux test for further diagnostic evaluation. The multiple puncture test is not recommended for TB screening. People with positive skin reactions should be evaluated further to assess whether they have active disease. This evaluation usually includes clinical examination, chest radiograph, and sputum smear examination. Based on this evaluation, decisions are then made about the need for antimicrobial prophylaxis or treatment. All cases of active tuberculosis should be reported to the local public health official according to state guidelines.

16. What about false-negative TB skin tests?

False-negative Mantoux TB skin tests may be caused by nonresponsiveness to delayed-type hypersensitivity-inducing antigens such as tuberculin; they are common in persons with impaired immunity (e.g., HIV-infected people). Delayed-type hypersensitivity responsiveness can be assessed with other antigens such as *Candida* sp. However, the scientific basis for such testing is tenuous, and most skin-test antigens have no standardization. Anergy testing, therefore, is usually not part of screening for TB infection.

17. Who should be screened for sexually transmitted diseases (STDs)?

DISEASE	POPULATIONS TO BE SCREENED
HIV	See question 12
Hepatitis B	Pregnant women at first prenatal visit; test may be repeated in the third trimester for high-risk women (injection drug use, exposure to hepatitis B).
Syphilis	Prostitutes, people with multiple sexual partners in areas where syphilis is prevalent, people undergoing treatment for STDs, sexual contacts of persons with syphilis, pregnant women at first prenatal visit with additional testing at 28 weeks or later for women at increased risk for acquiring syphilis during pregnancy. Depending on local prevalence rates, other high-risk populations also may benefit from screening, such as jail or prison inmates.

(Table continued on next page.)

DISEASE	POPULATIONS TO BE SCREENED
Gonorrhea	Prostitutes, people with multiple sexual partners, sexual contacts of people with gonorrhea, people with history of repeated episodes of gonorrhea, people undergoing treatment for other STDs, pregnant women at first prenatal visit with repeat testing later in pregnancy if the woman is at increased risk for acquiring gonorrhea during the pregnancy.
Chlamydial infection	People who attend clinics for STDs, people who attend other high-risk health care facilities (e.g., adolescent and family planning clinics) or have other risk factors (age < 20, multiple sexual partners, sexual partners with multiple sexual contacts). Pregnant women with other risk factors should be screened at the first prenatal visit.

To ensure adequate partner notification, all newly identified cases of STDs should be reported to the local public health officials according to state guidelines.

18. Which tests should be used for screening for syphilis?

Tests used for screening for syphilis include both treponemal tests, which detect antibodies against *Treponema pallidum* or its components, and nontreponemal tests, which detect antibodies directed against lipoidal antigens. The main nontreponemal tests are the Venereal Disease Research Laboratory (VDRL) and rapid plasma reagin (RPR) tests. The main treponemal tests are the fluorescent treponemal antibody absorption test (FTA-ABS) and microhemagglutination test (e.g., MHA-TP). The VDRL or RPR tests usually become reactive during primary syphilis, remain at a peak in the first year of infection, and then fall slowly thereafter. After adequate treatment, the patient usually becomes seronegative after 6–12 months, depending on the duration of infection. The FTA-ABS and MHA-TP tests usually become reactive during primary syphilis and remain reactive for the patient's lifetime, regardless of treatment. For asymptomatic persons, screening is usually done with the VDRL or RPR tests with confirmation of positive tests by a treponemal test.

19. For which infectious diseases should pregnant women be screened?

Screening during pregnancy should take into account the particular risk profile of the patient. Routine screening for certain STDs is recommended because of the potential risk for the newborn, including hepatitis B, syphilis, and gonorrhea. Voluntary HIV testing after appropriate counseling is also recommended for all pregnant women. Screening for other STDs, such as chlamydial infection, should be undertaken if the woman has specific risk factors. In addition to STDs, pregnant women also should routinely be screened for rubella. If the woman is seronegative, the vaccine should be administered after delivery but before discharge from the hospital (such women should be counseled to avoid conception for 3 months after vaccination).

BIBLIOGRAPHY

General information
1. Advisory Committee on Immunization Practices: General recommendations on immunization. MMWR 43(RR-1), 1994.
2. Advisory Committee on Immunization Practices: Update: Vaccine side effects, adverse reactions, contraindications, and precautions. MMWR 45(RR-12), 1996.
3. Advisory Committee on Immunization Practices: Immunization of adolescents. MMWR 45(RR-13), 1996.
4. American College of Physicians Task Force on Adult Immunization and Infectious Diseases Society of America: Guide for Adult Immunizations, 3rd ed. Philadelphia, American College of Physicians, 1994.
5. Benenson AS (ed): Control of Communicable Diseases in Man, 16th ed. Washington, DC, American Public Health Association, 1995.
6. Centers for Disease Control and Prevention: Assessing adult vaccination status at age 50 years. MMWR 44:561–563, 1995.
7. Centers for Disease Control and Prevention: Immunization of health care workers: Recommendations of the Advisory Committee on Immunization Practices. MMWR 46(RR-18), 1994.
8. Fedson DS, for the National Vaccine Advisory Committee: Adult immunization. Summary of the National Vaccine Advisory Committee Report. JAMA 272:1133–1137, 1994.

9. Gardner P, Eickhoff T, Poland GA, et al: Adult immunizations. Ann Intern Med 12(1 Pt 1):35–40, 1996.
10. Immunization Practices Advisory Committee: Update on adult immunization. MMWR 40(RR-12), 1991.
11. Peter G (ed): 1997 Red Book. Report of the Committee on Infectious Diseases, 24th ed. Elk Grove Village, IL, American Academy of Pediatrics, 1997.
12. U.S. Preventive Services Task Force: Guide to Clinical Preventive Services, 2nd ed. Baltimore, Williams & Wilkins, 1996.

Specific topics
1. Advisory Committee on Immunization Practices: Use of vaccines and immune globulins for persons with altered immunocompetence. MMWR 42(RR-4), 1993.
2. Advisory Committee on Immunization Practices: Update: Recommendations to prevent hepatitis B virus transmission—United States. MMWR 44:574–575, 1995.
3. Advisory Committee for the Elimination of Tuberculosis: Screening for tuberculosis and tuberculous infection in high-risk populations. MMWR 44(RR-11), 1995.
4. Advisory Committee on Immunization Practices: Prevention of varicella. MMWR 45(RR-11), 1996.
5. Advisory Committee on Immunization Practices: Prevention of hepatitis A through active or passive immunization. MMWR 45(RR-15), 1996.
6. Advisory Committee on Immunization Practices: Prevention of pneumococcal disease. MMWR 46(RR-8), 1997.
7. Advisory Committee on Immunization Practices: Pertussis vaccination: Use of acellular pertussis vaccines among infants and young children. MMWR 46(RR-7), 1997.
8. Advisory Committee on Immunization Practices: Prevention and control of influenza. MMWR 47(RR-6), 1998.
9. Advisory Committee on Immunization Practices: Poliomyelitis prevention in the United States: Introduction of a sequential vaccination of inactivated poliovirus vaccine followed by oral poliovirus vaccine. MMWR 46(RR-3), 1997.
10. Advisory Committee for the Elimination of Tuberculosis: Prevention and control of tuberculosis in U.S. communities with at-risk minority populations and prevention and control of tuberculosis among homeless persons. MMWR 41(RR-5), 1992.
11. Advisory Committee for the Elimination of Tuberculosis: Prevention and control of tuberculosis in migrant farm workers. MMWR 41(RR-10), 1992.
12. American Thoracic Society: Diagnostic standards and classification of tuberculosis, 1990. Am Rev Respir Dis 142:725–735, 1990.
13. Centers for Disease Control: Vaccine Adverse Event Reporting System—United States. MMWR 39:730–793, 1990.
14. Centers for Disease Control: Recommendations for HIV testing and services for inpatients and outpatients in acute-care hospital settings. MMWR 42(RR-2):1–6, 1993.
15. Centers for Disease Control and Prevention: U.S. Public Health Service recommendations for human immunodeficiency virus counseling and voluntary testing for pregnant women. MMWR 44(RR-7), 1995.
16. Centers for Disease Control and Prevention: Averaging(?) shift(?) testing and preventive therapy for HIV-infected persons: Revised recommendations. MMWR 46(RR-15), 1997.
17. Centers for Disease Control and Prevention: 1998 guidelines for treatment of sexually transmitted diseases. MMWR 47(RR-1), 1998.
18. Centers for Disease Control and Prevention: Measles, mumps and rubella—Vaccine use and strategies for elimination of measles, mumps, rubella, and congenital rubella syndrome and control of mumps: Recommendations of the Advisory Committee on Immunization Practices (ACIP). MMWR 47(RR-8), 1998.
19. Hart G: Syphilis tests in diagnostic and therapeutic decision making. Ann Intern Med 104:368–376, 1986.

5. ETHNIC DIVERSITY AND DISEASE

Irene Aguilar, M.D.

1. What is an ethnic group?

An ethnic group is an aggregate of people who share a real or presumed common origin, a mutual historical past, and cultural symbols or social norms that shape the thought and behavior of individual members. Examples include values (family dynamics), beliefs (religion), customs (food preferences, holidays), behaviors (sex roles), and language or distinctive dialects. Ethnic groups usually have a shared sense of identity within the larger social system.

2. What is the difference between behavioral and ideologic ethnicity?

Behavioral ethnicity values, such as beliefs, behavioral norms, and language, are learned during growth and development. Ethnicity permeates all interactions. In the United States behavioral ethnicity is seen primarily in first- and second-generation residents and ethnic minorities with a history of exclusion from the mainstream (e.g., African-Americans, Hispanics, and Native Americans). Ideologic ethnicity is based mainly on customs that are not central to a person's daily functioning but are symbols of their cultural heritage. It involves voluntary identification, such as observance of holiday customs and celebrations among third- or fourth-generation white ethnic immigrants (e.g., Germans).

3. How commonly are ethnic minority groups encountered in primary care settings?

The 1990 census demonstrates significant changes in the population of the United States. The white majority is shrinking and aging; many of the minority ethnic populations are young and growing. California is expected to have a "minority majority" by 2005.

	% TOTAL POPULATION	% POPULATION BELOW POVERTY
African-American	12.1	31
Hispanic	9	21.5
Asian and Pacific	2.9	12.2
Native Americans	0.8	19–45
Whites	80.3	10

The African-American population increased by 13.2% from 1980–1990. There is no breakdown by country of origin. African-Americans have been in the U.S. since as early as 1619.

The Hispanic population, which includes Spanish-speaking people of any race (black or white), increased by 53% from 1980–1990. The greatest numbers of the Hispanic population are of Mexican-American descent (62.6%); Puerto Rican (11.1%), Cubans (4.9%), and Central and South Americans (13.7%) make up most of the remainder.

Asian and Pacific populations increased by 108% from 1980–1990. Of these, 24% are Chinese, 21% Filipino, 10% Japanese, 10% Asian Indian, 10% Korean, 7% Vietnamese, 3.4% Hawaiian, 1.2% Samoan, and 1% Guamians.

The Native American, Eskimo, and Aleut populations in the United States increased by 37.7% from 1980–1990. The majority (96%) are American Indians, 3% are Eskimos, and 1% are Aleuts. The percentage of people who fell below the poverty level in 1980 varied from a high of 44.8% for reservation Indians to a low of 19.5% for Aleuts.

By contrast, the white population in the United States (including Hispanics, who may be of any race) constitutes 80.3% of the total population. This figure represents a population increase of 6% from 1980, but an overall 3% decrease of the total population. Ten percent of white persons were below the poverty level in 1990.

4. Why is it difficult to study health patterns or clinical research in ethnic groups?

Although technically different, ethnicity and social class are closely interrelated in the United States, making it difficult to interpret clinical research about health patterns of ethnic groups.

5. Why is it important to recognize ethnic diversity in the care of patients?

1. Ethnic groups may vary in rates of morbidity and mortality for specific diseases. These differences may result from biases in vital statistics; nonbehavioral factors, such as genetic predisposition; shared risk factors (largely due to class membership), such as poverty, poor nutrition, or exposure to different pathogenic agents; or ethnically patterned pathogenic cultural standards or behaviors. Specific diseases may have different prognosis dependent solely on ethnic status.

2. Ethnicity influences concepts of disease and illness, which in turn influence other aspects of health behavior, such as how symptoms are perceived, evaluated, and acted upon (or not acted upon). An understanding of traditional beliefs may ameliorate problems in patient interactions or compliance. Fundamental differences often exist between the health beliefs of health care providers and patients. Understanding the patient's behavior and beliefs may allow physicians to ask comfortably about patients' interpretation of symptoms and potential remedies. Such recognitions allow the health care provider to meet the patient's needs more effectively.

3. Ethnicity affects utilization of mainstream medical services. An obvious factor is the location of mainstream care (e.g., emergency department, hospital, clinic). Ethnic residential segregation may result in patient populations in hospitals, clinics, or private practices composed predominantly of specific local ethnic groups. Alternative providers of health care may be used before, during, or after access of mainstream care. Providers should be familiar with formal and informal sources of help outside the traditional medical community.

4. Ethnicity often dictates styles of interaction. Attitudes toward authority figures, gender roles, and ways of expressing emotion and asking for help are carried into health-care situations. For example, Southeast Asians expect health professionals to be experts and consequently tend not to contribute much information and not to question or oppose authority figures openly.

By knowing and respecting ethnically determined factors, physicians can tailor interventions to meet the patient's needs.

6. A 62-year-old Native American with constipation has seen a medicine man and was prescribed medicinal herbs, but his wife insisted that he see you. Should you change his treatment?

Recognition of the health beliefs and practices of local ethnic groups permits the physician to gain patient trust and to avoid creating a feeling of alienation. Every effort should be made to combine folk treatment with standard Western treatment as long as the two are not antagonistic and as long as the patient will come to no harm with the prescribed folk therapy. If the regimen is harmful, you may suggest that because this treatment has not seemed to work, something else may be tried.

7. A 28-year-old Mexican-American woman comes to see you for the sixth time in 3 months, complaining of restlessness, insomnia, anorexia, anergia, and anhedonia. After a comprehensive evaluation, you treat her for depression with little apparent improvement in symptoms. To which specialist should you refer her?

She should be referred to a traditional Mexican-American healer, a *curandero*. Curanderos believe in both natural and supernatural illness and often refer patients to traditional physicians if they feel that they are unable to diagnose and treat a natural illness. Curanderos deal with problems of a social, psychological, and spiritual nature as well as physical ailments.

The most likely diagnosis here is *susto*, which involves "soul loss" and is a folk illness believed to arise from fright. The soul is believed to have left the body to wander freely as a result of a dream or a particularly traumatic event. The symptoms of the disease, listed above, also may include hallucinations and various painful sensations. The curandero coaxes the soul back into the body, using prayer, *barridas* (sweeping over the body), and herb teas. Other common Mexican-American folk illnesses are listed below.

Empacho: an illness caused by a ball of food sticking to the wall of the stomach. Symptoms include stomachache, cramps, anorexia, diarrhea, and vomiting. Massaging the stomach, pinching the spine, and drinking a purgative tea are commonly prescribed by the curandero.

Mal ojo (evil eye): an illness to which all children are susceptible. It results from an admiring or covetous look from a person with a "strong" eye. Symptoms are vomiting, fever, crying, and restlessness. The evil eye may be prevented if the person with the strong eye touches the child while admiring him or her or by wearing protective amulets. The illness is treated by a curandero with a barrida and prayer.

Envidia (envy): cause of illness and bad luck. If success provokes the envy of friends and neighbors, misfortune may befall the person and his or her family.

8. An elderly Cambodian woman presents with diarrhea. On physical examination you notice cigarette burns on her abdomen. She is not a smoker. Should you report her family to adult protective services?

No. Cigarette burns are a traditional method of folk healing in Asian populations. Moxibustion and dermabrasive practices are among the Chinese folk remedies widely practiced among Vietnamese, Khmer, Hmong, and Mien peoples. The dermal methods are seen as ways to relieve headaches, muscle pains, sinusitis, colds, sore throat, coughs, difficulty with breathing, diarrhea, or fever. A cigarette or piece of burning cotton may be touched to the skin, usually the abdomen, to compensate for "heat" lost through diarrhea. Cupping involves placing a heated cup on the skin; as it cools, it contracts and draws the skin and excessive energy ("wind") or toxicity into the cup. This procedure leaves circular ecchymoses on the skin. Pinching produces bruises or welts at the site of treatment. Rubbing of skin with a spoon or coin is done to bring the toxic "wind" to the body surface and also produces bruises or welts. Other traditional practices used by Asians include acupuncture, massage, and herbal concoctions and poultices, which rarely present a threat to the person and often nurture a sense of being cared for and the ability to alleviate bothersome symptoms.

Such remedies relate to Chinese theories of health as a state of balance among the different components of the body and of the body with its environment. Therapeutic diets require considerations of the "hot" or "cold" natures of foods, cooking methods, and the person's ailment. The various parts of the human body correspond to the dualistic principles of "yin" and "yang" and must be kept in harmony.

9. How do you recognize jaundice in a dark-skinned person?

Few signs cannot be recognized in a dark-skinned person with proper technique. Lighting (nonglare daylight), positioning (examination of the part of the body at heart level), environmental temperature, and the patient's emotional state contribute to an accurate exam in any patient. Color changes are best observed at sites where pigmentation from melanin, melanoid, and carotene is least: sclera, conjunctiva, nailbeds, lips, buccal mucosa, tongue, palms, and soles (unless heavily calloused). African-Americans commonly have brown, freckle-like pigmentation of the gums, buccal cavity, border of the tongue, and even the nailbeds.

Jaundice is best seen in sclera. However, many darkly pigmented patients have heavy deposits of subconjunctival fat, which may mimic jaundice. Therefore, if inspection of the portion revealed naturally by the lid slit demonstrates icterus, the edges of the cornea and the posterior portion of the hard palate should be inspected.

Pallor is best diagnosed by the absence of underlying red tones; brown skin appears more yellowish brown and black skin appears ashen gray. The conjunctiva are also an excellent site to assess pallor.

Petechiae are more easily seen on the abdomen, buttocks, and volar surface of the forearm. In dark brown skin they may be more difficult to see except in mucous membranes.

Cyanosis is the most difficult to diagnose. The mucous membranes show bluish discoloration. Applying light pressure to create pallor, observing for return of color, and following the exam serially over time are helpful approaches.

10. A 24-year-old Laotian woman presents for a physical examination before getting pregnant. How does her ethnic background influence your search for possible disease or prevention considerations?

Knowledge of an ethnic group's genetic disorders and disease prevalence strongly influences evaluation. The following six potential diagnoses should be considered in light of her desire to become pregnant:

1. Hemoglobinopathies. Microcytosis in people of Southeast Asian origin is most commonly related to alpha- and beta-thalassemia and hemoglobin-E carrier states. A study of Southeast Asians in California found that 8% from Vietnam and 3% from Cambodia and Laos have the beta-thalassemia trait; 36% of refugees from Cambodia and 28% of refugees from Laos

were carriers of the hemoglobin-E trait. Correct diagnosis is necessary to provide genetic counseling and to avoid inappropriate treatment of carriers with iron (risking iron overload) for microcytic anemia.

    2. G6PD deficiency

    3. Lactose intolerance

    4. Hepatitis B carrier state. The carrier state for hepatitis B was as high as 8.6% in one study of Southeast Asians.

    5. Parasitic infection. As many as 35% of Southeast Asian refugees have positive stool for parasites.

    6. Tuberculosis. Up to 52% have a positive PPD, and the age-specific incidence of tuberculosis is 14–70 times higher than that for the U.S. population as a whole. Drug resistance is common.

11. Which chronic illness disproportionately affects Hispanics? Why?

The prevalence of diabetes is 1.7–2.4 times higher in Hispanics at all age groups than in non-Hispanic whites. Diabetes is present in 33% of Hispanics aged 65–74 years compared with 17% of non-Hispanic whites and 25% of non-Hispanic blacks. The age-adjusted death rate from diabetes is twice as high in Hispanics as in non-Hispanic whites. The excessive prevalence is believed to be related to multiple factors, including the high incidence of obesity, hyperinsulinemia, positive family history, and high frequency of Native American genes in Hispanics. Despite the excessive prevalence, macrovascular complications are not increased in Hispanics. However, microvascular complications of retinopathy, nephropathy, and neuropathy have been found to be increased in Mexican-Americans.

12. How has AIDS affected ethnic minorities?

AIDS disproportionately affects many ethnic minority populations. In 1996 African-Americans represented 41% of AIDS cases, up from 33.3% in 1991. Hispanics represented 18.9% of AIDS cases compared with 14.7% in 1991. Non-Hispanic whites represented 38.3% of AIDS cases, down from 50.9% in 1991. This disparity is even larger among women and children. Hispanic and African-American women of childbearing age represent 75.7% of all reported AIDS cases in women through 1996. Hispanic and African-American children account for 81% of all childhood AIDS cases through 1996. Intravenous drug use represents the primary route of HIV transmission in these populations. In 1991 HIV disease became the leading cause of death for African-American men between the ages of 25 and 44. In 1994 it became the leading cause of death for African-American women in the same age group.

13. What is the major health problem of Native Americans?

Alcohol abuse is the major cause of morbidity and mortality in the Native American community. Alcohol abuse contributes to death and illnesses from accidents, suicide, homicide, diabetes, congenital anomalies in infants, pneumonia, heart disease, and cancer. Alcoholism has been implicated in 50% of adult crime on Indian reservations. There is a high rate of unintentional injuries as well as chronic liver disease and cirrhosis-related deaths in Native Americans. The incidence of fetal alcohol syndrome is 4 per 1000 live births in Native Americans and Alaska Natives compared with 0.8 per 1000 live births in African-Americans.

14. What factors contribute to alcoholism in American Indians?

The multifactorial etiology of alcohol abuse includes genetic, physiologic, and social factors. Native Americans may be genetically predisposed to crave ever-increasing doses of alcohol during rapid loss of control of the senses. There are differences in alcohol absorption and metabolism between Native Americans and whites. Passive aggressiveness and emotional repression as well as socioeconomic conditions and failure to develop social sanctions regulating drunkenness contribute to alcoholism. Self-esteem of Native Americans is often low, perhaps related to inadequate formal education, poverty, and a traditional value system ignored by the dominant society.

15. Are African-Americans at increased risk for cardiovascular morbidity and mortality?

Many recent articles have addressed racial disparity in morbidity and mortality from heart disease. African-American men and women have a higher death rate from heart disease, stroke, and hypertensive heart disease. In addition, they have had a slower rate of decline in cardiovascular morbidity and mortality. Between 1970 and 1989 there was a 39% reduction in mortality from heart disease for white U.S. citizens compared with a 30% reduction for African-Americans.

16. Why do African-Americans have excessive cardiovascular morbidity and mortality?

Multiple reasons are likely to contribute:

1. Reduced access to health care. African-Americans are less likely to have medical insurance. Other financial barriers disproportionately affect African-Americans because of their poverty rate. African Americans are more often treated in public facilities that may be understaffed and underequipped in terms of the needs of the patient base. In addition, reduced geographic access or lack of transportation to facilities that offer invasive procedures may contribute. An absence of trust in the health-care system also limits access to medical care.

2. Increased prevalence of cardiovascular risk factors. African-Americans are more likely to have diabetes, hypertension, obesity, left ventricular hypertrophy, and tobacco dependence. Yet they make fewer office visits to physicians.

3. Limited knowledge of signs, symptoms, and available treatment of cardiovascular disease. African-Americans are less likely to go to an emergency department within 6 hours of an acute myocardial infarction, resulting in poor outcome of therapy. African-Americans are less familiar with revascularization procedures.

4. African-American patients are less likely to be aggressively evaluated and treated for cardiovascular disease. African-Americans are less likely than whites to undergo a wide range of major medical procedures, including cardiac catheterization, percutaneous transluminal coronary angioplasty, and coronary artery bypass grafting. African-Americans are less frequently seen by a cardiovascular specialist. Age, sex, variable disease severity, type of hospital, insurance, and socioeconomic status have not explained this difference. The black-white disparity in the use of procedures is greatest when decision making is less clearly dictated by the clinical situation. Poor communication about treatment options between physicians and African-American patients may contribute. African Americans are up to twice as likely to refuse an invasive procedure. The willingness of African-American patients to participate in treatment has been shown to be greater when they are asked by other African-Americans. Physicians must make an effort to explain and offer choices in a nonbiased, ethnically accessible way.

CONTROVERSY

17. Should antihypertensive therapy be chosen on the basis of ethnicity?

The use of a specific drug class for a particular ethnic group should be made only after considering other concomitant risks and diseases. No data suggest a hierarchy of response in Hispanics, but their increased risk of diabetes should encourage use of the lowest possible dose of diuretic or beta blocker. In addition, reports have shown a decline in hyperlipidemia and hyperglycemia in Hispanics taking angiotensin-converting enzyme (ACE) inhibitors and calcium channel blockers.

Some evidence indicates that Asian Americans respond more favorably to calcium channel blockers than to ACE inhibitors. In China, hypertensive patients taking hydrochlorothiazide had dose-related hypotensive responses without a plateau effect. There was also a high incidence of ACE inhibitor-induced cough, which has not been reported in the United States. Although some evidence suggests that African-Americans respond less favorably to beta blockers and ACE inhibitors compared with diuretics and calcium channel blockers, the reduction in blood pressure is still significant. In addition, African-Americans are at increased risk of diabetes, cardiovascular disease, left ventricular hypertrophy, and end-stage renal disease. The concomitant presence of any of these illnesses should guide the choice of therapy.

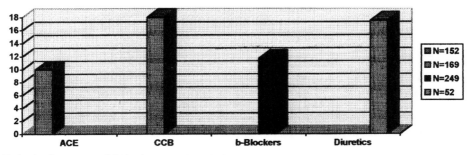

Reduction in mean arterial blood pressure (mmHg) in response to antihypertensive therapy in 13 prospective trials for treatment of hypertension in African Americans. (From Jamerson K, DeQuattro V: The impact of ethnicity on response to antihypertensive therapy. Am J Med 101(Suppl 3A):28S, 1996, with permission.)

BIBLIOGRAPHY

1. Ayanian JZ: Heart disease in black and white. N Engl J Med 329:656, 1993.
2. Becker LB, et al: Racial differences in the incidence of cardiac arrest and subsequent survival. N Engl J Med 329:600, 1993.
3. Buchwald D, Carolis PV, Gany F, et al: Five vignettes of cross-cultural care. Pat Care 28:120–123, 1994.
4. Centers for Disease Control: HIV/Aids Surveillance Report, 1996. Atlanta, Centers for Disease Control and Prevention, 1996.
5. Centers for Disease Control: Update: Mortality attributable to HIV infection among persons aged 25–44—United States, 1994. MMWR 45:121–125, 1996.
6. Chesney AP, et al: Mexican American folk medicine: Implications for the family physician. J Fam Prac 11(4):567, 1980.
7. Ford E, Cooper RS: Racial/ethnic differences in health care utilization of cardiovascular procedures: A review of the evidence. Health Serv Res 30:237–250, 1995.
8. Harwood A (ed): Ethnicity and Medical Care. Cambridge, Harvard University Press, 1981.
9. Henderson G, Primeaux M (eds): Transcultural Health Care. Menlo Park, NJ, Addison-Wesley, 1981.
10. Jamerson K, DeQuattro V: The impact of ethnicity on response to antihypertensive therapy. Am J Med 101(Suppl 3A):22S–32S, 1996.
11. Johnson PA, et al: Effect of race on the presentation and management of patients with acute chest pain. Ann Intern Med 118:593, 1993.
12. Lamarine R: The dilemma of Native American health. Health Educ 20(5):15, 1989.
13. Lamarine R: Alcohol abuse among Native Americans. J Community Health 13(4):143, 1988.
14. Lin-Fu JS: Population characteristics and health care needs of Asian Pacific Americans. Publ Health Rep 103(1):18, 1988.
15. Muecke MA: Caring for Southeast Asian refugee patients in the USA. Am J Publ Health 73:431, 1983.
16. Roach LB: Color changes in dark skin. In Henderson G, Primeaux M (eds): Transcultural Health Care. Menlo Park, NJ, Addison-Wesley, 1981.
17. Shea S, et al: Predisposing factors for severe, uncontrolled hypertension in an inner city minority population. N Engl J Med 327:776, 1992.
18. Smith DK: HIV disease as a cause of death for African Americans in 1987 and 1990. J Natl Med Assoc 84(6):481, 1992.
19. Spector RE: Cultural Diversity in Health and Illness. Stamford, CT, Appleton & Lange, 1996.
20. Stern MP, Haffner MP: Type II diabetes and its complications in Mexican Americans. Diabetes Metab Rev 6(1):29, 1990.
21. Thomson GE: Discrimination in health care. Ann Intern Med 126(11):910–912, 1997.
22. Trotter RT II, Chavira JA: Curanderismo: An emic theoretical perspective of Mexican-American folk medicine. Med Anthropol (Fall):423, 1980.
23. U.S. Congress, Office of Technology Assessment: Indian Health Care. OTA-H-290. Washington, DC, U.S. Government Printing Office, 1986.
24. Whittle J, et al: Racial differences in the use of invasive procedures in the Department of Veterans Affairs Medical System. N Engl J Med 329:621, 1993.
25. Whittle J, et al: Do patient preferences contribute to racial differences in cardiovascular procedure use? J Gen Intern Med 12:267–273, 1997.
26. 1990 Census of Population and Housing. Summary tape file 1c (computer file). Washington, DC, Bureau of the Census, Data Users Services Division, 1992.

6. ALTERNATIVE MEDICINE

Lisa Corbin Winslow, M.D.

1. What is alternative medicine?

Alternative medicine is a broad term which includes any treatment used for healing that is not widely taught in United States medical schools or widely available in United States hospitals. Frequently used equivalent terms are complementary medicine (often combined as complementary/alternative medicine or CAM) and unconventional medicine.

2. How many patients use alternative medicine?

A study in the *New England Journal of Medicine* found that one-third of adults in the United States use CAM, as defined above. In 1994, there were 425 million visits to alternative providers in the United States, which is more than the number of visits to primary care physicians over the same period.

3. What are the typical demographics of an alternative medicine user?

The typical CAM user is white, aged 25–49 years old, college-educated, and from a higher socioeconomic status. Most CAM users also see a conventional practitioner for the same problems. People with chronic health problems (such as cancer, arthritis, and AIDS) are also more likely to try CAM.

4. Why do people use CAM?

Patients perceive CAM to be a healthier alternative to conventional medicine, often because of reports in the lay press of toxicities of conventional treatments and the lack of such reporting on alternative treatments. Many people mistakenly believe that alternative treatments are natural and thus safe. In addition, patients often turn to CAM as a way to regain a sense of control of their own health care; they choose the treatment instead of their physician. When conventional options truly have run out, patients with chronic health problems may turn to CAM as a last-ditch effort.

5. What are the most popular alternative treatments?

The *New England Journal of Medicine* study found relaxation techniques, chiropractic therapy, and massage therapy to be the most frequently used. Other studies have found the use of other treatments to be much higher. The differences are probably due to how the questions were phrased and how treatments were defined. For example, one study found that 95% of patients in a Kaiser system were using herbal medicine.

6. Why should the primary care physician ask all patients about their use of CAM?

Primary care providers need to know all of the treatments their patients are using, because they may affect conventional treatments. A treatment may cause direct drug-drug or drug-treatment interactions, or the alternative treatment in fact may be the cause of the condition. In addition, a patient who is using CAM may have misconceptions about the utility of conventional treatment; for example, the patient may be using CAM because she or he believes that no conventional treatment exists for a certain condition or that the conventional treatment is unsafe. By asking all patients about CAM use, misconceptions about conventional treatments may be discussed.

7. In evaluating any treatment, alternative or conventional, what three questions should the physician try to answer before recommending for or against the treatment?

1. What is the safety of the treatment (what are the risks)?
2. What is the efficacy of the treatment (what are the benefits)?
3. Is the treatment cost-effective?

8. What is meant by primum non nocere? How does it relate to unconventional medicine?
First, do no harm. If you do not know much about an alternative treatment, your first priority and obligation is to make sure that your patient will not be harmed by it.

9. Which alternative treatments, when practiced by trained practitioners, are generally accepted to be safe?
The treatments listed below have few risks. However, the use of any alternative treatment can be harmful to the patient's health when it is used in place of a known, effective conventional treatment. The most obvious examples are alternative treatments for a cancer that can be cured by resection or when a patient forgoes insulin treatment in favor of an alternative treatment for type I diabetes.
- Chiropractic therapy. Despite concern about damage to the spinal cord or nerve roots with chiropractic therapy, such damage is exceedingly rare, especially with manipulation of the lower back. Manipulation of the cervical spine carries a higher risk and probably should be discouraged.
- Acupuncture. Risk of infection is basically negated by the use of disposable, sterile needles. Risk of pneumothorax is real but small.
- Relaxation techniques
- Therapeutic massage. Relatively contraindicated in patients with soft tissue infection, because of the theoretical risk of spreading infection, but otherwise generally safe.
- Yoga
- Homeopathy
- Aromatherapy
- Reflexology

10. Which alternative treatments have been shown to be beneficial?
First of all, few alternative treatments have been extensively studied in scientific fashion because funding for such studies is difficult to obtain, it is hard to recruit patients (who are drawn to CAM because they want to control their health care and thus do not want a 50/50 chance of receiving a placebo), and alternative providers do not often have a background in the scientific method. In addition, there are currently *no requirements* for proof of the safety and efficacy of herbal medicine and other dietary supplements before marketing (in contrast to conventional medications, which must go through rigorous testing and ongoing quality control). Thus, manufacturers do not feel the need to do studies. Despite these limitations, some good studies have shown benefit for the following conditions with certain alternative treatments:
- Chiropractic therapy for acute low back pain
- Acupuncture for chronic pain, addiction, and nausea
- Relaxation techniques for insomnia and behavioral problems
- Biofeedback for mild hypertension and irritable bowel disease
- Certain herbs for certain illnesses (e.g., St. John's Wort for depression and valerian to induce sleep)

11. Why are herbs and supplements not routinely recommended?
The use of herbs and supplements should not be recommended for patients because of the lack of quality control and standardization within the industry. The Dietary Supplement and Health Education Act of 1994 requires no proof of safety, efficacy, or quality control for this category of medications; thus, consumers cannot be sure of the following:
1. The actual content of the product (adulterants, such as antibiotics, steroids, tranquilizers, heavy metals, and NSAIDs are not uncommon).
2. Whether the right part of the plant has been picked (harvesters are often not well trained and toxic parts of the plant or the wrong plant entirely may have been used).
3. The right dosage of the supplement (without industry standardization, the amount of active ingredient varies up to 10,000-fold in various preparations of the same product; what may be safe or effective in one dosage may be frankly toxic in another).

In the future, it may be possible for conventional physicians to encourage the use of certain supplements in certain conditions, if requirements are made for standardization and quality control, and if information about proper dosing can be more easily obtained. Good quality control and extensive studies of herbs exists in Germany, where supplements are regulated like conventional medications. The German "commission E monographs" are being translated and will be available in the next few years.

12. Which alternative therapies have a risk of harm high enough to dissuade the patient from their use?
- Coffee or other "cleansing" enemas. The volume of infused hypotonic solution may cause massive fluid and electrolyte imbalances, bowel perforation, and gut flaccidity.
- Herbal medicines (see discussion above; in the future, we may be able to recommend certain agents with confidence because some appear safe and effective).
- Chelation therapy
- Intensive, restrictive diet therapy or megavitamin therapy (the patient may become malnourished or toxic).
- Certain Chinese patent medicines (herbs are often adulterated with steroids or heavy metals).

13. What is the placebo response?
When any treatment is studied against a placebo, a reproducible, measurable 20–30% placebo response rate is found. In other words, patients who receive a placebo instead of the active treatment show an improvement about 30% of the time. They also have side effects. Thus, in evaluating the efficacy (or side effect profile) of any given treatment, it is important to know how it compares with placebo. No one knows why the placebo effect exists, but it seems to support the idea of a mind-body connection. In other words, if a patient (or physician) perceives that a treatment will work, it is more likely to have an effect, perhaps related to release of endorphins and other chemicals. This also underscores the importance of a good doctor-patient relationship as the foundation of any medical treatment and may explain why some alternative treatments appear to work.

14. How much money is spent on CAM? How do CAM users pay for their treatments?
In 1994, $13.7 billion were spent in the United States on CAM. This amount is more than the costs of hospitalizations for a year in the United States. Most of the costs are paid directly out of pocket by consumers, but insurance plans are beginning to offer coverage for certain treatments, and coverage of certain CAM practices is mandated by law in some states.

15. How should a patient who inquires about the use of CAM be advised?
First, the patient should be cautioned about any treatments that are known to be unsafe. Next, the condition or symptom for which the patient is interested in trying CAM should be well-defined by both patient and clinician, and the risks and benefits of all possible conventional options should be discussed. If the patient does not want to try these options or has already exhausted them, it may be advisable to encourage the use of CAM. Both patient and physician should research the particular method in which the patient is interested and try to find and interview reliable providers in the area (see below). The patient should define the symptom or problem for which he or she is seeking treatment and keep a symptom diary before, during, and after the treatment to allow a more objective assessment of response, including side effects. The primary physician should communicate with the provider of the treatment as with any referral to ensure the best continuity of care.

Many providers of alternative treatments are required to be licensed in certain states. Your state's local organizations or national organizations can be contacted for this information. The provider should be asked about his or her experience with the problem in question, and if the provider has had good luck in treating it, the patient should talk with a former patient. The patient also should ask the provider how many visits the treatment will take, how much it will cost, and how soon the patient should expect a response. Potential side effects should be explored. All conversations with the patient and any other providers should be documented in the chart as with any patient encounter.

16. Does the primary care physician need to worry about being sued for referring to an alternative provider?

According to Eisenberg: "Although physicians have been prosecuted for malpractice when they have personally delivered alternative treatments, no cases have involved conventionally trained physicians who have advised patients about alternative medical therapies."

BIBLIOGRAPHY

1. Brown JS, Marcy SA: The use of botanicals for health purposes by members of a prepaid health plan. Res Nurs Health 14:339–350, 1991.
2. Eisenberg DM: Advising patients who seek alternative care. Ann Intern Med 127:61–69, 1997.
3. Eisenberg D, Kessler RC, Foster C, et al: Unconventional medicine in the United States. N Engl J Med 328:246–252, 1993.
4. Gevitz N: Three perspectives on unorthodox medicine. In Gevitz N (ed): Other Healers: Unorthodox Medicine in America. Baltimore, Johns Hopkins University Press, 1988.
5. Herbal Roulette. Consumer Reports, November 1995.
6. Rosenfeld I: Dr. Rosenfeld's Guide to Alternative Medicine. New York, Random House, 1996.
7. Winslow LC, Kroll DC: Herbal medicine. Arch Intern Med In press, 1998.

7. PHYSICAL EXAM CORRELATES

Andrew R. Robinson, M.D.

1. What is the correct method for measuring blood pressure?

The patient should be seated in a quiet environment, and a properly sized cuff should be wrapped around the bare arm 2 cm above the brachial pulse and held at the level of the heart. The radial pulse should be palpated during inflation until it disappears; this maneuver provides an estimate of the systolic pressure and prevents missing an auscultatory gap (see below). The bell of the stethoscope is then held over the brachial pulse, and the cuff is deflated at a rate of 2 mm/sec. The appearance of the first sound corresponds to systolic blood pressure. The disappearance of the sounds, not their muffling, correlates with diastolic pressure. In hypertensive patients, two separate measurements should be taken at least 30 seconds apart, and measurement should be done in each arm on at least one occasion.

2. What are the most common errors in measuring blood pressure?

Probably the most common error in auscultating blood pressure is the use of an improperly sized cuff. Too large a cuff underestimates true blood pressure, and too small a cuff overestimates it. Other errors include failure to palpate the radial artery during inflation, which may miss an auscultatory gap, and overly rapid cuff deflation, which underestimates true blood pressure. The use of faulty equipment is also probably common.

3. What is the significance of an auscultatory gap?

An auscultatory gap occurs when the Korotkoff sounds temporarily disappear during deflation of the blood pressure cuff, usually during phase II. A gap is reported to be present in up to 21% of hypertensive patients. If the gap is undetected and the point at which Korotkoff sounds resume is assumed to be the systolic pressure, there may be significant underestimation

and undertreatment of true blood pressure. The presence of an ausculatory gap is associated
with a 2-fold increase in the incidence of carotid artery atherosclerosis and an increase in arterial
wall stiffness and pulse velocity.

4. If you detect an abdominal bruit in a hypertensive patient, what should you do?

Although abdominal bruits are relatively common in young, healthy individuals, their
presence in hypertensive patients is suggestive of renovascular disease. In one study, the presence of a systolic bruit in hypertensive patients increased the likelihood of renovascular disease 6.4-fold; in another, the presence of a systolic-diastolic bruit increased the likelihood
39-fold. However, the absence of a bruit is not sufficiently sensitive to rule out renovascular
disease.

5. If you detect a carotid bruit on exam, what should you do?

It depends on the age of the patient. In asymptomatic patients younger than 50, no further
work-up is indicated. In men 50 and older, there is an increased risk of transient ischemic attack
(TIA) or stroke (3-fold relative risk; absolute risk 1.5%/yr vs. 0.5%/yr). However, in asymptomatic patients with carotid artery stenosis, with the exception of one study, no benefit to endarterectomy has been found. Thus, referral for carotid assessment may be deferred and medical
therapy for stroke prevention initiated. Of interest, beyond the age of 75, an increased risk of
stroke is no longer associated with an asymptomatic carotid bruit. In symptomatic patients (i.e.,
those with TIA or stroke in the ipsilateral distribution), the presence of a bruit increases the likelihood of high-grade stenosis, but its absence does not rule out stenosis and does not obviate the
need for further evaluation.

6. How should jugular venous pressure be measured? How accurate is it in assessing central venous pressure?

Jugular venous pressure (JVP) should be measured with the relaxed neck positioned 30–45°
above horizontal. The vertical distance from the sternal angle of Louis (which lies 5 cm above the
right atrium, regardless of the angle at which the patient is reclining) to the highest point of jugular venous pulsation (which usually occurs during expiration) should be measured. Adding 5 cm
to this number gives a rough estimate of central venous pressure (CVP).

In general, JVP is best used as an estimate of low, normal, or high CVP rather than as an
exact measurement. Overall, clinical studies show that physicians' assessments of CVP are correct around 55% of the time. In one study, the sensitivity of JVP for determining low, normal, or
high CVP was 0.33, 0.33, and 0.49, respectively, with a specificity of 0.73, 0.62, and 0.76. In another study, the JVP was found to be more accurate as an assessment of low or high CVP than of
normal CVP (an estimate of low or high JVP increased the likelihood of a correspondingly low
or high CVP 4-fold and was never mistaken for the opposite situation; but an estimate of a normal
JVP did not predict low, normal, or high CVP). Thus, the overall accuracy of JVP in determining
CVP may be questionable, but it is probably more helpful when CVP is thought to be abnormally
low or high.

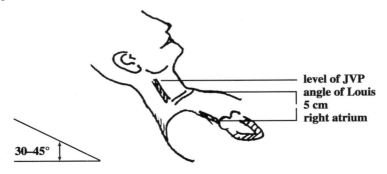

level of JVP
angle of Louis
5 cm
right atrium

30–45°

7. How do we test for abdominojugular reflux? What does a positive test mean?

The test for abdominojugular reflux is performed by measuring JVP, then by applying firm pressure to the patient's abdomen with an open hand for 15–30 seconds (the recommended pressure is 20–35 mmHg, which can be estimated by a partially inflated blood pressure cuff under the examiner's hand) with the patient breathing through his or her mouth. The test is considered positive if there is a *sustained* (> 10 sec) increase in JVP of 4 cm or more. The test is quite specific for increased right-sided pressure and, in the absence of isolated right-sided heart disease, is highly suggestive of congestive heart failure. The test is also positive in tricuspid stenosis, constrictive pericarditis, pulmonary hypertension, cardiac tamponade, and right ventricular infarction.

8. If you detect a systolic murmur on exam, how can you determine whether it is left- or right-sided in origin?

In a study by Lembo et al. using cardiologists as evaluators, an increase of murmur intensity during inspiration or a decrease during expiration occurred with all right-sided murmurs but in only 12% of other murmurs, giving these findings a sensitivity of 100%, specificity of 88%, and LR+ of 8.0. All patients in the study had known valvular abnormalities; thus these data may not be as applicable in unselected patients. In another study, increased murmur intensity with the application of sustained abdominal pressure significantly increased the likelihood that the murmur was due to tricuspid regurgitation (LR+ ∞, LR– = 0.20).

9. Which characteristics of a systolic murmur increase or decrease the likelihood that it is due to aortic stenosis (AS)?

The murmur of AS is typically a crescendo-decrescendo murmur best heart at the second right intercostal space. On physical examination, the following findings have been shown to increase significantly the likelihood of AS: decreased or absent S_2 (LR+ = 3.1–50), peak murmur intensity in mid or late systole (LR+ = 8.0–101), slow rate of rise in the carotid pulse (LR + = 2.8–130), apical-carotid delay (LR+ = 2.4–∞), or brachioradial delay (LR+ = 6.8). Lack of radiation to the right carotid artery significantly decreases the likelihood (LR– = 0.05–0.10). Effort syncope is the only historical item found to increase the likelihood of AS, but many patients with significant AS have no symptoms; thus, the absence of symptoms does not exclude significant AS.

10. Which characteristics of a systolic murmur increase the likelihood that it is due to hypertrophic cardiomyopathy (HCM)?

In the study by Lembo et al., two maneuvers were found to be helpful in distinguishing the murmur of HCM. Passive leg elevation, with the examiner elevating the patient's legs to 45°, increases both venous return and arterial resistance. A decrease in murmur intensity 20–30 seconds after elevating the legs had 85% sensitivity, 91% specificity, and an LR+ of 8.0. If it did not change or increase, the likelihood decreased (LR– = 0.22). Having the patient move from a standing to a squatting position (while breathing normally to avoid the Valsalva maneuver) has similar hemodynamic effects, and a decrease in murmur intensity during this maneuver had 95% sensitivity, 85% specificity, and LR+ of 4.5 for HCM. An increase in intensity with standing to squatting had an LR– of 0.13. Conversely, having the patient squat for 30 seconds and then stand rapidly decreases both venous return and arterial resistance. An increase of murmur intensity after this maneuver had 95% sensitivity and 84% specificity for HCM.

11. Is the physical exam useful for detecting obstructive airway disease?

Physical exam findings that are purported to signify decreased airflow include a barrel chest, hyperresonance or decreased diaphragmatic movement on percussion, and medial and inferior displacement of the apical impulse. Auscultatory findings may include decreased breath sounds, a prolonged expiratory phase, or wheezing. Other tests of airflow include forced expiratory time and the match test. Forced expiratory time is measured by auscultating over the larynx while the patient exhales completely after taking a deep breath; exhalation must be done with the patient's mouth fully open. The match test is performed by having the patient attempt to extinguish a match held 10 cm from the mouth; again, the patient's mouth must be completely open.

The presence of wheezing on unforced expiration is the best predictor of airflow limitation (LR+ = 36.0), although its absence is not helpful (LR– = 0.85). A subxyphoid apical impulse or hyperresonance increases the likelihood of obstruction nearly 5-fold, but their absence is not helpful. A positive match test increases the likelihood 7.1-fold, but a negative test only moderately decreases the likelihood of disease. A forced expiratory time of less than 6 seconds significantly decreases the likelihood (LR+ = 0.45), whereas a time of 6–9 seconds slightly increases the likelihood (LR+ = 2.7), and a time of > 9 sec increases the likelihood almost 5-fold. The clinical judgment of a barrel chest by clinicians has not been shown to be a reliable assessment of increased anteroposterior diameter in adults (although its presence in children increases the likelihood of obstructive disease). Although usually subjective, assessment of a decrease in lung sounds has been shown to correlate well with obstructive disease, and a judgment of "normal" amplitude makes severe obstruction much less likely. Another infrequently used test is assessment of the loudness of breath sounds heard at the mouth, which has been reported to have a reasonable relationship to airflow, although it too is subjective and not well studied.

12. Is the physical exam useful for detecting ascites?

The traditional physical exam for ascites includes inspection for bulging flanks, percussion for shifting dullness or flank dullness, and testing for a fluid wave. The presence of a fluid wave, shifting dullness, or peripheral edema significantly increases the likelihood of ascites (LR+ = 9.6, 5.8, 3.8, respectively), but bulging flanks or flank dullness does not. However, the absence of bulging flanks, flank dullness, shifting dullness, or edema significantly decreases the likelihood of ascites (LR– = 0.12, 0.17, respectively), as does a negative history for subjective increase in abdominal girth or ankle swelling (LR– = 0.10, 0.17). Of interest, a history of alcoholism has not been shown to affect the likelihood of ascites. Overall, clinicians are quite good at detecting ascites but are not as good at excluding it.

13. Are any physical exam findings useful for diagnosing alcoholic liver disease?

Although data are limited, one study by Espinoza et al. found that the presence of spider angiomata, splenomegaly, and abdominal wall collateral veins was helpful in diagnosing alcoholic liver disease but that liver examination itself was not. Other findings, such as palmar erythema, gynecomastia, and Dupuytren's contractures, are not helpful.

14. Is the gallbladder palpable in healthy people?

No.

15. How useful is the physical exam for detecting abdominal aortic aneurysms (AAA)?

In one study of high risk patients (men 60–75 years old with a history of hypertension or coronary artery disease), palpation of the abdomen for a pulsatile mass had a sensitivity of 0.80 for detecting AAA ≥ 5 cm. The finding of a definite or possible pulsatile mass had a sensitivity of 0.50, a specificity of 0.91, and a positive predictive value (PPV) of 0.35. In patients with an abdominal girth at the umbilicus of < 100 cm (39 in), no AAAs were missed. The presence of abdominal or femoral bruits or unequal femoral pulses was not helpful in detecting AAA. However, another study of patients referred for ultrasound to rule out AAA found that clinical suspicion of AAA had a PPV of only 0.15. The PPV increased to 0.24 if other macrovascular disease was present and decreased to 0.08 in its absence. Thus, the physical exam may be most helpful as a screening tool in thin, higher-risk patients.

16. What physical findings may be helpful in diagnosing appendicitis?

Elicitation of the psoas and obturator signs are useful findings supporting a diagnosis of appendicitis. The psoas sign is elicited by having the patient lift the right thigh against pressure applied by the examiner just above the knee. It also may be performed by having the patient lie in the left lateral decubitus position and extend the right leg at the hip. It is positive if it elicits pain in the right lower quadrant (RLQ). The obturator sign is elicited by internally rotating the hip with the knee and hip flexed, producing similar pain. Both maneuvers cause pain by stretching the respective muscles, which are irritated by the adjacent inflamed appendix. The reported sensitivity and specificity of the psoas sign are 0.16 and 0.95, respectively. The obturator sign has not been examined independently, but it is thought to have similar sensitivity and specificity because of its similar mechanism of eliciting pain.

Multiple other physical examination maneuvers have been shown to be helpful in diagnosing or excluding appendicitis. Of these, palpation of the right lower quadrant is clearly the most beneficial. The presence of pain and tenderness greatly increases the likelihood of appendicitis (sensitivity = 0.81, specificity = 0.53, positive LR = 7.3–8.5), whereas its absence strongly decreases the likelihood (negative LR = 0–0.3). However, the low specificity of this finding reflects the multiple other possible etiologies of RLQ tenderness. The presence or absence of fever also makes appendicitis more or less likely (LR+ = 1.9, LR– = 0.6). Other beneficial findings include the presence of abdominal rigidity (LR+ = 3.8), a positive psoas (and presumably obturator) sign (LR+ = 2.4), or rebound tenderness (LR+ = 1.1–6.3); however, the absence of these findings is less helpful.

17. How is transillumination of the sinuses best performed? Is it helpful in diagnosing sinusitis?

It is essential to perform transillumination of sinuses in a completely darkened room, and the examiner's eyes must be allowed time to adapt. To examine the maxillary sinuses, the light source is placed over the infraorbital ridge, directing it downward while transmission of light through the hard palate is observed; this procedure is done on each side. The frontal sinuses are examined by placing the light under the supraorbital ridge and directing it upward. Transillumination of the maxillary sinuses as a single diagnostic test is of limited usefulness, but it becomes helpful when combined with other historical features and physical findings. Williams et al. found that abnormal transillumination along with maxillary tooth tenderness, poor response to decongestants, and purulent nasal discharge by history or on examination increased the likelihood of sinusitis 6.4-fold; the absence of all of these signs essentially rules it out (LR– = 0.1). Because the frontal sinuses are often asymmetric in normal people, the usefulness of transillumination of the frontal sinuses is limited.

18. How useful is the physical exam for diagnosing anemia?

Findings proposed as useful in the diagnosis of anemia include pallor of the conjunctivae, oral mucosa, or nailbeds; decreased or absent blanching of nailbeds; and loss of erythema in the palmar creases with hyperextension of the hand and fingers. However, few rigorous studies have been done. Classic teaching has often been that loss of palmar creases correlates with a hemoglobin level of 7 gm/dl or less, but this finding has been reported in series of patients with higher (but still anemic) hemoglobin levels.

19. What are Kernig's and Brudzinski's signs? And how useful are they in the diagnosis of meningitis?

Kernig's sign is elicited by having the patient lie supine, flex the hip to 90°, and then extend the knee; it is considered positive if there is hamstring spasm at knee flexion of < 135° (pain is often considered an endpoint also). Brudzinski's sign (he actually described several) is elicited by forward flexion of the neck in a supine patient causing flexion at the hips and knees. One or both of these signs is reportedly positive in around 80% of patients with acute bacterial meningitis but less frequently in infants or patients with tuberculous meningitis. Thus, positivity of either should increase clinical suspicion of meningitis in the appropriate clinical setting, but further data about their sensitivity and specificity are not available.

20. Which physical exam maneuvers have been shown to be useful in diagnosing carpal tunnel syndrome?

Commonly used maneuvers include checking for Tinel's and Phalen's signs, assessment of thenar muscles for weakness and atrophy, and testing of two-point discrimination in the distribution of the median nerve. Tinel's sign is elicited by repetitive tapping (5 or more times) on the ventral aspect of the wrist, usually with a reflex hammer or the examiner's finger, which causes pain or paresthesias in the fingers in the distribution of the median nerve. Its sensitivity has been estimated at around 0.60 and its specificity at around 0.70, with a PPV of 0.25–0.60 and a negative predictive value (NPV) of 0.70–0.90, depending on the clinical setting. Phalen's sign is elicited when the patient flexes both wrists to 90° and holds them in apposition for 60 seconds, which causes symptoms similar to Tinel's sign. Its sensitivity is somewhat higher in most studies (around 0.75) with a lower specificity (around 0.50), a PPV of 0.20–0.50, and an NPV of 0.75–0.90. The presence of weakness or atrophy in the thenar muscles is neither sensitive nor specific for CTS. Loss of two-point discrimination (measured with caliper points 4 mm apart) is relatively specific (around 0.85) but not sensitive and occurs late in the disease.

BIBLIOGRAPHY

1. Cavallini MC, Roman MJ, Blank SG, et al: Association of the auscultatory gap with vascular disease in hypertensive patients. Ann Intern Med 124:877–883, 1996.
2. Etchells E, Bell C, Robb K: Does this patient have an abnormal systolic murmur? JAMA 277:564–572, 1997.
3. Holleman DR, Simel DL: Does the clinical examination predict airflow limitation? JAMA 273:313–319, 1995.
4. Lederle FA, Walker JM, Reinke DB: Selective screening for abdominal aortic aneurysms with physical examination and ultrasound. Arch Intern Med 148:1753–1756, 1988.
5. Lembo NJ, Del'Italia LJ, Crawford MH, O'Rourke RA: Bedside diagnosis of systolic murmurs. N Engl J Med 318:1572–1578, 1988.
6. Perloff D, Grim C, Flack J, et al; Human blood pressure determination by sphygmomanometry. Circulation 88:2460–2470, 1993.
7. Sauve J, Laupacis A, Ostbye T, et al; Does this patient have a clinically important carotid bruit? JAMA 270:2843–2845, 1993.
8. Simel DL, Halvorsen RA, Feussner JR: Quantitating bedside diagnosis: Clinical evaluation of ascites. J Gen Intern Med 3:423–428, 1988.
9. Wagner JM, McKinney WP, Carpenter JL: Does this patient have appendicitis? JAMA 276:1589–1594, 1996.
10. Williams JW, Simel DL, Roberts L, Samsa GP: Clinical evaluation for sinusitis: Making the diagnosis by history and physical examination. Ann Intern Med 117:705–710, 1992.

II. Behavioral Medicine

8. DEPRESSION

Edmund Casper, M.D., and Allan Liebgott, M.D.

1. How frequently does the primary care provider encounter patients with clinically relevant depression?

The prevalence of depressive disorders in primary care practice may be greater than 25% and even higher in patients with chronic medical illnesses. Among adolescents, the prevalence is approximately 15%. Thus, the primary care provider must recognize depressive disorders, be comfortable providing the first level of care, and recognize danger signs and symptoms that require referral to a psychiatrist.

2. Describe the spectrum of depression.

Depression ranges from normal signs of bereavement to major depression accompanied by frank psychoses. Major depression is usually an episodic illness, often beginning in adolescence, with remissions and exacerbations throughout life. A chronic form of less severe depression without acute major episodes is termed dysthymia. Patients with depression may have a bipolar manic-depressive disorder.

3. What is the epidemiology of depression?

Depression occurs more frequently in women than men. The incidence decreases with age in women but increases with age in men and is higher among single people. Depression is inversely related to social class but shows no racial, urban, or rural predilection. Major depressive episodes frequently follow a stressful life event in predisposed people.

4. How can the primary care provider recognize depression?

1. By recognition of classic symptoms: depressed mood accompanied by changes in sleep patterns, weight, and/or energy level and feelings of hopelessness, loss of self-worth, and/or disinterest in usual activities.

2. By the responses to screening questionnaires on routine physician visits. Routine questionnaires for new patients should include items related to depression or a standard depression screening test (such as the Center for Epidemiologic Studies Depression Scale).

3. By carefully pursuing concomitant depression in patients who abuse alcohol or drugs. Up to one-third of substance abusers have concurrent mood disorders.

4. By suspecting depression in patients who somaticize. Patients who are depressed may present with physical symptoms that cannot be supported by the diagnosis or severity of a physical disorder. Such vague symptoms as dizziness, headache, palpitations, or other complaints that result in multiple physician visits should suggest depression.

5. By being alert to medical conditions with a high rate of accompanying depression (see question 8).

5. What criteria lead to a diagnosis of a major depressive episode?

The diagnosis requires the 2-week presence of depressed mood and/or disinterest, accompanied by four of the following:

- Weight changes
- Sleep disturbances
- Daily fatigue
- Feelings of wothlessness or guilt
- Poor concentration
- Thoughts of death
- Observed psychomotor agitation or retardation

The depression should not be due to loss of a loved one or other organic causes. The patient should not carry a diagnosis of schizophrenia or other psychotic disorder. Although severe depression may be accompanied by psychotic symptoms (e.g., delusional thinking—hallucinations), such symptoms should not be seen in the absence of depression.

6. Describe manifestations of depression in the child or adolescent.

Children and adolescents may have symptoms similar to adults, including substance abuse and hypochondriasis. Depression also should be suspected with mood irritability, difficulty in family relationships or with the law, or fall in school grades.

7. How does one distinguish between normal depressive reaction to loss of a loved one and a major depressive episode?

Definitive distinction between bereavement and major depression may be difficult, because grieving may result in all of the symptoms of a major depression. However, prolonged symptoms that lead to a significant threat to health should be treated similarly to a major depressive episode.

8. Which medical diseases are associated with a high incidence of depression?

Disease	Approximate Prevalence (%)
1. Stroke	50
2. Chronic fatigue syndrome	50
3. Diabetes mellitus	30
4. Malignancies (especially of the pancreas or lung)	25
5. Myocardial infarction	25
6. Rheumatoid arthritis	20

From Katon W, Sullivan MD: Depression and chronic medical illness. J Clin Psychiatry 51(Suppl 6):3–11, 1990.

9. Which drugs are particularly likely to induce depression?

Drugs that may frequently precipitate depression include the phenothiazines, steroids, propranolol, cimetidine, levodopa, indomethacin, isotretinoin, and withdrawal from CNS stimulants.

10. Which persons are at highest risk for suicide?

1. Persons who have developed a specific plan for suicide
2. Persons who are socially isolated
3. Elderly men
4. Substance abusers
5. Persons with terminal malignancies

11. How does the patient's personal or family history aid in the diagnosis of depression?

A history of mood disorder in a first-degree relative or a major previous depression predisposes the patient to depression.

12. How should patients with major depression be treated?

Patients with a major depressive episode should be treated pharmacologically. Although many drugs are available, the primary care physician should restrict therapy to widely accepted agents. Although selective serotonin reuptake inhibitors are the current drugs of choice, the physician also should consider agents that have resulted in improvement in previous episodes. Therapy should be continued for 6–12 months; the highest risk of recurrence is within 2 months of tapering off medication. Drug therapy for patients with less severe depression or dysthymia has been less effective. Behavior therapy and/or self-help groups may be as effective as antidepressants in patients with mild-to-moderate depression.

13. Does therapy for depression differ in patients with comorbid medical illness and other patients with major depression?

Aggressive therapy of the underlying illness and return to function may ameliorate depression caused by illness. However, specific therapy for depression may be needed to allow complete return to health.

14. What response is anticipated with treatment?

Approximately 65% of patients with depression respond to therapy with one or more agents. However, the chance of recurrence is high; the majority of patients experience a recurrent episode, and one-fourth follow a chronic course with debilitating symptoms.

15. Describe the mortality and morbidity associated with major depression.

Up to 15% of patients with recurrent major depressive disorders die of suicide, and over three-fourths of completed suicides occur in patients with major mood disorders. In medical patients major depression or dysthymia causes greater disability than hypertension, diabetes, arthritis, and chronic lung disease. In addition, untreated patients with chronic depression often function poorly.

16. Which patients with major depression should be referred to a psychiatrist?
1. Patients who are suicidal
2. Patients who have a history of mania or who become manic on antidepressant therapy
3. Patients with accompanying psychosis
4. Patients who show no response to treatment after 4 weeks

17. What are the side effects of tricyclic antidepressant drugs (TCAs)?

As a class, TCAs cause sedation, postural hypotension, and anticholinergic effects (dry mouth, urinary retention, tachycardia, constipation). Newer TCAs (such as nortriptyline or desipramine) have fewer side effects than older TCAs (amitriptyline, imipramine, doxepin) and may be less expensive than second-generation antidepressants. Before beginning therapy patients should undergo a physical exam and have normal values on hemogram, liver function tests, and electrocardiogram. Side effects may be minimized by initiating therapy with lower doses and slowly reaching therapeutic doses by 7–10 days. Elderly patients should be treated with 30–50% of recommended doses. Full therapeutic efficacy is not reached for up to 28 days.

18. When are TCAs contraindicated or likely to prove problematic?
Contraindicated
1. In patients with cardiac conduction defects, TCAs have a quinidinelike effect and may induce arrhythmias; thus, alternative drugs should be used.
2. In patients with narrow-angle glaucoma, because of the anticholinergic effects of TCAs.
Problematic
1. In patients with preexisting conditions that may be exacerbated by TCAs. Prostatism and mild congestive heart failure may worsen because of the anticholinergic effects (urinary retention and tachycardia, respectively).
2. In patients taking phenothiazines, cimetidine, and other anticholinergics (e.g., antihistamines), TCAs should be used cautiously and at lower doses. Patients also should be instructed to refrain from alcohol.

19. What is the advantage of newer second-generation antidepressants?

Newer agents include drugs that are tricyclic derivatives or inhibit uptake of serotonin and have fewer anticholinergic side effects, including less effect on the cardiac conduction system. Examples include fluoxetine, bupropion, sertraline, and paroxetine. Several of the newer agents have demonstrated an efficacy similar to that of TCAs. Despite their cost, these medications have become the primary drugs of choice in depression because of decreased side effects and greater margin of safety compared with TCAs.

BIBLIOGRAPHY

1. Frank E, Prien RF, Jarrett RB, et al: Conceptualization and rationale for consensus definitions of terms in major depressive disorder. Arch Gen Psychiatry 48:851, 1991.
2. Judd LL, Britton KT, Braff DL: Mental disorders. In Isselbacher KJ, et al (eds): Harrison's Principles of Internal Medicine, 13th ed. New York, McGraw-Hill, 1994, pp 2400–2420.
3. Katon W, Sullivan MD: Depression and chronic medical illness. J Clin Psychiatry 51(Suppl 6):3–11, 1990.

4. McGreery JF, Franco K: Depression in the elderly: The role of the primary care physician in management.
    J Gen Intern Med 3:498–507, 1988.
5. Michaels R, Marzuk PM: Progress in psychiatry. N Engl J Med 329:552, 628, 1993.
6. Stewart AI: Functional status and well-being of patients with chronic conditions. Results from the medical
    outcomes study. JAMA 262:907, 1989.

9. SLEEP DISORDERS

Lisa Corbin Winslow, M.D., and Eric T. McFarling, M.D.

1. Describe the stages of normal sleep.

By monitoring sleep in a laboratory, using electroencephalography (EEG), electrooculography (EOG), electromyography (EMG), and other recording methods, normal sleep patterns have been described. Sleep is divided into rapid eye movement (REM) sleep and non-REM sleep. REM sleep is characterized by eye movement bursts, a high-frequency EEG with low voltage, and atonia of skeletal muscles. In addition, REM is the stage of sleep during which most dreams occur.

Non-REM sleep is divided into four stages based on EEG patterns and accounts for the majority of time spent sleeping. Stages 1 and 2 (light sleep) are identified by a low-amplitude, high-frequency EEG tracing and stages 3 and 4 (deep sleep) by a high-amplitude, slow (delta wave) pattern. Initial sleep is non-REM sleep.

A period consisting of stages 1 through 4 and REM sleep is a sleep cycle, and a night's sleep commonly consists of 3–5 cycles. As waketime nears, deep sleep is less prevalent, and a greater proportion of sleep is spent in REM.

2. How common are problems with sleep patterns in an otherwise healthy population?

Surveys show that approximately 1 in 3 people had problematic insomnia at some time during the past year. Prevalence is higher among women, elderly people, and people of high socioeconomic status. Approximately 1 in 20 adults complain of problems with excessive daytime sleepiness, which may include falling asleep at inappropriate times (e.g., during conversations, during work, or while driving).

3. Is insomnia a natural consequence of aging?

Older patients complain more about sleep difficulties than younger ones for a variety of reasons. The sleep/wake cycle changes with age, with less deep sleep, less REM sleep, and more nocturnal awakenings. The circadian rhythm advances so that older adults tend to get sleepier earlier in the evening and to wake up earlier in the morning. In addition, older people are more likely to have medical and psychiatric disorders that interfere with sleep. Patients tend to make up for less nocturnal sleep with daytime naps, preserving the overall amount of sleep time. Special attention to medical disorders and sleep hygiene (see question 7) and the use of sunlight or bright lights late in the afternoon may help elderly insomniacs.

4. What questions should be asked in taking a sleep history?

Primary care physicians often fail to ask patients about sleep problems, although they are common and often readily treatable. A sleep history results in diagnosis of the majority of sleep disorders. Useful adjuncts to the sleep history include talking to a sleep partner and having the patient keep a 1- or 2-week sleep log. The following specific questions supplement the medical and psychiatric history:

- Do you fall asleep during the day, or do others notice that you are excessively sleepy?
- Do you have problems getting enough sleep?
- When did the symptoms begin?
- What is your daily schedule, including work, meals, exercise, and naps?

- What is your bedtime routine?
- What medications are you taking?
- Do you know of unusual movements, abnormalities in breathing, or snoring during sleep?
- What treatments have been tried in the past? Which were effective?

5. How does the time course of insomnia help with classification?

Insomnia is classified as recent onset (i.e., less than 3 weeks ago) or chronic. Insomnia of recent onset is usually transient and may develop in patients with previously normal sleep due to a stressful life change. Examples are hospitalization, bereavement, academic exams, and disturbance of circadian rhythms because of air travel across time zones or shift changes at work. Chronic insomnia of months' or years' duration has a poorer prognosis and a high association with psychiatric or medical disorders.

6. Which medical disorders commonly interfere with sleep?

Many medical disorders cause symptoms that interfere with sleep (e.g., nocturia, pain, or dyspnea). Examples of medical conditions that specifically disrupt sleep include the following:

Respiratory disease, including asthma, emphysema, and cystic fibrosis	Rheumatoid arthritis (pain)
Congestive heart failure	CNS neoplasms
Gastroesophageal reflux	Headaches, especially cluster headaches
End-stage renal disease	Seizure disorders
Endocrine disease	Parkinson's disease
Hypo- or hyperthyroidism	Fibromyalgia (associated with nonrestorative sleep)
Addison's or Cushing's syndrome	Alzheimer's disease
Diabetes mellitus (due to nocturnal hypoglycemia)	

Therapy directed specifically at the medical problem may relieve the insomnia. In addition, prescription and over-the-counter medications may interfere with sleep, either as a direct effect (e.g., certain antidepressants, theophylline, corticosteroids, decongestants, histamine-2 blockers, stimulants) or indirectly (e.g., diuretics may cause nocturia).

7. What is "sleep hygiene"?

Sleep hygiene is a set of behaviors used to promote sleep and improve sleep quality. The following measures are recommended:

- The bedroom should be dark, quiet, and comfortable in temperature.
- Reading, watching TV, or working in the bedroom should be avoided. Only sleep and sexual relations should occur there.
- Caffeine (present in tea, chocolate, some soft drinks, and some analgesic preparations) should be restricted for at least 8 hours before bedtime. Nicotine also should be minimized.
- Patients should attempt to keep a regular sleep-wake schedule with consistent bed and wake times, regardless of the amount of sleep achieved. Naps should be avoided.
- Regular exercise, finished at least 3–4 hours before bedtime, appears to promote sleep.
- Heavy meals at dinner should be avoided. A light snack before bedtime may aid sleep.
- Alcohol may hasten sleep onset, but its metabolites may cause sleep interruption later in the night, and its use should be avoided.
- If sleep is not achieved 10–20 minutes after bedtime, the patient should leave the bedroom and do a quiet activity such as reading. When sleepiness occurs, the patient returns to bed. If sleep is again not achieved, the cycle is repeated.
- Illuminated bedroom clocks (the insomniac's nemesis) should be removed.

The goal of sleep hygiene is to associate the bedroom with falling asleep quickly, minimizing frustration and anxiety.

8. What medications are used for the treatment of insomnia?

Commonly used prescription hypnotics are benzodiazepines and sedating antidepressants. Barbiturates have a high incidence of tolerance, addiction, and death (if overdosed) and should not be used as hypnotics. Chloral hydrate (a "Mickey Finn," when mixed with alcohol) may be safer than barbiturates but can cause gastritis. Nonprescription medications sold as hypnotics include antihistamines, scopolamine (an anticholinergic), and salicylates. Tryptophan, in high doses, was used as a "natural" hypnotic before it was associated with the eosinophilia-myalgia syndrome. Melatonin is an endogenous hormone secreted by the pineal gland in concordance with the circadian sleep cycle in humans. It is sold as a supplement in health food stores, derived from bovine brains or chemically synthesized. Small trials have presented subjective evidence that melatonin may have modest efficacy in sleep disorders due to jet lag, shift work, and neurologic impairment, but no long-term studies have documented either efficacy or safety, including drug interactions. The Food and Drug Administration does not review drugs classified as "supplements," nor is their production regulated or standardized. For these reasons, melatonin cannot be routinely recommended.

9. When are medications appropriate in the treatment of insomnia?

All patients with short- or long-term insomnia should be instructed in good sleep hygiene as first-line therapy. Relaxation techniques and biofeedback also have been suggested, but clinically significant improvement in sleep has not been demonstrated. Sleep medications may be a useful adjuvant to good sleep hygiene in the management of short-term insomnia but should not be prescribed for chronic insomnia or used for more than 3–4 weeks; they should be prescribed only in the context of a secure doctor-patient relationship.

10. If medications to promote sleep are needed, which are most appropriate to prescribe?

The benzodiazepines are most commonly used and have a reasonable safety record. Benzodiazepines currently marketed as hypnotics are triazolam (Halcion), temazepam (Restoril), and flurazepam (Dalmane). They vary chiefly in rates of absorption and elimination, with triazolam having the shortest half-life and flurazepam the longest; temazepam has an intermediate duration.

Antihistamines are not as potent as benzodiazepines and may have anticholinergic side effects, such as urinary retention. Low-dose sedating antidepressants (e.g., amitriptyline or trazodone) have advantages in that they are nonaddictive and safe in sleep apnea, but data about safety and efficacy for chronic insomnia are unavailable.

Agitation and insomnia in hospitalized elderly patients ("sundowning") may be paradoxically worsened by benzodiazepines; low-dose haloperidol is a more effective treatment.

11. What precautions must be observed when benzodiazepines are used for insomnia?

Most importantly, the insomnia should be fully investigated before prescribing sleep medications. Many medical and psychiatric disorders can present as insomnia and can be masked or worsened with benzodiazepines. They may depress respiratory drive and can worsen sleep apnea and emphysema. Rebound insomnia (worsening of sleeplessness after discontinuation of hypnotics) may occur after only one dose. It should also be kept in mind that any benzodiazepine can be addictive. Short-acting drugs (e.g., triazolam) may reduce sleep latency, but unwanted effects include early-morning awakening, anterograde amnesia, and increased daytime anxiety. Long-acting benzodiazepines (e.g., temazepam) may prevent early-morning awakening but can result in daytime sleepiness. Flurazepam has a long-acting metabolite that may cause daytime sedation after multiple doses, especially in the elderly. Drug interactions (e.g., alcohol, phenobarbital) may be dangerous. Tolerance to benzodiazepines is the rule, and no study shows a difference between hypnotics and placebo after 3–4 weeks of therapy.

12. My patient complains of falling asleep during the day. What diagnoses should be considered?

For patients with excessive daytime sleepiness, sleep apnea, narcolepsy, and idiopathic hypersomnolence (sleepiness of unknown cause but not meeting criteria for narcolepsy) should be considered. Medical disorders (e.g., thyroid disease, anemia, hydrocephalus) and medications (e.g., clonidine, antihistamines, neuroleptics, tricyclic antidepressants) cause sleepiness. Schizophrenia and depression may present with somnolence. Patients with transient hypersomnia have excessive daytime sleepiness and loss of energy, usually due to a stressful event, and recover in

less than 3 weeks. Also, some patients are simply getting insufficient amounts of sleep to participate in their daily schedules.

13. Describe classic narcolepsy.

Narcolepsy is characterized by the sudden onset of daytime sleep with abnormally prompt
entry into REM sleep. Classic narcolepsy includes the following:

Cataplexy—the sudden, temporary loss of skeletal muscle tone, often following excitement
or fear.

Sleep paralysis—a transitory but frightening inability to move or speak occurring at transitions between wakefulness and sleep.

Hypnagogic hallucinations—dreamlike visual or auditory hallucinations at the transitions
of wakefulness and sleep.

Abnormal nocturnal sleep—with frequent awakenings.

The diagnosis is confirmed in the sleep lab by repetitively measuring the time from attempting sleep to sleep onset (multiple sleep latency testing, or MSLT). Sleep latency is usually less
than 5 minutes in narcolepsy and greater than 10 minutes in normal persons. The majority of nar-
coleptics also are found to have direct entry from wakefulness into REM sleep.

Current therapy includes stimulants to prevent daytime sleepiness, tricyclics such as
imipramine or protriptyline to control cataplexy, and scheduled daytime naps.

14. What is sleep apnea?

Sleep apnea is the repetitive cessation of airflow through the nose or mouth for at least 10
seconds during sleep. Apnea may occur hundreds of times per night and result in partial arousal
from sleep. Sleep apnea may result from obstruction of the upper airway (obstructive sleep
apnea), failure of respiratory drive (central sleep apnea), of a combination of the two.

15. When should sleep apnea be suspected?

Sleep apnea should be considered in any patients with excessive daytime sleepiness and a
history of snoring. Suspicion is heightened in males, the elderly, the obese, and probably alcoholics. Other clues include long pauses without audible respirations (reported by bed partner),
frequent arousals, and early-morning headaches. Patients with obstructive sleep apneas may have
large necks and a narrow upper airway on physical exam.

16. How is sleep apnea syndrome diagnosed?

Sleep apnea is diagnosed in a sleep laboratory. Polysomnographic monitoring for sleep
apnea includes nasal and oral thermistors to measure airflow, chest and abdominal strain gauges
to measure respiratory effort, ear oximetry to follow arterial oxygen saturation, EKG to detect
heart rhythm abnormalities, and monitoring to determine sleep stage. Simple ear oximetry is
used by some centers for screening, but a normal study does not rule out significant sleep apnea.

Patients having more than five apneas per hour are abnormal. Hypopneas (a decrease in ventilation severe enough to cause a fall in arterial oxygen saturation without complete cessation of
ventilation) are also quantitated. Results of polysomnography must be interpreted in the context
of signs and symptoms before the diagnosis of sleep apnea syndrome can be considered certain.

17. What are the consequences of sleep apnea?

Complications of sleep apnea are believed to result from cessation of ventilation with acute
oxygen desaturation and carbon dioxide retention. The immediate consequence is sleep disruption
due to intermittent nocturnal asphyxiation. Resulting daytime sleepiness may impair the ability to
stay awake while working or driving. Short-term consequences also may include personality
changes, intellectual deterioration, memory impairment, and impotence.

Systemic blood pressure rises during apneas, and sustained daytime hypertension, often refractory to medicines, is commonly found. Some studies have shown that treatment of sleep apnea can
lower systemic blood pressure. Effects on cardiac rhythm during sleep are commonly noted and

probably contribute to the overall decrease in survival in patients with sleep apnea. Sleeping EKG may show bradycardia, sinus pauses, atrioventricular block, and ventricular premature beats. Chronic sleep apnea, usually in concert with primary pulmonary disease or severe obesity, may result in pulmonary hypertension and right-sided heart failure.

18. How is obstructive sleep apnea treated?

Conservative measures include weight loss (when modest weight loss may be effective), abstinence from alcohol and other sedatives, oxygen therapy to prevent severe desaturation, and training patients to sleep on their side rather than supine. **Drugs** result in mild, if any, improvement in obstructive sleep apnea. The tricyclic antidepressant protriptyline appears to be the most effective. It appears to reduce REM sleep, during which the upper airway muscles are most relaxed. **Mechanical measures** are indicated for more severe cases. Nasal continuous positive airway pressure (CPAP) used during sleep appears to "splint" the upper airway and prevents soft-tissue collapse during inspiration. CPAP is delivered through a close-fitting nasal mask used at home. Although successful when used, patients often find the device uncomfortable, and long-term compliance is variable. Removals of parts of the soft palate (uvulopalatopharyngoplasty [UPPP]) results in improvement in approximately one-half of those treated, but it is currently difficult to predict who will benefit. Experience with prostheses designed to hold the pharynx open during sleep has been limited. Tracheostomy remains the definitive therapy for severe obstructive sleep apnea refractory to other therapies.

19. My patient complains that his legs jerk and keep him awake. How can I help?

Periodic leg movements of sleep are stereotypical leg jerks that occur after sleep onset and may cause frequent awakenings in the patient. They occur more commonly with age and are rare before age 40. They may be worsened by tricyclic antidepressants. Short-acting benzodiazepines do not reduce twitching but suppress arousal from sleep.

Restless leg syndrome is a waketime disorder consisting of unpleasant "crawling" muscular sensations in the legs that cause an almost irresistible urge to move the legs. This condition makes sleep onset difficult. Small doses of the antiparkinsonian drug Sinemet (carbidopa/L-dopa, 25/100) may enable sleep onset.

Hypnic jerks are sudden movements involving all extremities and occur in the transition from wakefulness to sleep. They are commonly experienced by normal people and seldom impair sleep.

20. What are parasomnias?

Parasomnias are unpleasant or undesirable behavioral phenomena that occur predominantly during sleep. **Disorders of arousal**, which include sleep walking and sleep terrors, are caused by rapid alternations between wakefulness and NREM sleep. The patient is awake enough to carry out activities but not enough to be aware of the actions. **REM sleep behavior disorder** is more common in older people, in whom the paralysis that normally accompanies REM sleep is absent. It results in "acting out dreams" and can be dangerous.

21. Who should have a sleep study?

Most patients with excessive daytime sleepiness should be studied in the sleep lab (polysomnography). The evaluation may include MSLT (usually on the day after polysomnography), during which the time from wakefulness to sleep during several daytime naps is measured. Patients with clinical suspicion of a parasomnia should have the diagnosis confirmed by sleep study. Insomnia has not routinely been an indication for polysomnography.

BIBLIOGRAPHY

1. Aldrich MS: Narcolepsy. N Engl J Med 323:389, 1990.
2. Ancoli-Israel S: Sleep problems in older adults: Putting myths to bed. Geriatrics 52:20–30, 1997.
3. Brownell LG, West P, Sweatmen P, et al: Protriptyline in obstructive sleep apnea. N Engl J Med 307:1037, 1982.
4. Chase J, Gidal B: Melatonin: Therapeutic use in sleep disorders. Am Pharmacother 31:1218–1226, 1997.

5. Fletcher EC, DeBehnke RD, Lovoi MS, Gorin AB: Undiagnosed sleep apnea in patients with essential hypertension. Ann Intern Med 103:190, 1985.
6. Gillin JC, Byerly WF: The diagnosis and management of insomnia. N Engl J Med 322:239, 1990.
7. Hauri JH, Esther MS: Insomnia. Mayo Clin Proc 65:869, 1990.
8. Hoffstein V, Szalai JP: Predictive value of clinical features in diagnosing obstructive sleep apnea. Sleep 16:118, 1993.
9. Kreuger BR: Restless leg syndrome and periodic movements of sleep. Mayo Clin Proc 65:999, 1990.
10. Kryger MH, Roth T, Dement WC: Principles and Practice of Sleep Medicine. Philadelphia, W.B. Saunders, 1989.
11. Mahowald M: Diagnostic testing for sleep disorders. Neurol Clin 14:183–200, 1996.
12. Nakra BRS, Groosberg GT, Peck B: Insomnia in the Elderly. Am Fam Physician 43:477, 1991.
13. NIH Technology Assessment Panel: Integration of behavioral and relaxation approaches into the management of chronic pain and insomnia. JAMA 276:313–318, 1996.
14. Reite MI, Nagel KE, Ruddy JR: The Evaluation and Management of Sleep Disorders. Washington, DC, American Psychiatric Press, 1990.
15. Shapiro CM, Devins GM, Hussain MRG: ABC of sleep disorders: Sleep problems in patients with medical illness. BMJ 306:1532, 1993.
16. Swift CG, Shapiro CM: ABC of sleep disorders: Sleep and sleep problems in elderly people. BMJ 306:1468, 1993.
17. Wiggins RV, Schmidt-Nowara WW: Treatment of the obstructive sleep apnea syndrome. West J Med 147:561, 1987.
18. Young T, Palta M, Dempsey J, et al: The occurrence of sleep-disordered breathing among middle-aged adults. N Engl J Med 328:1230, 1993.

10. ALCOHOL AND SUBSTANCE ABUSE

Mary Chri Gray, M.D., and Philip S. Mehler, M.D.

1. What are the societal implications of alcoholism?

Alcohol abuse and its sequelae present some of the most serious social and medical problems in the United States. The toll on human life is staggering: approximately 70,000 Americans died in 1990 as a result of alcohol abuse. After heart disease and cancer, alcoholism is America's third largest health problem. Up to 25% of patients admitted to community teaching hospitals have alcohol dependence. Approximately 12 million are hospitalized annually with manifestations of alcohol abuse. Moreover, the alcohol trauma syndrome is an enormous problem; 41% of patients experiencing trauma have measurable blood alcohol levels on initial evaluation in the emergency department. Alcohol is also involved in about 25% of suicides. The annual cost to society is estimated to be $136 billion.

2. Given the magnitude of alcohol abuse and the paramount importance of early detection, what types of screening instruments are available?

Two types of screening instruments are available: (1) self-report questionnaires and structured interviews and (2) clinical laboratory tests that detect pathophysiologic changes associated with excessive alcohol usage.

The CAGE questionnaire is a self-report screening instrument that appears to be suited to a busy medical practice in which time for patient interviews is limited. Two "yes" answers correctly identify 75% of alcoholics. The specificity of the test is 95%. The sensitivity of the CAGE questionnaire is dramatically enhanced by an open-ended introduction as opposed to questions about the frequency and amount of drinking. Another questionnaire, the Michigan Alcoholism Screening Test (MAST), is a formal 25-item test that requires 25 minutes to complete. A shortened 10-item MAST (B-MAST) has been constructed with items from the original test that are highly discriminating for alcoholism. A cut-off score of 6 is suggestive for the B-MAST.

CAGE Questionnaire

Have you ever felt you ought to	**C**ut down on your drinking?
Have people	**A**nnoyed you by criticizing your drinking?
Have you ever felt bad or	**G**uilty about your drinking?
Have you ever had a drink first thing in the morning to steady your nerves or get rid of a hangover?	**E**ye-opener

Brief MAST

POINTS	
(2)	*1. Do you feel you are a normal drinker?
(2)	*2. Do friends or relatives think you are a normal drinker?
(5)	3. Have you ever attended a meeting of Alcoholics Anonymous?
(2)	4. Have you ever lost friends or girlfriends/boyfriends because of drinking?
(2)	5. Have you ever gotten into trouble at work because of drinking?
(2)	6. Have you ever neglected your obligations, your family, or your work for two or more days in a row because you were drinking?
(2)	7. Have you ever had delirium tremens (DTs), severe shaking, heard voices, seen things that weren't there after heavy drinking?
(5)	8. Have you ever gone to anyone for help about your drinking?
(5)	9. Have you ever been in a hospital because of drinking?
(2)	10. Have you ever been arrested for drunk driving or driving after drinking?

* Negative responses are alcoholic responses.
Scoring: ≤ 3 points, nonalcoholic; 4 points, suggestive of alcoholism; 5 indicates alcoholism.

Clinical laboratory tests frequently are used to corroborate results of questionnaires. Several tests provide objective evidence of problem drinking, especially in patients who deny an alcohol problem. Increased levels of serum gamma-glutamyl transferase (GGT) are a relatively sensitive index of alcohol use. Although serum GGT is the most widely used laboratory screening test for alcoholism, it lacks diagnostic specificity. Results are more specific in conjunction with elevated mean corpuscular volume (MCV), which increases with excessive alcohol intake. The ratio of the liver enzyme aspartate aminotransferase (AST) to alanine aminotransferase (ALT), if greater than 1, may be a useful marker of alcoholic liver disease.

3. What major organ systems are affected by alcohol abuse?

Alcohol affects almost every organ system in the body.

Cardiovascular system
Hypertension
Cardiomyopathy
Atrial and ventricular dysrhythmias
Endocrine system
Testicular atrophy
Feminization
Amenorrhea and premature menopause
Pseudo-Cushing's syndrome
Gastrointestinal system
Hepatitis and cirrhosis
Esophagitis and gastritis
Peptic ulcer disease
Esophageal carcinoma
Malabsorption with diarrhea
Pancreatitis

Hematologic system
Anemia due to folate deficiency or sideroblastosis
Thrombocytopenia
Diminished neutrophil migration
Nervous system
Cognitive impairment
Dementia
Korsakoff's psychosis
Wernicke's encephalopathy
Peripheral neuropathy
Musculoskeletal system
Osteoporosis
Avascular necrosis
Skin
Telangiectasias
Palmar erythema

4. Are gender differences observed in alcohol-related liver disease?

Yes. Although the cirrhosis-induced death rate is higher for men than women, women are more susceptible to alcohol-related liver damage and develop liver disease with shorter durations of alcohol abuse.

5. What are the consequences to the fetus of alcohol use during pregnancy?

Alcohol is a teratogen. Although a critical dosage or exposure level has not been determined, observations of human infants and experimental animals make clear that a mother who drinks heavily during pregnancy may severely damage her fetus. The distinct pattern of birth defects, known as the fetal alcohol syndrome, includes growth retardation, a characteristic constellation of craniofacial anomalies, central nervous system dysfunction, and malformations of major organ systems.

6. Describe the manifestations of alcohol withdrawal syndrome.

Alcohol withdrawal may have several different and occasionally overlapping manifestations. The clinical spectrum ranges from a "hangover" to life-threatening delirium tremens. Minor withdrawal may begin 6–12 hours after a significant decrease or cessation of drinking in heavy, chronic drinkers despite significant blood levels of alcohol. This stage may last 3–5 days and is characterized by tremors, sweating, anxiety, diarrhea, nausea, and insomnia. Patients may not require pharmacologic therapy. The degree of autonomic hyperactivity may progress to marked tremulousness, tachycardia, hyperactivity, and agitation after 12–24 hours. The patient may have visual and auditory hallucinations. The hallucinations are usually unpleasant and separated by a lucid interval.

Alcohol withdrawal seizures are not uncommon and usually occur within the first 48 hours. They are grand mal seizures without focality. Multiple seizures may occur in 2–5% within a 6–10-hour period. Any focal findings on exam, seizures occurring during delirium tremens, and seizures occurring over several days or accompanied by fever should prompt a further neurologic evaluation.

7. Outline the principles of management in patients with alcohol withdrawal symptoms.

Although outpatient treatment of minor alcohol withdrawal has its place, patients with hyperactivity of the sympathetic nervous system, concurrent medical problems, lack of a social support system, and history of complications during previous withdrawal episodes require inpatient treatment. Delirium tremens requires management in the intensive care unit. Although patients experiencing mild withdrawal symptoms can be managed without adjunctive pharmacologic therapy, current guidelines recommend medicinal treatment for most patients experiencing alcohol withdrawal.

The proper management of alcohol withdrawal is aimed at alleviating patient suffering and preventing minor symptoms from progressing to major symptoms. Normalization of vital signs and moderate sedation are two desired endpoints of treatment. Sedation is accomplished by substituting for alcohol another sedative hypnotic agent, such as a benzodiazepine, in a gradually tapering dose. The dosage of benzodiazepine for alcohol withdrawal is larger than usually given for anxiety or panic disorder. The patient should be carefully assessed to ensure adequate dosing to achieve sedation and amelioration of the hyperautonomic state. In patients with significant liver disease, lorazepam (Ativan) or oxazepam (Serax) should be used because neither is extensively oxidized by the liver. Intravenous use of benzodiazepines until mild sedation occurs prevents the physiologic storm that may be seen with delirium tremens. Whether symptom-triggered benzodiazepines are preferable to a fixed dosing schedule that is tapered over time is currently under debate.

Adjunctive therapy also may be used. Haloperidol (Haldol) may be used to control agitation and belligerence, but only after benzodiazepines have been given, because haloperidol lowers the seizure threshold. In all stages of alcohol withdrawal, compulsive attention to fluid and electrolyte status is required. Beta blockers such as atenolol (Tenormin) also have been used successfully to reduce the adrenergic signs of withdrawal. A daily dose of 50 mg during the withdrawal period shortens hospital stays and reduces the total dose of benzodiazepine required for treatment. In addition to beta blockers, alpha$_2$-receptor agonists, such as clonidine (Catapres), also have been used to treat alcohol withdrawal because of their sedative as well as blood pressure- and pulse-lowering properties. The usual dosage is 0.2 mg twice daily. It is important not to use these adjunctive treatments without benzodiazepines because they do not prevent withdrawal seizures.

8. What pharmacotherapies are available to deter alcoholism?

Traditionally, **disulfiram** has been used to deter alcohol use. It blocks the enzyme aldehyde dehydrogenase, which results in an increased concentration of acetaldehyde. Therefore, patients who ingest alcohol while taking disulfiram get palpitations, dyspnea, headache, tachycardia, and flushing. The alcohol-disulfiram reactions are usually self-limiting; severe reactions are associated with doses greater than 500 mg/day. Data about the efficacy of disulfiram in preventing relapse are scant, despite its widespread use. **Selective serotonin reuptake inhibitors** (SSRIs) have been investigated for their potential to decrease the desire for alcohol. Studies have shown some benefit in patients with coexisting depression. Buspirone has been noted to decrease alcohol craving in alcoholics with coexisting anxiety. The newest pharmacologic treatments center on narcotic antagonists that reduce alcohol craving and use. **Naltrexone** is the only one approved by the FDA. In one 12-week study naltrexone compared favorably with placebo. There was a 23% relapse rate with naltrexone compared with a 54% relapse rate in the placebo group. Naltrexone should not be given to patients taking narcotics. It may result in narcotic withdrawal symptoms. During routine use the most common side effects are nausea, headache, constipation, fatigue, and somnolence. Elevations in liver enzymes may occur, but levels return to baseline after the drug is stopped.

9. Which patients may benefit from disulfiram?

The ideal patient for disulfiram therapy is a daily rather than binge drinker who is committed to treatment but prone to relapse. The main contraindications to its use are heart disease, history of seizures, cirrhosis, diabetes, pregnancy, and significantly elevated levels of transaminases.

10. Which classes of drugs are characterized by potentially dangerous withdrawal syndromes?

Drugs of abuse are generally divided into the following categories: sedatives, stimulants, opiates, psychedelic agents, and phencyclidine (PCP). Withdrawal is defined as the predictable development of physical and psychologic signs and symptoms in response to the abrupt discontinuation of a drug in dependent people. The only class of drugs connected with dangerous withdrawal syndromes is the central nervous depressants, which include alcohol, benzodiazepines, barbiturates, chloral hydrate, and meprobamate.

11. Characterize the opiate withdrawal syndrome.

Mild withdrawal is characterized by yawning and dilated pupils. In more severe cases, vomiting, diarrhea, piloerection, rhinorrhea, and lacrimation are seen. Symptoms include anxiety, insomnia, abdominal cramping, irritability, and leg spasms. Withdrawal usually begins 6–12 hours after the last use of narcotics. Heroin withdrawal symptoms generally peak within 36–72 hours and may last 7–10 days. Most of the withdrawal syndrome is effectively mitigated through the use of two medications: (1) clonidine, in doses of 0.8–1.2 mg/day in divided increments for a total of 10–14 days, with ancillary medications for pain and sleep, or (2) methadone, a longer-acting opioid that, in doses of 15–20 mg/day, is substituted for the opioid of abuse, whether it is heroin, meperidine, or codeine. This dose is maintained through the second or third day and then slowly tapered by 10–15% per day as guided by the patient's symptoms. Recently, buprenorphine hydrochloride has been shown to reduce heroin intake sharply in abusers. Because it is a mixed agonist-antagonist, it has a low potential for abuse and overdose.

12. Does discontinuance of hallucinogens result in withdrawal?

No. Hallucinogens and PCP do not produce withdrawal symptoms, although drug craving is present.

13. Describe characteristic syndromes associated with particular drugs of abuse or their withdrawal.

Severe depression	→	Cocaine
Panic attacks	→	Lysergic acid diethylamide (LSD)
Flashbacks ("bad trips")	→	Hallucinogens

| Psychoses | → | PCP, cocaine, amphetamines |
| Chronic organic brain syndrome | → | Alcohol, solvents, PCP |

14. What are the physiologic effects of cocaine?

Cocaine is obtained by adding hydrochloric acid to cocoa leaves. The water-soluble crystal that forms may be absorbed through the nasal mucosa or injected intravenously. "Crack" is a highly purified form of the cocaine free base that makes a popping sound when heated. When smoked, it produces immediate euphoria, but the effects last only for minutes, prompting repeated, frequent administration. The resulting craving makes it difficult for patients to abstain from cocaine use. The physiologic responses to cocaine are primarily related to excessive cate-cholamine discharge: hypertension, tachycardia, hyperthermia, agitation, and seizures.

15. What medications are available to treat cocaine addiction?

No medication is currently approved for the treatment of cocaine addiction. Retrospective data suggest that tricyclic antidepressants, SSRIs, and dopamine agonists, such as bromocriptine, may have some efficacy in reducing craving.

16. Why must chest pain related to cocaine be seriously evaluated?

Cocaine is one of the most dangerous illicit drugs because of its association with acute myo-cardial infarction in young people with normal coronary arteries. The cause of myocardial infarc-tion is multifactorial but includes vasoconstriction of large epicardial coronary arteries and thrombosis, most commonly involving the left anterior descending artery. Recent evidence indi-cates that cocaine changes endothelium vasodilator capacity, exerts a potent myocardial depressant effect on myocytes, and may directly constrict vascular muscle, independently of alpha-adrenergic stimulation. Although chest pain is frequently encountered after cocaine use, the actual incidence of acute myocardial infarction is low, especially when the initial electrocardiogram is normal. Most patients can be safely managed in a nonintensive care setting.

17. Which drug is contraindicated in cocaine-related chest pain?

If the chest pain is believed to indicate myocardial ischemia, beta blockers are contraindi-cated because they result in unopposed coronary vasoconstriction mediated by alpha-adrenergic agents and may actually exacerbate cocaine-related cardiovascular toxicity. Nitroglycerin and calcium channel blockers are the mainstay of therapy along with the mixed alpha- and beta-adrenergic blocker, labetolol. Heparin, aspirin, and thrombolytic agents also have a role because of experimental evidence of cocaine-enhanced platelet aggregation and thrombosis.

18. Bidirectional nystagmus should suggest abuse of which recreational drug?

PCP is the only drug of abuse that produces bidirectional nystagmus; it has dopaminergic, anticholinergic, and adrenergic activities. Intoxicated patients present with hypertension, tachy-cardia, bidirectional nystagmus, hyperthermia, hallucinations, and marked agitation. The combi-nation of a comalike state with open eyes, diminished pain perception, intermittent periods of excitation, and severe muscle rigidity indicates a PCP reaction. Patients are at risk for hyperten-sive crisis, rhabdomyolysis, seizures, and bizarre, often violent behavior. PCP is abused because of the sense of invisibility and power that it produces. It is most often smoked but also may be taken intravenously or orally. Management of acute PCP intoxication may be extremely chal-lenging. The patient should be placed in a quiet environment; in most instances, this suffices. Patients who are severely agitated, however, should be sedated adequately with benzodiazepines, cooled rapidly if indicated, and hydrated. Drugs such as haloperidol are effective for treatment of terrifying hallucinations.

19. What drug of abuse imposes the largest health and economic burden on society?

The surprising answer is nicotine, one of the major preventable nemeses of public health. The 1989 Surgeon General's report estimated that 1 in 6 deaths in the United States was caused by ciga-rettes. Almost 400,000 deaths were directly attributable to smoking. Only recently have efforts been made to portray tobacco smoking as an addictive disease. Nicotine is a psychoactive drug associated with definite dependence, tolerance, and withdrawal syndrome. The withdrawal process is characterized by dysphoria, craving, irritability, and nervousness. Tobacco addiction is a complex process involving nicotinic-cholinergic receptors in the brain. Because of the complexity of the addiction, many smokers are not able to quit by themselves. The pharmacotherapy of tobacco addiction involves maintaining a fairly consistent level of nicotine in the body through nicotine-substitution therapy. Thus, symptoms of abstinence are relieved. Nicotine chewing gum and transdermal delivery systems are available to achieve this end. However, without some form of concomitant behavioral support from a physician or other caregiver, substitution therapy is frequently unsuccessful. Reports about the effects of clonidine on decreasing cigarette usage are encouraging.

20. Although the margin of safety with benzodiazepines is reassuring compared with other central nervous system sedatives, which addiction issues should the health care provider consider?

Benzodiazepines produce significant physical and psychological dependence as well as a potentially dangerous withdrawal syndrome after prolonged use. In 1990, 60 million benzodiazepine prescriptions were dispensed. The effects are additive with other central nervous system depressants, such as alcohol and barbiturates. Certain medications, such as cimetidine and disulfiram, and certain conditions, such as older age and hepatic impairment, impede the metabolism of benzodiazepines. Medications such as phenytoin and carbamazepine enhance the metabolism of benzodiazepines.

21. Characterize benzodiazepine withdrawal and its therapy.

Benzodiazepines are divided into short-acting agents, such as temazepam (Restoril) and triazolam (Halcion); intermediate-acting agents, such as alprazolam (Xanax), lorazepam (Ativan), and oxazepam (Serax); and long-acting agents, such as clorazepate (Tranxene), diazepam (Valium), and clonazepam (Klonopin). Dependence may develop rapidly, often within a few weeks. In general, the shorter the half-life, the more intense the withdrawal syndrome. Signs and symptoms of withdrawal occur within 24 hours of cessation with a short-acting benzodiazepine and by the fifth day with longer-acting drugs. Benzodiazepine withdrawal produces a highly excitable state that is contrary to the usual sedative effects and may include palpitations, diarrhea, polyuria, tremor, and seizures. Detoxification is predicated on the premise that benzodiazepines have mutual cross-tolerance. Conversions for equivalent doses are easily calculated. In general, a long-acting benzodiazepine is preferable for suppressing withdrawal symptoms. A schedule of 7–10 days of gradual tapering is set up if the abused benzodiazepine is short-acting; a schedule of 10–14 days is used for longer-acting drugs.

Dose Conversions for Sedative Hypnotic Drugs

DRUG	DOSE (mg)	DRUG	DOSE (mg)
Barbiturates		Benzodiazepines	
Pentobarbital	100	Alprazolam	1
Secobarbital	100	Chlordiazepoxide	25
Butalbital	100	Clonazepam	4
Amobarbital	100	Clorazepate	15
Phenobarbital	30	Diazepam	10
Nonbarbiturates		Flurazepam	15
Nonbenzodiazepines		Lorazepam	2
Ethchlorvynol	300	Oxazepam	10
Glutethimide	250	Quazepam	15
Methyprylon	200	Temazepam	15
Methaqualone	300	Triazolam	0.25
Meprobamate	400		
Carisoprodol	700		
Chloral hydrate	500		

22. How accurate is urine drug testing?

Because of a determined effort to reduce drug abuse, drug testing has become more common. Most urine drug panels screen for marijuana, cocaine, opiates, PCP, and amphetamines. The cost of such tests is $50–100. Positive results are confirmed by gas chromatography-mass spectrometry (GC-MS). Almost one-third of positive results on initial screening tests are found to be false. For example, sympathomimetic agents in over-the-counter decongestants test positive for amphetamines; confirmatory testing, however, is negative for the D-isomer of abused amphetamines.

In general, marijuana is detected for 1–3 days after occasional use and for up to 3–4 weeks in a heavy smoker because of accumulation in fatty tissues. The major metabolite of cocaine, benzoylecgonine, may be detected for 2–3 days after use. A positive test for PCP usually indicates drug use within the previous week.

23. What is a medical review officer (MRO)?

Another caveat with drug testing is that poppy seeds on baked goods contain sufficient amounts of morphine to produce a positive urine test. The result is not a false positive, because the drug is actually present. Errors in handling or analysis also may result in false-negative results. Therefore, decision making in drug testing requires the expertise of a medical review officer (MRO) with specific training in addiction medicine. MROs help to protect the rights of a patient while contributing to the effort to reduce drug abuse.

CONTROVERSY

24. What is the role of anticonvulsants in preventing alcohol withdrawal seizures?

A seizure may herald the onset of a major withdrawal syndrome, and one-third of patients with alcohol withdrawal seizures may later develop delirium tremens. Nonetheless, the routine use of phenytoin to prevent seizures in patients withdrawing from alcohol is controversial. Three studies have focused on this issue: two do not support the use of phenytoin, whereas one does. The efficacy of phenytoin in combination with a benzodiazepine thus remains uncertain. Current practice is to give phenytoin only to withdrawing patients with a documented history of nonalcohol-related seizures or a history of withdrawal seizures.

BIBLIOGRAPHY

1. Alldredge BK, Simon RP: Placebo-controlled trial of IV diphenhydantoin for short-term treatment of alcohol withdrawal seizures. Am J Med 87:645–648, 1989.
2. Baldridge BE, Bessen HA: Phencyclidine. Emerg Clin North Am 8:541–549, 1990.
3. Everett WD, Linden N: Drug testing in the workplace. Postgrad Med 91:164–170, 1992.
4. Ewing JA: Detecting alcoholism: The CAGE questionnaire. JAMA 252:1905–1907, 1984.
5. Gorelick DA: Overview of pharmacologic treatments for alcohol and other drug addictions: Intoxication, withdrawal, and relapse prevention. Psychiatr Clin North Am 10:171–179, 1994.
6. Hayner G, Galloway G, Wiehl WO: Haight-Ashbury clinic's drug detoxification protocols: Benzodiazepines and other sedatives. J Psychoact Drugs 25:331–335, 1993.
7. Has AA, Tavassoli M: Laboratory markers of alcohol intake and abuse. Am J Med Sci 303:415–428, 1992.
8. Henry JA, Jeffrey KJ, Dawling S: Toxicity and death from methamphetamine. Lancet 340:384–387, 1992.
9. Lee EW, D'Alonzo GE: Nicotine addiction and its pharmacologic treatment. Arch Intern Med 153:34–48, 1993.
10. Ling W, Wesson DR: Drugs of abuse—opiates. West J Med 152:565–572, 1991.
11. Mayo-Smith MF: Pharmacological management of alcohol withdrawal. JAMA 278:144–151, 1997.
12. Mynor RL, Scott BD, Brown DP, Windford MD: Cocaine-induced myocardial infarction and patients with normal coronary arteries. Ann Intern Med 115:797–806, 1991.
13. O'Connor PG, Schottenfeld RS: Patients with alcohol problems. N Engl J Med 338:592–602, 1998.
14. O'Connor RG, Selwyn PA, Stein MD: Management of the hospitalized intravenous drug users. Am J Med 96:551–558, 1994.
15. Saitz R, Mayo-Smith MF, Roberts MS: Individualized treatment of alcohol withdrawal: A randomized double-blind controlled trial. JAMA 272:519–523, 1994.
16. Swift RM: Effect of naltrexone on human alcohol consumption. J Clin Psychiatry 56(Suppl 7):24–29, 1995.
17. Volpicelli JR, Alterman AI, Hayashida M, O'Brien CP: Naltrexone in the treatment of alcohol dependence. Arch Gen Psychiatry 49:876–880, 1992.

18. Warner E: Cocaine abuse. Ann Intern Med 119:226–235, 1993.
19. Zitten RZ, Allen JP: Pharmacotherapies for alcoholism. Alcohol Clin Exp Res 15:623–633, 1991.

11. ANXIETY

Joyce Seiko Kobayashi, M.D.

1. Why does the primary care physician need to be knowledgeable about the evaluation and management of anxiety in the medical setting?

Frequently anxiety is accompanied by specific physical symptoms that may trigger a major diagnostic work-up. The astute clinician can avoid this pitfall. Early diagnosis of anxiety spares expense and protects the patient from unnecessary distress. Furthermore, a number of primary medical disorders may present with anxiety. In this case the physician should avoid premature diagnosis of an emotional disorder, which may delay proper medical treatment until the disease process worsens.

Many patients react to a range of medical illnesses with significant anxiety, particularly in relationship to the acute diagnosis or later as symptoms become more severe or the illness becomes more life-threatening. Management of anxiety as part of the adjustment to medical illness is best done by the primary care physician, who has a long-term relationship with the patient, and should be considered one of the most important tasks affirming the doctor-patient relationship in comprehensive primary care. Patients who either express their anxiety through somatic symptoms or experience significant anxiety in reaction to medical illness frequently prefer to share their feelings with their primary care physician and may feel abandoned if referred to a psychiatrist or other specialist. If the physician judges that a referral is necessary because of the severity of symptoms, suicidal ideation, acuity of presentation, or comorbid disorders, the patient should be assured that the physician will work closely with the psychiatrist and continue to follow the patient.

2. What are the three most common errors that a primary care practitioner can make with a patient who presents with significant anxiety?

1. The physician may be too quick to consider anxiety a psychiatric problem and either refer the patient to a mental health professional prematurely or rush to prescribe benzodiazepines. Routine treatment of anxiety with benzodiazepines is no more appropriate than routine treatment of fever with penicillin. Anxiety is often treated as the diagnosis rather than a signal to pursue the source of the anxiety or to attempt to understand its meaning. The physician should not prematurely close the diagnostic evaluation and should learn to feel comfortable with exploring the patient's feelings with a few open-ended questions.

2. The physician may assume that he or she knows what the patient "must" be anxious about. A classic example is assuming that the patient about to undergo a course of chemotherapy is most concerned about the medically serious side effects rather than, for example, about losing hair or some other side effect that may feel more immediately threatening.

3. The physician may rush to reassure the patient that "there is really nothing to worry about." Instead, the physician should allow the patient to express his or her feelings, acknowledge that the patient must feel some reason to be anxious, and ensure the patient continued support as well as collaboration to identify and manage the source of anxiety.

3. What are the primary causes of anxiety in the medical setting?

1. Anxiety as a normal alerting response to the perceived threat of medical illness and treatment interventions
2. Anxiety as a symptomatic manifestation of medical illness
3. Anxiety as a symptom of intoxication or withdrawal syndromes
4. Anxiety disorders or other psychiatric disorders

4. What physical symptoms frequently associated with anxiety disorders may be confused with medical illness?

The variety of physical symptoms associated with anxiety may be classified in three general categories:

1. **Motor tension:** trembling, twitching, feeling shaky, muscle tension or aches, restlessness, easy fatigability.

2. **Autonomic hyperactivity:** shortness of breath or smothering sensations, palpitations or tachycardia, sweating or clammy hands, dry mouth, dizziness or lightheadedness, nausea, diarrhea or other abdominal distress, hot flashes or chills, frequent urination, trouble with swallowing, or "lump in throat."

3. **Vigilance of scanning:** feeling keyed-up or on edge, exaggerated startle response, difficulty in concentrating or "mind going blank," trouble with falling or staying asleep, irritability.

Symptoms associated with panic attacks commonly precipitate major medical work-ups.

5. What aspects of medical illness and treatment are common sources of anxiety?

Many aspects of medical illness and treatment may cause anxiety depending on the patient's history, capacity to cope, support network, and specific tasks of adjustment associated with a particular disease or its treatment. It is essential to start by asking several open-ended questions about reactions to diagnosis, experiences with proposed or related therapies, and major current concerns. Some patients may feel that the illness is a punishment; others may use it as an organizing focus for unmet dependency needs. The physician should attempt to understand the meaning of illness to each person.

A number of predictable, deeper concerns are common, and the physician should listen for them in the patient's discussions. Examples include fears of pain, abandonment, dependency, disfigurement, or social unacceptability; loss of control or function; and death. Asking about such deeper concerns too directly or prematurely, however, may increase the patient's anxiety; clinical judgment must be exercised. Reassuring the patient that he or she will not be abandoned, for example, does not require specific acknowledgment of this fear.

The physician also should assess whether the level of anxiety is adaptive or signals the patient's need for further treatment and whether it is pathologic and out of proportion to the situation. Reassurance focused on the medical aspects of the illness in patients with pathologic anxiety does not address their underlying concerns; psychiatric consultation may be considered, with reassurance that the physician will continue to be involved.

Finally, patients also may feel anxious about the doctor-patient relationship or unable to trust the efficacy of medical treatment or the health care system in general because of prior experiences, sociocultural barriers, or personal histories of abuse or neglect. Such patients often feel less anxious as the physician gains their trust through consistent caring and compassionate interaction.

6. List the medical disorders that may present with anxiety as a primary symptom.

Endocrine disorders: hyperthyroidism, pheochromocytoma, hypoglycemia, hypo/hypercalcemia

Cardiac disorders: hypoxia, angina, arrhythmias, congestive heart failure, mitral valve prolapse

Pulmonary disorders: hypoxia, chronic obstructive pulmonary disease, pneumonia, hyperventilation, pulmonary embolism

Neurologic disorders: partial complex seizures, encephalitis, postconcussion syndrome, sleep disorders

Metabolic disorders: vitamin B_{12} deficiency, porphyria

Stimulant toxicity: caffeine, sympathomimetic medications or drugs

Withdrawal syndromes: alcohol, benzodiazepines, barbiturates, opiates, or delirium of any etiology. The reader also is referred to chapter 12 on psychoses.

7. Which psychiatric disorders present with anxiety as a major symptom?

Several categories of psychiatric disorders may present with anxiety, including adjustment disorders, generalized anxiety, posttraumatic stress disorders, substance-induced anxiety disorder, and intoxication/withdrawal disorders (see chapter 10 on substance abuse). Less common underlying disorders include phobias, obsessive-compulsive disorder, and complicated bereavement. In addition, patients with somatoform, conversion, and certain personality disorders often seek help in the primary care setting with similar presentations. Finally, comorbid disorders are quite common. Generalized anxiety disorder, for example, does not commonly occur in isolation (current and lifetime prevalence: 1.2–6.6%) but has a lifetime comorbidity rate of 90%. One of the most common and treatable comorbid diagnoses that should always be kept in mind when anxiety is the presenting symptom is major depressive disorder. The reader is referred to the fourth edition of the Diagnostic and Statistical Manual of the American Psychiatric Association (DSM-IV) for a more specific listing of the diagnostic criteria of the above disorders.

8. What is a panic attack? What other disorders may be associated with panic attacks?
Patients with panic attacks often seek help first from their primary care physician. The essential element of a panic attack is a discrete period of intense fear or discomfort, in which four (or more) of the following symptoms develop abruptly and reach a peak within 10 minutes:

Palpitations	Feeling dizzy or faint
Sweating	Derealization (feelings of unreality)
Trembling	or depersonalization (being detached
Sensation of shortness of breath	from oneself)
or smothering	Fear of losing control or sanity
Feeling of choking	Fear of dying
Chest pain or discomfort	Paresthesias
Nausea or abdominal distress	Chills or hot flushes

Because such patients often feel as if they are going to have a heart attack or stroke or fear that they are dying, they are seen frequently in emergency departments. Some patients fear catastrophic outcomes from minor physical symptoms or medication side effects and may be mislabeled as histrionic or hypochondriacal, when direct reassurance and continuity of care may lessen their fears over time. They may receive multiple major medical work-ups (often at multiple sites) when an initial exclusionary work-up, thorough review of past records and careful history, may suffice. Accurate diagnosis and stabilization and continuity of care with a primary care physician and psychiatrist may prevent further mismanagement of panic disorder.

9. What clues help the primary care physician to recognize other common psychiatric disorders that present with anxiety?
1. **Major depressive disorder** is one of the most common and readily treatable disorders that may present with clinically significant anxiety, with or without panic attacks. Depressive disorders are easily overlooked when anxiety and/or anhedonia (loss of pleasure) is more prominent than sadness.
2. **Bipolar disorder (manic phase)** may present with agitation and irritability that often may be differentiated from anxiety by the sense of pressured speech and easy provocation to anger.
3. **Adjustment disorder** with anxiety may be an acute or chronic condition and is characterized by the development of emotional or behavioral symptoms in response to an identifiable stressor(s) occurring within 3 months of the onset of symptoms. The degree of distress exceeds what normally would be expected, or social or occupational functioning is significantly impaired.
4. A **substance-induced anxiety disorder** is diagnosed when the anxiety is judged to be due to the direct physiologic effects of an illicit drug, medication, or toxin.
5. **Posttraumatic or acute stress disorders** are diagnosed by characteristic symptoms in response to an extreme traumatic stressor.
6. **Phobias** are common in the general population but rarely reach the level of clinical significance. Lifetime prevalence of diagnosable specific phobias is around 10%. However, specific phobias (categorized as animal, natural environment, blood-injection injury, situational, and other types) may have significant effect on health care behavior (e.g., fears of blood, needles, and choking [medications]) and should be consciously assessed for clinical severity with an in-depth

history. Patients with such disorders are aware that their fears are out of proportion to the situation but may not say so unless asked.

7. **Obsessive-compulsive disorders** are important to note (lifetime prevalence of 2–5%), because they are more common than is realized, effective pharmacologic treatments are available, they are often disabling, and fears of contamination may bring a patient to the primary care physician.

DSM-IV provides a more specific listing of the diagnostic criteria of the above disorders.

10. What is DSM-IV?

DSM-IV, published in 1994, is the fourth edition of the American Psychiatric Association's Diagnostic and Statistical Manual of Mental Disorders. This manual was the product of 13 work groups whose comprehensive literature reviews were critiqued by 50–100 advisers representing a diversity of clinical and research expertise; two methods conferences; 40 data reanalyses; and 12 field trials of the revised diagnostic criteria, involving 70 sites and more than 6000 subjects. The APA acknowledges the limitations of any categorical approach, given the heterogeneity of human behavior, but the DSM-IV has begun to incorporate different cultural perspectives and represents a major step in standardizing clinical diagnosis, communication, and research about mental disorders.

11. Which medications, substances, and toxic agents may cause anxiety as a symptom in either intoxication or withdrawal?

Although the term "intoxication and withdrawal syndromes" (see chapter 10) appropriately brings to mind street drugs and alcohol, excessive caffeine ingestion and nicotine withdrawal are two of the most commonly overlooked causes or contributors to anxiety. Caffeine is frequently underestimated as a toxic agent, and a careful history of all sources of caffeine (coffee, sodas, chocolate) should be included in the evaluation of the anxious patient. Symptoms may occur with 200 mg of caffeine daily (less than 2 cups of coffee), and individuals vary in susceptibility. Minor withdrawal from nicotine is usually self-medicated with more cigarettes, but patients who gradually increase tobacco consumption may not be conscious of withdrawal effects.

Withdrawal from benzodiazepines, barbiturates and other sedative/hypnotics, opiates, and alcohol commonly cause anxiety with or without tremulousness. Despite awareness of these pharmacologic effects, the physician may prescribe anxiolytics to a person who presents in great distress, without considering the possibility of a minor withdrawal syndrome.

Cocaine, phencyclidine, amphetamine, metamphetamine, and other stimulants, such as over-the-counter alpha-adrenergic medications (e.g., phenylpropanolamine, ephedrine, phenylephrine, and pseudoephedrine) may cause varying degrees of anxiety, irritability, agitation, and restlessness.

Among the major offending agents in causing anxiety, however, are commonly prescribed medications. The akathisia of neuroleptics is frequently accompanied by a subjective feeling of restlessness and anxiety that may be profoundly disturbing to the sensitive patient. Antidepressants, such as fluoxetine or imipramine; xanthines, such as theophylline and other bronchodilators (epinephrine, isoproterenol, metaproterenol, albuterol, isoetharine); and calcium channel blockers (verapamil, nifedipine, diltiazem) may cause anxiety at therapeutic doses.

Other medications that have been reported to cause anxiety as a side effect include antihistamines, baclofen, cycloserine, indomethacin, oxymetazoline, and quinacrine.

12. For what reasons may the primary care physician be hesitant to discuss an issue that causes anxiety in a particular patient?

1. The busy physician is sometimes concerned that such discussions will take too much valuable time. More often, however, they save time over the long term, because some patients escalate their presenting symptoms (somatic, interpersonal, emotional) to ensure that they will be heard.

2. The conscientious physician may feel "responsible" for solving the problem. Few patients, however, expect the physician to find a solution; they are nevertheless profoundly grateful that someone is willing to listen. Often the more "helpless" the circumstances, the smaller the number of people who will listen; therefore, the patient is even more appreciative (and comforted) if the physician takes a few minutes to do so.

13. What clinical approaches to anxious patients may be useful?

The maxim, "Don't just do something, stand there," is important. Therefore, after ruling out medical etiologies, medication toxicity, and intoxication/withdrawal syndromes and reviewing psychiatric history, the following guidelines may be considered for approaching the anxious patient:

1. **Listen**, using a calm, responsive, but nondirect approach; do not rush to "solve" or "fix" the problem.

2. **Explore** the meaning of the illness, treatment, or situation for the patient.

3. **Target** the conscious reasons for the anxiety (such as fears of abandonment, dependency, and pain) by direct reassurance, while continuing to listen for other concerns.

4. **Understand** that it may be difficult for the patient to identify the immediate cause of anxiety, but that the physician's willingness to listen may be directly calming.

5. **Assess** whether the anxiety is out of proportion to the situation, and consider psychiatric consultation.

6. **Support** through continued discussions, marshalling the natural support network of friends and family or other support groups, trying to address concerns once they are identified, and considering pharmacologic approaches when indicated.

14. What conservative pharmacologic approaches may be safely used for anxiety?

When medical etiologies and intoxication/withdrawal syndromes have been ruled out, medication may be considered for a short time, along with supportive psychosocial and adjunctive approaches, such as meditation and relaxation exercises. Benzodiazepines are highly effective agents, and patients should not be denied their benefits in bona fide circumstances. They are also problematic because of their significant potential for tolerance and dependence. Thus, they should be used only after extensive patient education.

Lorazepam (Ativan), 0.5–1.0 mg; clorazepate (Tranxene), 7.5–15 mg; and diazepam (Valium), 2–5 mg—all up to 3 times/day as needed for anxiety—may be considered when the severity of the anxiety or circumstances warrants. Lorazepam has the advantage of a short half-life. Alprazolam (Xanax), 0.5 mg, has a relatively short half-life, and patients occasionally experience minor withdrawal anxiety before the next scheduled dose. Alprazolam may be more difficult for the patient to discontinue, although studies have shown that discontinuance is facilitated by sufficient patient education about withdrawal effects. It may be considered specifically for panic attacks. If the panic attacks are in the context of depressive symptoms, however, antidepressant medication such as imipramine (Tofranil) in the range of 100–150 mg, or one of a variety of selective serotonin reuptake inhibitors such as paroxetine (Paxil), 20–60 mg, or sertraline (Zoloft), 50–150 mg, should be tried first. Clonazepam (Klonopin), 0.5 mg, is more useful for severe insomnia and agitation because of its relative potency and long half-life.

Buspirone (Buspar), 5–20 mg 3 times/day, is a nonbenzodiazepine anxiolytic and may be tried before the benzodiazepines because of its lack of sedation and low abuse potential. However, the patient must follow a regular dosage pattern (3 times/day) for a full month before noticing significant results; frequently there is a lag of at least several weeks before full efficacy is reached. Buspirone is not useful on an as-needed basis and should not be used with inhibitors monoamine oxidase because of the possibility of hypertensive crisis. It is often effective in combination with a serotonin reuptake inhibitor for combined anxiety and depression.

Low-dose neuroleptics (such as trifluoperazine [Stelazine], 1 mg; loxapine [Loxitane], 5 mg; or liquid perphenazine [Trilafon], 2–4 mg) may be helpful for the patient with organic or extreme, disorganizing anxiety, for some personality disorders with significant anxiety, or anxiety associated with significant posttraumatic symptoms. If patients experience extrapyramidal symptoms even at these very low doses, newer antipsychotic agents, although expensive, may be beneficial, primarily as nighttime doses. Examples include risperidone (0.5–1.0 mg) or olanzaprine (2.5–5.0 mg).

Barbiturates are no longer indicated for anxiety or associated insomnia. A small dose of benzodiazepines to promote sleep in patients suffering acute grief, on as as-needed basis for a few days, is often helpful.

Once medications have been used, exploration of issues to identify sources of anxiety should continue, and nonpharmacologic approaches, such as meditation, self-relaxation exercises, support groups, or counseling should be encouraged.

BIBLIOGRAPHY

1. American Psychiatric Association: Diagnostic and Statistical Manual of Mental Disorders, 4th ed. Washington, DC, American Psychiatric Press, 1994.
2. Dubovsky S, Thomas M: Psychotic depression: Advances in conceptualization and treatment. Hosp Commun Psychiatry 43:1189–1218, 1992.
3. Fennig S, Bromet E, Jandorf L: Gender differences in clinical characteristics of first-admission psychotic depression. Am J Psychiatry 150:1734–1736, 1993.
4. Frank JB, Weihs K, Minerva E, Lieberman DZ: Women's mental health in primary care. Depression, anxiety, somatization, eating disorders, and substance abuse. Med Clin North Am 82:359–389, 1998.
5. Gater R, Tansella M, Korten A, Tiemens BG, et al: Sex differences in the prevalence and detection of depressive and anxiety disorders in general health care settings: Report from the World Health Organization Collaborative Study of Psychological Problems in General Health Care. Arch Gen Psychiatry 55:405–413, 1998.
6. Goldberg TE, Gold JM, Greenberg R, et al: Contrasts between patients with affective disorders and patients with schizophrenia on a neuropsychological test battery. Am J Psychiatry 150:1355–1362, 1993.
7. Hales RE, Yodofsky SC (eds): Textbook of Neuropsychiatry, 2nd ed. Washington, DC, American Psychiatric Press, 1992.
8. Kessler RC, McGonagle KA, Zhao S, et al: Lifetime and 12-month prevalence of DSM-III-R psychiatric disorders in the United States. Arch Gen Psychiatry 51:8–19, 1994.
9. Leon AC, Olfson M, Portera L: Service utilization and expenditures for the treatment of panic disorder. Gen Hosp Psychiatry 19:82–88, 1997.
10. Lipowski ZJ: Delirium. Springfield, IL, Charles C Thomas, 1980.
11. Nisenson LG, Pepper CM, Schwenk TL, Coyne JC: The nature and prevalence of anxiety disorders in primary care. Gen Hosp Psychiatry 20:21–28, 1998.
12. Popkin MK, Tucker GJ: Secondary and drug-induced mood, anxiety, psychotic, catatonic, and personality disorders: A review of the literature. J Neuropsychiatry Clin Neurosci 4:369–385, 1992.
13. Rickels K, Schweizer E: The clinical presentation of generalized anxiety in primary-care settings: Practical concepts of classification and management. J Clin Psychiatry 58:4–10, 1997.
14. Roy-Burne PP, Katon W: Generalized anxiety disorder in primary care: The precursor/modifier pathway to increased health care utilization. J Clin Psychiatry 58:34–38, 1997.
15. Severino S, Yonkers KA: A literature review of psychotic symptoms associated with the premenstruum. Psychosomatics 34:299–314, 1993.
16. Stoudemire A, Fogel BS (eds): Principles of Medical Psychiatry. New York, Grune & Stratton, 1987.
17. Tsuang D, Coryell W: An 8-year follow-up of patients with DSM-III-R psychotic depression, schizoaffective disorder and schizophrenia. Am J Psychiatry 150:1182–1188, 1993.
18. Ziedonis D, Brady K: Dual diagnosis in primary care. Detecting and treating both the addiction and mental illness. Med Clin North Am 81:1017–1036, 1997.

12. PSYCHOSES

Joyce Seiko Kobayashi, M.D.

1. What are the common symptoms of a psychosis?

Psychotic symptoms generally reflect thinking that is out of touch with reality. Psychotic symptoms are often divided into "deficit" symptoms, which are discussed in relationship to schizophrenia (see question 9), and "positive" symptoms, which include the following:

• Auditory or visual hallucinations
• Delusions (paranoid, grandiose, romantic, mistaken identities)
• Ideas of reference (e.g., a radio or television carrying a special message for an individual)

- Thought insertion
- Thought broadcasting
- Thought control
- Loosening of associations and disorganized thought process

2. How should the primary care provider identify and assess positive psychotic symptoms?

Patients often refer to positive symptoms in colloquial terms, and frank psychotic symptoms may go unrecognized if patients are not specifically asked about them. Questions should be simple and nonthreatening:

- Do you find that your thoughts sometimes feel like they are racing or come so fast that they feel out of control?
- Have you ever felt like you have special powers, such as being able to read other peoples' minds, or that your life has a special purpose?
- Do you ever feel that other people can control your thoughts or read your mind?
- Do you ever hear voices or see things that are not there? Have you ever heard your name called, turned around, and no one was there?
    - Do you ever feel that the television or radio is talking directly to you or that they have special messages intended just for you?

3. What are the most common diagnoses of patients with psychotic symptoms in the primary care setting?

Delirium or dementia	Mood disorders
Intoxication or withdrawal syndromes	Schizophrenia

4. Define delirium.

Delirium is an acute change of mental status with primary disturbance of attention and cognition. It has an organic cause and is characterized by abrupt onset (hours or days) and fluctuating course. It may be associated with rambling, incoherent, or muttering speech, perceptual disturbances, disruption of sleep-wake cycle, increased or decreased psychomotor activity, disorientation, or memory impairment.

5. Why should delirium be the first diagnosis considered in a patient with psychotic symptoms?

1. It is often iatrogenic (related to medications or to fluid and electrolyte disturbances).
2. Is is the initial presentation of many serious and treatable medical disorders.
3. It is very common, particularly in high-risk populations. An elderly patient may be unaware of any symptoms from a urinary tract infection but present with delirium. A demented patient or a patient with an extensive history of alcohol abuse may become acutely delirious after taking a narcotic or anticholinergic medication. In one study, up to 85% of terminally ill patients with cancer manifested delirium.

6. How useful are the terms toxic psychosis, ICU psychosis, organic psychosis, and organic mental syndrome?

Delirium should replace these earlier terms, which reflect the presumed causes of the delirium. Many medications, substances, and other toxins may cause delirium. Theories about the causes of delirium in the intensive care unit (ICU) include sensory deprivation and sensory overload with sleep deprivation as well as the other medical causes to which such patients are susceptible. Psychoses caused by identifiable biologic factors were historically termed "organic" to differentiate them from the "functional" psychoses such as schizophrenia. This distinction is no longer useful. Although the term "organic" may be helpful as a description of the range of possible causes of delirium (physiologic, metabolic, and structural), the general terms "organic mental syndrome" and "organic brain syndrome" should be discarded for a specific diagnosis of delirium or dementia.

7. What are the most common medications that may cause toxic psychosis or delirium in the medically ill patient?

Although any centrally active medication has the potential for toxicity in some patients or at high levels, the most common offenders should be kept in mind:

Narcotics

Benzodiazepines

Anticholinergics (or drugs with anticholinergic side effects, such as amitriptyline, thioridizine, antihistamines)

Antidepressants

Barbiturates

Steroids

Anticonvulsants

Antihypertensives

Cimetidine

Propranolol

Digoxin

Theophylline

Antibiotics such as cephalosporins, aminoglycosides, and metronidazole (less common)

8. Which conditions predispose a patient to the development of delirium?

Head injury, mental retardation, dementia, or other neurologic disorders may predispose a patient to delirium of any etiology. Other patients at high risk for psychotic symptoms associated with delirium include:

1. Patients over 65 years old with no prior psychiatric history

2. Patients with a history of significant substance abuse

3. Patients who have advanced medical illness or organ failure or are easily susceptible to infection

4. Patients who may be transiently vulnerable to psychotic symptoms because of other specific medical circumstances (e.g., postpartum delirium)

A good history is necessary to determine exposure to medications, substances, or toxins; both intoxication and withdrawal syndromes should be considered. It is also important to determine the premorbid level of function, psychiatric history, and timing of onset in relation to acute events, such as trauma or hypoxia. Common additional etiologies that should be assessed include infection, metabolic or fluid and electrolyte disturbances, vitamin deficiencies, endocrinopathies, cerebrovascular events (strokes, hemorrhage), and other pathology of the central nervous system such as tumors, seizures, abscesses, cerebritis, encephalitis, and hydrocephalus.

Finally, the physician should consider a summation effect, in which factors such as sleep deprivation, dehydration, anemia, or stress may precipitate delirium in conjunction with other conditions, such as a low-grade infection in an elderly patient.

9. How is delirium differentiated from schizophrenia?

	DELIRIUM	SCHIZOPHRENIA
Age at onset	> Fifth decade	< Fifth decade
Speech	May be dysarthric	Usually clear articulation
Hallucinations	Visual > auditory	Auditory > visual
Disorientation	Frequent	Uncommon
Memory	Often abnormal	May be normal
Diurnal variation	May be worse at night (sundowning)	No change
Misinterpretation	Unfamiliar as familiar	Familiar as unfamiliar

The positive psychotic symptoms observed in schizophrenia usually occur in the context of a deteriorating level of function and are frequently associated with a more extensive course of deficit symptoms, such as marked social isolation or withdrawal, peculiar or bizarre behavior, marked impairment in personal hygiene, blunted or inappropriate affect, poverty of speech or speech content, or marked lack of initiative. Formal diagnosis generally requires at least 1 week of positive psychotic symptoms within a 6-month period of deficit symptoms. If psychotic symptoms are not a result of delirium but part of a schizophrenic or other formal psychiatric disorder, optimal management includes close collaboration with a psychiatrist, case manager, and outpatient treatment program.

10. When are psychotic symptoms seen in a patient with dementia?

The diagnosis of dementia requires a primary disturbance in memory and new learning as well as secondary disturbances in higher cortical functions such as abstract reasoning, judgment, language, or personality. Patients are generally diagnosed with dementia before they experience frank psychotic symptoms. However, a surprisingly high percentage of patients with moderate-to-severe dementia of all etiologies may experience psychotic symptoms at some point in their illness, most commonly auditory or visual hallucinations or paranoid delusions.

Patients who are very forgetful or feel vulnerable because of becoming more disorganized may begin to believe that someone is taking their (misplaced) possessions or intends to harm them. Others who have difficulty hearing or who have little social contact may begin to talk to themselves or imagine visits from dead relatives. Diminished cognitive capacity may result in diminished ability to distinguish the real from the imaginary.

The possibility of superimposed delirium must always be considered in a demented patient with psychotic symptoms, particularly if the symptoms have an acute onset. In addition, many disorders that were historically described as secondary dementias because the cognitive symptoms are due to a treatable or identifiable disease may present with mild cognitive dysfunction and prominent psychotic symptoms. Examples include porphyria, Huntington's chorea, endocrinopathies, nutritional deficiencies, temporal lobe epilepsy, and heavy metal toxicity.

Treatment of the delirium or secondary dementias obviously requires treatment of the underlying disorders, but psychotic symptoms of any etiology are often ameliorated by very low doses of neuroleptics.

11. In which medical conditions may a mood disturbance be a prominent manifestation of delirium?

Steroid toxicity, hypo- and hypercalcemia, thyroid disease, and tertiary syphilis may result in prominent mood disturbances, although any delirious patient may intermittently manifest emotional lability.

12. What disorders in addition to schizophrenia or delirium may present with psychotic symptoms?

1. **Mood disorders** such as major depressive disorder or bipolar (manic-depressive) disorder may or may not be associated with psychotic symptoms during an episode of depression or mania. Psychotic symptoms usually are congruent with the mood, such as delusions of guilt and punishment in depression or grandiose delusions in mania. Episodes frequently recur at variable intervals, but functioning generally returns to normal between episodes.

2. If psychotic symptoms also occur in the absence of a mood disorder (mood-incongruent positive psychotic symptoms), the diagnosis is usually a **schizoaffective disorder**.

3. The symptoms of a **brief reactive psychosis** are indistinguishable from psychotic symptoms that may occur in schizophrenia, but they appear in relationship to one or more markedly stressful events and resolve within a short period (usually within hours to a few weeks). Reactive psychosis is usually accompanied by significant emotional turmoil and is not associated with the gradual deterioration of function that often precedes a schizophrenic psychosis. A brief reactive psychosis may be observed in a patient who has been sexually assaulted, for example.

Formal diagnostic criteria for these and less common psychotic disorders may be found in the fourth edition of the Diagnostic and Statistical Manual of the American Psychiatric Association (DSM-IV). (See chapter 11 for a description of DSM-IV.)

13. What behavioral, environmental, and pharmacologic approaches are useful in treating the psychotic patient with delirium?

Interventions that help to orient the patient, structure activities, and make the environment feel more familiar are helpful. Strategies include introducing anyone who enters the patient's room and reminding the patient of the date and purpose of the visit; maintaining a regular daily schedule without abrupt changes in location; keeping a diary, appointment book, or calendar visible in the patient's room; having a night light, clock, and familiar objects nearby; asking friends or relatives to accompany or visit the patient frequently; keeping information and discussions simple, with frequent repetition; and writing down specific instructions about medications or activities.

The most useful pharmacologic treatment for the delirious patient, besides treating the underlying disorder, is a trial of low-dose neuroleptic medication. High-potency antipsychotic medication in divided doses, such as haloperidol (0.5–4 mg/day) or trifluoperazine (1–4 mg/day), may have a remarkable effect on agitation and behavioral confusion, without significant orthostatic hypotension. Lower-potency medications, such as trifluoperazine (2–8 mg/day), thiothixene (2–10 mg/day), or loxapine (5–10 mg/day) may be substituted in the presence of extrapyramidal side effects rather than treating the side effects with anticholinergic agents or using thioridazine. Newer antipsychotic medications that have fewer extrapyramidal side effects, such as risperidone (0.5–1.0 mg) and olanzapine (Zyprexa), 2.5–5.0 mg, also may be useful.

Benzodiazepines may be useful in the acute management of significant physical agitation but risk further confusion. In an emergency situation, lorazepam also may be administered intramuscularly (1.0–2.0 mg as needed for severe agitation). The newer antipsychotics (e.g., resperidone, olanzapine, quetiapine) may be associated with significant weight gain, agitation, or mood swing.

14. What are the common side effects of antipsychotic medication in medically ill patients?
The most common side effects of antipsychotic medications are due to their effect on the extrapyramidal system. Short-term effects include akathisia (physical and/or subjective restlessness) and dystonia (stiffness) of the jaw, tongue, extraocular muscles, neck, back, or extremities. The primary long-term side effect is the risk of tardive dyskinesia, choreoathetoid movements of the fingers, mouth, and feet. Patients may complain of dry mouth, sialorrhea, or other anticholinergic side effects; orthostatic hypotension; diminished range of affect; or cognitive dysfunction. Less commonly, phenothiazines have been associated with hepatic dysfunction, agranulocytosis, gynecomastia and/or lactation, and pigmentary retinopathy. High-potency neuroleptics have been associated in rare cases with neuroleptic malignant syndrome. The newer antipsychotics (e.g., risperidone, olanzapine, quetiapine) may be associated with significant weight gain, agitation, or mood swings.

BIBLIOGRAPHY

1. American Psychiatric Association: Diagnostic and Statistical Manual of Mental Disorders, 4th ed. Washington, DC, American Psychiatric Press, 1994.
2. Barsky AJ, Cleary PD, Sarnie MK, et al: The course of transient hypochondriasis. Am J Psychiatry 150: 484–488, 1993.
3. Brawman-Mintzer O, Lydiard RB, Emmanuel N, et al: Psychiatric comorbidity in patients with generalized anxiety disorder. Am J Pyschiatry 150:1216–1218, 1993.
4. Bridges K, Beresford F: The systematic review in primary care of patients with chronic psychotic illnesses. J Mental Health (UK) 3:507–512, 1994.
5. Chignon JM, Lepine JP, Ades J: Panic disorder in cardiac outpatients. Am J Psychiatry 150:780–785, 1993.
6. Clark DA, Beck AT, Beck JS: Symptom differences in major depression, dysthymia, panic disorder, and generalized anxiety disorder. Am J Psychiatry 150:205–209, 1994.
7. Coryell W, Endicott J, Winokur G: Anxiety syndromes as epiphenomena of primary major depression: Outcome and familial pyschopathology. Am J Psychiatry 149:100–107, 1992.
8. Fricchione GL, Howanitz E, Jandorf L, et al: Psychological adjustment of end-stage renal disease and the implications of denial. Psychosomatics 33:85–93, 1992.
9. Hales RE, Yudofsky SC (eds): Textbook of Neuropsychiatry, 2nd ed. Washington, DC, American Psychiatric Press, 1992.
10. Kendrick T, Tylee A, et al (eds): The Prevention of Mental Illness in Primary Care. Cambridge, England, Cambridge University Press, 1996, pp 246–262.
11. Jarboe KS, Kilts CD: Diagnosis, neurobiology, and treatment of first-episode schizophrenia. J Am Psychiatr Nurs Assoc 4:S1–S9, 1998.
12. Kessler RC, McGonagle KA, Zhao S, et al: Lifetime and 12-month prevalence of DSM-III-R psychiatric disorders in the United States. Arch Gen Psychiatry 51:8–19, 1994.
13. Kirmayer LJ, Robbins JM: Somatization and the recognition of depression and anxiety in primary care. Am J Psychiatry 150:734–741, 1993.
14. Lydiard RB, Brady K, Ballenger JC, et al: Anxiety and mood disorders in hospitalized alcoholic individuals. Am J Addict 1:325–331, 1992.

15. Massion AO, Warshaw MG, Keller MB: Quality of life and psychiatric morbidity in panic disorder and generalized anxiety disorder. Am J Psychiatry 150:600–607, 1993.
16. Pardis CM, Friedman S, Lazar RM, et al: Anxiety disorders in a neuromuscular clinic. Am J Psychiatry 150:1102–1104, 1993.
17. Popkin MK, Tucker GJ: Secondary and drug-induced mood, anxiety, psychotic, catatonic, and personality disorders: A review of the literature. J Neuropsychiatry Clin Neurosci 4:369–385, 1992.
18. Smith SL, Colenda CC, Espeland MA: Factors determining the level of anxiety state in geriatric primary care patients in a community dwelling. Psychosomatics 35:50–58, 1994.
19. Stoudemire A, Fogel BS (eds): Principles of Medical Psychiatry. New York, Grune & Stratton, 1987.
20. Wald TG, Kahol RG, Noyes R, et al: Rapid relief of anxiety in cancer patients with both alprazolam and placebo. Psychosomatics 34:324–338, 1993.

13. THE DIFFICULT PERSONALITY

John F. Bridges, M.D.

1. What is personality?

Although it is a common and intuitive concept, personality is a difficult term to define with specificity and completeness. Personality encompasses both internal perceptions of the self and the world and and the activity of the self in the world (as objectively experienced and described by others). In addition, personality describes perceptions and actions that are consistent through time and characterize an individual with both biologic inborn traits and capacities (temperament) and acquired learned responses (character).

Most current understandings of personality suggest that inborn capacities and limitations interact with the accidents of environmental advantages and deficiencies to unfold the internal psychological structures and externally revealed patterns of behavior that we call personality.

2. When do personality traits become a personality disorder?

Constellations of personality traits that assume enduring, rigid patterns of maladaptive response to the stressors of life form the bases of a personality disorder.

3. Describe the salient features of the three major groups of personality disorders.

Ten personality disorders are grouped into three clusters (A–C). Disorders within clusters appear to share common features that suggest relationships among them. The clustering also acknowledges a high degree of overlap in symptomatology.

Cluster A: Persons who are unusual, odd, or eccentric in their thinking and appearance

• *Paranoid Personality Disorder*—characterized by a perception of others as motivated by a desire to harm or demean, a questioning of the trustworthiness of others, the bearing of grudges, and a tendency to be easily slighted and to find hidden meanings in the actions or words of others, confirming suspicions and mistrust.

• *Schizoid Personality Disorder*—characterized by a restriction in the capacity for social connection and an inability to feel or express emotions, the choice of solitary lifestyle, denial of the subjective experience of strong emotions, little affect expression, and apparent indifference to social, sexual, and emotional intimacy.

• *Schizotypal Personality Disorder*—characterized by the deficits in interpersonal connection of schizoid personality disorder with the additional features of oddities in thinking and behavior that share common themes with schizophrenia (though not as severe) and paranoid personality disorder, such as suspiciousness, ideas of reference, magical thinking, and additionally displaying quirky modes of speech, dress, and manner.

Cluster B: Persons who are dramatic, highly emotional, and engage in erratic behaviors

• *Antisocial Personality Disorder*—characterized by irresponsible behaviors, beginning in adolescence and carrying through to an adulthood of inconsistent work and social relationships, failure to conform to social norms, disregard for truth, impulsiveness, aggression, reckless behaviors, and lack of remorse for injuries to others.

• *Borderline Personality Disorder*—characterized by unstable moods, relationships, and identify; impulsiveness, with intense emotional reactions leading to reckless self-damaging behaviors, suicide threats and attempts, an impaired ability to regulate moods and mood-dictated expressions of anger and other strongly felt feeling states, and transient paranoid ideation.

• *Histrionic Personality Disorder*—characterized by extreme and inappropriate emotionality, with seductive sexualized interactions with others, fluctuating extremes of feeling states often dramatically demonstrated, low frustration tolerance and preoccupation with immediate gratification, and vague, shallow, impressionistic speech.

• *Narcissistic Personality Disorder*—characterized by imagined or enacted grandiosity in the absence of empathic connection with others, an easily injured and highly overvalued sense of self-importance, an unrealistic sense of uniqueness in a context of interpersonal callousness, entitlement, and demand for attention.

Cluster C: Persons with excessive fearfulness and anxiety

• *Avoidant Personality Disorder*—characterized by social discomfort based on a pervasive fear of being negatively judged, an inability to tolerate disapproval, a need for guarantees of acceptance, and an unwillingness to engage in social and interpersonal engagements that risk exposure to these fearsome situations.

• *Dependent Personality Disorder*—characterized by pervasive dependent behavior and fear of interpersonal loss leading to an unwillingness to take chances, express opinions, make decisions, or undertake projects for fear of severing overvalued connections with others, with attendant feelings of abandonment and loss when even small rifts occur in relationships.

• *Obsessive-Compulsive Personality Disorder*—characterized by inflexible demands for perfectionism that interfere with functioning, demands for submission by others to unreasonable standards, preoccupation with rules, details, right and wrong, and a marked lack of generosity in dealing with others.

Personality disorders under investigation for inclusion

• *Passive-Aggressive Personality Disorder* (Negativistic Personality Disorder)—characterized by a passive opposition to the demands of life, leading to an impaired capacity to work and accomplish goals, with irritable and oppositional responses to authority, deliberate procrastination, protestations of unreasonable expectations and personal misfortune, overevaluation of actual performance, and a concerted critical obstructionist stance to undertakings involving others coupled with feelings of being unappreciated.

• *Depressive Personality Disorder*—characterized by pervasive and nearly continuous feelings of gloom and hopelessness, low self-concept with a critical attacking attitude toward the self; persistent worry, blaming of others and self, and overall harboring a guilty, sad, unhappy view of life.

4. Are children and adolescents diagnosed with personality disorders?

Not usually. Because personality is presumed to be determined only partly by inborn traits or temperament, psychiatrists are wary of applying personality disorder diagnoses to youngsters. As defining criteria, such disorders have maladaptive long-term functioning and inflexible traits. It is the nature of human development over the entire life-span, and perhaps most prominently during the first 20 years of life, to try various methods of responding to and exploiting the world. This process necessarily involves many responses that are less than ideally adaptive and fruitful.

5. Do excessive characteristics in childhood herald adult personality disorders?

Perhaps. Certain childhood disorders, diagnosed in persons under 18 years of age, appear to bear some relationship to the later development of personality disorders.

Disorder of childhood/adolescence	Personality disorder
Conduct disorder	Antisocial personality disorder
Avoidant disorder of childhood	Avoidant personality disorder
Identity disorder	Borderline personality disorder

6. What overall characteristics suggest the possibility of a personality disorder?

One of the hallmarks of a personality disorder is that the patient does not accept personal responsibility for the subjective distress that he or she experiences. A second hallmark is that the disorder is observable within the context of human relationships. The invisibility of the source of the problems to the patient is called ego syntonicity. To the patient, the problem lies not with the self but with others. Thus, the paranoid patient does not see suspicion and mistrust as excessive, out of context, or causing repeated failures in relationships. Such perceptions appear justified and reasonable responses to the measureless potential for injury in everyday life. Similarly, the narcissistic patient does not complain about the relentlessly alienating effects of grandiose and unempathic exploitation of others; rather, the patient complains about the infuriating and hurtful sense of living in a world of persons who do not afford him or her appropriate credit and admiration.

7. What reactions in the caregiver may suggest that the patient has a personality disorder?

Clinicians usually discover the presence of a personality disorder in the context of attempting to provide care for the patient. They find unexpectedly that delivery of care becomes increasingly difficult, apparently troublesome for both physician and patient. Such patients engender powerful responses from the caregivers, as they have from families, friends, and employers; they are irritating, frustrating, and maddening and evoke exaggerated responses from others. In addition, given the ego syntonicity of the symptoms, the caregiver may frequently be seen as the source of the patient's distress.

8. Before diagnosing a personality disorder, what common organic causes of abnormal behavior should be considered?

Personality disorders may be mimicked by various organic disorders as well as by other mental illnesses. Three common medical conditions may cause symptoms that appear similar to those described for personality disorders:

1. **Dementias of senile or presenile onset.** Such patients frequently present with behavioral problems, including irritability, paranoia, anger, and impulsiveness. They may demonstrate the exact symptoms of a disordered personality and elicit from family and friends the same avoidance and anger. The insidious onset masks such dementias, as does the tendency of patients, at least initially, to become exaggerated versions of their former selves. For example, the man who was occasionally irritable and picky gradually becomes an angry, hypercritical caricature of himself, or the sentimental, easily injured woman evolves into a weepy, irrationally inconsolable burlesque of her former self.

2. **Chronic use of certain prescribed medicines.** Chronic changes in mood and attitude may result from certain long-term drug therapies to which both patient and family have become inured. For example, even digitalis may induce chronic depression and paranoia. The differential diagnosis may require subtle questioning about the onset and progression of changes that are nearly invisible to patient or family.

3. **Substance abuse.** Substance abuse, especially alcohol abuse, in a patient or perhaps even in a patient's family may distort personality development and alter long-term patterns. Some research suggests that commencement or cessation of substance use, over time, may radically alter personality style and functioning.

9. What classic patient-caregiver difficulties may occur with patients who have personality disorders or certain personality traits?

Patients with personality disorders can be extremely exasperating to treat. They approach the physician with admixtures of deep-seated fears and suspicions, unbounded wishes for dependency and caretaking, and profoundly distorted views of themselves and their doctors. Although the problems may not be appreciated by the clinician at the onset of the doctor-patient relationship, they soon manifest as characteristic and unwanted feelings and responses from the physician.

The hostile patient. Hostility from a patient is a surprise to clinicians accustomed to grateful and obedient responses. Patients who are paranoid or worried about their vulnerability easily perceive the doctor-patient relationship as unequal (as, in fact, it is) and compromising. They see the physician's ministrations as intrusive and threatening. Such anxiety is rationalized by attacking the physician, devaluing his or her motives, and questioning every decision. This response at first puzzles and later angers the doctor. It flies directly in the face of how physicians see themselves and prefer to be seen by others. Actual care for the patient quickly withers under the barrage of implied or expressed accusation. The doctor soon feels reluctant to pursue appropriate follow-up or to recommend difficult treatments, because he or she no longer wishes to be subjected to hostility and misunderstanding.

The dependent, demanding patient. Dependent patients with powerful wishes for unlimited nurturing initially may be welcomed by the physician, who is perceived as extremely competent and uniquely helpful. The physician responds by returning the patient's admiration and offering more explanations and thoroughness in treatment. Soon, however, such patients reveal an inexpressibly great need for attention. They increase their demands for time, advice, and contact. The physician begins to feel hounded and guilty for not responding wholeheartedly to the increasing demands. Eventually the physician withdraws, puts up barriers, and finds ways to avoid the patient. The patient responds with intensified demands for care and anger at the (accurate) perception of rejection. Thus rigorous medical care falters and fails.

The doctor defeater. Such patients may display paranoia, an exaggerated sense of self-worth, or wildly fluctuating attitudes toward themselves and the caretaker. Some patients seem to choose behaviors obviously in direct opposition to their own best interests. The common thread in their relations with physicians is the unremitting demand for care and the adamant refusal to acknowledge that any treatment is adequate or helpful. The physician becomes increasingly angry at such patients, often expressing the anger as jokes about the patient or benign neglect of the patient's complaints. The wish that the patient "just go away" may be contrary to the physician's ideal self-image and may even result in stubborn attempts to "save" the patient.

In all of these cases—and their many permutations—the patient's mode of interaction is unexpected and misunderstood by the physician. The patient unknowingly frustrates and alienates the physician. The physician, also unknowingly, may take countermeasures in an attempt to proceed with "business as usual," not recognizing that medical reasoning and delivery of care are hampered by the deterioration in the relationship itself.

10. What guidelines should the physician use in caring for the patient with difficult personality traits or a frank personality disorder?

Dealing with patients whose illness manifests in the doctor-patient relationship is not easy. Nor is it easy for the patient, who has a lifetime of failed attempts to relate and to satisfy needs and whose pain over time is enormous. The following guidelines are useful:

1. Recognize the problem by using your own feelings as guides. Take note when you find yourself dreading a patient, imagining the patient on someone else's service, joking about the patient, or arguing with yourself about whether it is necessary to like a patient in order to provide adequate care.

2. Identify what behaviors are affecting the patient's medical care. Discuss the patient with a colleague. Step outside the dysfunctional relationship, and apply diagnostic thinking to the relationship itself. For example, the patient's relentless telephone contact may cause you to pull away, or the insistent demand for ever more and better tests to prove you "wrong" ("I'm sure you're hiding something from me, doctor") or the patient "right" ("I'm just another check in the mail for you, doctor, so I've got to watch out for myself") may force you into practicing defensively and therefore inefficiently.

3. Determine the best way to confront the patient's behavior and spell out its consequences. It is advisable to be consistent with your diagnosis of the problem. For example, the dependent worrier who fears abandonment may be told: "All of these phone calls are making it hard to determine when you really need my help, and they come at times when I cannot think as clearly as I'd like about your problems. I think it best if you save your unscheduled calls for clear medical emergencies, but why don't you give me a call each week when I can make sure that I will have time to talk with you? Wednesdays after my clinic hours make the most sense."

For the hostile patient whose angry accusations and demeaning attacks betray a fear of dependency and damage, a realistic and reassuring approach that shares control may help the relationship: "It can be very hard to feel that you are putting yourself in someone else's hands when you are ill. I want to make certain that you clearly understand what I'm recommending and that you have as much time as you need to ask questions about how the treatment will work. I want you to feel free to tell me what your worries are. We will need to work together closely on this."

For the self-defeating obstructor, awareness of his or her control and the physician's relative lack of power is essential. The approach to such patients must be both humble and frank with change in behavior couched as a choice rather than a demand: "Drinking as much and as often as you do puts you at great risk. I think that you understand by now how dangerous it is. I can offer some suggestions again for what measures you can take to stop drinking and offer my support, but finally you will have to decide whether or not to do what is best for your health."

11. Is it appropriate for a physician to refer to a colleague a patient who evokes irreconcilable conflict?

Yes. Patients are best treated by physicians who can care about them in a genuine way. This caring may find its highest expression in the ability to tolerate the patient's behavior without becoming personally upset. Each physician has certain strengths and weaknesses in this regard. Part of delivering the best possible care is recognizing limitations and the point at which the ability to offer thoughtful, objective care has become compromised. Just as physicians cannot expect to give good care when they are deprived of sleep, or in the midst of a personal crisis, so they cannot expect to be capable of caring for every sort of problem patient.

If a patient presents impossible conflicts for the physician, it is the physician's right and responsibility to refer the patient to another practitioner from whom the patient may expect medical care uncompromised by negative feelings. This transfer should be undertaken openly, and the physician to whom the patient is referred should be told of the problems in advance. Alternatively, it may be helpful to share the care of such patients in an attempt to dilute the intensity of the conflicts.

12. Is referral to a psychiatrist appropriate in the care of patients with difficult personalities?

Yes. Although such patients frequently resent, and recoil from, referral to psychiatrists, it often is profitable to obtain a psychiatric consultation for the patient with a personality disorder or a difficult personality. A psychiatrist may be able to clarify the patterns of the patient's undermining of the relationship and offer suggestions about ways to deal with the conflicts.

BIBLIOGRAPHY

1. American Psychiatric Association: Diagnostic and Statistical Manual of Mental Disorders, 4th ed. Washington, DC, American Psychiatric Association, 1994.
2. Cloninger CR, Svrakic DM, Przybeck TR: A psychobiological model of temperament and character. Arch Gen Psychiatry 50:975–990, 1993.
3. Groves JE: Taking care of the hateful patient. N Engl J Med 298:893–897, 1978.
4. Kaplan HI, Freedman AM, Sadock BJ (eds): Comprehensive Textbook of Psychiatry III. Baltimore, Williams & Wilkins, 1980.
5. Morey L: Personality disorders in DSM-III and DSM-III-R: Convergence, coverage, and internal consistency. Am J Psychiatry 145:573–577, 1988.
6. Nestadt G, Romanoski AJ, Samuels JF, et al: The relationship between personality and DSM-III axis I disorders in the population: Results from an epidemiological survey. Am J Psychiatry 149:1228–1233, 1992.
7. Oldham JM (ed): Personality Disorders: New Perspectives on Diagnostic Validity. Washington, DC, American Psychiatric Press, 1991.
8. Perry JC: Problems and considerations in the valid assessment of personality disorders. Am J Psychiatry 149:1645–1653, 1992.
9. Stone MH: Abnormalities of Personality. New York, W.W. Norton, 1993.
10. Svrakic DM, Whitehead C, Przybeck TR, Cloninger CR: Differential diagnosis of personality disorders by the seven factor model of temperament and character. Arch Gen Psychiatry 50:991–999, 1993.
11. Valliant GE: Adaptation to Life. Boston, Little, Brown, 1977.
12. Widiger TA, Frances A, Spitzer RL, Williams JBW: The DSM-III-R personality disorders: An overview. Am J Psychiatry 145:786–795, 1988.

III. Primary Disorders of the Cardiovascular System

14. HYPERTENSION

Stuart L. Linas, M.D.

1. When is a patient hypertensive?

A patient is considered to be hypertensive when the average of two or more measurements over 4 weeks detects systolic blood pressure of 140 mmHg and/or diastolic blood pressure of 90 mmHg or greater. Patients with blood pressure ≥ 210 mmHg and diastolic blood pressure ≥ 120 mmHg should be evaluated or referred for care immediately.

2. Why should hypertension be treated?

Hypertension is a major risk factor for coronary, cerebral, and renal vascular disease. The Framingham heart study cohort demonstrated a statistically significant, progressive increase in coronary heart disease with increases in either systolic or diastolic blood pressure. Considerable evidence suggests that therapy reduces stroke and renal disease. In addition, hypertension clearly increases the risk of left ventricular hypertrophy (LVH), retinal changes (Keith-Wagener-Barker classification), and central nervous system injury (cerebral infarction and hemorrhage).

3. Does treatment of systolic hypertension alter outcome in elderly patients?

Yes. The Systolic Hypertension in the Elderly Program (SHEP), a large multicenter, randomized, placebo-controlled, and blinded study, followed patients with a mean age of 72 years, an average systolic blood pressure of 170 mmHg, and diastolic blood pressure less than 90 mmHg. Patients were randomized to treatment aimed at reducing systolic blood pressure to less than 160 mmHg. Results showed a 36% reduction in the incidence of stroke and a 27% reduction in the incidence of nonfatal myocardial infarction and death in the treatment versus placebo groups.

4. What is the combined effect of elevated levels of serum cholesterol, smoking, and hypertension on the rate of death from coronary heart disease (CHD)?

In the 316,099 men screened in the Multiple Risk Factor Intervention Trial (MRFIT), the rate of death from CHD was 230 times greater among smokers with a cholesterol level and systolic blood pressure in the highest quintile than in nonsmokers with a systolic pressure and cholesterol level in the lowest quintile. The study found a strong graded relationship between death due to CHD and an increase in systolic and diastolic blood pressure or cholesterol levels above 4.65 mmol/L (180 mg/dl).

5. Does therapy for hypertension influence LVH?

Yes. Major advances in understanding the relationship between hypertension and LVH have been made. LVH, found in 50% of all hypertensive patients by echocardiography (5% by electrocardiogram), is a major risk factor for adverse cardiovascular outcomes, such as myocardial ischemia and infarction, congestive heart failure, and sudden death. LVH regresses after the use of calcium blockers, beta blockers, and angiotensin-converting (ACE) inhibitors. No regression of LVH has been seen after treatment with vasodilator agents.

6. Describe the relationship between hypertension and abnormal carbohydrate metabolism.

Essential hypertension is associated with insulin resistance, glucose intolerance, and hyper-insulinemia; thus, it may be an insulin-resistant state. In addition, hyperinsulinemia is a risk factor for coronary artery disease (CAD). However, depending on the choice of drugs, treatment of hypertension may worsen (diuretics or beta blocker) or have no effect on insulin resistance.

7. When should secondary hypertension be suspected?

At least 95% of hypertensive patients have primary or essential hypertension. Secondary hypertension should be suspected in (1) patients < 35 years of age, (2) patients with no family history of hypertension, and (3) patients with an abrupt onset or unexplained change in hypertension on maximal medical management. In addition, secondary causes should be considered in patients with resistant hypertension (i.e., poor blood pressure control with maximal drug therapy).

8. How may the history, physical examination, and initial laboratory data provide clues to the possible etiology of secondary hypertension?

A thorough history, physical examination, and laboratory studies should be performed to look for causes of secondary hypertension. Renovascular hypertension should be suspected in patients less than 35 years old or older patients with an abrupt worsening of blood pressure, especially in the presence of an abdominal bruit. Oral contraceptives are the most common cause of secondary hypertension in women. Symptoms in the history may indicate pheochromocytoma (flushing, palpitation), drug-induced hypertension (e.g., cocaine), or hyperthyroidism. Cushing's syndrome is easily identified by centripetal obesity, moon face, and striae. Coarctation of the aorta may be diagnosed through comparison of arm and leg blood pressures. Diminished clearance of creatinine suggests renal parenchymal disease, the most common cause of secondary hypertension in an unselected population of hypertensive adults. Unprovoked hypokalemia suggests aldosteronism.

9. When should the diagnosis of renovascular hypertension be pursued?

The prevalence of renovascular hypertension among a general population of hypertensive patients is 0.5%, a rate much lower than prior estimates of 5%, but rises with increasing clinical suspicion. Six situations suggest renovascular hypertension: (1) severe hypertension (diastolic blood pressure > 120 mmHg), (2) hypertension refractory to treatment, (3) abrupt onset of sustained moderate-to-severe hypertension at an age < 20 or > 50 years, (4) hypertension with an abdominal bruit, (5) elevation of creatinine after initiation of ACE inhibitors, and (6) flash pulmonary edema in patients with occlusive vascular disease. In these subsets of patients the incidence of renovascular hypertension is as high as 15%.

10. How should renovascular hypertension be evaluated?

Noninvasive tests have a high predictive value in diagnosing renovascular hypertension. Plasma renin activity after administration of captopril and captopril renography have a sensitivity and specificity of > 90%. Random plasma renin activity (PRA), intravenous pyelography (IVP), and renography have not been shown to be useful.

11. Describe the most cost-effective evaluation of hypertension associated with hypokalemia.

The most common cause of hypokalemia in the hypertensive patient is diuretic therapy. Thus, patients receiving thiazide diuretics should receive potassium supplementation if the level falls below 3.0 mmol/L. In patients requiring large amounts of potassium supplementation, diuretics should be discontinued, and serum and urine concentrations of potassium should be determined 4–5 days later. Hypokalemia in the setting of urinary potassium wasting (urine K^+ > 30 mEq/L) is highly suggestive of aldosteronism.

The next test is paired measurement of upright plasma aldosterone concentration (PAC) and PRA. The screening is positive if PRA is less than 3.0 ng/ml/hr or if the PAC-PRA ratio is less than 20. Primary aldosteronism is confirmed when plasma aldosterone levels remain increased (> 10 mg/dl) after volume expansion with 2 liters of normal saline given over 4 hours. Subsequent evaluation should be done under the guidance of a nephrologist or endocrinologist.

12. What is the significance of borderline hypertension?

Patients with borderline hypertension are at increased risk for developing hypertension in the near future. Patients with blood pressure > 130/85 should be rechecked in 2 years, whereas patients whose blood pressure ranges from 130–139 systolic or 85–89 diastolic should be rechecked at 1 year.

13. When and how should one initiate therapy for hypertension?

Treatment of mild-to-moderate hypertension in an ambulatory setting follows a slow, deliberate course. Patients with mild-to-moderate hypertension should attempt to modify their lifestyle. Important modifications include weight reduction, moderation of alcohol intake to less than 2 drinks/day, regular mild or moderate physical activity 3 times/week, reduction of sodium intake to less than 2000–3000 mg/day, and smoking cessation. If the blood pressure remains at or above 140/90 mmHg over a 3–6-month period or if the patient has an initial systolic blood pressure of 180–210 mmHg and/or diastolic blood pressure of 110–120 mmHg, pharmacologic therapy should be initiated at lower doses and increased as necessary. In geriatric patients approximately one-half of the usual starting dose should be used. Drug treatment should follow an organized regimen of "stepped" care. For each medication that is chosen, the patient should be reevaluated within a few days to months, depending on the stage of hypertension. If the response is inadequate, the dose may be doubled. If control is inadequate, a second agent is added. If the blood pressure is controlled to less than 140/90 mmHg, therapy is continued and assessed at appropriate intervals. At least some therapy for hypertension is usually required for the remainder of the patient's life.

14. What is the single most important cause of inadequate blood pressure control?

The major cause of poor control is patient noncompliance. Fewer than 50% of patients with high blood pressure keep follow-up appointments, and fewer than 60% take their medications as prescribed. Barriers to adequate medical compliance include poor doctor-patient communication, cost of medications, and side effects. Care providers must consider all of these factors to improve the outcome of hypertensive therapy.

15. How do lifestyle modifications improve hypertension?

Lifestyle modifications may be used as primary treatment for mild hypertension. Such approaches have not definitively reduced morbidity or mortality but often lower blood pressure, reduce the number and dosage of medications, and improve the risk profile for cardiovascular disease.

16. Which hypertensive patient requires hospitalization?

When the diastolic blood pressure is > 140 mmHg and/or evidence suggests hypertensive encephalopathy, hypertension should be treated with careful inpatient monitoring, using parenteral therapy when needed.

17. What laboratory evaluation should all hypertensive patients undergo?

All newly diagnosed hypertensive patients should undergo basic laboratory studies, including urinalysis for protein, glucose, and blood; assessment of serum levels of creatinine, potassium, glucose, calcium, and uric acid; and a lipid profile. Further studies may be added at a later date either to evaluate the possibility of secondary hypertension or to analyze the effect of therapeutic trials. Electrocardiograms should be performed on all hypertensive patients to exclude CAD, LVH, and other nascent heart diseases and to establish baseline values.

18. How do age and race affect the choice of antihypertensive agents?

Two groups have been well studied: African-American men and elderly patients. African-American men are responsive to diuretics in major randomized, controlled trials. Diuretics may have added benefits in this population because they are inexpensive and compliance rates are high. Additional small studies suggest that calcium channel blockers also benefit African-American men. Hypertension in elderly patients is effectively controlled with low-dose diuretics. Three recent major clinical trials show that diuretics particularly reduce geriatric cardiovascular morbidity and mortality. Beta blockers also reduce hypertension in elderly patients; however, they have not significantly reduced cardiovascular mortality.

19. How do concomitant medical conditions affect the choice of antihypertensive drugs?

Antihypertensive Drugs in Patients with Additional Medical Illnesses

CONDITION	PREFERRED AGENT	NOT RECOMMENDED
Asthma with chronic obstructive pulmonary disease	ACE inhibitor Calcium antagonist Thiazide diuretic	Beta blocker
Coronary artery disease	Beta blocker Calcium antagonist	Vasodilators
Left ventricular dysfunction (systolic)	ACE inhibitor	Beta blocker Calcium antagonist
Left ventricular hypertrophy	ACE inhibitor Calcium antagonist	Vasodilators Thiazide
Diabetes mellitus	ACE inhibitor	Beta blocker Thiazide
Chronic renal failure (creatinine > 3 mg/dl)	Loop diuretics Calcium antagonist	ACE inhibitor
Renovascular hypertension	Calcium antagonist	ACE inhibitor

20. When should diuretics *not* be used in the treatment of high blood pressure?
    Diuretics are well tolerated, inexpensive, safe, and effective. However, they may be relatively contraindicated in patients with CAD, arrhythmia, gout, glucose intolerance, dyslipidemia, or neuropathy with orthostasis.

21. When is an ACE inhibitor contraindicated?
    Rarely. The primary contraindications include angioedema related to ACE inhibitor treatment, pregnancy, a creatinine level greater than 3 mg/dl, or potassium greater than 5 mmol/L. ACE inhibitors also may be contraindicated in patients with a history of angioedema unrelated to ACE inhibitors, because there may be an increased risk of angioedema while taking an ACE inhibitor. ACE inhibitors may cause fetal or neonatal morbidity or mortality primarily in the second or third semester. Thus, treatment with ACE inhibitors should be discontinued immediately after a patient learns that she is pregnant. An ACE inhibitor may worsen azotemia or hyperkalemia by reducing the glomerular filtration rate.

22. List indications for ambulatory or continuous blood pressure monitoring.
    • Discrepancy between home and office blood pressure readings
    • Persistent elevation of blood pressure in the office without target organ disease
    • Episodic elevation of blood pressure
    • Hypertension resistant to treatment
    • End-organ disease in the face of normal office blood pressure
    • Evaluation of efficacy of treatment

23. Does smoking cessation influence hypertension?
    Smoking cessation does not directly improve hypertension but profoundly reduces cardiovascular mortality.

24. How do calcium antagonists differ in their hemodynamic effects?
    Calcium antagonists lower blood pressure by decreasing either cardiac output (CO) or systemic vascular resistance (SVR). Some calcium antagonists reduce SVR with little (isradipine) or

no (felodipine, amlodipine) decrease in CO. Others (verapamil, diltiazem) have major cardiac effects, whereas nifedipine and nicardipine are predominantly vasodilators but decrease CO in the presence of underlying systolic dysfunction. Thus, the choice of calcium channel blocker is determined by additional underlying disease and cost effectiveness.

25. Other than noncompliance with antihypertensive therapy, what are the most common causes of drug-resistant hypertension?

The major cause of resistant hypertension is **salt and water retention**. With the exception of diuretics and possibly calcium channel blockers, all classes of antihypertensive therapy cause salt retention and tolerance to antihypertensive drug therapy. Although the role of salt retention in primary therapy of high blood pressure is highly controversial, salt should be restricted in hypertensive patients on all forms of antihypertensive therapies, especially patients who become resistant to antihypertensive therapy. In addition, in patients treated with agents other than diuretics as initial therapy for hypertension, diuretics should be included as part of the two-drug therapy. **Alcohol consumption** is also a frequent cause of drug-resistant hypertension. Studies have shown that reduction in alcohol consumption to less than two drinks per day is associated with better blood pressure control and reduction in the total number of antihypertensive drugs by one drug.

26. When should hypertension be treated in diabetic patients?

There are differences in the onset of hypertension in insulin-dependent and non–insulin-dependent diabetics. The natural history of insulin-dependent diabetes is well known. Microalbuminuria is followed by macroalbuminuria, hypertension, and then nephrotic syndrome, loss of glomerular filtration rate (GFR), and end-stage renal disease. ACE inhibitors have been shown to delay the progression of this process. Thus, ACE inhibitors should be instituted at the time of development of microalbuminuria.

In non–insulin-dependent diabetes, hypertension often precedes the development of diabetes. Antihypertensive therapy should be increased aggressively at the time of diagnosis of non–insulin-dependent diabetes. In patients with kidney disease (proteinuria or decreases in GFR), LVH, or heart failure, ACE inhibitors are the class of drugs of choice.

BIBLIOGRAPHY

1. Clark LT: Improving compliance and increasing control of hypertension: Needs of special hypertensive populations. Am Heart J 121:664, 1991.
2. Dunn FG, Burns JM, Hornung RS: Left ventricular hypertrophy in hypertension. Am Heart J 122:312, 1991.
3. Hansson L, Zanchetti A, Carruthers SG, et al: Effects of intensive blood pressure lowering and low-dose aspirin in patients with hypertension: Principal results of the hypertension optimal treatment (hot) randomized trial. Lancet 351:1755–1762, 1998.
4. Kaplan NM: Management of hypertension. Dis Mon 38:76, 1992.
5. Kaplan NM: Systemic hypertension: Mechanisms and diagnosis. In Braunwald E (ed): Heart Disease: A Textbook of Cardiovascular Disease. Philadelphia, W.B. Saunders, 1992, pp 817–874.
6. McCarron DA, Haber E, Slater EE: Hypertension. Sci Am Med 7:1, 1993.
7. Neaton JD, Wentworth D, for the Multiple Risk Factor Intervention Trial group: Serum cholesterol, blood pressure, cigarette smoking, and death from coronary heart disease. Arch Intern Med 152:56–64, 1992.
8. Schwartz GL: Initial therapy for hypertension-individualizing care. Mayo Clin Proc 65:73, 1990.
9. SHEP Cooperative Research Group: Prevention of stroke by antihypertensive drug treatment in older persons with isolated systolic hypertension: Final results of the Systolic Hypertension in the Elderly Program (SHEP). JAMA 26:3255, 1991.
10. Sixth Report of the Joint National Committee on Prevention, Detection, Evaluation, and Treatment of High Blood Pressure (JNC VI). Arch Intern Med 157:2413–2446, 1997.
11. Weinberger MH, Grim CE, Hollifield JW, et al: Primary aldosteronism. Ann Intern Med 55:86, 1979.

15. CHEST PAIN

Valerie K. Ulstad, M.D., M.P.A., M.P.H.

1. What is the most important tool in distinguishing the cause of chest pain?
The history taken by the health care provider is without question the most valuable tool. It is important to have a systematic way in which to obtain the history.

2. What are the important components of the history in the evaluation of chest pain?
The two Cs should be remembered in evaluating chest pain or discomfort—characterize and categorize.
1. **Characterize.** You are seeking a thorough description of the pain, including the *quality* of the sensation (crushing, burning, stabbing, tearing), the *location* and *radiation* of the pain, the *temporal intensity* of the discomfort, including how it begins (starts abruptly or builds up insidiously) and the *duration* (second, minutes, hours, days); the sources of *provocation* (exercise, emotional stress, eating, inhalation/exhalation, changing position); the *palliative features* (rest, nitroglycerin, food, change of position); and other *associated features* (pallor, diaphoresis, dyspnea, palpitations).
2. **Categorize.** What organ systems are you dealing with? Is there more than one type of pain? Is the discomfort cardiac, pulmonary, gastrointestinal, breast, musculoskeletal, neurologic, or psychological?

3. Name the most common cardiovascular causes of chest pain.
Common causes include atherosclerosis manifesting as ischemic heart disease (angina pectoris) and acute ischemic heart disease (myocardial infarction), pericarditis, dissecting aortic aneurysm, valvular heart disease, and hypertrophic cardiomyopathy. A careful history and physical exam are important in differentiating these individual and sometimes coexistent problems.

4. Describe typical angina pectoris.
Angina pectoris is a clinical syndrome characterized typically by a deep retrosternal pressurelike sensation that occurs during physical exercise (particularly in the cold), eating, or emotional excitement. Patients in fact may protest at the word "pain" and prefer "discomfort" as a suitable descriptor. When the patient places a clenched fist over the sternum to describe the chest discomfort, angina is strongly suggested (Levine sign). The discomfort usually builds up gradually to its peak. Anginal discomfort usually does not radiate, but when it does, it may radiate to a variety of locations: the neck, jaw, teeth, left or right arm, or back. The ulnar aspect of the left arm is a particularly common site of radiation. There may be accompanying symptoms such as pallor, diaphoresis, nausea, dyspnea, and fatigue. The discomfort usually lasts 5–15 minutes and disappears with rest and/or sublingual nitroglycerin. The frequency of discomfort and level of exertion that precipitates the angina are important in determining the urgency for further diagnostic and therapeutic interventions.

5. List the risk factors for atherosclerotic cardiovascular disease.

Hypertension	Family history
Diabetes	Hyperlipidemia
Smoking	Obesity
Male > 40 years of age	Type A personality
Postmenopausal female	

6. What physical findings support the presence of coronary artery disease?
The physical examination in a patient with severe angina may be completely normal. Relatively subtle findings such as an S4, a mitral regurgitation murmur, and/or a sustained apical impulse may occur during an ischemic episode. Hypertension also may be present during pain.

7. Does a normal EKG rule out coronary artery disease as the cause of chest pain?

Absolutely not. The EKG may be normal even during an acute myocardial infarction in up to 10% of patients. The history is more sensitive than the EKG. A normal EKG should never dissuade you from pursuing a worrisome history. Certainly evidence of ST-T changes during an episode of pain can support the clinical diagnosis already made by the history, as would Q waves suggesting previous myocardial infarction.

8. How does the chest pain associated with acute myocardial infarction differ from that of angina pectoris?

The only real difference between these two syndromes is that angina pectoris is relieved relatively promptly with rest and/or nitroglycerin, whereas in acute myocardial infarction the pain may be prolonged (> 30 minutes), lasting potentially for hours. The pain of acute myocardial infarction also tends to radiate more widely.

9. What are anginal equivalents?

Anginal equivalents are symptoms that may occur in place of typical anginal chest pain but represent the same pathophysiologic process. Examples include dyspnea; discomfort along the ulnar aspect of the left forearm; lower jaw, teeth, neck, or shoulder pain; nausea; indigestion; diaphoresis; or the development of gas or belching. The clinician should initially consider ischemic heart disease in the differential of these symptoms.

10. When is chest pain called "atypical"?

Atypical chest pain has only two of the three following characteristics: (1) substernal location, (2) precipitation by exertion, or (3) relief by rest or nitroglycerin in 10 minutes or less.

11. What is Prinzmetal's angina?

Prinzmetal's angina occurs at rest or with ordinary activity and is precipitated by exercise. The discomfort tends to occur at night or in the early morning. The episodes may be severe and longer in duration than those of typical angina pectoris. This relatively rare situation is thought to be due to coronary spasm. The clinician would be unable to distinguish between Prinzmetal's angina and an acute ischemic syndrome (such as unstable angina or acute myocardial infarction) while actually observing a patient having pain. A history that suggests recurrence, particularly at the same time of day, is suggestive of Prinzmetal's angina.

12. How does typical pericardial pain differ from angina?

Pericardial pain is sharper than angina. The patient may describe the pain as stabbing. The discomfort is often located on the left side of the chest and may radiate to the neck and left trapezius ridge. Leaning forward may alleviate pericardial pain by causing the pericardium to fall away from the heart and worsen when the patient lies flat on the back. Breathing, swallowing, and twisting the upper body may increase discomfort. The pain of pericarditis lasts for hours to days and is unaffected by exercise.

13. What physical findings support the diagnosis of pericarditis?

A low-grade fever may be present. High spiking fevers and a toxic-appearing patient should alert the clinician to possible purulent pericarditis that requires urgent draining. The classic cardiac exam in acute pericarditis is characterized by tachycardia and a friction rub. The rub may come and go. It is more likely to be heard with the patient lying on his or her back. Having the patient exhale and suspend respirations while one quickly listens maximizes the chances that the rub will be heard. Of course, one should look for evidence of systemic diseases that may be associated with pericarditis.

14. What are the causes of pericarditis?

Most commonly pericarditis is idiopathic. Other etiologies include viral infection, myocardial infarction, aortic dissection rupturing into the pericardium, blunt chest trauma, malignancy, radiation, uremia, surgery, drugs (procainamide and hydralazine are the most common), and various connective tissue diseases.

15. Is an abnormal echocardiogram necessary to make the diagnosis of pericarditis?

No. Pericarditis is a clinical diagnosis. The absence of an effusion on the echocardiogram means just that. The echocardiogram is insensitive to inflammation. On the other hand, it is capable of detecting a very small amount of pericardial fluid.

16. What are the characteristic symptoms of aortic dissection?

The most striking feature of the classic presentation is abrupt onset with sudden severe pain. The pain is of maximal intensity immediately (as opposed to the crescendo nature of angina) and may be waxing and waning or unrelenting. The pain is frequently described as ripping or tearing. It commonly radiates from the anterior chest to the back, sometimes following the path of the dissection. The patient also may present with neurologic symptoms or limb ischemia, suggesting compromise of vessels leaving the aorta.

17. What are the risk factors for aortic dissection?

Hypertension is present in 70–90% of persons who develop dissection of the aorta. Other risk factors include Marfan syndrome, pregnancy, coarctation of the aorta, and trauma.

18. What types of valvular heart disease may present with chest pain?

An important valvular cause of chest discomfort is significant aortic stenosis. The pain is a typically anginal discomfort, probably due to inability to augment coronary blood flow to the hypertrophied myocardium. Angina is one of the classic symptoms of severe aortic stenosis.

Chest pain is no more frequent in patients with mitral valve prolapse than in healthy controls. When chest pain is present with documented mitral valve prolapse, it is most commonly stabbing and unrelated to exertion. The discomfort, however, may mimic angina pectoris.

19. How does hypertrophic cardiomyopathy cause chest pain?

This typical anginal pain is related to subendocardial ischemia with or without coexisting coronary artery disease. The demand of the hypertrophied myocardium outstrips the available myocardial oxygen supply, and ischemia results.

20. What features suggest a pulmonary or pleural etiology of chest pain?

An increase in chest discomfort with inspiration and sharp, well-localized pain with sudden onset of dyspnea should point to the lungs or pleura as the source of chest pain.

21. What features of the history suggest a musculoskeletal cause of chest pain?

Aggravation by moving or coughing suggests such a cause. Discrete superficial chest pain probably arises from a musculoskeletal injury. Pain lasting constantly for days or weeks suggests a musculoskeletal etiology, although space-occupying malignant processes in the mediastinum also should be considered.

22. What is Tietze syndrome?

Tietze syndrome consists of discomfort localized to swollen costochondral and costosternal joints that are painful on palpation.

23. Describe the chest pain associated with Da Costa syndrome or neurocirculatory asthenia.

This pain is functional or psychogenic. It is localized in the area of the cardiac apex, is dull and persistent, and lasts for hours with associated intervals of lancinating inframammary pain that lasts seconds. The pain may be associated with palpitations, hyperventilation, lightheadedness, dyspnea, weakness, generalized numbness and tingling, and emotional instability.

24. How may gastrointestinal pathology masquerade as cardiac disease?

Esophageal spasm may closely mimic angina pectoris. The discomfort may be substernal, brought on by eating, and relieved by nitroglycerin; it also may radiate to the back. Relief of the discomfort with antacids, a water brash taste in the mouth, or dysphagia help point to the esophagus as the cause. Stooping or bending tends to provoke esophageal reflux. Indigestion due to peptic ulcer disease may imitate angina. Pain due to pancreatitis or cholecystitis may resemble acute myocardial infarction. Generally there is no relationship between exercise and GI causes of chest pain.

25. How often can the clinician determine a specific cause of chest discomfort?

Chest pain or discomfort is a common clinical problem. The priority is to rule out life-threatening causes promptly, realizing that after this is done no definite etiology for chest pain is found in as many as 50% of cases. Serial observation may provide other clues or simply resolution of the discomfort.

26. What is the immediate goal in the evaluation of the patient with acute chest pain?

Risk stratification into high, intermediate, or low risk for acute ischemic syndrome is the immediate goal. An ischemic cause of chest pain should always be considered first because the importance of early treatment of patients with acute MI is well documented.

27. How does one assess the likelihood of significant coronary artery disease in patients with chest pain suggestive of unstable angina?

The majority of predictive information comes from the symptoms and the EKG. The likelihood of significant coronary disease is **high** with any of the following features:
- Known history of CAD
- Classic angina in men ≥ 60 or women ≥ 70
- EKG or hemodynamic changes with pain
- ST segment increase or decrease ≥ 1 mm
- Marked symmetrical T-wave inversion in multiple precordial leads
- Variant angina

The likelihood of significant coronary disease is **intermediate** with absence of high-risk features and presence of any of the following features:
- Classic angina in men ≤ 60 or women ≤ 70
- Probable angina in men > 60 or women > 70
- Nonspecific chest pain in diabetic patients or nondiabetic patients with two or more other risk factors
- Evidence of other vascular disease
- ST depression of 0.05–1.0 mm
- T-wave inversion ≥ 1 mm in leads with dominant R waves

The likelihood of significant coronary disease is **low** with absence of any high- or intermediate-risk features:
- Chest pain probably not angina
- One risk factor but not diabetes
- Normal EKG
- T-wave flat or inverted < 1 mm in leads with dominant R waves

28. What characteristics suggest high, intermediate, and low short-term risk of death or nonfatal MI?

High risk of death or nonfatal MI (at least one of the following must be present)
- More than 20 minutes of ongoing rest pain
- Pulmonary edema
- Angina with new or worsening MR murmur
- Rest angina with dynamic ST changes ≥ 1 mm
- Angina with S3 or rales
- Angina with hypotension

Intermediate risk of death or nonfatal MI (no high-risk features but any of the following)
- Rest angina now resolved but not a low likelihood of CAD
- Rest angina (> 20 minute or relieved with rest or nitroglycerin)
- Angina with dynamic T-wave changes
- Nocturnal angina
- New-onset angina with walking < 2 blocks or at rest in past 2 weeks (but not a low or high likelihood of CAD)
- Q waves or ST depression ≥ 1 mm in multiple leads
- Age > 65 years

Low risk of death or nonfatal MI (no high or intermediate features)
- Increased angina in frequency, duration, or severity
- Angina provoked at a lower threshold
- New angina within 2 weeks to 2 months
- Normal or unchanged EKG

BIBLIOGRAPHY

1. American College of Emergency Physicians: Clinical policy for the initial approach to adults presenting with a chief complaint of chest pain, with no history of trauma. Ann Emerg Med 25:274–299, 1995.
2. Braunwald E (ed): Heart Disease: A Textbook of Cardiovascular Medicine, 5th ed. Philadelphia, W.B. Saunders, 1997.
3. Braunwald E, Jones RH, Mark DB, et al: Diagnosing and managing unstable angina. Agency for Health Care Policy and Research. Circulation 90:613–622, 1994.
4. Christie L, Conti CR: Systematic approach to the evaluation of angina-like chest pain. Am Heart J 102:897, 1981.
5. Constant J: The clinical diagnosis of nonanginal chest pain: The differentiation of angina from nonanginal chest pain by history. Clin Cardiol 6:11, 1983.
6. Duprez DA: Angina in the elderly. Eur Heart J 17(Suppl G):8–13, 1996.
7. Gomez MA, Anderson JL, Karagounis LA, et al: An emergency department-based protocol for rapidly ruling out myocardial ischemia reduces hospital time and expense: Results of a randomized study (ROMIO). J Am Coll Cardiol 28:25–33, 1996.
8. Herlitz J, Karlson BW, Hjalmarson A: Ten-year mortality rate among patients in whom acute myocardial infarction was not confirmed in relation to clinical history and observations during hospital stay: Experiences from the Goteborg Metroprolol Trial. Int J Cardiol 44:217–224, 1994.
9. Hurst JW, Logue RB: Angina pectoris: Words patients used and overlooked precipitating events. Heart Dis Stroke 2:89–91, 1993.
10. Levine HJ: Difficult problems in the diagnosis of chest pain. Am Heart J 100:108, 1980.
11. Markiewicz W, Stoner J, London E, et al: Mitral valve prolapse in 100 presumably healthy young females. Circulation 53:464–473, 1976.
12. Matthews MB, Julian DG (eds): Angina Pectoris. New York, Churchill Livingstone, 1985.
13. Miller A: Diagnosis of Chest Pain. New York, Raven Press, 1988.
14. Norell M, Lythall D, Coghlan G, et al: Limited value of the resting electrocardiogram in assessing patients with recent onset chest pain. Br Heart J 67:53–56, 1992.
15. Sampson JJ, Cheitlin MD: Pathophysiology and differential diagnosis of cardiac pain. Prog Cardiovasc Dis 13:507, 1971.
16. Shima MA: Evaluation of chest pain: Back to the basics of history and physical examination. Postgrad Med 91:155–158, 161–164, 1992.
17. Stubbs P, Collinson P, Moseley D, et al: Prospective study of the role of cardiac troponin T in patients admitted with unstable angina. BMJ 313:262–264, 1996.
18. Tarum JL, Jesse RL, Kontos MC, et al: Comprehensive strategy for the evaluation and triage of the chest pain patient. Ann Emerg Med 29:116–125, 1997.
19. Tibbing L: Issues in the treatment of noncardiac chest pain. Am J Med 92(5A):84S–87S, 1992.

16. EDEMA

Valerie K. Ulstad, M.D., M.P.A., M.P.H.

1. Name the signs and symptoms of edema.
- Unexplained weight gain
- Tightness of a ring or shoe
- Puffiness in the face and eyelids, especially in the morning
- Swollen extremities
- Enlarged abdominal girth
- Persistence of indentation of the skin following pressure

2. What is the pathogenesis of edema?
Edema is not a disease but rather a sign suggesting abnormal fluid shifts within the body. Edema forms when the production of interstitial fluid exceeds its removal through the lymphatic and/or venous system. The overproduction or decreased removal of fluid from the interstitium results in edema.

3. Classify the pathophysiologic differential diagnosis of edema.

Increased fluid accumulation	**Decreased fluid removal**
• Hypoalbuminemia	• Mechanical obstruction
Decreased synthesis	Clot
Increased loss	Tumor
• High hydrostatic pressure	• Poor venous or lymphatic return
Systemic venous hypertension	Infection
• Increased capillary permeability	Varicosities
Immunologic injury—vasculitis	Neuropathy
Idiopathic cyclic edema of women	
Postanoxic syndrome	

4. What factors perpetuate the edematous state?
Edema due to abnormal production of interstitial fluid may cause a drop in the effective circulating blood volume. Underperfusion of the kidney triggers retention of salt and water in an attempt to augment tissue perfusion. Thus, despite massive interstitial edema, salt and water are retained.

5. What is lymphedema?
Painless swelling of the lower extremity(ies) due to obstruction of the lymphatic capillaries and larger lymphatic vessels is termed lymphedema. This condition may be primary (congenital) or secondary. Secondary causes include infection (streptococci, tuberculosis, filariasis), inflammation (chronic dermatitis), and obstruction (tumors, especially of the prostate, and lymphoma).

6. List the causes of venous hypertension that result in peripheral edema.
- Congestive heart failure—right ventricular or biventricular
- Constrictive pericarditis
- Tricuspid regurgitation
- Hemodynamically significant pericardial edema
- Restrictive cardiomyopathy

7. How can one use the pit recovery time as a clue to the cause of edema?
The pit recovery time is the length of time (in seconds) required for the pit made by one's finger to refill. This simple test is a crude measure of the protein content in the edema fluid.

Classically this test is performed by applying firm pressure to the bone, usually pretibially. Osmotic forces act quickly to draw the fluid back into the microvasculature of the pit, once pressure is released. In patients with hypoalbuminemia or early lymphedema, the pit recovery time is short (< 40 sec); with increased venous pressure or capillary leak of protein, the recovery time is > 40 seconds. The protein concentration in the interstitial fluid is lower in hypoalbuminemia than in the other states. Thus, fluid reequilibrates rapidly, and the pit disappears. This test applies only to acute edema (< 3 months' duration). Chronic edema causes interstitial scarring and fibrosis and thus results in a prolonged pit recovery time.

8. Distinguish among stasis dermatitis, brawny edema, and myxedema.

Stasis dermatitis results from edema due to venous incompetence. Initially, a mild, pruritic erythema begins over a varicosity, which becomes hyperpigmented with time as blood extravasates and hemosiderin accumulates.

Brawny edema results from chronic stasis dermatitis that has led to dermal fibrosis. Thus, brawny edema does not pit easily and may lead to ulceration.

Myxedema is the dermopathy associated with Graves' disease. It is pretibial and demarcated from normal skin by its thickened "peau d'orange" appearance, hyperpigmentation, and pruritus.

9. What conditions predispose patients to form edema from venous insufficiency?
- History of phlebitis
- Obesity
- Extensive varicosities
- Peripheral neuropathy

10. Should diuretics be used in the edematous patient?
When the primary cause cannot be reversed, diuretics may be used cautiously to help to mobilize the peripheral edema. However, because diuretics block sodium reabsorption, leading to renal compensation in the face of reduced intravascular volume, diuretics may worsen the condition.

11. When are diuretics of no use in edema?
Lymphedema and edema due to mechanical obstruction do not respond to diuretics.

12. Which processes should be considered in asymmetric unilateral edema?
Local: allergic reaction, infection, myxedema

Generalized: inguinal or retroperitoneal lymph node or other mechanical obstruction in the deep venous system or a past injury to the extremity

13. What simple advice may help patients with lower extremity edema of any cause?
1. Practice meticulous skin care: emollients, aggressive care of fungal and potential bacterial infections
2. Avoid prolonged sitting and binding garments.
3. Use mechanical methods to reduce edema: elevation, graduated compression hose.

14. What is an appropriate evaluation for a patient with suspected venous or lymphatic obstruction that results in lower extremity edema?
Abdominal and pelvic ultrasound examinations, along with computed tomography, are used to clarify the etiology of obstruction. Lymphangiography is rarely indicated.

15. Is peripheral edema an early or late finding in congestive heart failure?
Fluid retention usually occurs early, before the clinical syndrome of heart failure.

BIBLIOGRAPHY

1. Anand IS, Ferrari R, Kalra GS, et al: Edema of cardiac origin: Studies of body water and sodium, renal function, hemodynamic indexes, and plasma hormones in untreated congestive heart failure. Circulation 80:299–305, 1989.
2. Henry JA, Altmann P: Assessment of hypoproteinemic oedema: A simply physical sign. BMJ i:890–891, 1978.

3. Kelly WN (ed): Textbook of Internal Medicine, 3rd ed. Philadelphia, Lippincott-Raven, 1997.
4. Little RC, Ginsburg JM: The physiology basis for clinical edema. Arch Intern Med 144:1661–1664, 1984.
5. Loscalzo J, Craeger MA, Dzau VJ (eds): Vascular Medicine: A Textbook of Vascular Biology and Diseases. Boston, Little, Brown, 1992.
6. Milroy WF: Chronic hereditary edema: Milroy's disease. JAMA 182:14–22, 1928.
7. Powell AA, Armstrong MA: Peripheral edema. Am Fam Physician 55:1721–1726, 1997.
8. Sapira JD (ed): The Art and Science of Bedside Diagnosis. Baltimore, Williams & Wilkins, 1990.
9. Schirger A, Harrison EG Jr, Janes JM: Idiopathic lymphedema: Review of 131 cases. JAMA 182:124–132, 1962.
10. Schrier R, Gottschalk GW (eds): Diseases of the Kidney, 4th ed. Boston, Little, Brown, 1988.
11. Thorn GW: Approach to the patient with "idiopathic edema" or "periodic edema." JAMA 206:333–338, 1968.

17. AORTIC VALVE DISEASE

Valerie K. Ulstad, M.D., M.P.A., M.P.H.

1. How does aortic stenosis result in cardiac failure?

Aortic stenosis presents a fixed obstruction to the forward flow of blood. Thus, cardiac output cannot be augmented in times of need, potentially leading to inadequate blood supply to important vascular beds. The left ventricle hypertrophies to normalize the increased wall tension created by the stenosis. Left ventricular hypertrophy (LVH) results in abnormal ventricular filling, because the ventricle is less compliant. Filling pressure must then be elevated to maintain adequate ventricular filling. Finally the ventricle dilates when the muscle fails.

2. What are the common age-related etiologies of aortic stenosis?

In adults, aortic stenosis is nearly always the result of progressive leaflet calcification. When aortic stenosis becomes apparent in the 30–50 age group, an underlying congenital bicuspid or unicuspid aortic valve is usually present. After age 50, calcification is usually due to degeneration of the leaflets. The incidence of degenerative aortic stenosis increases with age. Rheumatic aortic stenosis is now relatively uncommon and is almost always accompanied by rheumatic mitral disease.

3. What is the pathophysiology of the symptoms in patients with severe aortic stenosis?

Patients with severe aortic stenosis are **SAD**. They have **s**yncope, **a**ngina, and **d**yspnea. Syncope is due to reduced cerebral perfusion during exercise. Because cardiac output across the obstruction cannot be increased, the vasodilatation of exercise results in systemic hypotension.

Angina occurs because the myocardial oxygen demand of the hypertrophied ventricle exceeds the oxygen supply available via the coronary arteries, which themselves may be compressed by the hypertrophied myocardium. The subendocardium is the major site of ischemia in patients with thick hypertrophied ventricles.

Dyspnea or other evidence of congestive heart failure may be due to diastolic or systolic ventricular dysfunction. Systolic dysfunction may develop secondary to coexisting coronary artery disease and/or subendocardial fibrosis from recurrent subendocardial ischemia of the hypertrophied ventricle. Diastolic dysfunction may result from impaired relation to the hypertrophied ventricle.

4. Does chest pain in aortic stenosis always imply associated coronary artery disease?

No. In 50% of patients with critical aortic stenosis, angina occurs in the absence of coronary artery disease. The most likely mechanism for angina pectoris in aortic stenosis is tachycardia associated with shortened diastolic perfusion time in the face of LVH, impaired ventricular relaxation, and high diastolic wall stress. The result is a delay in the rise of diastolic perfusion to the endocardium.

5. List eight classic findings in aortic stenosis.

   1. Narrow pulse pressure.

   2. Sustained apical impulse, which results from sustained outflow obstruction.

   3. Parvus et tardus pulse contour, which is small in volume and late in peaking. It results in a delayed carotid upstroke.

   4. Systolic ejection murmur, which is heard best at the right second intercostal space and often at the left sternal border, with radiation to the neck.

   5. Systolic ejection click, which may be heard at the moment of termination of the abnormal valve opening and is not heard when the aortic valve is no longer mobile.

   6. Paradoxically split S2. Because emptying of the left ventricle is delayed, the aortic component now comes at the last part of the second heart sound. In aspiration, filling of the right side of the heart is augmented so that the two heart sounds are concordant.

   7. Soft S2, which occurs when the valve moves very little.

   8. S4, which occurs with active diastolic filling into a hypertrophied ventricle.

6. Does the intensity of murmur help in assessing aortic stenosis?

One should not be fooled by the intensity of the murmur, either soft or loud. However, the duration of the murmur and a later peak of intensity suggest more severe aortic obstruction.

7. How does the physician know when aortic stenosis has become critical?

The development of symptoms in a patient with aortic stenosis portends a poor prognosis. The average survival of patients with untreated aortic stenosis is 2–3 years after the development of angina or syncope and 1.5 years after congestive heart failure ensues. The natural history of aortic stenosis is characterized by a long asymptomatic period followed by a much shorter period. Although the rate of progression of aortic stenosis is unpredictable, once the valve is calcified, progression tends to become more rapid.

8. How should the physician follow patients with aortic stenosis?

By Doppler echocardiography. Noninvasive assessment of the severity of obstruction should be carried out after a murmur radiating to the carotids is detected to establish the baseline degree of severity. Patients with mild aortic stenosis should have echo-Doppler every 2 years in anticipation of disease progression.

9. What should you tell the patient who has asymptomatic or mild aortic stenosis?

   1. Become familiar with the possible symptoms.

   2. Avoid vigorous physical activity.

   3. Schedule regular yearly follow-up with the physician, and undergo echocardiography as directed.

   4. Request subacute bacterial endocarditis prophylaxis for invasive and dental procedures.

10. What is the Gallavardin murmur?

It is a murmur of aortic stenosis heard best at the apex and left sternal border. Although it is ejection in quality, it has a high-pitched musical sound that may be confused with mitral regurgitation because of its location. It is associated with aortic stenosis in the elderly. It should not radiate to the axilla, as mitral regurgitation classically may do.

11. When is aortic valve replacement indicated in aortic stenosis?

When the patient starts to become symptomatic, aortic valve replacement is indicated. Aortic valve surgery is usually not indicated in asymptomatic patients even when the valve becomes critically stenosed, because the operative risk exceeds the nonoperative risk.

12. What are the indications for percutaneous balloon valvuloplasty of the aortic valve?

This technique is of limited value in adults. Restenosis occurs in one-half of patients within 6 months. The procedure may have a role in patients with severe aortic stenosis who are not operative candidates; in patients with cardiogenic shock due to critical aortic stenosis as a bridge to eventual surgery; for palliation of symptoms in selected nonoperable patients; or for pregnant patients with critical aortic stenosis.

13. How does chronic aortic insufficiency cause left ventricular failure?

In aortic insufficiency the entire stroke volume is ejected into a high-pressure system (the aorta). The increase in diastolic volume due to regurgitation leads to ventricular dilatation. Ventricular hypertrophy occurs to normalize wall stress. The increased stroke volume causes enlargement of the left ventricle and the aortic root. Ventricular compliance is increased so that end-diastolic pressure does not become elevated until the ventricle can no longer keep up with the extra volume. End-diastolic volume then increases without an increase in the regurgitant fraction. End-systolic volume also increases, but both ejection fraction and forward stroke volume decrease. As the compliance of the ventricle falls, diastolic pressure rises and dyspnea occurs.

14. What are the most common causes of chronic aortic insufficiency?

- **Cusp abnormality**
  Perforation from endocarditis
  Scarring from rheumatic disease
  Bicuspid aortic valve
- **Loss of valvular support**
  Aortic dissection
- **Aortic root distortion (aortitis)**
  Ankylosing spondylitis
  Syphilis
  Rheumatoid disease
- **Aortic root dilatation**
  Marfan syndrome

15. Describe the potential physical findings in chronic aortic insufficiency.

1. Hyperdynamic apical impulse displaced laterally and inferiorly
2. Signs associated with the wide pulse pressure of aortic regurgitation (diastolic runoff into the left ventricle)
   - Head bobbing—de Musset's sign
   - Vigorous collapsing pulse—Corrigan's pulse
   - Pulsations in capillary beds of nails—Quincke's pulse
   - Systolic pulsations of the uvula—Müller's sign
   - Femoral artery murmurs in systole when compressed proximally and diastolic murmur when compressed distally—Duroziez's sign
3. Murmurs
   - High-pitched, blowing, decrescendo diastolic murmur immediately after S2 heard best at the second right intercostal space, on expiration with the patient leaning forward
   - Systolic ejection murmur due to increased flow across the aortic valve
   - Mid-diastolic rumble—the Austin Flint murmur, due to vibration of the anterior leaflet of the mitral valve in the regurgitant jet, may be heard at the apex

16. Once the diagnosis of aortic insufficiency is confirmed, what are the appropriate advice and follow-up?

Aortic insufficiency can be well tolerated for many years. Asymptomatic patients with severe aortic insufficiency and normal left ventricular function have been shown to remain symptom-free for long periods. In addition to subacute bacterial endocarditis prophylaxis, patients required serial clinical exams, periodic echocardiographic exams to detect early heart failure or deterioration in left ventricular function, and periodic exercise tests to confirm their asymptomatic status.

17. When should you consider referral for aortic valve replacement in aortic insufficiency?

Asymptomatic patients with depressed left ventricular (LV) function need to be watched closely. If progressive deterioration in LV function is seen, aortic valve replacement should be considered. If LV dysfunction is truly present, most patients have symptoms. Exercise testing may be useful to unmask the presence of symptoms in a sedentary individual.

Symptomatic patients should undergo valve replacement to improve ventricular function and survival. Patients with severe LV dysfunction are very high-risk surgical candidates, but the prognosis is dismal with medical therapy. It is impossible to predict which patients will have persistent LV dysfunction after surgery.

18. Can the rate of hemodynamic progression of aortic stenosis be predicted in asymptomatic patients?

Yes. Progression of clinical disease may be predicted by the aortic jet velocity, as assessed by Doppler echocardiography. Patients with an aortic jet velocity > 4.0 m/s have a > 50% likelihood of death or onset of symptoms in the next 5 years compared with patients with a jet velocity < 3.0 m/s, who are unlikely to develop symptoms due to aortic stenosis within the next 5 years. Patients with a jet velocity of 3–4 m/s have an intermediate time to onset of symptoms.

BIBLIOGRAPHY

1. Bonow RO, Lakatos E, Maron BJ, Epstein SE: Serial long-term assessment of the natural history of asymptomatic patients with chronic aortic regurgitation and normal left ventricular systolic function. Circulation 84:1625–1635, 1991.
2. Braunwald E (ed): Heart Disease: A Textbook of Cardiovascular Medicine, 4th ed. Philadelphia, W.B. Saunders, 1992.
3. Elayda MA, Hall RJ, Reul RM, et al: Aortic valve replacement in patients 80 years and older: Operative risks and long-term results. Circulation 88(Pt 2):11–16, 1993.
4. Faggiano P, Aurigemma GP, Rusconi C, Gaasch WH: Progression of valvular aortic stenosis in adults: Literature review and clinical implications. Am Heart J 132(Pt 1):408–417, 1996.
5. Gould KL: Why angina pectoris in aortic stenosis? Circulation 95:790–792, 1997.
6. Greenberg B, Massie B, Bristow JD, et al: Long term vasodilator therapy of chronic aortic insufficiency: A randomized double-blinded controlled trial. Circulation 78:92–103, 1988.
7. Kennedy KD, Nishimura RA, Holmes DR Jr, Bailey KR: Natural history of moderate aortic stenosis. J Am Coll Cardiol 17:313–319, 1991.
8. Lombard JT, Selzer A: Valvular aortic stenosis: A clinical and hemodynamic profile of patients. Ann Intern Med 106:292–298, 1987.
9. Oakley CM: Management of valvular stenosis. Curr Opin Cardiol 10:117–123, 1995.
10. Otto CM, Burwash IG, Leggett ME, et al: Prospective study of asymptomatic valvular aortic stenosis: Clinical, echocardiographic, and exercise predictors of outcome. Circulation 95:2262–2270, 1997.
11. Rahimtoola SH: Perspective on valvular heart disease: An update. J Am Coll Cardiol 14:1–23, 1989.
12. Ross J: Afterload mismatch in aortic and mitral valve disease: Implications for surgical therapy. J Am Coll Cardiol 5:811–826, 1985.
13. Selzer A: Changing aspects of the natural history of valvular aortic stenosis. N Engl J Med 317:91–98, 1987.
14. Siemienczuk D, Greenberg B, Morris C, et al: Chronic aortic insufficiency: Factors associated with progression to aortic valve replacement. Ann Intern Med 110:587–592, 1989.
15. Sprigings DC, Forfar JC: How should we manage symptomatic aortic stenosis in the patient who is 80 or older? Br Heart J 74:481–484, 1995.
16. Stone PH: Management of the patient with asymptomatic aortic stenosis. J Card Surg 9(2 Suppl): 139–144, 1994.

18. MITRAL VALVE DISEASE

Valerie K. Ulstad, M.D., M.P.A., M.P.H.

1. What causes mitral valve prolapse (MVP)?

MVP occurs when part of a leaflet or both leaflets of the mitral valve extend above the plane of the atrioventricular junction during ventricular systole. The usual cause is an inherent abnormality of the leaflets and supporting chordae. Normal valves may demonstrate prolapse during conditions that make the left ventricle small, such as the Valsalva maneuver, dehydration, atrial septal defect (blood shunted to the right atrium away from the left atrium leads to underfilling of the left ventricle), and hypertrophic cardiomyopathy. Conditions in which the mitral valve is intrinsically abnormal are most likely to produce significant adverse consequences.

2. How common is mitral valve prolapse?

By strict echocardiographic criteria, approximately 2–5% of the population of the United States has MVP. Myxomatous degeneration of the mitral valve is hereditary as an autosomal dominant trait. Gene penetrance is stronger in women than in men, leading to the predominance of MVP in women.

3. What is MVP syndrome?

Most patients with MVP are asymptomatic. However, the MVP syndrome applies to patients with low body weight, low blood pressure, minor skeletal abnormalities (pectus excavatum, scoliosis, joint laxity), orthostatic hypotension, palpitations, and mild mitral regurgitation.

The pathogenesis of the symptoms is poorly understood but probably is related to autonomic dysfunction. Papillary muscle tension from billowing redundant leaflets may play a role in chest discomfort and development of certain arrhythmias. Patients tend to develop MVP syndrome in the second or third decade of life. Anxiety and panic attacks are no more common in patients with MVP than in the general population. Other names for MVP syndrome include Da Costa's syndrome, soldier's heart, effort syndrome, and neurocirculatory asthenia.

4. Does therapy always help patients with MVP syndrome?

Beta blockers slow the heart rate and increase diastolic filling, thereby increasing left ventricular size and reducing the degree of prolapse. The relief of symptoms with beta blockers is variable. Aerobic exercise has been shown to provide symptomatic improvement for some patients.

5. How is the diagnosis of MVP made?

The diagnosis is largely clinical; the hallmark is a midsystolic click with or without a late systolic murmur. The click occurs when the elongated chordae are snapped tight at the maximal excursion of the valve during closure in early systole. The regurgitant murmur most commonly is produced by abnormal coaptation of the leaflet edges. The Valsalva maneuver and the upright standing position make the ventricle smaller and thus may lead to a louder click earlier in systole and a longer, louder murmur. The auscultatory features may vary from day to day, according to changes in ventricular size.

Once the clinical diagnosis is made, an echocardiogram establishes baseline values and assesses the degree of prolapse, extent of leaflet thickening, and degree of mitral regurgitation. The echocardiographic diagnosis of MVP depends on the criteria used by the echocardiographer. Because the mitral anulus is shaped like a saddle, only in certain echocardiographic views can the prolapse be interpreted as genuine.

6. What risks are associated with MVP?

The major potential complications of MVP are (1) endocarditis, (2) development of severe mitral regurgitation, (3) significant arrhythmias, (4) stroke due to thromboemboli, and (5) orthostatic syncope.

Endocarditis is more likely to occur in patients with thickened, deformed valves. The incidence of endocarditis in this subset of patients is 3.5–6%. Antibiotic prophylaxis for subacute bacterial endocarditis is recommended, especially if thick mitral leaflets and mitral regurgitation murmur are present on physical examination or echocardiogram.

Significant mitral regurgitation (MR) develops in 9–12% of patients with severely deformed valves. Progressive MR is related to various combinations of mitral anulus dilatation, chordal elongation, or chordal rupture. The risk of developing severe MR increases with age in men more than in women. Patients who develop significant MR should be followed echocardiographically. Once symptoms develop and the ventricular end-systolic dimension increases, surgery for mitral valve repair or replacement should be considered.

The incidence of **serious arrhythmia** is low enough that screening for arrhythmias is not indicated.

The abnormal surface of the myxomatous valve potentially predisposes to the development of **thromboemboli.** The presence of MVP increases the risk of stroke and transient ischemic attacks in patients under 45 years of age. Aspirin therapy is rational but unproved.

The risk of **sudden death** is slightly higher in patients with MVP than in the normal population. Ventricular fibrillation appears to be the mechanism of death.

The cumulative risk of all complications of MVP is 5–10% by age 75 in affected men and 2–5% by age 75 in affected women. Patients with MVP who have no auscultatory or Doppler evidence of MR should be reassured that their condition is benign.

7. **List the causes of mitral regurgitation.**
   Primary mechanisms
   Abnormalities of the leaflets
      Rheumatic valvulitis
      Endocarditis
      Myxomatous degeneration
   Abnormalities of the chordae tendinae
      Spontaneous rupture from myxomatous degeneration
      Elongation from myxomatous degeneration
      Scarring and fusion from rheumatic inflammation
   Abnormalities of the papillary muscles
      Ischemic dysfunction—disruption secondary to infarction
   Secondary mechanisms
   Left ventricular dysfunction and dilatation leading to malalignment of the mitral apparatus

8. **Which cause of chronic MR most commonly requires surgery?**
   Myxomatous degeneration of the mitral valve.

9. **What is the pathophysiology of chronic MR?**
   In MR a portion of the left ventricular stroke volume is ejected backward into the relatively low-pressure left atrium. This part of the stroke volume is ineffective because it does not perfuse the body and deleterious because it adds works for the left ventricle. Increased diastolic stress produced by volume overload triggers myocyte hypertrophy and thus increases end-diastolic volume. Increased diastolic volume leads to an augmentation of stroke volume with a preservation of net forward flow. Eventually constant severe volume overload leads to left ventricular systolic dysfunction. Reduced emptying of the ventricle leads to pulmonary congestion and symptoms of dyspnea.

10. **How does MR manifest itself?**
    MR presents with symptoms of left-sided heart failure, including dyspnea, orthopnea, and paroxysmal nocturnal dyspnea. In advanced disease right heart failure also may be present.

11. **What are the classic physical findings of chronic MR?**
    1. The apical impulse is diffuse and laterally displaced.
    2. The intensity of the first heart sound is reduced, because the leaflets float relatively near the atrioventricular ring just before the onset of isovolumic contraction as a result of the large volume of blood entering the ventricle.
    3. The second heart sound may be widely split, because the aortic valve closes early as a result of reduced stroke volume.
    4. A holosystolic murmur, heard best over the apex, radiates to the axilla. A click and a late systolic murmur may be present with MVP. Loudness does not correlate with severity.
    5. A third heart sound indicates a large left ventricular filling volume propelled into the left ventricle under higher than normal left atrial pressure. The absence of an S3 suggests that the MR is not severe.

12. When is the optimal time for consideration of surgical intervention in patients with MR?
The correct timing for mitral valve surgery is immediately before the ejection fraction begins to fall, which is usually before the patient develops symptoms. It is hard for the clinician to anticipate the exact time. Close follow-up of patients with significant MR is important, because it is easy to wait too long, leaving the patient with heart failure even after surgery. The normal ejection fraction in MR is > 65%, with a hyperdynamic left ventricle emptying into the low-pressure left atrium. A "normal" ejection fraction in such patients is not normal. Regular echocardiographic evaluations are a reasonable way to follow ventricular function.

Regular exercise testing also may be indicated to uncover early symptoms of exercise intolerance. The mildest symptoms of dyspnea on exertion are an indication to consider surgery. It is currently unclear whether vasodilators retard the progression of MR.

13. Why is mitral valve repair preferable to replacement?
- Better durability
- Lower risk of endocarditis
- Lower incidence of postoperative thromboembolism
- Better postoperative ventricular function
- Anticoagulation may be avoided
- Better operative and long-term survival

14. What is the most common cause of mitral stenosis?
Rheumatic heart disease is the cause of nearly all cases of mitral stenosis in the United States. In patients without a history of rheumatic fever, it is assumed that the acute episode was mild or misdiagnosed. The valvular stenosis results from the initial inflammation of the heart. Thickening of the leaflets and fusion and shortening of the chordae produce the stenosis several decades after the initial insult. The greater the original inflammation of the heart, the more likely the person is to develop significant valvular sequelae.

15. What is the pathophysiology of mitral stenosis?
The narrowed mitral orifice limits inflow into the left ventricle. The resulting elevation of left atrial pressure leads to pulmonary venous congestion and reactive pulmonary hypertension, which in turn may lead to right ventricular pressure overload and clinical right-heart failure.

16. What are the symptoms of mitral stenosis?
- Dyspnea
- Orthopnea
- Paroxysmal nocturnal dyspnea
- Hemoptysis, when high left atrial pressure causes rupture of the small bronchial veins
- Systemic embolism in patients with atrial fibrillation secondary to atrial dilation
- Hoarseness, when the enlarged left atrium impinges on the left recurrent laryngeal nerve

17. Describe the physical examination in patients with mitral stenosis.
- Normal left ventricular apical impulse
- Possible atrial fibrillation
- Loud first heart sound (S1). The pressure gradient across the mitral valve holds the leaflets in a position deep into the ventricle throughout diastole. The leaflets close through a relatively wide excursion, with onset of isovolumic contraction giving a loud S1. S1 may become soft or absent when the valve becomes so diseased that it does not move at all in systole or diastole.
- Opening snap in diastole. The diseased valve reaches its maximal excursion in diastole and is stopped short by the valvular thickening.
- Diastolic rumbling murmur immediately after the opening snap. The murmur may become louder at the end of diastole in the patient still in sinus rhythm. The accentuation of the murmur is due to increased flow secondary to atrial coarctation. Such an increase in intensity is not heard in patients with atrial fibrillation.

18. What are the two common complications of mitral stenosis?

1. **Atrial fibrillation.** With an associated rapid ventricular response, atrial fibrillation is poorly tolerated, because shortened diastole limits the time for blood to cross the stenotic valve. Such patients may experience sudden onset of pulmonary edema, requiring prompt cardioversion. Medical therapy to achieve rate control is needed if the atrial fibrillation becomes chronic.

2. **Systemic embolization.** Chronic anticoagulation of patients with atrial fibrillation and mitral stenosis is clearly indicated to prevent systemic embolization of atrial mural thrombi. Many experts advocate anticoagulation for all patients with mitral stenosis, regardless of the rhythm, because 25% of nonanticoagulated patients with mitral stenosis suffer a systemic embolus.

19. What interventions are available for the patient with disabling symptoms due to mitral stenosis?

Patients who are asymptomatic can be managed medically with careful use of diuretics and control of heart rate. Once mild-to-moderate symptoms occur, three options are available:

1. **Percutaneous balloon valvuloplasty** is limited to patients with commissural fusion and noncalcified, pliable leaflets without evidence of left atrial thrombi (which may be dislodged during the procedure) or significant MR. Procedural morbidity is < 1%. This is a good option in pregnant women.

2. **Surgical commissurotomy** has the same indications as balloon valvuloplasty. Procedural mortality is < 1%. This option offers the opportunity for valve reconstruction.

3. **Mitral valve replacement** results in excellent long-term survival rates.

20. What preoperative clinical factors are associated with suboptimal outcomes (death, CHF) after mitral valve surgery?

• Advanced age
• Poor functional class
• Coronary artery disease
• Abnormal renal function
• Atrial fibrillation

21. Do marked pulmonary hypertension and right ventricular dysfunction preclude repair of the stenotic mitral valve?

No. Patients are at increased risk, but advances in perioperative management with the use of selective pulmonary vasodilators to improve right ventricular function have improved outcomes.

BIBLIOGRAPHY

1. Angell WW, Oury JH, Shah P: A comparison of replacement and reconstruction in patients with mitral regurgitation. J Thorac Cardiovasc Surg 93:665–674, 1987.
2. Antunes MJ, Franco CG: Advances in surgical treatment of acquired valve disease. Curr Opin Cardiol 11:139–154, 1996.
3. Ben Farat M, Maatouk F, Betbout F, et al: Percutaneous balloon mitral valvuloplasty in eight pregnant women with severe mitral stenosis. Eur Heart J 13:1658–1664, 1992.
4. Benjamin EJ, Plehn JF, D'Agostino RB, et al: Mitral annular calcification and the risk of stroke in an elderly cohort. N Engl J Med 327:374–379, 1992.
5. Boudoulas H, Kolibash AJ, Baker P, et al: Mitral valve prolapse and the mitral valve prolapse syndrome. Am Heart J 118:796–818, 1989.
6. Carabello BA: Mitral valve disease. Curr Probl Cardiol 18:421–480, 1993.
7. Cohen DJ, Kuntz RE, Gordon SPF, et al: Predictors of long-term outcome after percutaneous balloon mitral valvuloplasty. N Engl J Med 327:1329–1335, 1992.
8. Dajani AS, Bisno AL, Chung KJ, et al: Prevention of bacterial endocarditis: Recommendations by the American Heart Association. JAMA 264:2919–2922, 1990.
9. Devereux RB: Recent developments in the diagnosis and management of mitral valve prolapse. Curr Opin Cardiol 10:107–116, 1995.
10. Devereux RB, Kramer-Fox R, Kligfield P: Mitral valve prolapse: Causes, clinical manifestations, and management. Ann Intern Med 111:305–317, 1989.
11. Duran CM, Gometza B, Saad E: Valve repair in rheumatic mitral disease: An unsolved problem. J Card Surg 9(Suppl 2):282–285, 1994.

12. Enriquez-Sarano M, Schaff HV, Orszulak TA, et al: Valve repair improves the outcome of surgery for mitral regurgitation: A mulitvariate analysis. Circulation 91:1022–1028, 1995.
13. Farb A, Tang AL, Atkinson JB, et al: Comparison of cardiac findings in patients with mitral valve prolapse who die suddenly to those who have congestive heart failure from mitral regurgitation and to those with fatal noncardiac conditions. Am J Cardiol 70:234–239, 1992.
14. Fenster MS, Feldman MD: Mitral regurgitation: An overview. Curr Probl Cardiol 20:1–280, 1995.
15. Galloway AC, Colvin SB, Bauman G, et al: Long-term results of mitral valve reconstruction with Carpentier techniques in 148 patients with mitral insufficiency. Circulation 78(Suppl I):I-97–I-105, 1991.
16. Hochreiter C, Niles N, Devereaux R, et al: Mitral regurgitation: Relationship of noninvasive descriptor of right and left ventricular performance to clincal and hemodynamic findings and to prognosis in medically and surgically treated patients. Circulation 73:900–912, 1986.
17. Horstkotte D, Niehues R, Strauer BE: Pathomorphological aspects, aetiology and natural history of acquired mitral valve stenosis. Eur Heart J 12:55–60, 1991.
18. Jung B, Cormick B, Ducimetiere P, et al: Functional results 5 years after successful percutaneous mitral commissurotomy in a series of 528 patients and analysis of predictive factors. J Am Coll Cardiol 27:407–414, 1996.
19. Lehman KG, Francis CK, Dodge HT: Mitral regurgitation in early myocardial infarction: Incidence, clinical detection, and prognostic implications. TIMI Study Group. Ann Intern Med 117:10–17, 1992.
20. Llaneras MR, Nance ML, Streicher JT, et al: Pathogenesis of ischemic mitral regurgitation. J Thorac Cardiovasc Surg 105:439–442, 1993.
21. Reyes VP, Raju BS, Wynne J, et al: Percutaneous balloon valvuloplasty compared with open surgical commissurotomy for mitral stenosis. N Engl J Med 331:961–967, 1994.
22. Turu ZG, Reyes VP, Raju S, et al: Percutaneous balloon versus surgical closed commissurotomy for mitral stenosis: A prospective randomized trial. Circulation 83:1179–1185, 1991.
23. Wooley CF, Baker PB, Kolibash A, et al: The floppy myxomatous mitral valve, mitral valve prolapse, and mitral regurgitation. Prog Cardiovasc Dis 33:397–433, 1991.

19. SUPRAVENTRICULAR ARRHYTHMIAS

Valerie K. Ulstad, M.D., M.P.A., M.P.H.

1. When does a rhythm fall into the category of a supraventricular tachycardia (SVT)?
When the heart rate is greater than 100 and there is a narrow QRS complex.

2. What are the two most common mechanisms of SVTs?
Abnormal automaticity and reentry.

3. Explain abnormal automaticity.
The sinoatrial (SA) node, elements of the atrioventricular (AV) node, and the His-Purkinje system spontaneously depolarize and thereby are said to demonstrate automaticity. These cells initiate the normal cardiac impulse and provide a hierarchy of subsidiary pacemakers ready to take over if the SA node fails. The SA node fires at the fastest rate and keeps the lower pacemakers suppressed. In certain pathologic situations, such as metabolic disturbances or certain drug toxicities, cells that do not usually exhibit spontaneous depolarization may become automatic and generate impulses that propagate through the heart.

4. What are the prerequisites for a reentry tachycardia?
Reentry is the most common mechanism producing SVTs. A reentrant rhythm develops when a region of the myocardium is reexcited by one electrical impulse that returns to a given area by a circuitous route. There are three requirements for reentry to take place:

1. Two distinct parts of the heart must have different conduction velocities: two areas within the AV node; the conduction system and an accessory pathway; or two areas of the ventricular myocardium.

2. The two parts or paths for propagation of an electrical impulse must have the potential to form a circuit. Because they are different, one must conduct more slowly than the other; the path that conducts more rapidly takes longer to recover.

3. A premature beat enters the potential circuit and finds one path ready to conduct, but the other blocked because it has not yet recovered. The impulse proceeds down one path and propagates through the tissue. At that point the second path may have recovered and is ready to conduct the propagated impulse. Thus the premature beat is the trigger. Under normal circumstances both pathways would have been ready to conduct the impulse. However, the premature beat exaggerated the difference between the two paths, finding one ready to conduct, the other still refractory. When the impulse comes around to the pathway that was initially refractory and finds it now ready to conduct, the reentrant circuit begins.

5. What are the five most common SVTs?
1. Atrial fibrillation
2. Atrial flutter
3. Multifocal atrial tachycardia (MAT)
4. Paroxysmal SVT
5. Sinus tachycardia

6. Which of the two major mechanisms accounts for each of the common SVTs?
1. **Reentry**
   Atrial fibrillation—multiple reentry circuits in the atrium
   Atrial flutter—reentry circuit within the atrium
   Paroxysmal SVT—reentry circuits within the AV node (AV node reentry) or via an accessory pathway (AV reentry as in Wolff-Parkinson-White syndrome [WPW])
2. **Accelerated automaticity**
   Sinus tachycardia
   MAT

7. What is paroxysmal SVT?
Paroxysmal SVT is a supraventricular rhythm that is regular at 120–130 beats/minute and has sudden onset and termination. The term is confusing, because it does not describe a specific arrhythmia mechanism but rather the clinical characteristics of the tachycardia. Paroxysmal SVT accounts for one-half of all patients with SVT. In the majority of patients, AV nodal reentry is the mechanism of the paroxysmal tachycardia. The second most common mechanism is AV reciprocating tachycardia via an extranodal bypass tract.

8. How may the P wave be helpful in diagnosing the type of SVT?
P-wave morphology is especially helpful in identifying the following SVTs:

No discreet P wave	Atrial fibrillation
Distinct sawtooth waves at 250-340 bpm (seen best in inferior leads)	Atrial flutter
P waves negative in inferior leads or buried within QRS	AV nodal reentry
Short PR and delta wave in sinus rhythm	WPW (potential for AV reentry)
Three different P-wave morphologies	MAT

9. Which rhythms usually have an irregular rate?
• Atrial fibrillation, even at a rapid rate
• Atrial flutter (which may be regular)
• MAT

10. The QRS is usually narrow in SVTs. When may the QRS be wide?
1. Aberrant conduction, such as preexisting right or left bundle-branch block.
2. When an accessory connection (as in WPW) conducts antegrade, the AV node conducts retrograde, and the ventricular myocardium is depolarized cell to cell rather than along the conduction system.

11. In evaluating a patient with SVT, what historical and other medical information should be sought?

- History of palpitations or syncope
- Symptoms of possible hyperthyroidism or pheochromocytoma
- Habits and drug use: alcohol, caffeine, inhaled or oral beta agonists, over-the-counter cold medicines, illicit drugs
- Effect of a possible SVT on the patient's lifestyle (e.g., airplane pilot)

12. What are palpitations? To what are they due?

Palpitations represent the patient's awareness of his or her own heart beat. The etiology of palpitations can be determined in a majority of patients. One-half of cases are due to cardiac disease, whereas one-third are due to psychiatric causes and a smaller number to other causes (habits, medicines, metabolic causes). Paroxysms of prolonged palpitations suggest a cardiac arrhythmia, either supraventricular or ventricular in origin.

13. How should patients with SVT be evaluated?

After a complete history and physical examination, the patient should have a chest radiograph and electrocardiogram (EKG); thyroid function tests, hematocrit, and echocardiography to look for mitral valve prolapse or other evidence of valvular disease should be considered.

14. How may carotid sinus massage or Valsalva maneuvers aid in the diagnosis and treatment of arrhythmias?

Carotid sinus massage and Valsalva maneuvers may have three major outcomes: abrupt cessation of the arrhythmia, slowing of heart rate during the maneuver, or no effect. Abrupt cessation of the arrhythmia with conversion to sinus rhythms is the most useful outcome. It may be seen when the arrhythmia is supraventricular and originates from an AV nodal reentrant or aberrant pathway mechanism. Sinus tachycardia slows during massage and subsequently regains speed. Other possible outcomes include accentuation of AV block or dissociation, atrial fibrillation in atrial flutter, and transient slowing of the ventricular rate.

15. When is carotid massage contraindicated?

In patients with possible digoxin toxicity, carotid massage may lead to fatal arrhythmias. Additional risks of carotid massage include stroke, syncope, seizures, asystole, or ventricular arrhythmias. Thus carotid massage should be avoided in elderly patients.

16. When should a patient with supraventricular arrhythmias be hospitalized?

Patients who present with hypotension, chest pain, congestive heart failure, or sustained tachycardia should be hospitalized.

17. When should strategies to provide chronic prophylaxis against paroxysmal SVT be considered?

If the episodes are relatively slow, infrequent, and well tolerated, no therapy may be necessary. Patients should be counseled to limit use of caffeine, alcohol, and other drugs. When symptoms are frequent and bothersome, drug therapy and radiofrequency ablation of the arrhythmogenic focus are options. Drugs should slow AV node conduction; the most common are beta blockers and calcium channel blockers.

18. When should drugs that block the AV node be avoided?

Beta blockers, calcium channel blockers, and digoxin are contraindicated in patients who may have tachycardias due to accessory pathways. In patients with MAT, digoxin may prove harmful.

19. When and why is it important to recognize WPW syndrome or accessory pathway arrhythmias?

WPW syndrome should be suspected in the presence of a delta wave on routine EKG or, more importantly, when the patient has atrial fibrillation that is conducted at a rapid rate (faster than the capability of the AV node), resulting in a rapid ventricular response > 280. Of patients with WPW syndrome, 50% experience atrial fibrillation, which may deteriorate to ventricular fibrillation or present as sudden death. Thus, recognition of this rare entity is life-saving and requires referral to a cardiologist for appropriate management.

20. Which patients should be referred to a cardiologist for possible electrophysiologic testing?

1. Patients with uncontrolled symptomatic tachycardias of unknown diagnosis after preliminary work-up.

2. Patients with symptomatic tachycardias with delta wave or other suspicion of aberrant conduction. The sole finding of delta waves is controversial.

3. Patients who respond poorly to initial medical management.

21. What features in WPW suggest a low risk of rapid ventricular conduction, if atrial fibrillation should occur?

Two EKG features in WPW suggest that the accessory pathway conducts relatively slowly:

1. Intermittent preexcitation on the resting EKG (delta wave comes and goes)

2. Disappearance of delta wave with exercise

22. Is radiofrequency ablation (RFA) standard therapy for any SVTs?

Yes. RFA is more cost-effective than life-long drug therapy for some SVTs and can be performed safely with little discomfort to the patient. The most common applications are in patients with AV node reentry or WPW.

23. Is there an advantage to using an event recorder instead of a 48-hour Holter monitor to assess the patient with palpitations?

Yes. Event recorders are more cost-effective and provide better data. Holter monitoring is a poor diagnostic test for the evaluation of intermittent palpitations.

BIBLIOGRAPHY

1. Benditt DG, Goldstein M, Reyes MJ, Milstein S: Supraventricular tachycardias: Mechanisms and therapies. Hosp Pract Aug:103–127, 1988.
2. Blackshear JL, Kopecky SL, Litin SC, et al: Management of atrial fibrillation in adults: Prevention of thromboembolism and symptomatic treatment. Mayo Clin Proc 71:150–160, 1996.
3. Camm AJ, Garratt CJ: Adenosine and supraventricular tachycardia. N Engl J Med 375:1621–1629, 1991.
4. Dreifus LS, Hessen S, Samuels F: Recognition and management of supraventricular tachycardias. Heart Dis Stroke 2:223–230, 1993.
5. Futterman LG, Lemberg L: Atrial fibrillation: An increasingly common and provocative arrhythmia. Am J Crit Care 5:379–387, 1996.
6. Ganz LI, Friedman PL: Supraventricular tachycardia. N Engl J Med 332:162–173, 1995.
7. Kalbfleisch SJ, El-Atassi R, Calkins H, et al: Differentiation of paroxysmal narrow QRS complex tachycardias using the 12-lead electrocardiogram. J Am Coll Cardiol 21:85–89, 1993.
8. Kinlay S, Leitch JW, Neil A, et al: Cardiac event recorders yield more diagnoses and are more cost effective than 48 hour Holter monitoring in patients with palpitations. A controlled clinical trial. Ann Intern Med 124(1 Pt 1):16–20, 1996.
9. Manolis AS, Wang PJ, Estes NA III: Radiofrequency catheter ablation for cardiac tachyarrhythmias. Ann Intern Med 121:452–461, 1994.
10. Reiffel JA, Estes NA III, Waldo AL, et al: A consensus report on antiarrhythmic drugs. Clin Cardiol 17: 103–116, 1994.
11. Waldo AL: An approach to therapy of supraventricular tachyarrhythmias: An algorithm versus individualized therapy. Clin Cardiol 17(9 Suppl 2):II-21–II-26, 1994.
12. Zimetbaum P, Josephson ME: Evaluation of patients with palpitations. N Engl J Med 338:1369–1373, 1998.

20. ATRIAL FIBRILLATION

Valerie K. Ulstad, M.D., M.P.A., M.P.H.

1. What are the common causes of chronic atrial fibrillation?
- Congestive heart failure
- Mitral stenosis
- Ischemic heart disease
- Hypertension
- Constrictive pericarditis

2. What evaluation should be performed in the patient with new-onset atrial fibrillation?
After a thorough physical examination most patients should have the following tests:
- Assessment of electrolytes
- Assessment of thyroid-stimulating hormone (TSH)
- 12-lead electrocardiogram (EKG)
- Chest radiograph
- Echocardiogram

3. What are the clinical consequences of chronic atrial fibrillation?
- Increased risk of embolic stroke
- Increased mortality
- Bothersome symptoms
- Progressive impairment of ventricular function
- Progressive atrial myopathy

4. What three therapeutic goals should be considered in patients with atrial fibrillation?
1. Rate control
2. Maintenance of sinus rhythm
3. Prevention of thromboembolism

5. What does rate control mean?
Cardiac output increases in most patients with atrial fibrillation to a mean rate of about 140 beats/min. At faster rates, cardiac output begins to fall. A resting rate of 90 beats/min is probably ideal, provided that it can be increased during exercise.

6. Which agents are available to control the rate in atrial fibrillation?
Rate control can be achieved with drugs that slow atrioventricular (AV) node conduction, such as beta blockers, calcium channel blockers, or digoxin. Sometimes combinations are necessary. These drugs rarely terminate atrial fibrillation. Digoxin provides good rate control at rest but poor rate control with exercise.

7. Which drugs are useful in pharmacologic cardioversion?
Procainamide has been the most frequently studied drug for cardioversion. Quinidine is also commonly used. Patients with recent-onset atrial fibrillation are more likely to be chemically converted. Digoxin does not influence conversion to sinus rhythm. Ibutilide (IV) has recently been released for the conversion of atrial flutter or atrial fibrillation to normal sinus rhythm.

8. Describe the practical guidelines for pharmacologic treatment of patients with atrial fibrillation.
1. Treat the symptomatic patient.
2. Treat underlying heart failure.
3. Correct metabolic disturbances.
4. The longer the patient has been in atrial fibrillation, the less likely a response to therapy will be seen.
5. The occurrence of proarrhythmia during therapy is impossible to predict.
6. Consider hospitalizing and monitoring the patient when therapy is started, particularly if the patient has underlying structural heart disease (including left ventricular hypertrophy [LVH]) or a prolonged QT interval.

9. Which drugs are available for maintenance of normal sinus rhythm after conversion of atrial fibrillation?

Pharmacologic options include class IA antiarrhythmics, such as quinidine or procainamide; class IC agents, such as flecainide and propafenone; and two class III drugs, sotalol and amiodarone. LVH or other structural heart disease increases the susceptibility to proarrhythmia from class I drugs. For example, in the CAST study, class IC drugs were associated with increased mortality in patients with previous myocardial infarction (MI). In patients with LVH, previous MI, or LV dysfunction, class III agents (sotalol or amiodarone) should be considered.

10. Will the patient maintained on quinidine after cardioversion stay in normal sinus rhythm?

A meta-analysis of the randomized control trials investigating the role of quinidine in the therapy of chronic atrial fibrillation demonstrated that quinidine was more effective than no treatment in maintaining normal sinus rhythm at 3, 6, and 12 months after cardioversion. About 50% of quinidine-treated patients were in sinus rhythm at 12 months after cardioversion compared with 25% of controls. Few data are available for procainamide and disopyramide.

At 1 year, sinus rhythm is maintained in more than of 50% of patients treated with flecainide, propafenone, or sotalol with fewer side effects than quinidine. Two-thirds of patients remain in sinus rhythm after 1 year on amiodarone, making it the most effective therapy for recurrent atrial fibrillation. Use of amiodarone is limited by its side-effect profile.

11. What is the rate of ischemic stroke in elderly patients with atrial fibrillation compared with elderly patients without atrial fibrillation?

The stroke rate is 6 times higher.

12. List 10 factors that increase the risk of stroke in patients with atrial fibrillation.

1. Mitral stenosis
2. Cardiomyopathy
3. Congestive heart failure
4. History of systemic emboli
5. Hypertension, including LVH
6. Mitral anular calcification
7. Left atrial size > 52 mm
8. Age > 60 yr
9. Hyperthyroidism
10. Cardioversion and postcardioversion

13. List five independent predictors of embolic risk in patients with atrial fibrillation.

1. History of hypertension
2. Prior stroke or transient ischemic attack (TIA)
3. Diabetes
4. Age > 65 yr
5. Recent heart failure

14. Is anticoagulation with warfarin effective in preventing stroke in patients with atrial fibrillation?

Yes. Five recent randomized clinical trials showed a 70% reduction in ischemic stroke when the international normalized ratio (INR) ranged from 1.8–4.2. In general, INR from 2.0–3.0 is recommended. The elderly may be at increased risk for major bleeding. In the elderly the INR should be particularly closely monitored.

15. Which low-risk patients with atrial fibrillation may be considered for treatment with aspirin instead of warfarin?

Patients without diabetes, hypertension, heart failure, or previous stroke/TIA who are under age 65 may be given 325 mg of aspirin/day to prevent stroke. It should be noted, however, that clinical trials in low-risk patients are ongoing and that clinicians often tend to anticoagulate patients with atrial fibrillation.

16. How should anticoagulation be managed at the time of cardioversion?

Patients with atrial fibrillation of unknown duration or for more than 48 hours should be anticoagulated for 3 weeks before electrical cardioversion. Anticoagulation should be continued for at least 4 weeks after successful cardioversion to allow atrial contractile function to return to normal. Patients should then be assessed for the need for long-term anticoagulation.

17. When is it too late to consider cardioversion for atrial fibrillation?

It is probably never too late to try cardioversion. Increasing evidence indicates the progression of atrial myopathy and LV dysfunction in patients with atrial fibrillation so that restoration of sinus rhythm is advantageous. Adequate anticoagulation before cardioversion is mandatory.

BIBLIOGRAPHY

1. Alber GW: Atrial fibrillation and stroke. Arch Intern Med 154:1443–1457, 1994.
2. Blackshear JL, Kopecky SL, Litin SC, et al: Management of atrial fibrillation in adults: Prevention of thromboembolism and symptomatic treatment. Mayo Clin Proc 71:150–160, 1996.
3. Boston Area Anticoagulation Trial for Atrial Fibrillation Investigators: The effect of low-dose warfarin on the risk of stroke in patients with nonrheumatic atrial fibrillation. N Engl J Med 323:1505–1522, 1990.
4. Cairns JA, Connolly SJ: Nonrheumatic atrial fibrillation: Risk of stroke and role of antithrombotic therapy. Circulation 84:469–492, 1991.
5. Connolly SJ, Laupacis A, Gent M: Canadian Atrial Fibrillation Anticoagulation (CAFA) study. J Am Coll Cardiol 18:349–355, 1991.
6. Coplen SE, Antman EM, Berlin JA, et al: Efficacy and safety of quinidine therapy for maintenance of sinus rhythm after cardioversion. A meta-analysis of randomized control trials. Circulation 82:1106–1116, 1990.
7. Ezekowitz MD, Bridgers SL, James KE, et al: Warfarin in the prevention of stroke associated with non-rheumatic atrial fibrillation. Veterans Affairs Stroke Prevention in Nonrheumatic Atrial Fibrillation Investigators. N Engl J Med 327:1406–1412, 1992.
8. Fiore LD: Anticoagulation: Risks and benefits in atrial fibrillation. Geriatrics 51:22–24, 27–28, 31, 1996.
9. Futterman LG, Lemberg L: Atrial fibrillation: An increasingly common and provocative arrhythmia. Am J Crit Care 5:379–387, 1996.
10. Juul-Moller S, Edvardsson N, Rehnquist-Ahlberg N: Sotalol versus quinidine for the maintenance of sinus rhythm after cardioversion of atrial fibrillation. Circulation 82:1932–1939, 1990.
11. Kahn ZU, Adolph RJ, Engel PJ: Persistent atrial mechanical dysfunction after spontaneous conversion of chronic atrial fibrillation to sinus rhythm. Am Heart J 131:606–608, 1996.
12. Klein AL, Grimm RA, Black IW, et al: Cardioversion guided by transesophageal echocardiography. The ACUTE Pilot Study. A randomized, controlled trial. Assessment of Cardioversion Using Transesophageal Echocardiography. Ann Intern Med 126:200–209, 1997.
13. Mackstaller LL, Alpert JS: Atrial fibrillation: A review of mechanism, etiology and therapy. Clin Cardiol 20:640–650, 1997.
14. Manning WJ, Silverman DI, Gordon SPF, et al: Cardioversion from atrial fibrillation without prolonged anticoagulation with use of transesophageal echocardiography to exclude the presence of atrial thrombi. N Engl J Med 328:750–755, 1993.
15. Man-Song-Hing M, Laupacis A, O'Connor A, et al: Warfarin for atrial fibrillation. The patient's perspective. Arch Intern Med 156:1841–1848, 1996.
16. Morley J, Marinchak R, Rials SJ, Kowey P: Atrial fibrillation, anticoagulation, and stroke. Am J Cardiol 77:38A–44A, 1996.
17. Pai SM, Torres V: Atrial fibrillation: New management strategies. Curr Probl Cardiol 18:233–300, 1993.
18. Petersen B, Boysen G, Godtfredsen J, et al: Placebo-controlled trial of warfarin and aspirin for the prevention of thromboembolic complications in chronic atrial fibrillation: The Copenhagen AFASAK Study. Lancet 1:175–179, 1989.
19. Prystowsky BN, Benson W, Fuster V, et al: Management of patients with atrial fibrillation: A statement for healthcare professionals from the Subcommittee on Electrocardiography and Electrophysiology, American Heart Association. Circulation 93:1261–1277, 1996.
20. Reardon M, Camm AJ: Atrial fibrillation in the elderly. Clin Cardiol 19:765–775, 1996.
21. Stein B, Halperin JL, Fuster V: Should patients with atrial fibrillation be anticoagulated prior to and chronically following cardioversion? Cardiovasc Clin 21:231–249, 1990.
22. Stroke Prevention in Atrial Fibrillation Investigators: Stroke Prevention in Atrial Fibrillation study: Final results: Circulation 84:527–539, 1991.

21. VENTRICULAR ARRHYTHMIAS

Valerie K. Ulstad, M.D., M.P.A., M.P.H.

1. Describe the electrocardiographic (EKG) characteristics of the premature ventricular contraction (PVC).

A PVC is an early (premature) QRS complex with a bizarre shape and a duration that exceeds the dominant QRS complex duration in the underlying rhythm. The T-wave deflection is large and in the opposite direction from the main QRS deflection. There is no preceding P wave.

The PVC is commonly conducted in a retrograde fashion toward the atria, but the sinoatrial (SA) node is rarely reset by the premature ventricular beat (in contrast to the premature atrial beat). A compensatory pause occurs after the premature beat until the next sinus beat arrives. The next sinus beat after the compensatory pause comes in time with the underlying sinus rhythm determined by the SA node. Another SA depolarization occurs simultaneously with the PVC, but its electrical activity is not seen on the EKG because it is hidden by the wide QRS complex.

2. How common are PVCs?

When a simple 12-lead EKG is used for screening, PVCs are documented in fewer than 1% of the population. If 24-hour Holter monitoring is used, PVCs are observed in 50–80% of normal people. The forms seen in normal people are usually single PVCs, but nonsustained ventricular tachycardia (NSVT) may be seen infrequently. The incidence of ventricular arrhythmias increases with age.

3. What is considered a normal number of PVCs?

Fewer than 100 PVCs /day or 5/hour is within normal limits for the healthy population. A higher number of PVCs or repetitive forms (NSVT) suggest electrical heart disease.

4. Which everyday substances should patients with PVCs avoid?

Caffeine, tobacco, and alcohol increase the number of PVCs.

5. What is complex ventricular ectopy?

Complex ventricular ectopy consists of more than 10–30 PVCs/hour and multiform or repetitive patterns of ventricular beats.

6. Defined NSVT.

NSVT is defined as 3 or more ventricular beats in a row at a rate of at least 100 beats/minute, lasting 15–30 seconds. Longer runs are called sustained ventricular tachycardia (VT).

7. List the three classes of ventricular arrhythmias.

1. Benign ventricular arrhythmias
2. Potentially malignant ventricular arrhythmias
3. Malignant ventricular arrhythmias

8. Why are some ventricular arrhythmias classified as benign?

Benign forms comprise one-third of all ventricular arrhythmias and are associated with a low risk of sudden cardiac death. They include PVCs of low-to-moderate frequency in persons with normal ejection fraction and no organic heart disease. Benign arrhythmias are usually asymptomatic and found on routine examination. Occasionally patients may present with mild dizziness or palpitations. The only indication for treatment is bothersome symptoms that Holter monitoring clearly demonstrates as due to arrhythmia. For bothersome benign ventricular arrhythmias, beta blockers are the drugs of choice.

9. When should potentially malignant ventricular arrhythmias be treated?

Potentially malignant forms are seen in 65% of patients with ventricular arrhythmias and are associated with a low-to-moderate risk of sudden death. They include PVCs of moderate-to-high frequency, common couplets, or NSVT in the presence of organic heart disease and moderately decreased left ventricular function. Potentially malignant arrhythmias may be symptomatic with mild hemodynamic impairment or completely asymptomatic. The only clear indication for antiarrhythmic treatment is patients with NSVT after myocardial infarction, in whom beta blockers have been shown to reduce mortality.

10. What are malignant ventricular arrhythmias?

Malignant forms are seen in 5% of patients with ventricular arrhythmias and are associated with moderate-to-high risk of sudden death. They include PVCs of moderate-to-high frequency, common couplets, NSVT, sustained uniform VT, sustained multiform VT, and ventricular fibrillation in the presence of organic heart disease and markedly reduced left ventricular ejection fraction. Patients with left ventricular ejection fraction less than 30% are at high risk for malignant arrhythmias. They often present with heart failure, myocardial ischemia, palpitations, syncope, or cardiac arrest. Therapy is indicated to control symptoms and to reduce the risk of sudden death. Patients need a thorough cardiac evaluation and careful choice and follow-up of antiarrhythmic therapy.

11. What is the prognosis for the patient with simple or complex ventricular ectopy and a structurally normal heart?

The prognosis in such patients is excellent, even with nonsustained VT. Exercise-induced ectopy is not associated with an increased risk of sudden death in the normal population. The presence of symptoms with the arrhythmia does not alter the prognosis.

12. What does the presence of a PVC on a routine EKG mean?

PVCs may be the first evidence of underlying congenital, hypertensive, ischemic, or myopathic heart disease. Observation of PVCs should prompt an evaluation for cardiac pathology. A thorough history and physical examination are the first steps. Further testing should be done only if certain aspects of the history and physical exam need clarifying.

13. How does the presence of PVCs in patients with mitral valve prolapse influence prognosis?

Such patients have more simple and complex PVCs than the general population, but the prognosis is excellent in persons with structurally normal hearts. Reassurance is the best therapy. Bothersome symptoms may be treated with beta blockers if other lifestyle modification fails. Class I agents are not advisable because of an unfavorable risk-benefit ratio.

The risk of sudden death is increased in the patient with a highly redundant mitral valve, severe mitral regurgitation, a history of syncope, a family history of sudden death, or a prolonged QT interval. In this small subgroup, runs of NSVT may be a marker of increased risk.

14. What is the risk associated with ventricular ectopy after myocardial infarction?

In the first weeks after an infarction, approximately 90% of patients have frequent PVCs. Complex forms have been documented in 20–40% during this period. Simple PVCs are not associated with an increased mortality, but complex ectopy, particularly runs of NSVT, independently increases the risk of sudden cardiac death 2- to 5-fold. Left ventricular (LV) function is another independent prognostic factor in the postinfarction patient. LV dysfunction increases the risk of sudden death by 2–3-fold. Patients with complex ventricular ectopy and LV dysfunction are at highest risk, with an incidence of sudden death in the first year after infarction as high as 35%.

15. What was the CAST study? What did it show?

The Cardiac Arrhythmia Suppression Test (CAST) was a long-term, multicenter, placebo-controlled study designed to test the hypothesis that antiarrhythmic drugs for suppression of asymptomatic or mildly symptomatic PVCs reduce the risk of sudden cardiac death in postin-farction patients. After a 10-month follow-up, excessive mortality among patients randomized to encainide and flecainide therapy led to the removal of both agents from the trial. Even though the agents were shown to suppress asymptomatic or mildly symptomatic PVCs, suppression was associated with increased mortality. The benefit of antiarrhythmic drugs other than beta blockers after myocardial infarction is unproved. Three placebo-controlled trials of amiodarone in postinfarction patients show no difference in mortality between treated patients and patients receiving placebo. Amiodarone does not increase mortality and may be advantageous in patients at high risk of sudden death. However, the routine use of amiodarone in postinfarction patients cannot be recommended.

16. Will treatment of postinfarction patients at high risk for sudden death improve survival?

No evidence suggests that suppression of arrhythmia reduces risk and improves survival. Data from the CAST trial indicate that antiarrhythmic therapy may be harmful in such patients.

17. Should patients with NSVT in the presence of dilated cardiomyopathy and congestive heart failure be treated with antiarrhythmic drugs?

We do not know. In patients with cardiomyopathy and clinical congestive heart failure, the 2-year mortality rate may be as high as 50%. Approximately 40% are sudden cardiac deaths, presumably due to a fatal arrhythmia. Ambulatory monitoring has shown that 70–95% of pa-tients have frequent PVCs and 60–80% have NSVT. This group requires further study to deter-mine whether antiarrhythmic agents offer a survival benefit. Unfortunately, no cohort of patients not receiving antiarrhythmic therapy for NSVT has been followed. The excessive mortality may be due to antiarrhythmic therapy rather than simply to the presence of the arrhythmia. Current evidence does not support the use of antiarrhythmic agents to suppress the ectopy in such patients. Angiotensin-converting enzyme inhibitors reduce mortality in patients with LV dysfunction and reduce the frequency of ventricular arrhythmias in patients with clinical heart failure. These drugs, therefore, are currently the best antiarrhythmic therapy for such high-risk patients. Amiodarone can be used to treat symptomatic arrhythmias. It does not improve sur-vival in mild CHF but may improve survival in patients with class III and IV congestive heart failure and NSVT.

18. Can antiarrhythmic therapy improve survival for patients with aborted sudden car-diac death?

Yes. In patients resuscitated from sudden cardiac death, the recurrence rate of sudden cardiac death is approximately 30% in the first year. Such patients require electrophysiologic evaluation. Several studies have shown improved survival after antiarrhythmic therapy is directed at the spontaneous arrhythmia documented with monitoring or at the induced arrhythmia in the electro-physiologic laboratory. This is the only group of patients in whom antiarrhythmic drugs have been reported to prolong life.

19. Is the implantable cardiac defibrillator (ICD) better than antiarrhythmic drugs in pa-tients with life-threatening ventricular arrhythmias?

Recently a large clinical trial (AVID) was stopped because of the significant reduction in deaths among patients whose arrhythmias were treated with a defibrillator. This was the first trial to show that ICDs improve overall survival in patients with a history of ventricular fibrillation or serious ventricular tachycardia.

20. How is the efficacy of antiarrhythmic therapy assessed?

Efficacy is assessed by clinical symptoms and objective means such as ambulatory monitor-ing. Because of the marked spontaneous variability in the frequency of ventricular arrhythmias, a 75–80% reduction in the frequency of PVC and a 90–100% reduction in the presence of NSVT is required to declare that the drug is effective in suppression of arrhythmia.

21. What is proarrhythmia?

Proarrhythmia is the appearance of a new arrhythmia or aggravation of an existing arrhythmia. In the broadest sense, the term refers to bradyarrhythmias, supraventricular tachycardias (SVTs), and VTs. Proarrhythmia is potentially seen with all antiarrhythmic agents; the incidence varies from 5–35%. The etiology is unclear, and occurrence is hard to predict. Proarrhythmia may be part of the mechanism of increased mortality in certain patients treated with antiarrhythmic drugs. The potential for proarrhythmia with antiarrhythmic agents must be considered whenever a patient is started on a new agent and each time the dose is adjusted. A fourfold increase in the number of PVCs and a 10-fold increase in repetitive forms fit the criteria for identifying proarrhythmia with ambulatory monitoring.

22. What are the major side effects of antiarrhythmic therapy?
- Noncardiac side effects specific to each agent
- Organ toxicity specific to each agent
- Proarrhythmia
- Conduction defects
- Precipitation of congestive heart failure

There are many antiarrhythmic drugs in part because they all pose potential problems. No antiarrhythmic drug is perfect. Beta blockers are probably the best. It is important to be completely familiar with the pharmacology of any prescribed antiarrhythmic drug.

23. When the physician is presented with a hemodynamically stable patient with a wide complex tachycardia, what is the likely diagnosis on the basis of statistics alone?

The differential diagnosis centers on VT or SVT conducted aberrantly through the heart. VT is more common by far and thus more likely.

24. What four clues does the electrocardiogram give to help differentiate VT from SVT with aberrancy?
1. Underlying heart disease favors VT.
2. Capture and fusion beats indicate VT.
3. AV dissociation indicates VT.
4. QRS width > 140 msec in the absence of preexisting bundle-branch block or accessory connection suggests VT.

25. What therapeutic considerations are important in patients with wide complex tachycardia?
1. Assume that the problem is VT, which is much more common.
2. Cardiovert the hemodynamically unstable patient.
3. Do not give verapamil, which may lead to profound hypotension and cardiovascular collapse in a patient with VT.
4. The drug of choice is probably procainamide, administered intravenously (loading dose followed by infusion).

BIBLIOGRAPHY

1. Braunwald E (ed): Heart Disease: A Textbook of Cardiovascular Medicine, 5th ed. Philadelphia, W.B. Saunders, 1997.
2. Brugada P, Brugada J, Mont L, et al: A new approach to the differential diagnosis of a regular tachycardia with a wide QRS complex. Circulation 83:1649–1659, 1991.
3. Chou T: Electrocardiography in Clinical Practice, 2nd ed. Philadelphia, W.B. Saunders, 1986.
4. Echt DS, Liebson PR, Mitchell LB, et al: Mortality and morbidity in patients receiving encainide, flecainide, or placebo. The Cardiac Arrhythmia Suppression Trial. N Engl J Med 324:781–788, 1991.
5. Ewy GA, Bressler R (eds): Cardiovascular Drugs and the Management of Heart Disease, 2nd ed. New York, Raven Press, 1992.
6. Horowitz LN: Current Management of Arrhythmias. Philadelphia, B.C. Decker, 1991.

7. Hsia HH, Buxton AE: Work-up and management of patients with sustained and nonsustained monomorphic ventricular tachycardia. Cardiol Clin 11:21–37, 1993.
8. Julian DG, Camm AJ, Frangin G, et al: Randomised trial of effect of amiodarone on mortality in patients with left-ventricular dysfunction after recent myocardial infarction: EMIAT. European Myocardial Infarct Amiodarone Trial Investigators. Lancet 349:667–674, 1997.
9. Moss AJ, Hall WJ, Cannom DS, et al: Improved survival with an implanted defibrillator in patients with coronary disease at high risk for ventricular arrhythmia. Multicenter Automatic Defibrillator Implantation Trial Investigators. N Engl J Med 335:1933–1940, 1996.
10. Rankin AC, Rae AP, Cobbe SM: Misuse of intravenous verapamil in patients with ventricular tachycardia. Lancet 1:472–474, 1987.
11. Richards DA, Byth K, Ross DL, Uther JB: What is the best predictor of spontaneous ventricular tachycardia and sudden death after myocardial infarction? Circulation 83:756–763, 1991.
12. Singh SN, Fletcher RD, Fisher SG, et al: Amiodarone in patients with congestive heart failure and asymptomatic ventricular arrhythmia. Survival Trial of Antiarrhythmic Therapy in Congestive Heart Failure. N Engl J Med 333:77–82, 1995.
13. Steinbeck G, Greene HL: Management of patients with life-threatening sustained ventricular tachyarrhythmias—the role of guided antiarrhythmic drug therapy. Prog Cardiovasc Dis 38:419–428, 1996.
14. Wellens JJ: The value of the electrocardiogram in the differential diagnosis of a tachycardia with a widened QRS complex. Am J Med 64:27–33, 1978.
15. Wilber DF: Evaluation and treatment of nonsustained ventricular tachycardia. Curr Opin Cardiol 11:23–31, 1996.

22. CORONARY ARTERY DISEASE

Valerie K. Ulstad, M.D., M.P.A., M.P.H.

1. What causes myocardial ischemia?

Myocardial ischemia is caused by an imbalance between myocardial oxygen supply and demand.

2. How may myocardial ischemia manifest?

Myocardial ischemia may manifest as angina pectoris, as ST-T changes on the electrocardiogram (EKG), and as left ventricular dysfunction due to inadequate supply of myocardial oxygen for normal contractile function.

3. What are the determinants of myocardial oxygen demand?

The need for oxygen delivery to the heart is increased when any of the following four conditions exist: (1) increased heart rate, (2) increased contractility of the heart, (3) increased afterload for the ejecting heart (crudely measured as the systolic blood pressure), and (4) increased preload (filling of the ventricles in diastole).

4. What are the most common clinical presentations of coronary artery disease (CAD)?

Typical angina pectoris, unstable angina pectoris, acute myocardial infarction, and sudden cardiac death.

5. What is the pathophysiology of typical angina pectoris?

In typical exertional angina pectoris, ischemia results when myocardial oxygen demand is increased but supply is relatively reduced because of atherosclerotic obstruction of 50–70% of the coronary lumen. The affected individual has exertional chest discomfort relieved by rest. Because coronary reserve is reduced most in the subendocardium, ischemia occurs first in this region. An EKG during an episode of pain would likely show ST depression, which is indicative of subendocardial ischemia.

Some patients with chronic stable angina develop ischemia because of dynamic coronary vasoconstriction in the setting of fixed atherosclerotic disease. The eccentric lesions of atherosclerosis leave muscle in the neighboring vessel wall; thus spasm in that area may suddenly worsen the stenosis. Such inappropriate coronary vasoconstriction has been shown to occur with cigarette smoking, exposure to cold, and exercise.

6. Describe the management of a patient with typical angina pectoris.

1. **Educate.** The patient needs to understand the disease process to be motivated to modify CAD risk factors and to seek medical attention promptly if symptoms worsen.

2. **Treat.** The patient should be started on therapy to relieve discomfort and to improve exercise tolerance. Sublingual nitroglycerin should be used as necessary.

3. **Evaluate.** An exercise stress test should be done to define objectively the level of exercise that precipitates myocardial ischemia and to provide the clinician with prognostic information. The patient who develops ischemia either clinically or on EKG during the first minutes of exercise has a poor prognosis. Such a patient should be referred for more invasive evaluation by coronary angiography.

7. What are the objectives in the medical treatment of angina?

1. Reduction of myocardial oxygen demand during exercise or stress: nitrates, beta blockers, calcium channel blockers.

2. Promotion of maximal vasodilation of the coronary arteries: nitrates, calcium channel blockers.

Severity of disease determines the amount of therapy. Usually nitrates are the first-line treatment, with other drugs added if more than episodic nitroglycerin is required.

Antianginal Therapy

AGENT	ACTION	IMPORTANT CONSIDERATIONS
Nitrates	Dilate coronaries Decrease preload	8–10 hr/day free of drug to avoid tolerance May cause headache
Beta blockers	Decrease heart rate Decrease contractility Decrease blood pressure	All agents potentially block $beta_1$ and $beta_2$ receptors; selective agents at low dose block $beta_1$ receptors more than $beta_2$ May precipitate CHF, bronchospasm, CNS side effects
Calcium channel blockers	Dilate coronaries Decrease contractility Decrease systolic pressure Decrease heart rate	Heterogeneous group Constipation

CHF = congestive heart failure; CNS = central nervous system.

8. What education should the patient receive about therapy with nitroglycerin?

Sublingual nitroglycerin prescriptions should be refilled every 6 months because the tablets become outdated. A patient who develops flushing or headache with sublingual therapy probably is using active nitroglycerin. Patients who use nitrates (either orally or by patch) to sustain blood levels must have a 10–12-hour nitrate-free period each day. This decreases the incidence of nitroglycerin tolerance and improves efficacy.

9. What is unstable angina?

The following situations suggest that the anginal pattern is unstable:
1. Rest angina or angina occurring with less effort than previously
2. More frequent angina with the same degree of exertion
3. More protracted discomfort that is less responsive to therapy or rest
4. Prolonged pain without evidence of myocardial infarction
5. Recent onset of angina

10. What is the pathophysiology of unstable angina?

Unstable angina is a clinical syndrome that falls between chronic stable angina pectoris and acute myocardial infarction. Studies suggest that myocardial oxygen supply is further reduced. The involved coronary artery in unstable angina tends to have an eccentric plaque with a fissure or crack and superimposed thrombus adherent to the site of the plaque crack or rupture. The precise factors that lead to plaque rupture are unknown. Platelets adhere to the disrupted thrombogenic intima and produce thromboxane A_2, which stimulates further platelet aggregation. The resultant thrombus is responsible for the sudden change in myocardial oxygen supply and subsequent change in symptoms. The thrombus may be intermittently occlusive, leading to waxing and waning discomfort at rest. If the thrombus completely occludes the vessel, a myocardial infarction follows, unless the vessel can be rapidly opened.

11. Describe the EKG in patients with unstable angina.

The majority of patients have transient ST-T changes (elevation or progression) and/or peaking or inverted T waves during pain. An EKG with ST-T segment deviation in two or more leads is highly predictive of adverse clinical events.

12. What therapy is indicated in patients with unstable angina?

Unstable angina is associated with a tendency to develop continually worsening pain, acute myocardial infarction, life-threatening ventricular arrhythmias, or sudden cardiac death. Patients should be promptly hospitalized for observation, monitoring, antianginal therapy (IV nitroglycerin and beta blockers), and antithrombotic therapy (heparin infusion and aspirin) to promote coronary artery patency. Thrombolytic therapy has no role in patients with unstable angina. Patients with EKG changes and chest pain may be referred for early catheterization, whereas patients without EKG changes may be risk-stratified with exercise testing.

13. Describe the presentation of the patient with acute myocardial infarction (AMI).

The patient with AMI usually presents with discomfort similar in character to angina pectoris. The discomfort does not resolve promptly with rest and nitroglycerin. Continued discomfort at rest distinguishes AMI from a simple episode of angina. The EKG in patients with AMI typically shows ST segment elevation, suggesting transmural ischemia usually due to obstruction of an epicardial coronary artery.

14. What is the pathophysiology of AMI?

An intracoronary thrombus develops because of atherosclerotic plaque disruption and fissure. When the thrombus totally occludes the vessel, myocardial ischemia begins. If the vessel remains closed, myocardial infarction occurs. In more than 85% of patients with AMI, occluding thrombus can be demonstrated angiographically.

15. Why is prompt recognition of AMI so important?

The obstruction of a coronary artery quickly leads to abnormal ventricular wall motion in the distribution of the affected coronary artery. If the vessel remains closed for longer than 20–40 minutes, the ventricular muscle in the distribution of the coronary artery begins to become necrotic (infarction); the deepest layers of the myocardium are affected first.

The highest priority is to open the coronary artery. Thrombolytic therapy to lyse the occluding thrombus should be considered in every patient with AMI as soon as the diagnosis is made; it is now considered standard therapy. When immediate percutaneous transluminal coronary angioplasty (PTCA) is available, immediate revascularization may be preferable to thrombolytic therapy.

16. What is thrombolytic therapy?

Thrombolytic agents are capable of causing clot lysis directly or indirectly by accelerating the conversion of plasminogen to plasmin. Plasmin is a proteolytic enzyme that acts on fibrin to cause fibrinolysis, which results in thrombolysis and reperfusion. The three agents approved by the Food and Drug Administration for coronary thrombolysis include streptokinase, alteplase (a recombinant tissue-type plasminogen activator [TPA]), and anistreplase (an acylated plasminogen-streptokinase complex [APSAC]).

17. Does thrombolytic therapy work?

Yes. Intravenous thrombolytic therapy reduces early mortality from AMI by 25%, leads to an increase in postinfarction left ventricular ejection fraction, and reduces the likelihood of postinfarction congestive heart failure. Survival rates with various agents have so far been similar, although the role of adjunctive heparin with each has not been well studied. Using early patency of the coronary artery as an endpoint, randomized trials have shown that TPA is superior to streptokinase. In the GUSTO study, differences in early patency translated into a greater reduction in mortality in patients given TPA vs. patients receiving streptokinase.

18. Who is the ideal candidate for thrombolytic therapy?

Ideal patients (who tend to be included in controlled trials) are younger than 75 years, with ST elevation in two or more contiguous leads, and present within 6 hours of the onset of chest discomfort. Many other patients may benefit from thrombolytic therapy, including patients with new left bundle-branch block, elderly patients with large infarctions, and patients presenting between 6 and 12 hours after the onset of pain.

19. What is the major side effect of thrombolytic therapy?

With all thrombolytic agents the major adverse effect is bleeding. Hemorrhage requiring transfusion occurs in 1–5% of patients and intracranial bleeding in 0.5–1.5%.

20. What is the role of aspirin in AMI?

Aspirin has been shown to reduce the incidence of reinfarction in patients treated with streptokinase and to double the reduction in mortality observed with streptokinase alone. Aspirin, 160–325 mg/day, should be started in the emergency department at presentation and continued indefinitely.

21. Should beta blockers be given after AMI?

Yes. Beta blockers have been shown to reduce mortality when started several days to several months after infarction. Both selective and nonselective forms of beta blockers reduce the incidence of sudden death after infarction.

22. Should beta blockers be started immediately upon presentation with AMI?

Yes. The immediate use of beta blockers, presumably to reduce myocardial oxygen demand by opposing the heightened adrenergic tone associated with AMI, has been shown to lead to a 13% reduction in 1-week mortality and a 19% reduction in nonfatal reinfarctions.

23. What is the role for angiotensin-converting enzyme (ACE) inhibitors in the postinfarction patient?

The Studies of Left Ventricular Dysfunction (SOLVD) and the Survival and Ventricular Enlargement (SAVE) trials suggest that postinfarction patients with an ejection fraction less than 40% have lower mortality, fewer hospitalizations for heart failure, and a lower incidence of recurrent infarction when treated with an ACE inhibitor.

24. What are the major complications of AMI?

Arrhythmias (particularly ventricular)
Systolic heart failure
Mechanical complications (free wall, septal, or papillary muscle rupture)
Left ventricular (LV) mural thrombus with embolization

25. What is the 1-year mortality rate after AMI?

The 1-year mortality rate after discharge is 4–7%. In patients younger than 70 years who are treated with thrombolytic therapy, the mortality rate may be as low as 3–5%.

26. List the factors associated with a poor prognosis after AMI.

1. Decreased LV ejection fraction— independent factor
2. Advanced age—independent factor
3. Female sex—independent factor
4. Complex or frequent PVCs— independent factor
5. Congestive heart failure
6. Postinfarction angina
7. Prior myocardial infarction
8. Large infarction
9. Atrial fibrillation
10. Extensive coronary artery disease
11. Diabetes
12. Hypertension
13. Continued smoking
14. Elevated serum cholesterol

27. What can be done to minimize the postinfarction risk?

1. Coronary angiography during acute hospitalization if the patient has continued ischemic symptoms in the hospital
2. Predischarge limited exercise testing to identify patients with residual ischemia for referral for coronary angiography and possible revascularization
3. Referral of patients with sustained ventricular tachycardia for coronary angiography and electrophysiologic evaluation
4. Smoking cessation (associated with a 40–60% decrease in mortality)
5. Lowering of cholesterol
6. Use of beta blocker
7. Aspirin
8. ACE inhibitor if ejection fraction is ≤ 40%
9. Referral to cardiac rehabilitation (may reduce mortality by 20–50%)
10. Hormone replacement therapy in women

28. Does lowering lipids in the patient with known CAD make a difference?

Yes. The Scandinavian Simvastatin Survival Study (4S) showed a 30% decrease in total mortality and a 42% reduction in cardiac mortality at 5 years in patients with known CAD and elevated total (= 261) and LDL (= 188) cholesterol. The Cholesterol and Recurrent Events (CARE) trial was an analysis of statin use in patients with known CAD and average cholesterol levels (mean total cholesterol = 209, LDL = 139). This study showed a 24% reduction in fatal CAD and nonfatal MI in the treated group after a follow-up of 5 years. The problem mechanism of the marked decrease in events is plaque stabilization.

BIBLIOGRAPHY

1. American College of Cardiology/American Heart Association Task Force on Assessment of Diagnostic and Therapeutic Cardiovascular Procedures (Subcommittee to Develop Guidelines for the Early Management of Patients with Acute Myocardial Infarction): Guidelines for the early management of patients with acute myocardial infarction. J Am Coll Cardiol 16:249–292, 1990.
2. ACC/AHA Guidelines for the Management of Patients with Acute Myocardial Infarction: A report of the American College of Cardiology/American Heart Association Task Force on Practice Guidelines (Committee on Management of Acute Myocardial Infarction). J Am Coll Cardiol 28:1328–1428, 1996.
3. Balady GJ, Fletcher BJ, Froelicher ES, et al: Cardiac rehabilitation programs: A statement for health care professionals from the American Heart Association. Circulation 90:1602–1610, 1994.
4. Bertolet BD, Dinerman J, Hartke R Jr, Conti CR: Unstable angina: Relationship of clinical presentation, coronary pathology, and clinical outcome. Clin Cardiol 16:116–122, 1993.
5. Braunwald E: Unstable angina: A classification. Circulation 80:410–414, 1989.
6. Braunwald E, Jones RH, Mark DB, et al: Diagnosing and managing unstable angina. Agency for Health Care Policy and Research. Circulation 90:613–622, 1994.
7. Chesebro JH, Zoldhelyi P, Fuster V: Pathogenesis of thrombosis in unstable angina. Am J Cardiol 68:2B–10B, 1991.
8. Conti CR, Hill JA, Mayfield WR: Unstable angina pectoris: Pathogenesis and management. Curr Probl Cardiol 14:549–624, 1989.
9. Eisenberg MS, Aghababian RV, Bossaert L, et al: Thrombolytic therapy. Ann Emerg Med 22(Pt 2):417–427, 1993.

10. Fuster V, Badimon L, Badimon JJ, Chesebro JH: The pathogenesis of coronary artery disease and the acute coronary syndromes: Part 1. N Engl J Med 326:242–250, 1992.
11. Fuster V, Badimon L, Badimon JJ, Chesebro JH: The pathogenesis of coronary artery disease and the acute coronary syndromes: Part 2. N Engl J Med 326:310–318, 1992.
12. Global Use of Strategies to Open Occluded Coronary Arteries in Acute Coronary Syndromes (GUSTO IIb) Angioplasty Substudy Investigators: A clinical trial comparing primary coronary angioplasty with tissue plasminogen activator for acute myocardial infarction. N Engl J Med 336:1621–1628, 1997.
13. Muller DW, Topol EJ: Selection of patients with acute myocardial infarction for thrombolytic therapy. Ann Intern Med 113:949–960, 1990.
14. Pearson T, Rapaport E, Criqui M, et al: Optimal risk factor management in the patient after coronary revascularization: A statement for health care professionals from an American Heart Association writing group. Circulation 90:3125–3133, 1994.
15. Popma JJ, Topol EJ: Adjuncts to thrombolysis for myocardial reperfusion. Ann Intern Med 115:34–44, 1991.
16. Pfeffer MA, Braunwald E, Moye LA, et al: Effects of captopril on mortality and morbidity in patients with left ventricular dysfunction after myocardial infarction: Results of the Survival and Ventricular Enlargement trial. The SAVE investigators. N Engl J Med 327:669–677, 1992.
17. Puleo P, Roberts R: Early biochemical markers of myocardial necrosis. Cardiovasc Clin 20:143–154, 1989.
18. Sacks FM, Pfeffer MA, Braunwald E, et al for the CARE investigators: Effect of pravastatin on coronary events after myocardial infarction in patients with average cholesterol levels. N Engl J Med 335:1001–1009, 1996.
19. Shah PK: Pathophysiology of unstable angina. Cardiol Clin 9:11–26, 1991.
20. SOLVD Investigators: Effect of enalapril on mortality and the development of heart failure in asymptomatic patients with reduced left ventricular ejection fractions. N Engl J Med 327:658–691, 1992.
21. Topol EJ: Which thrombolytic agent should one choose? Prog Cardiovasc Dis 34:165–178, 1991.
22. Wenger NK, Froelicher ES, Smith LK, et al: Cardiac rehabilitation as secondary prevention. Clinical Practice Guideline. Quick Reference Guide for Clinicians, no. 17. Rockville, MD, U.S. Department of Health and Human Services, Public Health Service, Agency for Health Care Policy and Research, and National Heart, Lung, and Blood Institute. AHCPR pub. no. 96-0673, 1995.
23. Yusuf S, Sleight P, Held P, McMahon S: Routine medical management of acute myocardial infarction: Lessons from overviews of recent randomized controlled trials. Circulation 82(Suppl II):II-117–II-134, 1990.
24. Yusuf S, Wittes J, Friedman L: Overview of results of randomized clinical trials in heart disease. I: Treatments following myocardial infarction. JAMA 260:2088–2093, 1988.

23. CONGESTIVE HEART FAILURE

Valerie K. Ulstad, M.D., M.P.A., M.P.H.

1. What is congestive heart failure (CHF)?

CHF is a clinical syndrome related to cardiac dysfunction (systolic and/or diastolic) and characterized by limited exercise tolerance, fluid retention, and reduced life expectancy.

2. What are the incidence and prevalence of CHF?

Three million people in the United States and 15 million people worldwide have CHF. There are approximately 400,000 new cases in the U.S. each year. The incidence is increasing despite the decline in mortality from cardiovascular disease, probably because an aging population has received benefit from improved therapies. CHF is the most common discharge diagnosis in patients 65 years or older.

3. Describe the New York Heart Association (NYHA) classification of heart failure.

Class I: No limitation of physical activity; no dyspnea, fatigue, or palpitations with ordinary physical activity.

Class II: Slight limitation of physical activity; patients have dyspnea, fatigue, or palpitations with ordinary physical activity but are comfortable at rest.

Class III: Marked limitation of activity; less than ordinary physical activity results in symptoms, but patients are comfortable at rest.

Class IV: Symptoms are present at rest, and any physical exertion exacerbates the symptoms.

4. Characterize low-output cardiac failure.

Low-output failure, the most common form of heart failure, is characterized by reduced stroke volume, peripheral vasoconstriction, reduced pulse pressure, and increased arteriovenous oxygen difference.

5. What are the most important causes of low-output CHF in the United States?

Coronary artery disease—underlying cause in 50–75% of cases	Hypertrophic cardiomyopathy
	Congenital heart disease
Hypertension	Cor pulmonale
Dilated cardiomyopathy	Toxins—alcohol, Adriamycin
Valvular heart disease	Infections

6. What is the most common cause of low-output CHF worldwide?

Chagas disease.

7. List five prognostic indicators in CHF.

1. Ventricular function measured by ejection fraction
2. Peak exercise oxygen consumption
3. NYHA class
4. Plasma norepinephrine levels
5. Ventricular arrhythmias

8. What is the mortality rate from CHF?

The 5-year mortality rate in men is 60%. Women do somewhat better, with a 5-year mortality rate of 45%. When the patient has symptoms of heart failure at rest (class IV), the 1-year mortality rate is about 50%. About 40% of deaths are sudden, presumably due to ventricular arrhythmias.

9. What is high-output cardiac failure?

High-output cardiac failure is characterized by widened pulse pressure, peripheral vasodilation, and an increased arteriovenous oxygen difference.

10. What conditions are associated with high-output heart failure?

Anemia	Paget disease
Hyperthyroidism	Hepatic disease
Systemic arteriovenous fistula	Dermatologic conditions causing high blood flow in skin
Beriberi	

11. Which symptoms of CHF are due to isolated left ventricular dysfunction?

Dyspnea on exertion	Wheezing
Paroxysmal nocturnal dyspnea	Hemoptysis
Orthopnea	Fatigue
Cough	Weakness

12. What are the clinical signs of isolated left ventricular dysfunction?

Hypotension	Cardiomegaly (systolic dysfunction)
Weak pulses	S3 gallop
Peripheral vasoconstriction	Rales
Cachexia	Pleural effusions
Cheyne-Stokes respirations	

13. Which symptoms of CHF are due to isolated right ventricular dysfunction?

Right upper quadrant discomfort	Early satiety
Abdominal distention	

14. What are the clinical signs of isolated right ventricular dysfunction?

Elevated jugular venous pressure	Ascites
Hepatomegaly	Peripheral edema
Splenomegaly	

15. What is the most common cause of right-heart failure?
Left-heart failure.

16. Contrast systolic and diastolic dysfunction.
    Systolic dysfunction occurs with a defect in the expulsion of blood from the ventricles or a decrease in ventricular contractility. Diastolic dysfunction occurs with abnormal resistance to ventricular filling in diastole.

17. How do Frank-Starling curves (stroke volume on the Y axis and end-diastolic volume on the X axis) differ for the normal heart and the heart with severe systolic dysfunction?
    Note the effect of increasing preload. The normal heart augments its output with increases in preload. The heart with systolic failure is unable to augment its output further by increasing preload.

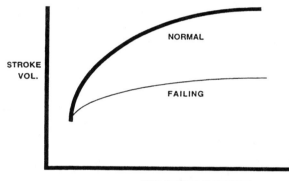

Frank-Starling curves for the normal heart and the heart with severe systolic dysfunction.

18. How do the function curves (stroke volume on the Y axis and afterload on the X axis) differ for the normal heart and the heart with severe systolic dysfunction?
    Note the effect of increasing impedance or afterload. The normal heart tolerates increased impedance well without a drop in stroke volume. The heart with systolic failure fails further (that is, stroke volume falls further) with increased impedance.

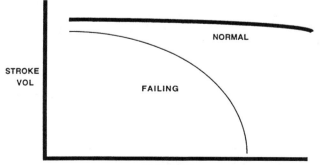

Function curves for the normal heart and the heart with severe systolic dysfunction.

19. Which is the more common cause of CHF syndrome, systolic or diastolic dysfunction?

Systolic dysfunction is the more common cause. As a result, the terms systolic and CHF syndrome tend to be used synonymously. Such usage is inaccurate.

20. Describe the vicious cycle of heart failure.

A particular cardiac problem causes a drop in cardiac output that leads to activation of the neurohormonal mechanisms, including the sympathetic nervous system, the renin-angiotensin-aldosterone system, and the arginine vasopressin system. The net effects are excessive vasoconstriction and increased sodium and water retention, which lead to increased vascular impedance to the already failing heart. Thus the patient's condition worsens.

21. List the three major goals of therapy for CHF.

1. Improved quality of life
2. Prolonged survival
3. Improved natural history

22. What are the principles of treatment of CHF?

1. Remove or correct the precipitating cause. Always consider whether ischemia plays a role.
2. Correct exacerbating factors.
3. Determine whether the dysfunction is predominantly systolic or diastolic by echocardiography.
4. Use vasodilators to reduce vasoconstriction in patients with systolic dysfunction.
5. Add diuretics and low-sodium diet to control salt and water retention.
6. Encourage weight loss (if the patient is overweight) and regular exercise.
7. Prescribe digoxin in patients with atrial fibrillation or patients in normal sinus rhythm who are still symptomatic on vasodilators and diuretics.

23. What common causes of cardiac decompensation should be considered in patients with previously stable CHF?

- Myocardial ischemia
- Mitral regurgitation
- Uncontrolled hypertension
- Increased dietary intake of sodium
- Superimposed medical illness, especially:
  Poorly controlled diabetes mellitus
  Pneumonia
  Pulmonary embolus

24. When should diuretic therapy be used in the treatment of CHF?

In chronic therapy of **CHF due to systolic dysfunction**, diuretics are used frequently, although in some cases they may not be necessary. Excessive diuresis may result in further activation of the neurohormonal system and intolerance of vasodilators (hypotension).

In chronic therapy of **CHF due to diastolic dysfunction**, diuretics may be needed to decrease pulmonary congestion and to improve dyspnea. Diuretics must be given carefully to avoid an excessive drop in preload, because patients have stiff ventricles with intrinsic resistance to diastolic filling.

Loop diuretics are needed when renal function is abnormal (creatinine = > 2.0 mg/dl), because thiazide diuretics are ineffective in such patients. In patients with mild CHF, thiazide diuretics may have a role if renal function is normal. In refractory heart failure a combination of thiazide and loop diuretics may be needed.

25. How should vasodilators be used in CHF due to systolic dysfunction?

Angiotensin-converting enzyme (ACE) inhibitors should be started in nearly all patients with symptomatic or asymptomatic left ventricular (LV) systolic dysfunction. Hypotension can be prevented by starting with low doses and by avoiding volume depletion before institution of therapy. Marked subsequent increases in blood urea nitrogen (BUN) and creatinine (Cr) suggest renovascular disease, and the ACE inhibitor should be stopped. Hydralazine and isosorbide dinitrate should be tried in patients intolerant of ACE inhibitors or patients with side effects.

26. Should the asymptomatic person with LV systolic dysfunction be treated with vasodilator therapy?

Yes. This recommendation is based on the outcome of two major trials. The SOLVD trial showed that enalapril reduced the incidence of heart failure and the rate of related hospitalizations in patients with asymptomatic decreased function (ejection fraction ≤ 35%). In the Survival and Ventricular Enlargement (SAVE) study, patients enrolled 3–17 days after infarction with ejection fractions of < 40% and no clinical heart failure were randomized to captopril or placebo. Captopril prevented further reduction in ejection fraction and reduced the rates of recurrent infarction and mortality.

27. What is the difference in treatment of systolic as opposed to diastolic failure?

A patient with **systolic dysfunction** should be treated with inotropes to improve contractility; with diuretics to decrease congestion due to increased preload; and with vasodilators to decrease afterload or impedance imposed on the left ventricle by vasconstrictors released by neurohormonal activation. A patient with **diastolic failure** should be treated with agents to improve relaxation (negative inotropes), gentle diuresis if congestion exists (because the ventricle does not fill well, excessive diuresis decreases cardiac output precipitously), and agents to slow the heart rate (so that diastole is longer and allows more time to fill). Patients with diastolic dysfunction may tolerate vasodilators poorly.

28. How does one distinguish between systolic and diastolic dysfunction as the cause of the clinical syndrome of CHF?

The clinical syndrome is the same in both types of dysfunction. Echocardiography is a useful test in any patient with new heart failure. This test may demonstrate any important valvular or pericardial disease. Systolic dysfunction is evident with decreased contractility of the heart. If both left and right ventricular systolic functions are normal, restricted ventricular filling or diastolic dysfunction may be the culprit. Echo-Doppler studies may be used to look more carefully for diastolic dysfunction.

29. What endpoints should be evaluated in drug trials for treatment of CHF?

Improved quality of life	Reversal of neurohormonal abnormalities
Improved exercise capacity	Reduction of mortality

30. Describe the common types of cardiomyopathy.

Cardiomyopathy is a condition of varying and frequently unknown etiology in which the dominant feature is cardiomegaly and low-output cardiac failure. Cardiomyopathies are categorized in three groups:

Dilated
- Most common type; dilation of all chambers
- Decrease in systolic function of the ventricles
- Causes include idiopathic factors, alcohol, Adriamycin, myocarditis, valve replacement, diabetes, thyroid disease, thiamine deficiency, pheochromocytoma, peripartum complications, and coronary artery disease
- Chest radiograph shows enlarged heart; echocardiography shows enlarged chambers and reduced contractility; radionuclide ventriculography shows reduced ejection fraction

Hypertrophic
- Less common; thickening of ventricular wall; small ventricular cavity
- Abnormal diastolic function
- Causes include genetic factors, hypertension, and acromegaly
- Chest radiograph shows normal to mildly enlarged heart size, echocardiography shows small ventricular chamber, increased wall thickness, and increased contractility

Restrictive (infiltrative)
- Rare
- Systolic and diastolic function affected; both ventricles affected equally
- Causes include amyloid and sarcoid disorders and hemochromatosis

• Diagnosis often found only with biopsy after hemodynamic evaluation shows equal diastolic filling pattern (square-root sign) on right and left sides of heart

31. Which patients should undergo cardiac transplantation?
Transplantation should be considered in patients who remain severely compromised despite
medical therapy. The 5-year survival rate for cardiac transplantation is 75–80%. Donor availability, however, limits widespread application.

**32. What factors are associated with increased morbidity or mortality from cardiac trans-
plant?**

Obesity	Previous cardiac or thoracic surgery
Diabetes with organ damage	Chronic lung disease
Pulmonary hypertension	Intrinsic hepatic or renal disease

33. What is the role of ACE inhibitors after myocardial infarction?
In the presence of symptomatic or asymptomatic LV dysfunction, ACE inhibitors provide
additional benefit to aspirin, beta blockers, and thrombolytic therapy. They should be given as
soon as the physician believes that the patient is stable with an adequate blood pressure. A reasonable time to start the ACE inhibitor is the morning after admission, if the patient is stable, and
certainly before discharge. A meta-analysis of the use of ACE inhibitors after MI suggests a 24%
reduction in mortality, a 27% reduction in hospitalization, and 20% reduction in recurrent MI.

BIBLIOGRAPHY

1. Captopril-Digoxin Multicenter Research Group: Comparative effects of captopril and digoxin in patients
   with mild to moderate heart failure. JAMA 259:539–544, 1988.
2. Captopril Multicenter Research Group: A placebo-controlled trial of captopril in refractory congestive
   heart failure. J Am Coll Cardiol 2:755–763, 1983.
3. Cohn J: The management of chronic heart failure. N Engl J Med 335:d490–498, 1996.
4. Cohn JN: Physiological variables as markers for symptoms, risks and interventions in heart failure.
   Circulation 87(Suppl VII):VII-110–VII-114, 1993.
5. Cohn JN, Archibald D, Ziesche S, et al: Effect of vasodilator therapy on mortality in chronic congestive
   heart failure: Results of a Veterans Administration Cooperative Study (V-HeFT). N Engl J Med
   314:1547–1552, 1986.
6. Cohn JN, Johnson GR, Shabeti R, et al: Ejection fraction, peak exercise oxygen consumption, cardiotho-
   racic ratio, ventricular arrhythmias, and plasma norepinephrine as determinants of prognosis in heart
   failure. Circulation 87(Suppl VI):VI-5–VI-16, 1993.
7. Cohn JN, Johnson GR, Ziesche S, et al: A comparison of enalapril with hydralazine-isosorbide dinitrate
   in the treatment of chronic congestive heart failure. V-HeFT II. N Engl J Med 325:303–310, 1991.
8. CONSENSUS Trial Study Group: Effects of enalapril on mortality in severe congestive heart failure:
   Results of the Cooperative North Scandinavian Enalapril Survival Study (CONSENSUS). N Engl J
   Med 316:1429–1435, 1987.
9. Fletcher RD, Clinton GB, Johnson G, et al: Enalapril decreases ventricular tachycardia in patients with
   chronic congestive heart failure. Circulation 87(Suppl VI):VI-49–VI-55, 1993.
10. Francis GS: Development of arrhythmias in the patient with congestive heart failure: Pathophysiology,
    prevalence, and prognosis. Am J Cardiol 57:3B–7B, 1986.
11. Goldman S, Johnson G, Cohn JN, et al: Mechanism of death in heart failure: The vasodilator-heart fail-
    ure trials. Circulation 87(Suppl VI):VI-24–VI-31, 1993.
12. Guidelines for the evaluation and management of heart failure. Report of the American College of
    Cardiology/American Heart Association Task Force on Practice Guidelines (Committee on
    Evaluation and Management of Heart Failure). J Am Coll Cardiol 26:1376–1398, 1995.
13. Latini R, Maggioni AP, Flather M, et al: ACE inhibitor use in patients with myocardial infarction.
    Summary of evidence from clinical trials. Circulation 92:3132–3137, 1995.
14. Lorell BH: Significance of diastolic dysfunction of the heart. Annu Rev Med 42:411–436, 1991.
15. McAlister FA, Teo KK: The management of congestive heart failure. Postgrad Med J 83:194–200, 1997.
16. McFate-Smith W: Epidemiology of congestive heart failure. Am J Cardiol 55:3A–8A, 1985.
17. Parmley WW: Pathophysiology and current therapy of congestive heart failure. J Am Coll Cardiol
    13:771–785, 1989.

18. Senni M, Redfield MM: Congestive heart failure in elderly patients. Mayo Clin Proc 72:453–460, 1997.
19. SOLVD Investigators: Effect of enalapril on survival in patients with reduced left ventricular ejection fractions and congestive heart failure. N Engl J Med 325:293–302, 1991.
20. SOLVD Investigators: Effect of enalapril on mortality and development of heart failure in asymptomatic patients with reduced left ventricular ejection fractions. N Engl J Med 327:685–691, 1992.
21. Stevenson LW: Therapy tailored for symptomatic heart failure. Heart Fail 11:87–107, 1995.
22. Vasan RS, Benjamin EJ, Levy D: Prevalence, clinical features and prognosis of diastolic heart failure: An epidemiologic perspective. J Am Coll Cardiol 26:1565–1574, 1995.

24. CARDIAC TESTING

Valerie K. Ulstad, M.D., M.P.A., M.P.H.

1. How often is the initial echocardiogram (EKG) diagnostic of myocardial infarction (MI)?

The initial EKG is diagnostic in 60% of patients. In 25% the EKG is abnormal but not diagnostic. In 15% the EKG is absolutely normal. Therefore, decisions about admission to the hospital should be based primarily on the history and current findings. The diagnostic accuracy of the EKG is enhanced by obtaining serial EKGs.

2. Does an EKG without Q waves rule out a previous MI?

No. A definitive diagnosis of a previous MI depends on the presence of pathologic Q waves. Within 6–12 months after an acute MI, about 30% of EKGs are still abnormal but no longer diagnostic for previous MI because the Q waves are absent. After 10 years 6–10% of EKGs are completely normal.

3. List eight contraindications to exercise testing.
1. Uncontrolled hypertension
2. Critical aortic stenosis
3. Hypertrophic cardiomyopathy with significant obstruction
4. Untreated life-threatening cardiac arrhythmias
5. Decompensated heart failure
6. Advanced atrioventricular (AV) block
7. Acute pericarditis or myocarditis
8. Other acute illness

4. When should a stress test be stopped?
1. **Patient signs and symptoms**
   - Severe fatigue
   - Severe dyspnea
   - Chest pain
   - Marked elevation in systolic blood pressure (> 250 mmHg)
   - Definite drop in systolic blood pressure (≥ 10 mmHg)
   - Patient request
   - Gait disturbance
2. **EKG changes**
   - ≥ 3-mm ST depression
   - ≥ 1-mm ST elevation in lead without abnormal Q wave
   - Ventricular tachycardia
   - Paroxysmal supraventricular tachycardia
   - Decrease in heart rate
3. **Noncardiac factors**
   - Technical problems interfering with test interpretation

5. In addition to exercise-induced chest pain, what signs and symptoms during an exercise test indicate an adverse prognosis and probable multivessel coronary artery disease (CAD)?
1. Inability to exercise to 6 metabolic equivalents (METS) in an otherwise healthy patient
2. Failure to increase systolic blood pressure ≥ 120 mmHg

3. Definite drop in systolic blood pressure ≥ 10 mmHg

4. ST depression > 2 mm

5. Downsloping ST depression under 6 METS in 5 or more leads or persisting more than 5 minutes into recovery

6. Exercise-induced ST elevation (excluding lead aVR)

7. Sustained ventricular tachycardia

6. What is the value of a stress test in patients with an uncomplicated MI before hospital discharge?

A low-level exercise test to 5–6 METS or 70–80% of the age-predicted maximal heart rate is frequently performed before hospital discharge to assess the patient's functional capacity and to test for residual provocable myocardial ischemia at a relatively low level of myocardial oxygen demand. A negative submaximal stress test is associated with a 1-year mortality rate of 1–2%. An ischemic response indicates a poorer prognosis. Cardiac catheterization before discharge should be considered in such patients to assess revascularization options.

7. What are the major general principles to consider for stress testing?

1. Stress testing gives physiologic information, whereas angiography gives anatomic information.

2. Interpretation of the stress test requires integration of clinical data from the history and physical exam with data from the stress test.

3. Stress testing is done to identify patients who have a high risk of severe coronary disease. Stress testing is not done to rule out the presence of coronary disease.

8. What stress tests are available to aid in the assessment of patients with known or suspected CAD?

1. Standard treadmill testing with EKG monitoring

2. Bicycle ergometer with EKG monitoring

3. Myocardial perfusion imaging with thallium-201 or 99mTc sestamibi

4. Radionuclide angiography

5. Stress echocardiography

6. Cardiopulmonary exercise testing

7. Pharmacologic stress with dobutamine, dipyridamole, or adenosine and perfusion or echocardiographic imaging

9. List four advantages of stress imaging in comparison with standard exercise electrocardiography.

1. Greater accuracy when resting EKG is abnormal

2. Higher sensitivity

3. Ability to localize and characterize the extent of ischemia

4. Direct measurement of ventricular function

10. Should regular stress testing be done in patients with an abnormal baseline EKG?

The clinician may gain useful information about functional capacity by watching the patient exercise, although the interpretation of the EKG is difficult. In patients with baseline EKG abnormalities, perfusion imaging is preferred to regular treadmill testing because of its increased diagnostic accuracy. Baseline abnormalities include ST-T abnormalities, left bundle-branch block, intraventricular conduction delay, paced ventricular rhythm, left ventricular hypertrophy, and Wolff-Parkinson-White syndrome.

11. Is a nondiagnostic treadmill study the same as a negative test?

No. It usually means (1) that the patient could not adequately exercise to address the clinical question or (2) that the baseline EKG was abnormal.

12. What is myocardial perfusion imaging?

Perfusion scanning provides physiologic information about coronary blood flow reserve, location of hypoperfusion, and extent and severity of the abnormality. Uptake of the agent by the myocardium is proportional to blood flow. Common perfusion agents include thallium-201 and the technetium agent, sestamibi. Perfusion imaging can be used with treadmill, bicycle, or pharmacologic stress testing to assess the patient for myocardial ischemia.

13. What are the important factors in selecting an imaging modality since the sensitivity for detecting CAD is similar for stress echocardiography and perfusion imaging?
   • Institutional expertise.
   • Body habitus of patient—can the heart be seen on echocardiography?
   • Perfusion imaging is more expensive than echocardiographic imaging.
   • Echocardiography provides other anatomic information.
   • Myocardial perfusion imaging can detect ischemia in segments with abnormal wall motion at rest, whereas the significance of a worsening wall motion abnormality on exercise echocardiography is not well understood.
   • Nuclear studies have been better validated for determining prognosis.

14. Which stress test should be used in patients with left bundle-branch block (LBBB)?

Exercise-induced ST depression cannot be used as a diagnostic or prognostic indicator in patients with LBBB. Most patients have ST depression with exercise, and the extent of ST depression is not meaningful. Pharmacologic stress testing is indicated in patients with resting or exercise-induced LBBB.

15. How should patients on digoxin be evaluated for CAD?

Digitalis glycosides may produce exertional ST depression even with no evidence of digitalis effect on the resting EKG. Absence of ST depression during an exercise test in a patient on digitalis glycosides is considered a valid negative response. Digitalis should be withheld 1–2 weeks before exercise testing if one plans to rely only on EKG data. Having the patient remain on the drug is an option if one uses thallium perfusion imaging or stress echocardiography instead.

16. What are the options for stress testing in the patient who cannot exercise?

Pharmacologic stress testing with echocardiographic or myocardial perfusion imaging is an option for the patient who cannot exercise. Pharmacologic agents include dobutamine, dipyridamole, and adenosine. Dobutamine increases cardiac contractility and heart rate, thereby increasing myocardial oxygen demand and simulating physical stress. Dipyridamole increases coronary blood flow and leads to redistribution of flow, producing a steal phenomenon in the distribution of significant coronary stenosis. Simultaneous echocardiographic imaging allows the detection, grading, and localization of wall-motion abnormalities due to ischemic provocation.

Dipyridamole thallium-201 imaging is also used in patients who cannot exercise. The most extensive experience with this test has been in the assessment of perioperative risk in patients requiring peripheral vascular surgery. Predictive value is greatest when the patient has clinical evidence of CAD, such as angina, previous MI, Q waves on the EKG, S3 gallop, congestive heart failure, or diabetes. The patient with none of the above features has a low perioperative risk, and the patient with three or more has a high risk, no matter what the dipyridamole thallium test shows. Adenosine may be used instead of dipyridamole. It is probably safer in patients with cerebral vascular disease because of its short half-life.

17. How does antianginal therapy affect the exercise treadmill test?

Nitrates, beta blockers, and calcium channel blockers prolong the time to the onset of ischemic ST segment depression and increase exercise tolerance. If the treadmill test is done for diagnostic purposes, cardiac drugs should be withheld for 3–5 half-lives. If the adequacy of drug therapy is being assessed, the test should be done with the patient taking the antianginal medication.

18. What diagnostic test should be ordered after a positive exercise treadmill test in a middle-aged woman with no risk factors and atypical chest pain to eliminate the diagnosis of significant CAD?

In this setting exercise-induced ST depression is more likely to be falsely positive for CAD. Myocardial perfusion imaging or stress echocardiography improves the diagnostic yield in patients with a suspected false-positive test.

19. What is the best way to assess the severity of aortic stenosis (AS)?

Two-dimensional echocardiography detects a thickened and calcified aortic valve with reduced opening. The LV size and wall thickness also can be assessed. Doppler echocardiography determines the transvalvular gradient and the valve area. AS is severe if the peak aortic flow velocity exceeds 4.5 m/sec, the aortic valve area is < 0.75 cm^2, and the LV outflow tract/aortic flow velocity is ≤ 0.25. A complete echocardiographic examination gives the clinician the necessary data to interpret the patient's complaints. Echocardiography can be done serially with minimal patient discomfort.

Before the refinement of echocardiographic technology, it was necessary to cross the aortic valve in a retrograde fashion in the catheterization laboratory to confirm the presence of severe AS. Now the only reason to catheterize a patient with AS before surgery is to perform coronary angiography when coincident CAD is suspected. Such a patient may receive bypass grafts at the time of valve surgery.

20. Is there a reliable test to assess the presence of left atrial clot before cardioversion of atrial fibrillation?

Successful cardioversion is associated with 5–7% incidence of embolism among patients who have not received anticoagulant therapy. Atrial thrombi are poorly detected by transthoracic echocardiography. A normal transthoracic echocardiogram does not rule out the presence of left atrial thrombi. The standard practice is several weeks of oral anticoagulation in patients with atrial fibrillation of unknown duration or duration > 2 days. Cardioversion of an anticoagulated patient carries an embolic rate of < 1.6%.

Transesophageal echocardiography (TEE) is a highly accurate method of detecting atrial thrombi. If TEE excludes the presence of thrombi, early cardioversion probably can be performed safely without preprocedure anticoagulation. However, skeptics point out that small thrombi potentially missed by TEE can have important consequences, that the risk of anticoagulation in most patients is low, and that larger studies are needed. Anticoagulation during and after the procedure is still recommended until atrial contractility returns to normal.

21. Which imaging modalities can be used in patients in whom aortic dissection is suspected?

Potential imaging modalities include aortography, CT, magnetic resonance imaging (MRI), and TEE. The choice of test depends on the precise information that is sought by the surgeon and the expertise available in acquiring the images. Potentially available diagnostic information includes presence of dissection, involvement of the aortic root, sites of entry, extent of dissection, branch-vessel involvement, thrombus in the false lumen, aortic insufficiency, pericardial effusion, and coronary artery involvement.

All modalities are similar in specificity, but MRI and TEE tend to be more sensitive. Sensitivity is most important because aortic dissection is a rapidly lethal condition. MRI is probably better at defining the site of the intimal tear and recognizing intraluminal thrombus. Both modalities are noninvasive and easily identify the presence of pericardial effusion; neither requires the use of intravenous contrast material. TEE is superior at detecting and quantifying the degree of aortic insufficiency and in detecting involvement of the proximal coronary arteries. TEE tends to be more readily available and more rapid, because it can be performed at the patient's bedside.

22. What is the best test for rapid evaluation of potential cardiac etiologies in a hypotensive patient?

As fluid support is initiated, a simple transthoracic echocardiogram rapidly reveals the status of ventricular function. A hyperdynamic left ventricle suggests hypovolemia or sepsis as a cause of the hypotension. A poorly contractile left ventricle suggests low-output heart failure as the cause. A large pericardial effusion causing right and left ventricular diastolic collapse indicates a hemodynamically significant pericardial effusion that needs emergent drainage. A markedly dilated right ventricle leads to consideration of right ventricular infarction or large pulmonary embolus as the culprit. With such information the physician can begin to tailor therapy. A Swan-Ganz catheter eventually may be in order, but it should not be the starting point.

23. What is a signal-averaged EKG? How is it used?

Signal-averaged EKG is a diagnostic test used to detect delayed, low-amplitude electrical activation in the terminal portion of the QRS complex. The signal-averaged EKG is an amplified representation of the QRS complex. The amplification allows the small late potentials to be seen. The late potential is a moderately sensitive and highly specific indicator for inducible ventricular tachycardia in the electrophysiology laboratory. The clinical application of signal-averaged EKGs is still under study.

24. What does rest radionuclide ventriculography evaluate?

Rest radionuclide ventriculography provides a quantitative measurement of left ventricular ejection fraction. The red blood cells are tagged with a radioactive label, and counts in the left ventricle are obtained by a gamma counter in systole and diastole. The fraction of counts lost from diastole to systole is the ejection fraction. It can be obtained simply and requires no artificial assumptions about geometry of the left ventricle. It is reproducible on serial measurements and is the desired test for accurate measurement of the ejection fraction. The accuracy of the test may be affected by frequent premature atrial or ventricular beats or by atrial fibrillation.

BIBLIOGRAPHY

1. Berman DS, Kiat H, Friedman JD, Diamond G: Clinical application of exercise nuclear cardiology studies in the era of health care reform. Am J Cardiol 75:3D–13D, 1995.
2. Braunwald E (ed): Heart Disease: A Textbook of Cardiovascular Medicine, 4th ed. Philadelphia, W.B. Saunders, 1992.
3. Bonow RO, Dilsizian V: Thallium-201 and technetium-99m-sestamibi for assessing viable myocardium. J Nucl Med 33:815–818, 1992.
4. Brown KA: Prognostic value of thallium-201 myocardial perfusion imaging: A diagnostic tool comes of age. Circulation 83:363–381, 1991.
5. Cerqueira MD: Diagnostic testing strategies for coronary artery disease: Special issues related to gender. Am J Cardiol 75:52D–60D, 1995.
6. Chang JA, Froelicher VF: Clinical and exercise test markers of prognosis in patients with stable coronary artery disease. Curr Probl Cardiol 19:533–587, 1994.
7. Cigarroa JE, Isselbacher EM, DeSanctis RW, Eagle KA: Diagnostic imaging in the evaluation of suspected aortic dissection: Old standards and new directions. N Engl J Med 328:35–43, 1993.
8. Douglas PS, Ginsburg GS: The evaluation of chest pain in women. N Engl J Med 334:1311–1315, 1996.
9. Eagle KA, Coley CM, Newell JB, et al: Combining clinical and thallium data optimizes preoperative assessment of cardiac risk before major vascular surgery. Ann Intern Med 110:859–866, 1989.
10. Ehman RL, Julsrud PR: Magnetic resonance imaging of the heart. Mayo Clin Proc 64:1134–1146, 1989.
11. Gajraj H, Jamieson CW: Coronary artery disease in patients with peripheral vascular disease. Br J Surg 81:333–342, 1994.
12. Gibbons RJ, Balady GJ, Beasley JW, et al: ACC/AHA guidelines for exercise testing: A report of the American College of Cardiology/American Heart Association Task Force on Practice Guidelines (Committee on Exercise Testing). J Am Coll Cardiol 30:260–315, 1997.
13. Hendel RC, Layden JJ, Leppo JA: Prognostic value of dipyridamole thallium scintigraphy for evaluation of ischemic heart disease. J Am Coll Cardiol 15:109–116, 1990.
14. Junega R, Wasir HS: Abnormal exercise electrocardiogram in an asymptomatic person—what next? Int J Cardiol 4:1–9, 1994.
15. Kahn JK, Sills MN, Corbett JR, Willerson JT: What is the current role of nuclear cardiology in clinical medicine? Chest 97:442–446, 1990.

16. Kotler TS, Diamond GA: Exercise thallium-201 scintigraphy in the diagnosis and prognosis of coronary artery disease. Ann Intern Med 113:684–702, 1990.
17. Manning WJ, Silverman DI, Gordon SPF, et al: Cardioversion from atrial fibrillation without prolonged anticoagulation with use of transesophageal echocardiography to exclude the presence of atrial thrombi. N Engl J Med 328:750–755, 1993.
18. Mayo Clinic Cardiovascular Working Group on Stress Testing: Cardiovascular stress testing: Description of the various types of stress tests and indications for their use. Mayo Clin Proc 71:43–52, 1996.
19. Nienabar CA, von Kodolistch Y, Nicolas V, et al: The diagnosis of thoracic aortic dissection by noninvasive imaging procedures. N Engl J Med 328:1–9, 1993.
20. Pellikka PA, Roger VL, Oh JK, et al: Stress echocardiography: Part II: Dobutamine stress echocardiography: Techniques, implementation, clinical applications, and correlations. Mayo Clin Proc 70:16–27, 1995.
21. Pina IL, Balady GJ, Hanson P, et al: Guidelines for clinical exercise testing laboratories: A statement for health care professionals from the Committee on Exercise and Cardiac Rehabilitation, American Heart Association. Circulation 91:912–921, 1995.
22. Schlant RC, Blomquist CG, Brandenburg RO, et al: Guidelines for exercise testing: A report of the American College of Cardiology/American Heart Association Task Force on Assessment of Cardiovascular Procedures (Subcommittee on Exercise Testing). J Am Coll Cardiol 8:725–738, 1986.
23. Schulman SP, Fleg JL: Stress testing for coronary artery disease in the elderly. Clin Geriatr Med 12:101–119, 1996.
24. Sox HC, Littenberg B, Garber AM: The role of exercise testing in screening for coronary artery disease. Ann Intern Med 110:456–469, 1989.
25. Tresch DD, Aronow WS: Clinical manifestations and diagnosis of coronary artery disease. Clin Geriatr Med 12:89–100, 1996.

IV. Disorders of the Eyes, Ears, Nose, and Throat

25. VISUAL IMPAIRMENT

Jon M. Braverman, M.D., and Thomas D. MacKenzie, M.D., M.S.P.H.

1. How is vision generally measured in the primary care office?

Most patients read an eye chart, which tests central visual acuity. Testing of standard acuity requires the equivalent of a 20-ft Snellen target. However, testing nearer vision in a patient who is farsighted or presbyopic (over 40 years of age) does not yield accurate results unless a near correction is used.

Peripheral vision can be tested grossly by confrontation. The examiner sits in front of the patient, and each closes the opposite eye to overlap respective fields. The examiner then asks the patient either to count the number of fingers presented within the field or to indicate when a finger is first seen entering the field. Most modern ophthalmologic practices use automated computerized perimeters to assess visual fields more accurately.

Several other components of vision can be measured, including color perception, dark adaptation, and contrast sensitivity. Changes in these parameters may occur secondary to eye disease; however, the tools and techniques required for evaluation are usually beyond the resources of a primary care provider.

2. What three levels of visual processing should be considered in evaluating the possible etiologies of diminished visual acuity?

1. Loss of the ability to form a clear image on the retina
2. Loss of the ability of the retina to process the image (retinal or nerve injury)
3. Loss of the ability to process the information from the retina to higher perceptual centers via the intracranial visual pathway

3. Which structures of the eye are required to produce a clear retinal image?

A clear retinal image requires three components: a clear cornea with a normal tear film, a clear lens, and a clear vitreous (intraocular) medium.

4. List the three most common causes of visual impairment in adults.

Cataracts, macular degeneration, and chronic glaucoma. Although presbyopia is the most common cause of reduced near acuity in adults, it is not regarded as a disease.

5. How can the ophthalmoscopic exam aid in defining the etiology of decreased visual acuity?

The direct ophthalmoscopic exam is initially all that is necessary to identify the characteristics of the three most common causes of visual loss in adults. If necessary, a 1% tropicamide solution should be used to dilate the pupil in order to optimize visualization. The three major diagnoses may be suggested by the following abnormalities:

Cataract: A developing cataract is suggested by a cloudy view of the optic nerve and retinal vessels, along with loss of brightness of the red reflex.

Chronic open-angle glaucoma: If the view of the optic nerve is clear but the ratio of the optic cup to the entire nerve head area (cup-to-disc) ratio is high, chronic open-angle glaucoma may be the cause.

Macular degeneration: In a patient with central visual impairment, the examiner has a clear view of the fundus details, and the optic nerve appears normal. Drusen of the retina (beige spots that may coalesce to cause pigment abnormalities in the macular region) are commonly seen in macular degeneration. Advanced cases demonstrate scarring and disorganization of the macular retina.

6. What causes vitreous opacification?

Vitreous opacification, as evidenced by poor visibility of the fundus on ophthalmoscopic exam (not caused by cataract), may result from hemorrhage, inflammatory or infectious infiltration, and rarely tumor (lymphoma). Common causes of hemorrhage include diabetic retinopathy and retinal tears. Infectious causes include endophthalmitis and parasitic infection (toxoplasmosis, toxocariasis).

7. What causes blurring of the optic disc?

- Papilledema due to increased central nervous system pressure
- Optic neuritis (papillitis)
- Arterial ischemia to the optic disc, resulting in pale color and an edematous disc
- Retinal vein occlusion, which is usually accompanied by hemorrhages and dilated veins.

8. When should cataract removal be considered?

In the United States, 70% of people over age 75 years have an opacification of the lens, referred to as a cataract. The degree of visual acuity loss is directly proportional to the density of the cataract, provided that no other ocular disease is present. However, much controversy surrounds the timing of cataract surgery, and the health care expenditure associated with removal is enormous. Detection of the cataract is not an indication for ophthalmologic surgery. Apparent premature surgery is best avoided by carefully determining the degree to which the cataract impairs the patient's activities and safety.

9. Can a cataract cause serious ocular problems other than visual limitations due to poor light transmission?

Yes. On occasion, cataracts may contribute to various secondary disorders, including intraocular inflammation due to leaking of lens material inside the eye; chronic glaucoma resulting from the inflammatory response to liberated lens material; and acute glaucoma due to the physical apposition of the swollen lens with the iris and subsequent closure of the filtering angle.

10. Which diseases interfere with the ability of the retina to process images?

Senile macular degeneration, retinal detachment, vascular ischemia, trauma, and certain acute infections of the retina (cytomegalovirus, herpes, especially in the immunocompromised host) can interfere with the processing of retinal images.

11. What is the natural history of macular degeneration?

Macular degeneration usually occurs in patients over the age of 50 and may progress with time. Patients may have no visual symptoms initially but may develop blurring and distortion gradually in the later stages of the disease. In 10–20% of cases, subretinal hemorrhage acutely compromises visual function and leads to scarring, causing permanent visual loss. Focal laser treatments have proved to be helpful in this subset of patients with the neovascular form of the disease. Currently there is no known effective treatment for the chronic or "dry" form of the disease. Anecdotal reports suggest than vitamin and antioxidant supplementation may help to stabilize vision in some patients.

12. Why should patients be screened for glaucoma?

Chronic glaucoma causes damage to the optic nerve fibers as a result of an abnormal relationship between intraocular pressure and blood circulation. In its most common form (primary open angle) it is painless and asymptomatic until late in the course of the disease. Early visual loss occurs in the visual periphery and is typically not noticed by the patient. For these reasons, it is vital that patients be referred for glaucoma screening as part of a regimen of routine eye health care.

13. Who should be screened for glaucoma?

Risk factors for open-angle glaucoma include age (over 40 yea
and family history of glaucoma. The American Academy of Ophth
mends routine yearly screening for patients at risk.

14. What is standard therapy for patients with chronic open-angle glaucoma.

Treatment of open-angle glaucoma begins with the use of topical agents to reduce intrav.
lar pressure. Oral carbonic anhydrase inhibitors are second-line agents because of systemic side
effects. Laser therapy and intraocular surgery are reserved for patients whose condition is not
controlled effectively by medical therapy, although studies to evaluate the efficacy of early surgical intervention are ongoing.

15. What causes floaters?

Opacities in the vitreous gel may throw shadows onto the retina, causing the patient to perceive dots or webs floating in space of front of the eye. Common causes of floaters include vitreous syneresis (mild degeneration of the vitreous collagen skeleton), hemorrhage, retinal tears,
and vitreous detachment (a consequence of aging). Often the cause of floaters is not visible to the
examiner. Acute onset of floaters, especially when associated with flashing lights (photopsia),
should be referred to an ophthalmologist to rule out retinal tears or detachments.

16. What diagnoses should be considered in a patient who experiences sudden, painless unilateral loss of vision?

- Central retinal artery occlusion, often due to an embolus or vasculitis
- Giant cell arteritis resulting in central retinal artery occlusion or ischemic optic neuropathy
- Central retinal vein occlusion
- Acute hemorrhage into the vitreous element
- Optic neuritis

17. What diagnoses should be considered in a patient who complains of sudden loss of vision in both eyes?

Sudden loss of vision in both eyes is an extremely uncommon event. If the fundi are normal,
one must consider toxic neuritis or a possible conversion reaction (diagnosis of exclusion).

18. What is the classic cause of a bitemporal hemianoptic visual defect?

Lesions, usually pituitary tumors, that involve the optic chiasm.

19. What is the most common cause of severe visual loss in adolescents and young adults?

Preventable ocular trauma remains a serious public health problem. The primary care physician should counsel patients about the importance of proper eye protection during high-risk
sports and other recreational or workplace activities.

BIBLIOGRAPHY

1. American Academy of Ophthalmology: 1989–1990 Public and Professional Information Catalog. San
    Francisco, American Academy of Ophthalmology, 1989, pp 9–13.
2. American Academy of Ophthalmology: Educational Programs 1990. San Francisco, American Academy
    of Ophthalmology, 1990, pp 16–17.
3. Berson EG: Basic Ophthalmology for Medical Students and Primary Care Residents, 6th ed. San
    Francisco, American Academy of Ophthalmology, 1993.
4. Kalina RE: Seeing into the future. Vision and aging. West J Med 167:253–257, 1997.
5. Newell W: Ophthalmology: Principles and Concepts, 5th ed. St. Louis, Mosby, 1992.
6. Sussman EJ, et al: Diagnosis of diabetic eye disease. JAMA 247:3231–3234, 1982.
7. Sweet EH, et al: Eye care by primary care physicians. Ophthalmology 98:1454–1460, 1991.

EYE PAIN AND INFLAMMATORY DISEASES

Jon M. Braverman, M.D., and Thomas D. MacKenzie, M.D., M.S.P.H.

1. What are the usual sources of eye pain?

The eyelid, cornea, conjunctivae, and uveal tract (iris, ciliary body, and choroid) are the most richly innervated structures of the eye; thus, lesions affecting these areas are the most painful. Pathology limited to the vitreous element, retina, or optic nerve is likely to be painless. Optic neuritis is an exception to this rule. Diseases of the sinuses and orbit also may cause referred pain to the eye.

2. Which diseases are associated with a red eye?

A red eye is the most common ocular complaint in the general population. The presence and severity of pain and visual changes are used to distinguish the many different entities that may account for this finding.

Possible Causes of Red Eye as Determined by Associated Findings

ETIOLOGY	PAIN	VISUAL CHANGES
Acute glaucoma	Yes, severe	Acute loss
Corneal inflammation (keratitis) or ulceration	Yes	Blurring
Uveal tract or scleral inflammation	Yes, with photophobia	Blurring
Vascular or retinal disease	No	Acute or subacute loss
Conjunctival inflammation (conjunctivitis)	Sometimes	Sometimes

3. Acute-angle closure glaucoma is an absolute ocular emergency. When should the primary care provider suspect this diagnosis?

Acute elevations in intraocular pressure are far more damaging than slowly and chronically acquired elevations. The clinical presentation reflects this basic difference. Acute-angle closure glaucoma presents as an extremely painful eye (unilateral) with loss of vision. The pupil is mid-dilated and nonreactive, and marked conjunctival injection is accompanied by clouding of the cornea due to edema. The fundus is poorly visualized. This constellation of symptoms and findings requires immediate referral to an ophthalmologist.

4. What is the significance of photophobia?

Photophobia, the avoidance of light due to pain, may result from ocular or nonocular processes. Ocular photophobia results from intraocular inflammation or congestion of the structures of the uveal tract, including the iris and ciliary body, and their associated contractile muscles. During exposure to light, pupillary constriction produces pain. Thus, inflammation in any of these structures (uveitis for all; iritis, cyclitis, choroiditis) is indicated by the complaint of photophobia. Nonocular processes resulting in photophobia include migraine, meningeal irritation, and certain drugs, particularly those that cause pupillary dilation via anticholinergic properties.

5. What are the usual causes of uveitis? How is uveitis treated?

Inflammation of the uveal tract, presenting as photophobia and injection, is usually idiopathic. Abnormal pupils that react poorly to light may result from adhesions, called posterior synechiae, of the iris tissue to the lens surface. Several systemic diseases also are associated with uveitis or variable inflammation of the components of the uvea, including rheumatoid arthritis, sarcoidosis, lupus erythematosus, ankylosing spondylitis, Reiter's syndrome, inflammatory bowel disease, and juvenile rheumatoid arthritis. Infectious causes include syphilis, herpes simplex, varicella zoster, cytomegalovirus (CMV), and Lyme disease.

Treatment ranges from topical cycloplegics to systemic steroids or other immunosuppressive agents. Referral to an ophthalmologist is appropriate for work-up and treatment.

6. What are the most common causes of conjunctivitis?

Bacterial, viral, allergic, and irritant etiologies are possible. Patients usually complain of red eyes and a sticky or watery discharge. Irritation is common, but severe pain and photophobia are not. Bacterial or viral conjunctivitis is usually self-limited, but it may be treated with a topical antibiotic without steroids, such as sulfacetamide (10% 3–4 times/day). Topical aminoglycoside should be reserved for more refractory disease. Allergic conjunctivitis may be effectively treated with a new class of nonsteroidal topical antiinflammatory agents. Irritant conjunctivitis, including dry eyes, may be treated with topical, nonpreserved lubricants.

7. When are topical steroids contraindicated in the treatment of eye disorders?

Topical steroids are absolutely contraindicated in patients who have a history of herpetic eye disease or who may have herpetic infection at presentation. Such patients require referral to an ophthalmologist.

8. What is ocular medicamentosis?

Ocular medicamentosis refers to iatrogenic or medication-induced conjunctivitis. Inflammation is a reaction to prescribed medication, any of its components or contaminants, or to over-the-counter medicines or home remedies used by the patient to relieve the original conjunctivitis. This entity is improved by discontinuing all medications and using topical, nonpreserved lubricants if needed.

9. What produces the sensation of a foreign body in the eye with blinking?

- Foreign body
- Corneal abrasion
- Eyelid injury or a turned-in eyelid (which may cause an abrasion)
- Keratitis

10. What are common infectious causes of keratitis?

Herpes simplex infection and zoster dermatomal infection cause keratitis, although other viral and bacterial infections are also possible. Steroids are contraindicated in acute herpes simplex infections. Accurate diagnosis and therapy with the consultation of an ophthalmologist are paramount.

11. What principles should guide therapy for a foreign body?

1. Attempt removal under topical anesthetic only with a cooperative patient and blunt-tip instruments (a cotton applicator moistened with anesthetic is best).

2. Ascertain the mechanism of injury. Any circumstance involving high-speed microprojectiles should be further evaluated by the ophthalmologist.

3. Patch the eye after treatment and refer the patient to an ophthalmologist. Topical 10% sulfa ointment is a well-tolerated medication.

12. What is the difference between a sty and a chalazion?

A sty is painful and usually due to a bacterial infection. A chalazion is a mildly painful swelling of the eyelid margin due to granulomatous inflammation and usually resolves spontaneously with warm soaks and time. Both are common inflammations of the sebaceous glands of the eyelid.

13. Name the potential eye diseases associated with acquired immunodeficiency syndrome (AIDS).

Over one-half of all patients with AIDS have ocular complications. Cotton wool spots, due to retinal microvascular disease, are the most frequent physical finding. Ocular complications include the following:
- CMV retinitis, as evidenced by hemorrhage and exudate on funduscopic examination
- Retinal/choroidal infections due to toxoplasmosis and *Pneumocystis carinii*
- Retinal necrosis due to herpetic infections (simplex and zoster), with or without keratitis or iritis

• Orbital Kaposi's sarcoma and non-Hodgkin's lymphoma
• Optic neuropathy, sometimes a side effect of antituberculous treatment

14. What common ocular complaints should be interpreted with increased scrutiny in patients with HIV/AIDS?

Chronic dryness and foreign body sensation may be the only symptoms of corneal microsporidosis, which is often a system-wide infestation when ocular infection is diagnosed. Floaters are also a common benign complaint of healthy patients. In the HIV population, these symptoms may represent the early stages of retinitis, often due to CMV.

15. What causes cotton wool spots in the fundus?

Cotton wool spots represent ischemic injury to the superficial nerve layer of the retina. Although frequently seen in severe hypertensive retinopathy, they are not pathognomonic and also may occur with diabetes mellitus, anemia, leukemia, collagen vascular disease, endocarditis, and AIDS.

BIBLIOGRAPHY

1. American Academy of Ophthalmology: 1989–1990 Public and Professional Information Catalog. San Francisco, American Academy of Ophthalmology, 1989, pp 9–13.
2. American Academy of Ophthalmology: Educational Programs 1990. San Francisco, American Academy of Ophthalmology, 1990, pp 16–17.
3. Berson FG: Basic Ophthalmology for Medical Students and Primary Care Residents, 6th ed. San Francisco, American Academy of Ophthalmology, 1993.
4. Morrow GL, Abbott RL: Conjunctivitis. Am Fam Physician 57:735–745, 1998.
5. Newell W: Ophthalmology: Principles and Concepts, 5th ed. St. Louis, Mosby, 1992.
6. Sussman EJ, et al: Diagnosis of diabetic eye disease. JAMA 247:3231–3234, 1982.
7. Sweet EH, et al: Eye care by primary care physicians. Ophthalmology 98:1454–1460, 1991.
8. Vaughan DG, et al: General Ophthalmology, 14th ed. Norwalk, CT, Appleton & Lange, 1995.

27. HEARING LOSS AND TINNITUS

Thomas D. MacKenzie, M.D., M.S.P.H., and Michael L. Lepore, M.D., FACS

1. What are the three types of hearing loss?

1. **Conductive hearing loss** is the most common type of hearing loss in children. It is manifested by a pathologic process blocking the transmission of sound from the external auditory canal to the cochlear. Examples include cerumen impaction, otitis media in children, and otosclerosis.

2. **Sensorineural hearing loss** is the most common type of hearing loss in the elderly population. It results from an abnormality affecting the sensory cells of the cochlea or involving the neural distributions of the eighth cranial nerve. Patients with prior exposure to loud noises are more susceptible to sensorineural hearing loss and may experience the loss at an earlier age.

3. **Mixed hearing loss** is not as common as the other types of hearing loss. It is a combination of the above types. The patient has a neurosensory component and a conductive component on hearing tests. Mixed hearing loss is commonly seen in patients with a long history of chronic otitis media with intermittent otorrhea and evidence of cholesteatoma.

2. What percentage of adults over the age of 65 years have a handicapping hearing loss?

Data from the National Health Interview Study in 1989 indicate that approximately 29% of people over age 65 years and 36% of people over age 75 years have a hearing loss severe enough to interfere with effective conversation. Presbycusis, the most common variety, may be defined as an unexplained, slowly progressive decline in aural sensitivity due to the aging process. The hearing loss is usually symmetric, as is noise-induced hearing loss.

3. Why does hearing loss progress to a severe state before the patient seeks assistance?

The aging process may be accompanied by a number of chronic physical conditions of which the patient is acutely aware. Hearing loss, however, most commonly develops over many years and is therefore overshadowed by the acuity of concurrent conditions. The patient unknowingly develops coping mechanisms and does not notice an acute change in hearing until a severe loss is present.

4. What psychological effects of hearing loss may offer clues to its presence?

Patients often withdraw from their surroundings. They may demonstrate conversational manipulation, phobic behavior, paranoia, and mood disorders. The most frequent symptoms are mood disorders, as manifested by insomnia, loss of appetite, guilt, fatigue, anxiety, and uncontrolled emotional outbursts.

5. How does one evaluate the patient with presbycusis?

A careful history and a high index of suspicion in particularly susceptible patients are extremely important to identify warning signs. All elderly patients should undergo evaluation of hearing. Particularly important signs are difficulty with hearing in a room with other people and turning up the sound on the television set. Tinnitus is also an early symptom of hearing loss. A careful history of previous exposure to loud noise is important to ascertain. If hearing loss is suspected, an audiometric evaluation should be performed to determine the type and quality.

6. What level of noise exposure may contribute to hearing loss?

Long exposure to noise over 90 dB SPL (sound pressure level) may cause progressive symmetrical hearing loss. Sources of chronic noise exposure with corresponding dB SPL levels are listed below:

Riveting steel tank	130	Boiler shop	100
Automobile horn	120	Hydraulic press	100
Sandblasting	112	Can manufacturing plant	100
Wood-working shop	100	Subway	90
Punch press	100	Average factory	80
Pneumatic drill	100		

7. How is sudden sensorineural hearing loss (sudden deafness) defined?

For research purposes, it is defined as sensorineural hearing loss of 30 dB or more over at least 3 contiguous audiometric frequencies within 3 days or less.

8. What is the most common cause of sudden deafness?

The incidence of sudden deafness is reported to be 5–20 per 100,000 persons per year. This figure, however, is probably higher because some patients recover so rapidly that they do not seek medical attention. The common etiology of sudden deafness is idiopathic sudden sensorineural hearing loss. Characteristically approximately one-third of patients develop hearing loss upon waking in the morning, and about one-half also notice disequilibrium or frank vertigo. The intensity of the vertigo usually corresponds to the severity of the hearing loss. Some of the predisposing factors associated with idiopathic sudden sensorineural loss include changes in the physical environment, such as altitude or atmospheric pressure; emotional disturbances; diabetes; atherosclerosis; pregnancy; use of contraceptive drugs; and stress of surgery, physical exertion, or general anesthesia.

9. What are the specific causes of acute hearing loss?

1. **Viral infections** may affect the cochlea by causing labyrinthitis or direct inflammation of the cochlear nerve. Measles, mumps, influenza, and adenoviruses have been associated with sudden deafness. Herpes zoster has been shown to produce a viral neuronitis or ganglionitis.

2. **Tumors** of the cerebellopontine angle may produce sudden deafness.

3. **Damage to the organ of Corti** may be induced by sneezing, coughing, bending, the Valsalva maneuver, or scuba diving.

4. **Rupture of the round or oval window** is usually accompanied by positional nystagmus. A positive fistula sign is demonstrated by applying positive pressure to the tympanic membrane, which causes ipsilateral nystagmus.

10. When should aggressive evaluation of a patient with sudden hearing loss be undertaken?

Initial evaluation of all patients should include a careful history, otologic and neurologic examination, audiologic testing, and routine laboratory studies. If hearing does not return in 1 month or if serial audiograms demonstrate progressive loss, computerized tomography (CT) or magnetic resonance imaging (MRI) with gadolinium of the internal auditory meatus should be performed to rule out the presence of an acoustic tumor.

11. What is the anticipated natural history of idiopathic sensorineural hearing loss?

Age appears to play a significant role in recovery. Patients under the age of 40 years recover normal hearing approximately 50% of the time. The more severe the hearing loss, the less likely the recovery. The presence of vertigo is a bad prognostic sign. Spontaneous recovery may occur within days or weeks; if the loss persists beyond 1 month, there is little likelihood for recovery.

12. Why should patients with an idiopathic sensorineural hearing loss without resolution be tested for syphilis?

In its late phase syphilis may cause sensorineural loss as the only manifestation of disease. Approximately 7% of patients with otherwise unexplained sensorineural hearing loss have a positive treponemal antibody test, as do 7% of patients with Ménière's disease. Thus, any patient with a positive treponemal antibody test and unexplained hearing loss should be treated for syphilitic otitis.

13. What other infectious disease may lead to hearing loss?

Tuberculosis may cause sensorineural and conductive hearing loss, although this is unlikely in the absence of pulmonary disease.

14. What commonly used medications may lead to hearing loss?

Aminoglycosides; loop diuretics, such as furosemide; salicylates; antineoplastic agents, such as cisplatin; interferon; and piroxicam.

15. How do the Weber and Rinne tests help in delineating the origin of hearing loss?

Both tests are used to determine whether hearing loss is conductive or sensorineural. The **Weber test** is done by placing the stem of the tuning fork midline on the skull and asking the patient whether the tone is heard in one ear better than in the other. The tone is louder on the side on which the balance of bone (sensorineural) to conductive hearing sensation is greatest. For example, if a patient has wax in the right ear, an ipsilateral conductive hearing loss causes a relative increase in bone (sensorineural) conduction. Thus, the Weber test lateralizes to the right. By contrast, an acoustic neuroma on the right side is accompanied by a relative decrease in bone conduction; thus, the Weber test lateralizes to the opposite side.

The **Rinne test** is done by placing the vibrating tuning fork on the mastoid process and asking the patient to acknowledge when the sound is no longer audible (bone conduction). At that point, the vibrating bells of the tuning fork are held at the external auditory canal. The patient normally should hear the tone better by air conduction than by bone conduction.

16. What precautions should be taken before removing impacted wax?

Before removing impacted ear wax by irrigation, the patient should be questioned about a history of perforated tympanic membrane or chronic otitis media. Care also must be exercised in the diabetic patient to avoid trauma to the ear canal and secondary external otitis. In patients with perforations or previously draining ears, the cerumen must be removed by using a microscope. To avoid complications, such patients should be referred to an otolaryngologist.

17. What potentially life-threatening disorder is heralded by new-onset tinnitus?

Tinnitus, a common symptom in primary care practice, is characterized by the complaint of ringing or any other abnormal sound in the ear. Most disorders associated with tinnitus are not life-threatening. However, tinnitus may be a prominent manifestation of one medical emergency: salicylate toxicity. Elderly patients who take aspirin chronically, as opposed to patients taking acute overdoses, experience the highest mortality rate from salicylism. One needs to ask specifically about aspirin intake, because many patients do not consider it a prescribed medicine. When in doubt, an aspirin level is appropriate. Other manifestations of salicylism should be sought.

18. What are the most common causes of tinnitus?

Tinnitus can be broadly divided into objective and subjective categories. **Objective tinnitus** is less common and often can be heard not only be the patient but also by the examiner. Causes of objective tinnitus include vascular abnormalities, such as arteriovenous shunts, arterial bruits, venous hums, and mechanical abnormalities, such as disorders of the eustachian tube and stapedial muscle spasm. This type of tinnitus may be pulsatile in the case of vascular disorders or may change character based on the position of the head, pharynx, or jaw. **Subjective tinnitus** is far more common and most likely arises from damaged cochlear hair cells that discharge discontinuously. The vast majority of patients with subjective tinnitus have an otologic disorder.

19. What categories of medication have been implicated in causing tinnitus?

Diuretics (Diamox), beta blockers (metoprolol), antibiotics (gentamicin), angiotensin-converting enzyme inhibitors (enalapril), antimalarials (chloroquine), narcotics (pentazocine), NSAIDs (diclofenac), antihistamines (promethazine), and anesthetics (lidocaine).

20. Which diseases are associated with unilateral tinnitus?

The majority of subjective tinnitus is bilateral. Unilateral tinnitus is usually due to an otologic disorder, such as chronic suppurative otitis, trauma, or Ménière's disease. In the absence of these diagnoses, work-up should include an MRI scan in search of a central auditory lesion.

21. Who should be involved in the diagnosis and management of severe tinnitus?

The primary care provider may need assistance from specialists in audiology, otolaryngology, neurology, and occasionally psychiatry. The audiologist localizes the pathology to the ear or to the central nervous system and through special testing detects the pitch and loudness of the tinnitus, the minimal masking level that eliminates the tinnitus, and the residual inhibition. An otolaryngologist or neurologist performs a thorough evaluation of the ears, nose, throat, head, and neck regions to determine the presence of any pathology that may explain the tinnitus. A neurologist may be required for diagnosis if a central lesion is suspected. In patients who are refractory to treatment or who have unexplained tinnitus, associated pyschologic disorders may require management.

22. How frequently can tinnitus be controlled?

About 30–40% of patients who report severe tinnitus may be treated, whereas 45–60% respond well to maskers or amplification instruments. Therefore, only 10–15% are refractory to therapy. In addition to addressing local otologic problems as an etiology, any eustachian tube dysfunction should be corrected, because it may significantly intensify tinnitus. Adequate ventilation of the eustachian tube and middle ear is achieved through the use of antihistamines and decongestants.

23. What advice should be given to patients with tinnitus?

1. Avoid loud noises, caffeine, drug use, alcohol excess, and tobacco.
2. Maintain an active lifestyle.
3. Join support groups such as the American Tinnitus Association (Portland, OR).

24. What is Ramsay Hunt syndrome?

Ramsay Hunt syndrome is a constellation of cranial nerve disorders resulting from recrudescence of latent varicella zoster virus infection of the facial nerve. The clinical presentation consists of severe otalgia associated with characteristic vesicular eruptions of the auditory canal and pinna. Complications of Ramsay Hunt syndrome arise from involvement of cranial nerves V, IX, and X and include facial paralysis, tinnitus, hearing loss, hyperacusis, vertigo, dysguesia, and decreased tearing. The syndrome is also called herpes zoster oticus. It is about one-fifth as common as Bell's palsy.

BIBLIOGRAPHY

1. Adour KK: Otologic complications of herpes zoster. Ann Neurol 35:S62–S64, 1994.
2. Barker RL, Burton JR, Zieve PD (eds): Principles of Ambulatory Medicine. Baltimore, William & Wilkins, 1991.
3. Bauer CA, Coker NJ: Update on facial nerve disorders. Otolaryngol Clin North Am 29:445–454, 1996.
4. Dobie RA: Noise-induced hearing loss. In Bailey BJ (ed): Head and Neck Surgery—Otolaryngology. Philadelphia, J.B. Lippincott, 1993, pp 1782–1792.
5. Hughes GB, Freedman MA, Haberdamp TJ, Guay ME: Sudden sensorineural hearing loss. Otolaryngol Clin North Am 29:393–403, 1996.
6. Kohut RI, Hinojosak R: Sudden hearing loss. In Bailey BJ, et al (eds): Head and Neck Surgery—Otolaryngology, vol 2. Philadelphia, J.B. Lippincott, 1993, p 1820.
7. Koopmann CF Jr: Otolaryngologic (head and neck) problems in the elderly. Med Clin North Am 75:1373–1388, 1991.
8. Lavizzo-Mourey RJ, Siegler EL: Hearing impairment in the elderly. J Gen Intern Med 7:191–198, 1992.
9. Lichtenstein MJ: Hearing and visual impairments. Clin Geriatr Med 8:173–182, 1992.
10. Mattox DE, Wilkins SA: Tinnitus. In American Academy of Otolaryngology—Head and Neck Surgery Self-Instructional Package. Rochester, NY, Mosby, 1989.
11. Nadol JB: Hearing loss. N Engl J Med 329:1092–1102, 1993.
12. Patt BS, Meyerhoff WL: Aging and auditory vestibular system. In Bailey BJ, et al (eds): Head and Neck Surgery—Otolaryngology, vol 2. Philadelphia, J.B. Lippincott, 1993, p 1843.
13. Pensak ML, Adelman RA: Conductive hearing loss. In Cummings DW (ed): Otolaryngology—Head and Neck Surgery, vol 4, 2nd ed. St. Louis, Mosby, 1993.
14. Schleuning AJ: Management of the patient with tinnitus. Med Clin North Am 76:1225–1237, 1991.
15. Seidman MD, Jacobson GP: Update on tinnitus. Otolaryngol Clin North Am 29:455–465, 1996.
16. Shikowitz MJ: Sudden sensorineural hearing loss. Med Clin North Am 75:1239–1250, 1991.
17. Shulman A: Electrodiagnostics, Electrotherapeutics and Other Approaches to the Management of Tinnitus. American Academy of Otolaryngology—Head and Neck Surgery Instructional Courses, vol 2. St. Louis, Mosby, 1989, p 137.
18. Vernon J, Schleuning AJ: Tinnitus: Its Care and Treatment. American Academy of Otolaryngology—Head and Neck Surgery Instructional Courses, vol 2. St. Louis, Mosby, 1989, p 131.
19. Vesterager V: Tinnitus—Investigation and management. BMJ 314:728–731, 1997.

28. EAR PAIN AND INFECTIONS

Thomas D. MacKenzie, M.D., M.S.P.H., and Michael L. Lepore, M.D., FACS

1. Which two cranial nerves are involved in the pathways for referral of ear pain?

Cranial nerves IX and X are the major nerves involved in causing referred ear pain (otalgia). The auricular nerve of Arnold and the internal branch of the superior laryngeal nerve provide sensory innervation from the ear and larynx, respectively; both are branches of the vagus nerve (cranial nerve X). The tympanic nerve (Jacobson's nerve), a branch of the glossopharyngeal nerve (cranial nerve IX) from the tympanic membrane and middle ear, and branches of the glossopharyngeal nerve from the oropharynx provide sensory innervation from their respective regions. Any pathologic condition involving the sensory innervations of these nerves may cause referred ear pain.

2. What entities cause ear pain?

Otalgia is a frequent complaint with multiple possible causes. Patients may have a pathologic process confined to the ear (primary origin), or the pain may be referred to the ear from another source (secondary otalgia). Because most of the ear develops embryonically from the first (mandibular) and second (hyoid) branchial arches, any process in the distribution of the two arches from the larynx and pharynx to the skull base may refer pain to the ear. Some of the common causes of primary otalgia are listed below.

Common Causes of Primary Otalgia

PINNA AND EXTERNAL CANAL	MIDDLE EAR AND MASTOID
Furunculosis	Acute otitis media
External otitis	Acute mastoiditis
Foreign body in the external canal	Acute eustachian tube obstruction
Impacted cerumen	
Acute myringitis and myringitis bullosa	
Trauma to tympanic membrane	
Perichondritis	

Causes of secondary otalgia include dental pathology, cancer of the larynx and piriform sinus, tonsillitis, peritonsillar abscess, arthritis of the cricoarytenoid joint, nasopharyngeal pathology, temporomandibular joint disease, and lesions of the esophagus.

3. What is swimmer's ear?

Swimmer's ear is otitis externa, an extremely painful inflammatory process of the external ear canal and auricle. It is often associated with swimming and is a frequent diagnosis in primary care, especially in children. The disease is usually highly responsive to otic antibiotic therapy. However, prevention of recurrence may require the use of ear protection with swimming.

4. Who is at risk for serious complications associated with otitis externa?

Patients over the age of 50 years and patients with diabetes are at risk for severe complications related to simple otitis externa. The disease may progress rapidly to a life-threatening condition of necrotizing (malignant) otitis externa. This syndrome is characterized by severe pain, purulent discharge, and progressive cellulitis of the ear and the base of the skull. If not adequately treated, otitis externa may be complicated by facial and other cranial nerve palsies, meningitis, mastoiditis, parotitis, osteomyelitis of the temporal bone or base of the skull, and death. It is frequently caused by *Pseudomonas aeruginosa*, and treatment requires specific oral antipseudomonal antibiotics. In the more severe forms complicated by cranial nerve involvement, hospitalization with intravenous antibiotics and surgical intervention may be required.

5. What causes otorrhea?

Otorrhea is a discharge from the ear canal associated with disease of both the middle ear and external canal. Disorders of the middle ear that result in otorrhea include acute otitis media with perforation (or the presence of a tympanostomy tube) and chronic suppurative otitis media. Disorders of the external canal that lead to otorrhea include otitis externa and necrotizing otitis externa.

6. How is otitis media classified?

For purposes of treatment and evaluation, otitis media is classified as acute (< 3 weeks' duration), subacute (3 weeks–3 months), and chronic (> 3 months).

7. Name the four pathogens most commonly identified in acute otitis media.

Streptococcus pneumoniae (most common)   Group A streptococci
Haemophilus influenzae   *Moraxella catarrhalis*

8. What is the most important factor in the pathogenesis of middle ear disease?

Abnormal function of the eustachian tube appears to be the most important pathogenic factor. The normal eustachian tube serves three functions: (1) it provides protection from nasopharyngeal secretions and sound pressure; (2) it acts to clear middle ear secretions by its mucociliary activity; and (3) it provides a ventilatory function for the middle ear. This function depends on gas absorption and on the characteristics of the mastoid air-cell system of the middle ear.

9. What is the most reasonable treatment approach to an acute episode of otitis media?

Uncomplicated otitis media should be treated with oral antimicrobials. Amoxicillin should be considered the drug of first choice; additional considerations include trimethoprim-sulfamethoxazole, erythromycin, sulfisoxazole, amoxicillin-clavulanate, and cefaclor. Clinical improvement should be evident in 72 hours, and a 10-day course is usually adequate. If no significant improvement is seen with amoxicillin, a beta-lactamase–producing organism should be suspected and antibiotic therapy should be changed. In refractory acute cases, tympanocentesis with or without myringotomy relieves pain, and culture of the middle ear effusion may yield the causative organism.

10. How does otitis media in neonates or young children differ from otitis media in older children or adults?

In neonates and young infants, the incidence of unusual organisms, particularly gram-negative bacilli and *Staphylococcus aureus*, is higher.

11. What is the incidence of persistent middle ear effusion after a 10-day course of antibiotics?

Up to 50% of patients are clinically well but have a persistent middle ear infection after a full course of antibiotics. Several options should be considered, because persistent effusions may lead to hearing loss with speech and language delay as well as provide a medium for bacterial growth. The patient should be treated for a longer time with the same antimicrobial agent, and systemic decongestants and/or antihistamines should be used to encourage evacuation of the eustachian tube. The Valsalva maneuver may be performed in the physician's office to inflate the eustachian tube.

A middle ear effusion may persist for approximately 3 months after an acute episode of otitis media resolves. However, if the patient is asymptomatic, watchful waiting is a reasonable approach. If the patient is continuously symptomatic, a more aggressive approach is necessary. In children with multiple episodes of acute otitis media with or without persistent middle ear effusions, speech and language delays may result from hearing loss.

12. What considerations must be given to adults who fail to resolve otitis media or a middle ear effusion?

In adults the nasopharynx must be examined carefully and repeatedly for pathology. Nasopharyngeal carcinoma and lymphoma may cause intermittent or persistent middle ear problems.

13. How is recurrent otitis media managed?

The development of recurrent otitis media should be considered an indication for intervention. Initially diseases that have a role in the etiology of recurrent episodes must be considered, including sinusitis, nasal allergy, immune deficiency, nasopharyngeal pathology, cleft palate, and submucosal palate. A child with recurrent episodes of otitis media and persistent middle ear effusion may be treated more aggressively. Chemoprophylaxis with chronic antibiotics may be used. Myringotomy, which may decrease the frequency of episodes and possible complications, should be considered carefully.

14. What are the consequences of untreated or inadequately treated acute otitis media?

Because of the widespread use of antimicrobial therapy, the incidence of complications from acute otitis media has decreased dramatically. However, because of the potential for serious morbidity, complications must be recognized early. Intracranial complications include lateral sinus thrombophlebitis, extradural abscesses, subdural abscesses, brain abscess, and meningitis. Local complications include conductive or sensorineural hearing loss; perforation of the tympanic membrane; chronic suppurative otitis media with or without cholesteatoma; atelectasis with retraction pockets and adhesions of the tympanic membrane; and erosion of the incus with ossicular discontinuity, labyrinthitis, and facial nerve paralysis.

15. What is Gradenigo's syndrome?

Gradenigo's syndrome is the triad of otalgia, otorrhea, and paralysis of the abducens nerve. It occurs as a complication of otitis media and requires immediate referral to an otolaryngologist.

16. What are the signs of coalescent mastoiditis in children?

With the emergence of antibiotic-resistant microorganisms, a slight increase in the number of children presenting with clinical signs and symptoms of acute mastoiditis has been noted. The presenting signs are varied and include any of the following: pain behind the ear, tenderness over the mastoid, persistent aural discharge, displacement of the auricle, fever, leukocytosis, and conductive hearing loss. The auricular displacement is characteristic in that the ear is pointing downward and outward as a result of a subperiosteal abscess that ruptures above the insertion of the sternocleidomastoid muscle. Occasionally, if the abscess breaks through the attachment of the posterior belly of the digastric muscle, the child presents with a neck mass signifying the presence of a deep neck abscess.

17. How is chronic otitis media manifested?

Chronic otitis media is an indolent inflammatory process involving the eustachian tube, middle ear, and mastoid air-cell system. Two varieties are commonly recognized: chronic suppurative otitis media (CSOM) and chronic otitis media with effusion (COME). Both conditions begin in childhood, usually in patients with a history of recurrent otitis media. In CSOM, hearing loss, painless otorrhea, and tympanic perforation are common. In COME, the hallmark is a 24–40 dB conductive hearing loss.

18. What is the most serious complication of chronic otitis media?

The development of cholesteatoma is the most serious complication of chronic otitis media. In the presence of chronic otitis media, retraction pockets or cysts form in the middle ear and are lined by skin. Desquamation leads to a build-up of keratin. Keratin-containing cysts, called cholesteatomas, invade the surrounding bone, leading to facial nerve paralysis, vertigo, and meningitis. As they grow in the middle ear, the cysts may cause destruction of the incus, stapes, and malleus, leading to severe conductive hearing loss. Cholesteatomas are often visible as a white ball in the middle ear. Their presence is usually an indication for surgery.

BIBLIOGRAPHY

1. Barker RL, Burton JR, Zieve PD (eds): Principles of Ambulatory Medicine. Baltimore, Williams & Wilkins, 1991.
2. Bartoshuk LM, Kveton JF, Karrer T: Taste. In Bailey J (eds): Head and Neck Surgery—Otolaryngology, vol 1. Philadelphia, J.B. Lippincott, 1993, p 520.
3. Bluestone CD, Klein JO: Otitis Media in Infants and Children. Philadelphia, W.B. Saunders, 1995.
4. Chartrand SA, Pong A: Acute otitis media in the 1990s: The impact of antibiotic resistance. Pediatr Ann 27:86–95, 1998.
5. Hirsh BE: Infections of the external ear. Am J Otolaryngol 13(3):145–155, 1992.
6. Jahn AF: Chronic otitis media: Diagnosis and treatment. Med Clin North Am 75:1277–1291, 1991.
7. Kenna MA: Otitis media with effusion. In Bailey BJ, et al (eds): Head and Neck Surgery—Otolaryngology, vol 2. Philadelphia, J.B. Lippincott, 1993, p 1592.
8. Lee KJ: Essential Otolaryngology. New Haven, CT, Medical Examination Publishing, 1995.
9. Paparella MM: Otalgia. In Paparella MM, et al (eds): Otolaryngology, vol 2. Philadelphia, W.B. Saunders, 1980, p 1354.
10. Pelton SI, Klein JO: The draining ear. Otitis media and externa. Infect Dis Clin North Am 2:117–129, 1988.
11. Rubin J, Yu VL: Malignant external otitis: Insights into pathogenesis, clinical manifestations, diagnosis, and therapy. Am J Med 85:391–398, 1988.
12. Shambaugh GE: Surgery of the Ear, 2nd ed. Philadelphia, W.B. Saunders, 1967, pp 251–255.

29. SORE THROAT AND HOARSENESS

Andrew W. Steele, M.D., M.P.H.

1. What are the main causes of sore throat?
About 50% of cases of sore throat are caused by viruses. The most common viruses include adenovirus, influenzavirus, parainfluenza virus, coxsackievirus, rhinovirus, coronavirus, and respiratory syncytial virus. About 20% of cases are caused by bacteria. Group A beta-hemolytic streptococcus (GAS) is the most common cause, accounting for about 10–20% of pharyngitis in adults. Other bacterial causes for pharyngitis include nongroup A streptococci (C and G), *Mycoplasma pneumoniae, Chlamydia trachomatis, Neisseria gonorrhoeae, Haemophilus influenzae,* and *Corynebacterium diphtheriae.* In about 30% of cases, no cause is found. The causes in such cases are believed to be a combination of environmental factors, allergies, and mouth-breathing. Common causes in immunocompromised hosts include *Candida albicans* (thrush), herpes simplex virus, and cytomegalovirus (CMV). Rare noninfectious causes of sore throat include tortuous carotid artery, thyroiditis, spontaneous pneumomediastinum, lymphoma, and leukemia.

2. What three life-threatening infections may present with severe sore throat in adults?
(1) Epigottitis, (2) peritonsillar abscess, and (3) retropharyngeal abscess are usually accompanied by evidence of pharyngitis, fever, and malaise. In all three cases clues may be provided by the presence of odynophagia, drooling, and voice changes. Epiglottitis is usually abrupt in onset in children; in adults it may be less acute, although still complicated by airway obstruction, especially when stridor and erect posture are evident. Peritonsillar and retropharyngeal abscesses may be insidious in nature. *Haemophilus influenzae* type b remains a cause of epiglottitis in adults, whereas peritonsillar and retropharyngeal abscesses are frequently polymicrobial (especially anaerobes); *Streptococcus pyogenes* is the most commonly isolated pathogen.

3. What presenting clinical features help to distinguish viral from bacterial pharyngitis?

Causes of Pharyngitis

SYMPTOM	VIRAL	BACTERIAL
Cough	Common	Rare
Rhinitis	Common	Occasional
Red throat	Common	Common
Fever (> 38.0° C)	Occasional	Common
Exudate	Occasional	Common
Tender anterior cervical nodes	Occasional	Common
Enlarged tonsils	Occasional	Common

4. Why should the primary care provider treat streptococcal infection?
1. Treatment prevents rheumatic fever.
2. Treatment prevents suppurative complications.
3. Treatment shortens the course of illness with decreased fevers and decreased pain by 24–48 hours.
4. Treatment decreases person-to-person spread of disease.

5. What is the probability that a person with streptococcal pharyngitis will develop acute rheumatic fever?

The probability of developing acute rheumatic fever depends on whether the patient has epidemic or endemic pharyngitis. For epidemic GAS, the probability of developing acute rheumatic fever is about 3%. In endemic areas the probability is about 0.3%. At least one-third of episodes of acute rheumatic fever result from unrecognized streptococcal infections.

6. Does treatment for GAS pharyngitis protect against poststreptococcal glomerulonephritis?

Most studies have not shown a protective effect of treatment on the development of poststreptococcal glomerulonephritis.

7. To what degree does antibiotic treatment lower the risk of developing acute rheumatic fever?

Treatment has been shown to decrease the risk of subsequent acute rheumatic fever by 90%. This effect may occur even if antibiotics are started later than 9 days after the onset of symptoms. To be fully effective, antibiotics should be given for 10 days.

8. How often do patients with acute rheumatic fever develop cardiac disease?

Assuming that patients with acute rheumatic fever receive appropriate prophylactic antibiotic therapy, about 1% subsequently develop severe cardiac disease (class IV rheumatic heart disease) and 4% develop debilitating rheumatic heart disease.

9. What are the main local suppurative complications of GAS?

The main complications are peritonsillar abscess (quinsy) and retropharyngeal abscess. Less common complications include suppurative otitis media and cervical lymphadenitis. It is estimated that antibiotic treatment decreases the suppurative complications from about 5% to less than 1%.

10. What is the recommended treatment for acute streptococcal pharyngitis?

The drug of choice is penicillin V with a newly recommended dose of 500 mg 2–3 times daily for 10 days. Benzathine penicillin G, given intramuscularly in a dose of 1.2 million units, is also effective. Amoxicillin also may be used but has a higher incidence of associated rashes. For penicillin-allergic patients, the first choice is erythromycin, 250 mg 4 times daily for 10 days. Azithromycin, clarithromycin, and oral cephalosporins also may be used, although they have not yet been proved in clinical trials to prevent acute rheumatic fever. The length of treatment is crucial; failure rate decreases when treatment is increased from 7 to 10 days. Recent meta-analysis has shown that cephalosporins may have higher eradication rates than penicillin, but concern still exists over higher costs and problems related to using broad-spectrum antibiotics.

11. Do you need to reculture after treatment to confirm eradication of GAS?

No. Treatment has been shown to be 85–90% effective in numerous studies. Patients with culture-positive GAS after treatment appear to have strains of streptococcus that are not associated with developing acute rheumatic fever. Follow-up cultures should be considered in patients with persistent or recurring symptoms or patients who have had rheumatic fever and are at high risk for recurrence.

12. How should the care provider decide when empirical treatment for suspected GAS is appropriate in a patient with sore throat?

1. Determine the clinical probability that the patient has GAS on the basis of the history and physical examination. The probability (%) of GAS pharyngitis based on prevalence and clinical findings is determined by the "strep score," which is derived by giving 1 point for each of the following: tonsillar exudate, anterior cervical lymphadenopathy, absence of cough, and presence of fever.

Strep Score	Prevalence	
	IN MOST OFFICE PRACTICES (%)	IN EMERGENCY DEPARTMENT (%)
0	1	3
1	4	8
2	9	18
3	21	38
4	43	63

Adapted from Centor RM, Meier FA, Dalton HP: Throat cultures and rapid tests for diagnosis of group A streptococcal pharyngitis. Ann Intern Med 105:892, 1986.

2. Use the predicted probability of GAS in the following evaluation and treatment algorithm:

< 5% (score < 1)	**5–40% (score = 2 or 3)**	**> 40% (score = 4)**
↓	↓	↓
No treatment	Rapid antigen test	Treat with antibiotics
Treat symptomatically	↓ ↓	No diagnostic test
No diagnostic tests	(−) (+)	
	↓ ↓	
	No treatment Treat with antibiotics	
	↓	
	Perform throat culture	
	(−) (+)	
	↓ ↓	
	No treatment Treat with antibiotics	

13. Should rapid strep test kits be used to guide the treatment of GAS?

Many rapid strep test kits or antigen detection tests (ADTs) are available to help in the diagnosis of GAS. In general, they have a sensitivity of about 70–90% and a specificity of 90–98%. The low sensitivity may be mainly operator-dependent, and newer optical immunoassay tests have shown sensitivities close to 95% when studied in pediatric populations. Currently, a positive rapid test is adequate to initiate treatment, but a negative test should be followed by a blood agar plate culture.

14. When should you refer recurrent sore throats to an ENT specialist?

In general, if a patient has three or more episodes in 1 year and has been appropriately treated, he or she should be referred for ENT evaluation.

15. What are the most common causes of hoarseness?

Hoarseness is due to abnormal vibration of the vocal cords, which may result from local disorders or paralysis of the laryngeal nerve. The most common cause of hoarseness is local inflammation of the vocal cords due to viral laryngitis or voice abuse. Other local causes result from laryngeal carcinoma, papillomas and polyps, trauma, or irritants. The common causes of laryngeal nerve paralysis in adults are carcinoma (20%), nerve injury from cardiomegaly, chest trauma, or other factors (23%); surgical damage (23%); and inflammatory lesions or lesions of the central nervous systems such as stroke (14%).

16. What is the best medical treatment for hoarseness?

The patient with hoarseness should rest the voice and stop smoking (if this applies). Humidifiers at home and work may help. Underlying diseases should be treated when possible (e.g., antibiotics for bacterial infections and thyroid hormone replacement for myxedema).

17. When should a complaint of hoarseness undergo more aggressive evaluation?

Hoarseness that persists for 6–8 weeks, especially in smokers, or that is accompanied by other symptoms suggestive of malignancy (mass, neck or chest pain, weight loss, shortness of breath, and aspiration) should be evaluated immediately.

18. What systemic medical diseases may be associated with hoarseness?

Hypothyroidism, rheumatoid arthritis (cricoarytenoid arthritis), and diabetes mellitus.

19. What is the initial evaluation of hoarseness?

After the history and physical examination, indirect laryngoscopy should be performed to evaluate voice quality, vocal cord mobility, and presence or absence of masses.

BIBLIOGRAPHY

1. Blumer JL, Goldfarb J: Meta-analysis in the evaluation of treatment for streptococcal pharyngitis: A review. Clin Ther 16:604–620, 1994.
2. Centor RM, Meier FA, Dalton HP: Throat cultures and rapid tests for diagnosis of group A streptococcal pharyngitis. Ann Intern Med 105:892, 1986.
3. Centor RM, Meier FA: Sore throat. In Dornbrand L, Hoole A, Fletcher R (eds): Manual of Clinical Problems in Adult Ambulatory Care, 3rd ed. Philadelphia, Lippincott-Raven, 1997, pp 76–82.
4. Dajani A, Taubert K, Ferrieri P, and other Committee Members: Treatment of acute streptococcal pharyngitis and prevention of rheumatic fever: A statement for health professionals. Pediatrics 96:758–764, 1995.
5. Frantz TD, Rasgon BM, Quesenberry CP: Acute epiglottitis in adults. JAMA 272:1358–1360, 1994.
6. Gerber MA, Tanz RR, Kabat W, et al: Optical immunoassay test for group A β-hemolytic streptococcal pharyngitis. JAMA 277:899–903, 1997.
7. Goldenberg D, Golz A, Joachims HZ: Retropharyngeal abscess: A clinical review. J Laryngol Otol 3:546–550, 1997.
8. Hillner BE, Centor RM: What a difference a day makes: A decision analysis of adult streptococcal pharyngitis. J Gen Intern Med 2:242, 1987.
9. Kline JA, Runge JW: Streptococcal pharyngitis: A review of pathophysiology, diagnosis, and management. J Emerg Med 12:665–680, 1994.
10. Komaroff AL, Pass TM, Aronson MD, et al: The prediction of streptococcal pharyngitis in adults. J Gen Intern Med 1:1, 1986.
11. Koster F: Respiratory tract infections. In Barker LR, Burton JR, Zieve PD (eds): Principles of Ambulatory Medicine. Baltimore, Williams & Wilkins, 1991, pp 303–320.
12. Maragos ND: Hoarseness. Primary Care 17:347, 1990.
13. Mayo-Smith MF, Spinale JW, Konskey CJ, et al: Acute epiglottitis. An 18 year experience in Rhode Island. Chest 108:1640–1647, 1995.
14. Millan SB, Cumming WA: Supraglottic infections. Prim Care 23:741–758, 1996.
15. Randolph MF, Gerber MA, DeMeo KK, Wright L: Effect of antibiotic therapy on the clinical course of streptococcal pharyngitis. J Pediatr 106:870, 1985.
16. Tompkins RK, Burnes DC, Cable BS: An analysis of the cost-effectiveness of pharyngitis management and acute rheumatic fever prevention. Ann Intern Med 86:481, 1977.

30. ORAL LESIONS

Thomas D. MacKenzie, M.D., M.S.P.H., and Michael L. Lepore, M.D., FACS

1. What is the most common cause of xerostomia (dry mouth)?

Medications are the most common cause of oral dryness, especially in older persons. In fact, increased use of medications in the geriatric population may explain the widely believed myth that salivary gland dysfunction is part of the normal aging process. The mechanisms by which medications may cause xerostomia include salivary gland hypofunction, mucosal dehydration, total body dehydration, altered sensory function, and cognitive disorders. Medications that frequently decrease salivary flow rates by blocking cholinergic activity are tricyclic antidepressants; antipsychotics; centrally acting antihypertensives such as clonidine; diphenhydramine; and the belladonna alkaloids, such as atropine, scopolamine, and hyoscyamine.

2. What medical conditions are commonly associated with xerostomia?

The two most common medical conditions associated with xerostomia are Sjögren's syndrome and radiation-induced salivary gland dysfunction. In its primary form Sjögren's syndrome is characterized by lymphocytic infiltration of the salivary and lacrimal glands, thus leading to dry mouth and dry eyes. It also may occur in association with another major rheumatologic disease, such as rheumatoid arthritis, systemic lupus erythematosus, primary biliary cirrhosis, or scleroderma. The vast majority of patients with radiation-induced salivary gland dysfunction have received ionizing radiation for head and neck carcinoma. A number of other disorders may lead to dysfunction of one or more of the major salivary glands (parotid, submandibular, and sublingual). Patients are rarely symptomatic because salivary flow must decrease by approximately 50% before xerostomia develops.

3. Why should salivary gland hypofunction raise concern?

Saliva contains various polypeptides and glycoproteins that have antimicrobial activity. In the absence of these elements, the patient is prone to recurrent oral candidiasis and dental decay.

4. What is the most common cause of recurrent painful mouth sores?

Aphthous ulcers are the most common type of nontraumatic mouth sores. In the general population, the incidence is 10–20%. Among professionals and upper socioeconomic groups the incidence is higher.

5. What causes aphthous ulcers?

The cause of aphthous ulcers is still unknown, but possibilities include (1) viral agents (herpes simplex virus), (2) bacteria (*Streptococcus sanguis*), (3) nutritional deficiencies (B12, folate, iron), (4) hormonal alterations, (5) stress, (6) trauma, (7) food allergies (nuts, chocolate, gluten), and (8) immunologic abnormalities.

6. Describe the three types of aphthous ulcers.

The three types of aphthous ulceration are minor, major, and herpetiform. In the **minor variety**, the patient usually notices a tingling or burning sensation before the ulcer appears. The ulcerations usually measure less than 1.0 cm and are localized to the freely movable keratinized gingiva. They are white in the center surrounded by a red border. They are extremely painful and usually resolve in approximately 7–10 days. The **major variety** may occur on the movable mucosa, soft palate, tongue, and tonsillar pillars. They are much more painful than the minor ulcers and also much larger, measuring 1–3 cm. From 1–10 ulcers may be present. **Herpetiform ulcers** are similar to herpetic lesions. Usually 10–100 ulcers are present, measuring 1–3 mm in diameter. The small ulcers may coalesce, forming larger ulcers. The minor and major types generally do not leave a scar, whereas the herpetiform variety may leave a scar if the ulcerations coalesce.

7. What is the current treatment for aphthous stomatitis?

Treatment includes both medical management and cauterization, if necessary. The ulcer bed may be cauterized either chemically or electrically. Silver nitrate is commonly used for chemical cauterization. After the application of silver nitrate the area should be swabbed with a cotton-tip applicator impregnated with sodium chloride, which converts the silver nitrate to silver chloride, thereby preventing a deep burn. Medical treatment includes oral antibiotics, antiinflammatory agents, or immunosuppressants. Local measures include the use of an oral suspension of tetracycline or topical steroids such as 0.5% fluocinonide ointment or a beta-methasone solution.

8. What is the significance of the presence of creamy white, curdlike lesions on the tongue and buccal mucosa?

Creamy white, curdlike lesions are likely due to oral candidiasis (thrush). *Candida* species are present in normal oral flora in 40–60% of the population. In certain immunocompromised states, candidal overgrowth may lead to thrush. The lesions represent patches of *Candida albicans* with leukocytes and desquamated epithelial cells. Common conditions that lead to thrush include inhaled corticosteroid use for reactive airways disease; debilitating systemic illnesses, such as cancer; and other immunocompromised states, such as acquired immunodeficiency syndrome (AIDS) and neutropenia. Less common etiologies include diabetes, pregnancy, adrenal insufficiency, systemic antibiotic or steroid use, nutritional deficiencies, and poor oral hygiene. The differential diagnosis includes leukoplakia and hyperkeratosis. Patients who have thrush for no obvious reason should be evaluated for infection with the human immunodeficiency virus (HIV).

9. How is thrush diagnosed?
The diagnosis can be made easily by scraping the lesions, which are easy to remove and have an erythematous base, and examining the scrapings in potassium hydroxide under the microscope. Characteristic hyphae and blastospores are easily recognized.

10. What is desquamative gingivitis?
Desquamative gingivitis, which affects women over the age of 30 years, is characterized by diffuse erythematous desquamation, ulceration, and at times bullae formation involving the free and attached gingiva. Associated conditions include lichen planus, cicatricial pemphigoid, bullous pemphigoid, pemphigus vulgaris, dermatitis herpetiformis, and drug reactions. Incisional biopsy is frequently necessary for diagnosis. Immunofluorescent studies may aid in differentiating the various entities.

11. How can one differentiate among the various white lesions of the oral cavity?
Lesions of the oral cavity may present acutely as red lesions, but during the course of the disease white elements appear and may predominate. White lesions of the mouth are often benign; however, 5–10% of oral malignancies present as white lesions. Thus the examining physician must always be concerned that the lesion in question is a possible malignancy. White lesions of the mouth may be separated into two broad clinical categories: keratotic and nonkeratotic. The most important clinical feature distinguishing the two groups is the ability of the lesion to adhere to the surface epithelium. Leukoplakia, carcinoma, and primary skin disease are usually keratotic. Infectious and bullous skin diseases usually present as nonkeratotic lesions.

Keratotic and Nonkeratotic Factors

KERATOTIC	NONKERATOTIC
Firmly adherent	Removed relatively easily
Usually of long duration	Usually of short duration
Usually change slowly	Frequently change rapidly
Surface is usually elevated and may be smooth, roughened, or even verrucous	Usually erosive or ulcerative

12. What are characteristically premalignant lesions?
Leukoplakia refers to a white patch or plaque of the mouth that cannot be removed by rubbing and cannot be ascribed to other apparent skin diseases, such as lichen planus. The incidence of malignancy may be as high as 30% in patients with leukoplakia; thus a biopsy is necessary. Asymptomatic, velvety red lesions of the mouth may be even more suspect for carcinoma in situ and should be biopsied.

13. What is "geographic" tongue?
Loss and regrowth of papillae lead to red patches on the tongue. This "geographic" appearance is asymptomatic and results from an idiopathic inflammatory condition.

14. What are the most common locations of squamous cell carcinoma of the mouth?
The most common locations are the lower lip, floor of the mouth, and tongue. Painless ulcers not healing in 1–2 weeks are highly suspect and should be biopsied.

15. What is the major differential diagnosis of an oral pigmented lesion?

The most worrisome diagnosis is malignant melanoma, but other possibilities include nevi and benign macules, lesions of Peutz-Jeghers disease, or Addison's disease. Any new suspicious lesion should be followed and biopsied early.

16. Who develops hairy leukoplakia?

White painless lesions that appear "hairy" are often found in patients with AIDS, usually on the lateral aspects of the tongue. They are caused by Epstein-Barr virus and may temporarily respond to high-dose acyclovir.

17. What is the difference between loss of taste (ageusia) and loss of flavor?

Smell and taste are separate senses. The combination of both produces the sensation of flavor, which is distinct from either sense alone. If the olfactory neurons are damaged (by head trauma or viral invasion) or if the nasal passages are blocked (by polyps or edema), the only sensation is produced by the taste buds. This loss of flavor is perceived by the patient as loss of taste.

18. How can taste and olfactory problems be differentiated?

If the patient can differentiate table salt, sugar, the sour taste of lemon juice, or the bitter taste of dark chocolate or coffee, the taste system is intact. Patients who lack the ability to smell state that they can taste the above but nothing else. Hence the problem is olfactory.

19. A 42-year-old woman presents with the chief complaint that sweet beverages taste bitter. Does this dysgeusia (abnormal taste) represent a true pathologic condition?

The effect of taste pleasure and displeasure is present at birth. Sugar produces a pleasurable response, whereas quinine produces a displeasurable response. Some patients may suffer from a chronic bitter taste in the mouth (bitter dysgeusia). To determine the possible origin of the dysgeusia, the mouth may be anesthetized with a topical anesthetic for 60 seconds. If a strong taste solution is given, the patient should not be able to taste. If the dysgeusia is not abolished, it does not originate in the mouth. Most patients usually complain that a sweet beverage, such as cola, tastes bitter. If topographic testing reveals that the patient has lost the ability to taste sweet, the residual taste of the cola is genuinely bitter. Various substances can alter taste because they affect the taste membrane.

1. The **orange juice effect**. Sodium laurel sulfate, the detergent in toothpaste and mouthwash, decreases the intensity of sweet tastes (orange juice) and adds bitter taste to acids.

2. The **artichoke effect**. If the tongue is exposed to artichoke, which contains chlorogenic acid, beverages such as milk, water, or wine taste as if they have been sweetened.

3. **Acetazolamide**, which is used to treat glaucoma, also may make substances taste bitter.

20. A 69-year-old man who drinks and smokes heavily presents with the chief complaints of difficulty tasting food and numbness on the anterior two-thirds of the tongue. What are the possible causes and sites of lesions?

Taste sensation in the anterior two-thirds of the tongue is supplied by a branch of the facial nerve called the chorda tympani nerve. This nerve travels along the posterior wall of the middle ear to the infratemporal fossa and the submandibular gland region, where it joins the lingual nerve to innervate the ipsilateral anterior two-thirds of the tongue. Pathology involving these regions must be carefully ruled out. Possible pathologic processes include neoplastic lesions in the floor of the mouth, submandibular gland region, or infratemporal fossa; acute and chronic otitis media; Bell's palsy; and Lyme disease.

21. During a routine physical examination, a 32-year man is noted to have a papillary lesion involving the uvula and anterior tonsillar pillar on the left. What is the significance of this finding?

Squamous papillomas are the most common benign tumors of the oral cavity and pharynx. These papillary growths are locally noninvasive like their laryngeal counterparts. Malignant degeneration of this benign tumor is rare. Polymerase chain reaction (PCR) studies of the DNA of the oral papilloma fail to demonstrate any human papillomavirus (HPV) type 6a or 11a, which is normally associated with the more aggressive types found in laryngeal papillomas of children.

22. What are torus mandibularis and torus palatinus?

Torus mandibularis is a benign bony enlargement on the lingual surface of the mandible opposite the cuspid and premolar teeth, above the insertion of the mylohyloid muscle. It is believed that this deformity is caused by an autosomal dominant trait with variable penetrance according to sex. It occurs in whites, 1:13; in African-Americans, 1:9; in American Indians, 1:7; and in Eskimos, 1:2.5. **Torus palatinus** is a benign bony enlargement that occurs on the hard palate at the junction of the midpalatal suture. The mass is normally covered by normal oral mucosa. The cause may be related to a dominant trait, but it is questioned whether autosomal dominant or X-linked dominance is a factor. It occurs in females more often than males. In both lesions surgical removal is indicated only if they interfere with function, particularly if dentures are needed.

23. How should severe toothaches be managed by the primary care provider?

Toothaches are most commonly a manifestation of inflammation of the pulp (pulpitis). They generally occur in the presence of a large dental caries or large restorations (fillings). Management depends greatly on the clinical presentation.

1. In the absence of fever and intraoral or extraoral swelling, patients can be managed with analgesics (acetaminophen with or without codeine) and a dental referral within 24 hours.

2. In patients with intraoral or extraoral swelling or with a low-grade fever, antibiotics (penicillin or erythromycin for penicillin-allergic patients) also should be given.

3. For patients with a fever above 101°F or with edema that causes facial asymmetry, an urgent dental referral is mandatory. Complications may include full-blown facial cellulitis or destruction of the alveolar bone that supports the teeth.

BIBLIOGRAPHY

1. Aragon SB, Jafek BW: Stomatitis. In Head and Neck Surgery—Otolaryngology, vol 1. Philadelphia, J.B. Lippincott, 1993, p 531.
2. Atkinson JC, Fox PC: Salivary gland dysfunction. Clin Geriatr Med 499–508, 1992.
3. Barker RL, Burton JR, Zieve PD (eds): Principles of Ambulatory Medicine. Baltimore, Williams & Wilkins, 1991.
4. English GM: Otolaryngology, vol 2. Philadelphia, J.B. Lippincott, 1991, pp 20, 22.
5. Epstein JB: The painful mouth: Mucositis, gingivitis, stomatitis. Inf Dis Clin North Am 2:183–200, 1988.
6. Krull EA, Fellman AC, Fabian LA: White lesions of the mouth. Ciba Clin Symp 25(2):1–32, 1973.
7. Lucente FE: Otolaryngologic aspects of acquired immunodeficiency syndrome. Med Clin North Am 75:1389–1398, 1991.
8. Mandell GL, Douglas RC, Bennett JE (eds): Principles and Practice of Infectious Disease. New York, Churchill Livingstone, 1990.
9. Nakamo K: Characteristics of human papillomavirus (HPV) infection in papilloma of the head and neck—detection of HPV according to clinical features and type specificity. Pippon Jibbinkoka Gakkai Kaiho 97:1381–1392, 1994.
10. Triantos D, Porter SR, Scully C, Teo CG: Oral hairy leukoplakia: Clinicopathologic features, pathogenesis, diagnosis, and clinical significance. Clin Infect Dis 25:1392–1396, 1997.

V. Endocrine and Metabolic Disorders

31. DIABETES MELLITUS

Terri L. Richardson, M.D., and Fred D. Hofeldt, M.D.

1. What end-organ damage is associated with diabetes mellitus?

Diabetes mellitus, a frequently occurring chronic disease, is associated with blindness, renal failure, myocardial infarction, amputation, stroke, and coma. Quality of life is diminished by impotence, bowel and bladder dysmotility, peripheral neuropathy, and neuropathic arthritis.

2. When is a person considered to be diabetic?

According to national guidelines, the diagnosis of diabetes in nonpregnant adults is made in any of the following scenarios: (1) plasma glucose > 200 mg/dl in patients with classic symptoms of polyuria, polydipsia, polyphagia, and weight loss; (2) fasting plasma glucose > 126 mg/dl on two occasions; and (3) two 75-gm oral glucose tolerance tests with fasting plasma glucose < 140 mg/dl, 2-hour plasma glucose ≥ 200 mg/dl, and one intervening value ≥ 200 mg/dl. With the new criteria for diagnosis of diabetes mellitus based on a fasting blood glucose of 126 mg/dl vs. 140 mg/dl, the number of diabetics in the U.S. population has doubled and is estimated to be 18 million persons.

3. Describe and characterize the three types of diabetes mellitus.

In **type 1 diabetes** endogenous insulin secretion is diminished. Type 1 diabetes has an autoimmune etiology and is associated with human leukocyte antigen (HLA) markers. Islet cell antibodies are present. Typically, type I diabetes has its onset during childhood, presenting with ketoacidosis. Patients always require exogenous insulin. They are usually lean and make up 10% of the diabetic population.

In **type 2 diabetes** endogenous insulin is produced, but cells are resistant to insulin action. Alterations in the insulin receptor or postreceptor function prevent normal cellular uptake of glucose. Persons with type 2 diabetes may not be prone to ketosis without insulin. Type 2 diabetes usually presents after age 30 years in genetically predisposed families. Often patients can be treated with diet alone or diet plus oral hypoglycemics, but exogenous insulin may be required to control hyperglycemia and associated microvascular complications. Such patients comprise 90% of diabetics and usually are obese.

A **third type of diabetes** is secondary to pancreatic compromise, drugs, or disease. Resection of the pancreas and recurrent bouts of pancreatitis in alcoholics are frequent causes of secondary diabetics. Drugs that induce diabetes include thiazides, hydantoins, and steroids.

4. Which syndromes include diabetes as part of their clinical presentation?

Hemochromatosis	Acromegaly	Glucagonoma
Cushing's disease or syndrome	Pheochromocytoma	Somatostatinoma

All of the above conditions are secondary causes of diabetes mellitus.

5. Who should be screened for diabetes?

Approximately 6% of the American population is diabetic. In addition, about 9 million adults with diabetes are undiagnosed. Although screening of the general population is not indicated, screening is of value in high-risk individuals with the following characteristics:

1. Obesity (> 20% over ideal body weight)
2. Family history of diabetes
3. American Indian, African-American, or Hispanic ancestry
4. Age > 40 years plus one other high-risk condition
5. Previously identified impaired glucose tolerance
6. Hypertension and hyperlipidemia, cholesterol ≥ 240 mg/dl, or triglycerides ≥ 250 mg/dl
7. History of gestational diabetes or delivery of infant weighing over 9 lb
8. Classic symptoms—polyuria, polydipsia, fatigue, weight loss
9. Recurrent skin, genital, or urinary tract infections

6. Describe the process of screening for gestational diabetes.

All pregnant women should be screened between 24–48 weeks' gestation with 50 gm of oral glucose at any time of day, followed by venous glucose sampling 1 hour later. If the plasma value is ≥ 140 mg/dl or ≥ 7.8 mM/dl, the 100-gm oral glucose tolerance test is performed. Diagnosis is based on two or more readings equal to or greater than the following values:

Fasting	105 mg/dl	(5.8 mM/dl)
1 hr	190 mg/dl	(10.6 mM/dl)
2 hr	165 mg/dl	(9.2 mM/dl)
3 hr	145 mg/dl	(8.1 mM/dl)

7. How should a patient newly diagnosed with diabetes be evaluated?

1. **History.** The initial history should include the date of onset of diabetes and presenting symptoms. It is also important to learn whether the patient has had ketoacidosis, hyperglycemia, or infections and with what frequency. The patient's attitude toward the disease should be evaluated. The history also should determine whether other endocrine, renal, or cardiovascular problems coexist and what medications are taken. In addition, the patient should be questioned about smoking, impotence, family planning, and a family history of diabetes.

2. **Laboratory evaluation.** Baseline laboratory studies should include a fasting glucose, fasting lipid profile, glycosylated hemoglobin, urinalysis, creatinine, electrolytes, thyroid-stimulating hormone (TSH), and electrocardiogram (EKG) in patients over 40 years of age. For patients over 30 years old at onset of diabetes, microalbumin should be measured annually. Physical examination must include height, weight, blood pressure, vision measurement, and examination of eye grounds. Baseline neurologic and cardiovascular examinations should be obtained. The foot examination should include peripheral pulses, sensation, and search for skin lesions and deformities.

3. **Follow-up.** Frequency of follow-up depends on the degree of hyperglycemia and related secondary problems, especially hyperlipidemia and hypertension. Hyperglycemic diabetic patients are seen at 1–2 week intervals until control is achieved.

4. **Education.** All patients must receive formal education about diabetes. The patient's education must include glucose monitoring, diet, exercise, foot care, sick-day rules, hypoglycemic reaction, use of insulin, and need for annual examination.

8. What are the goals of diabetic therapy, as suggested by the Diabetes Control and Complications Trials (DCCT)? Why?

In view of the DCCT results, improved glucose control must be the goal in all diabetic persons, with the expectation that long-term outcome will be measurably improved. In patients with type 1 diabetes, the method of intensive insulin therapy implies at least 3 injections of insulin daily and 4 measurements of glucose/day. Intensive insulin therapy improves hemoglobin A_1C and reduces the first appearance of retinopathy by 27%; severe nonproliferative and proliferative retinopathy requiring laser treatment by 45%; and expected progression of clinically meaningful retinopathy by 34–46%. Intensive insulin therapy reduces the development of microalbuminuria by 35%, clinical grade albuminuria by 56%, and clinical neuropathy by 60%. Any reduction in the hemoglobin A_1C is associated with improved long-term outcome.

9. What are the risks of intensive insulin therapy?

Drawbacks of intensive insulin therapy include a 3-fold increase in severe hypoglycemia and weight gain. However, major macrovascular events, worsened neurobehavioral status, and diminished quality of life were not found.

10. Which patients may be at greater risk for an adverse outcome during intensive therapy?

The risk-benefit ratio for use of intensive insulin therapy may be less favorable in the following groups: children under 13 years of age, patients with known coronary artery or cerebrovascular disease, patients with far-advanced complications, such as renal failure, and patients with recurrent severe hypoglycemia or hypoglycemic unawareness.

11. Which patients have the greatest risk of severe hypoglycemia?

Elderly patients on longer-acting oral hypoglycemics may experience episodes of hypoglycemia, especially in the setting of renal insufficiency or acute illness. The diabetic patient with loss of glucose counterregulatory hormone response or autonomic neuropathy and patients on intensive insulin therapy also are at increased risk of hypoglycemia. Patients with hypoglycemic unawareness do not have warning symptoms or reflex hormonal mechanisms to stimulate glucose production to reverse the hypoglycemia.

12. What advice should be given to patients about hypoglycemia?

At all times, diabetic persons must carry glucose snacks to treat hypoglycemic symptoms. Identification cards help to direct treatment if the individual is found unconscious. Frequent home glucose monitoring may avoid hypoglycemia by therapeutic alterations.

13. Describe the process of screening for and monitoring diabetic retinopathy.

Diabetes is the leading cause of adult blindness. Screening examinations for diabetic retinopathy should begin in patients with type 1 diabetes after 5 years of disease or after puberty. In patients with type 2 diabetes, retinal screening should begin at the time of diagnosis. Examinations should be repeated annually by an ophthalmologist. The 7-field stereophotography of the retina is one method, but annual dilated retinal examination by an ophthalmologist is most often done. The use of panretinal photocoagulation in proliferative retinopathy or severe nonproliferative retinopathy has been shown to save vision, as has focal argon laser therapy in patients with macular edema.

14. What are the basic principles for screening and follow-up of diabetic nephropathy?

Screening for diabetic nephropathy includes taking a family history for hypertension, measuring blood pressure, and checking urinalysis and serum creatinine. If these screens are normal, only an annual urinalysis is required. After 5 years of disease, a 24-hour urine specimen can be collected to assess microalbumin in patients who remain urine protein-negative. Angiotensin-converting enzyme (ACE) inhibitors are indicated in diabetic patients with proteinuria.

15. Characterize the three types of diabetic neuropathy.

1. **Focal neuropathies** involve sensory or motor loss of a particular nerve; for example, wrist or foot drop or diplopia due to cranial nerve palsy.

2. **Distal symmetric polyneuropathy** is most commonly manifest as stocking/glove paresthesias.

3. **Autonomic neuropathy** manifests as distal anhidrosis with compensatory increased sweating on face and trunk; gastrointestinal dysmotility; bladder overfilling with incomplete emptying; impotence, impaired glucose counterregulation; hypoglycemic unawareness; orthostatic hypotension; and loss of cardiac rate deceleration.

16. What are the macrovascular complications of diabetes? What can be done about them?

Diabetic persons are at increased risk for myocardial infarction, stroke, peripheral vascular disease, and amputation. They should be screened for arteriosclerotic disease at presentation with a vascular and cardiac history, physical examination for pulses and blood flow, a fasting lipid profile, and an EKG if ≥ 40 years of age. Proteinuria should be assessed, because it may indicate increased cardiovascular risk. Aggressive control of weight, physical activity, and treatment of hypertension and dyslipidemia are mandatory. Above all, smoking cessation reduces the morbidity of macrovascular complications. To prevent amputation, the high-risk foot should be identified. All feet must be examined annually, but the high-risk foot demands careful examination at each visit. Any of the following characteristics result in a high-risk foot: abnormal gait, neuropathy, peripheral vascular disease, structural deformity, history of foot ulcers, abnormal skin or nails, and history of skin infections.

17. How can the level of glycemic control be determined?

The level of glycemic control is best measured by using the hemoglobin A_1C (HgbA$_1$C) or the fructosamine assay. The Hgb A_1C reflects the mean glycemia over the preceding 2–3 months. For stable diabetes the HgbA$_1$C may be checked every 6–12 months, and diabetics with poor glycemic control should be checked every 3 months. The fructosamine assay, which reflects glucose control during the previous 3–6 weeks, is useful in monitoring glycemic control in pregnant women and patients on intensive insulin therapy. The patient's education must include glucose monitoring appropriate to intensity of therapy.

18. What is included in the annual evaluation of a patient with diabetes?

Secondary morbidity from renal, ocular, neurologic, and cardiovascular sources should be monitored annually. British authorities suggest the following comprehensive list for annual review:

1. Weight
2. Hemoglobin A_1C
3. Blood pressure
4. Smoking
5. Visual acuity and optic fundi
6. Feet
7. Lipid assessment
8. Proteinuria
9. Creatinine
10. Peripheral neuropathy, vibratory sense, light touch, pain
11. Impotence
12. Family planning advice about glycemic control during conception
13. Annual review of educational concepts

Patients need ready access to their health care team (e.g., physician, nurse, diabetes educator, dietician, podiatrist).

19. What are current recommendations for a diabetic diet?

In general, the diet should contain 25–30 kcal/kg of nonobese body weight or the number of calories needed to achieve normal body weight. Thirty percent or less of the calories should be in the form of fat with 8–10% saturated fat and generous use of monounsaturated fat. The proportion of fat and carbohydrate calories depends on dietary goals. Fat calories are restricted for weight loss and hypercholesterolemia. Simple carbohydrates can be substituted for more complex carbohydrates. Cholesterol should be < 200 mg/day. Meals and snacks should be eaten at the same time each day and contain the same proportion of total daily calories. Patients need education from a professional to implement this diet in practical and inexpensive terms. In developing any dietary plan, consideration must be given to cultural and ethnic factors.

20. What are the beneficial effects of exercise? What advice should be given to patients?

Exercise has beneficial effects on insulin receptor function and glycemic control. It increases cardiovascular fitness, decreases risk for macrovascular complications, helps to maintain ideal body weight, and complements dietary compliance. Patients with well-controlled diabetes should avoid hypoglycemia by snacking before exercise. Runners should be advised to use the abdomen rather than the legs as in the injection site, because the leg muscle group does the largest amount of exercise, which increases the absorption and bioavailability of insulin.

Patients with poorly controlled diabetes and plasma glucose values in the range of 300–400 mg/dl should not exercise. Because of insufficient bioavailable insulin, exercise may worsen their condition by increasing hyperglycemia and promoting ketosis. Exercise can be undertaken after glycemic control is improved.

21. What is the initial therapy for patients with type 2 diabetes?

Diet is the cornerstone of treatment for diabetes mellitus. Mild type 2 diabetes is often controlled with diet alone. Weight loss of as little as 10 pounds improves metabolic control in type 2 diabetes; therefore, normal weight must always be stressed as a therapeutic goal.

If type 2 diabetes is not controlled by diet, the second line of treatment includes an oral sulfonylurea agent, metformin, or combination sulfonylurea-metformin. The sulfonylureas stimulate beta cells to produce insulin in a more timely response to eating and increase the number and efficiency of insulin receptors, thereby improving peripheral insulin resistance. With the use of oral sulfonylurea hepatic glucose production is decreased, and fasting hyperglycemia improves. Metformin decreases hepatic glucose production, increases peripheral glucose utilization, and decreases insulin levels. It does not cause hypoglycemia but on rare occasions causes lactic acidosis. Its use is discouraged in patients with liver or renal disease.

22. Compare the oral hypoglycemic agents currently available.

It is important to note the individual characteristics of hypoglycemic agents before prescribing them. They differ in site of metabolism, half-life, activity of hepatic metabolites, and side effects. Chlorpropamide may cause the syndrome of inappropriate secretion of antidiuretic hormone (SIADH or hyponatremia) and has Antabuse-like effects.

Comparison of Oral Hypoglycemic Agents

FIRST GENERATION	HALF-LIFE	HEPATIC METABOLISM
Chlorpropamide	36 hr	No
Tolbutamide	4 hr	Yes
Tolazamide	7 hr	Yes—active metabolites
Glyburide	10 hr	Yes—weak metabolites
Glipizide	4 hr	Yes—weak metabolites (M1)
Glimepiride	9 hr	Yes

23. Which agents are safest in elderly patients?

Tolbutamide and glipizide. They have inactive metabolites (see table in question 22).

24. What is the role of acarbose in diabetic management?

Acarbose primarily decreases postprandial glucose bioavailability and absorption. Its major effect is to interfere with the absorption of disaccharides and hydrolysis products of complex carbohydrates. The malabsorption of carbohydrate fragments leads to significant GI side effects; hence, acarbose must be started at a low dose and slowly titrated to tolerance. Hypoglycemia in acarbose-treated patients must be treated with oral glucose (dextrose) instead of sucrose (cane sugar).

25. How is insulin therapy initiated in patients with type 2 diabetes?

Patients with type 2 diabetes who need exogenous insulin may begin with a morning injection that combines neutral protamine hagedorn (NPH) and regular insulin. A second injection can be added before supper, if needed. A reasonable starting dose is 0.5 U/kg body weight. It is best to adjust the dose with patients at their usual level of physical activity while consistently following their diet and doing home glucose monitoring. Intervals of 2–4 days between dosage changes are best. The addition of a small dose of sulfonylurea, metformin, or troglitazone may improve glucose control. Liver function tests must be monitored closely in patients treated with troglitazone, because it has been implicated in 26 deaths worldwide due to liver failure. Establishing normoglycemia may temporarily improve insulin secretion and insulin action so that the need for exogenous insulin is reduced and the patient's condition improves (glucotoxicity).

26. How should patients with type 1 diabetes be treated?

Insulin is needed in all patients with type 1 diabetes. The total insulin dose is lower than in patients with type 2 diabetes, who are more insulin-resistant.

Two insulin regimens are recommended in patients with type 1: (1) two injections (in the morning and before supper) of combined NPH/regular insulin (starting ratio = 70/30) with a third injection of regular insulin before lunch; (2) Ultralente insulin in the morning or evening with Semilente insulin before breakfast, lunch, and dinner. An arbitrary starting dose of a total of 24 U/day can be divided into separate doses, with two-thirds given before breakfast and one-third before supper. Some physicians start insulin at 0.5 U/kg as a total daily insulin dose. Adjustments are best done every 2–4 days on an outpatient basis in patients who have a consistent diet and exercise pattern. When diabetic control is erratic, ultra lente combined with three injections of Humalog (LISPRO), a rapid-acting insulin, may be effective. Decisions about dosage changes initially can be managed by the doctor or nurse specialist, but once the patient is educated and confident, the patient can make the decisions. Strict home glucose monitoring is essential in these types of patients.

27. What is the approach to diabetic dyslipidemia?
   1. Patients with diabetic dyslipidemia should avoid drugs that aggravate the dyslipidemia, such as beta blockers and thiazides, and choose lipid-neutral antihypertensive agents. Typically diabetics have a combined hyperlipidemia with elevated total cholesterol and triglycerides and low levels of high-density lipoprotein.
   2. Glucose must be controlled aggressively with optimal diet, exercise, oral agents, or insulin.
   3. A low-cholesterol diet, combined with increased physical activity, should be tried aggressively for 6 months before the addition of lipid-lowering drugs.
   4. Because diabetes and hypothyroidism often coexist, TSH should be checked in the dyslipidemic diabetic in good glycemic control.
   5. Lipid values meeting guidelines of the National Cholesterol Education Program (NCEP) require appropriate lipid-lowering therapy, which usually is gemfibrozil alone or in combination with an HMG-CoA reductase inhibitor.

BIBLIOGRAPHY

 1. American Diabetes Association: Practice guidelines. Diabetes Care 20(Suppl):S5–S63, 1997.
 2. Diabetes Control and Complications Trial. N Engl J Med 329:977–986, 1993.
 3. Diabetes mellitus. In Wilson JD, Foster DW (eds): Williams' Textbook of Endocrinology. Philadelphia, W.B. Saunders, 1992, pp 1255–1333.
 4. Hofeldt F: The office management of diabetes mellitus. Mod Med 58:36–58, 1990.
 5. Screening for diabetes. Diabetes Care 16(2):8, 1993.
 6. Summary of the NCEP Adult Treatment Panel II Report. JAMA 209:3015–3023, 1993.
 7. Glimepiride for NIDDM. Med Lett 38:47–48, 1996.
 8. Metformin for non–insulin-dependent diabetes mellitus. Med Lett 37:41–42, 1995.

32. ABNORMALITIES OF LIPIDS

Raymond Estacio, M.D., and Robert H. Eckel, M.D.

1. Name the two major classes of lipoproteins.
   Lipoproteins are carrier vehicles for the solubilization and subsequent transport of lipids in plasma. All lipoproteins consist of cholesterol (ester and unesterified), triglyceride (TG), phospholipid, and apoprotein (the protein component). The two major classes of lipoproteins are distinguished by a change in the relative proportion of these components as the lipoprotein becomes progressively smaller and more dense:
   1. TG-rich lipoproteins: chylomicrons and very-low-density lipoproteins (VLDL)
   2. Cholesterol-rich lipoproteins: low- and high-density lipoproteins (LDL and HDL, respectively). Intermediate-density lipoproteins are present in very small quantities in fasting plasma; however, they may be related to the pathogenesis of atherosclerosis.

2. Which lipoprotein is most important in the pathogenesis of atherosclerosis?

LDL. Current evidence suggests that LDL moves into the subintimal space, becomes oxidized, and thus is no longer recognized by the normal LDL receptor. As part of this process, circulating monocytes and T lymphocytes are attracted, and the oxidized LDL is taken up by tissue macrophages to form foam cells. Subsequently, arterial wall injury induced by smoking, hypertension, and hypercholesterolemia leads to platelet aggregation and release of mitogens, such as platelet-derived growth factor. Ultimately, smooth muscle cell proliferation and fibrosis occur.

3. What is the importance of HDL in atherosclerosis?

There appears to be an inverse relationship between the levels of HDL and atherosclerosis. Although HDL may be important in the early reversibility of LDL-induced damage, the mechanism explaining the inverse relationship remains unclear. One theory is that HDL mediates the process of reverse cholesterol transport. Although this theory is not entirely consistent with known biochemical data, it suggests that when HDL binds to cell surfaces, it is not internalized and degraded like LDL. In addition, HDL may promote cellular efflux of cholesterol and diminish the extrahepatic tissue burden of excessive cholesterol.

4. What is the definition of significant hyperlipidemia?

As defined by the National Cholesterol Education Program (NCEP) Adult Treatment Panel II Recommendations for Consideration of the Diagnosis of Hyperlipidemia, the following levels, when consistently determined after a 12-hour fast, should be considered for treatment:

Total cholesterol > 200 mg/dl
LDL cholesterol > 130 mg/dl
TG > 250 mg/dl

5. Who should be screened for hyperlipidemia?

The recommendations for screening are controversial and variable.

1. The **NCEP Adult Treatment Panel II** recommends that all adults over 20 years of age and children of dyslipidemic parents should be evaluated at least every 5 years. Screening may occur without fasting and should include a total cholesterol and HDL cholesterol.

2. The **Canadian Task Force** on the Periodic Health Examination concluded that there was insufficient evidence to recommend routine cholesterol screening but endorsed case-finding in men 30–59 years old.

3. The **American College of Physicians** concluded that screening serum cholesterol was appropriate but not mandatory for asymptomatic men aged 35–65 and women aged 45–65; screening is not recommended for younger persons unless they are suspected of having a familial lipoprotein disorder or have multiple cardiac risk factors. The ACP concluded that evidence was not sufficient to recommend for or against screening asymptomatic persons between the ages of 65 and 75, but it recommends against screening after age 75.

6. What are the caveats of screening for nonfasting cholesterol?

1. False-positive result: the increased level of cholesterol may be secondary to increases in VLDL or HDL rather than LDL.

2. False-negative result: people with reduced levels of HDL may be missed by this procedure. Thus, adequate evaluation and work-up before therapy requires several determinations of cholesterol, triglycerides, and HDL cholesterol after a 12-hour fast.

7. How does the provider determine the level of LDL cholesterol?

Currently, tests for cholesterol, triglycerides, and HDL cholesterol are readily available in standard laboratories. When triglyceride levels are less than 400 mg/dl, VLDL cholesterol is well approximated by the total triglycerides divided by 5. When the triglycerides are higher than 400 mg/dl, VLDL becomes TG-enriched and the denominator becomes larger. Thus, when triglycerides are less than 400 mg/dl, one may easily calculate the LDL from these measurements as follows:

$$\text{Cholesterol} = (\text{LDL} + \text{HDL} + \text{VLDL})\ \text{cholesterol}$$
$$\text{LDL cholesterol} = \text{cholesterol} - (\text{HDL cholesterol} + \text{TG}/5)$$

LDL cholesterol may be measured, but the available laboratory test is time-consuming and costly.

8. How can the physical manifestations of the dyslipidemias be more easily remembered?

Relating the physical manifestations of dyslipidemia to the lipoproteins important in normal metabolism may help to recall physical abnormalities more easily.

Physical Manifestations of Dyslipidemias

METABOLISM	ABNORMALITY OF METABOLISM	ELEVATED LEVELS	PHYSICAL MANIFESTATION
TG-rich particles (chylomicrons from dietary fat and VLDL synthesized from liver) from the plasma are presented to peripheral tissues for utilization. Lipoprotein lipase at the capillary endothelium removes some TG and other surface components.	Increased chylomicrons (+ VLDL)	Severe hypertriglyceridemia Mild hypercholesterolemia	Eruptive xanthomas Lipemia retinalis Pancreatitis Hepatosplenomegaly (LPL deficiency)
After TG removal, remnants of chylomicrons and VLDL are taken up by the liver. Chylomicron remnants are completely metabolized by the liver, whereas some VLDL remnants give rise to LDL.	Increased remnants	Both hypertriglyceridemia and hypercholesterolemia (usually TG > cholesterol)	Plantar xanthomas Tuberous xanthomas Atherosclerosis
LDLs are formed only from the metabolism of VLDL (mostly small remnants)	Increased LDL	Hypercholesterolemia	Tendinous xanthomas Xanthelasma Arcus cornealis Atherosclerosis
HDLs are secreted by the liver and intestine. Cholesterol ester transfer protein (CETP), which facilitates movement of cholesterol from HDL to other lipoproteins, also controls HDL composition and metabolism.	Decreased HDL	Hypercholesterolemia	Atherosclerosis (decreased HDL)

9. Which conditions cause hypertriglyceridemia?

Hypertriglyceridemia may result from an increase in VLDL production or a decrease in triglyceride (TG) metabolism. Severe hypertriglyceridemia may occur when two disorders are simultaneously present and fat remains in the diet.

Decreased VLDL (and chylomicron) metabolism
Acquired: insulin deficiency
Inherited: LPL deficiency, deficiency of apo-CII activator

Increased VLDL production
Acquired: insulin resistance, alcohol
Inherited: autosomal dominant familial disorders

10. Which single disease causes abnormal lipid remnant catabolism?

Abnormal lipid remnant catabolism is caused by familial dysbetaliproteinemia (broad beta disease), which results in part from abnormalities in the apo E gene. Although this genetic predisposition occurs in 1% of the population, it becomes clinically expressed only when acquired forms of VLDL metabolism are also present. Lipoprotein electrophoresis is indicated to distinguish this disease from combined defects of VLDL and LDL.

11. Which diseases or medications cause combined hyperlipidemia (increases in cholesterol and triglycerides)?

Diseases: hypothyroidism, nephrotic syndrome, diabetes mellitus, and liver disease (parenchymal or obstructive)

Medications: diuretics and glucocorticoids

12. What is the beneficial effect of estrogen on lipid profiles?

Although oral estrogens increase triglycerides, they have a beneficial effect by decreasing LDL and augmenting HDL.

13. Name the two autosomal dominant inherited defects in cholesterol metabolism that lead to premature cardiac death.

1. Increased cholesterol (LDL) production: familial combined hyperlipidemia. This disorder of VLDL production results in a threefold increase in the risk of coronary artery disease. Despite the abnormality in VLDL, the disease often presents as isolated LDL elevation.

2. Decreased LDL catabolism: familial hypercholesterolemia. This disorder results from complete or partial absence of or defects in the LDL receptor. An increase in LDL production is also present. Patients have a twofold (heterozygotes) or fourfold (homozygotes) increase in cholesterol levels; premature death from atherosclerosis is common (even before age 20 years in homozygotes)

14. When do defects in HDL occur?

Defects in HDL may occur because of alterations in the composition of HDL due to other dyslipidemias or reduction in HDL particle number. Most defects are acquired; the factors that decrease HDL cholesterol are listed below:

Genetic: male gender (rare: hypoalphalipoproteinemia, CETP deficiency)

Acquired: diet—decreased fat (high carbohydrate), obesity; drugs—beta blockers, diuretics, progestins, androgens; hypertriglyceridemia; sedentary lifestyle; smoking

15. Provide three lines of clinical evidence that support the treatment of hyperlipidemia for the prevention, arrest, and reversibility of atherosclerosis.

1. The incidence of morbid and fatal coronary artery disease is decreased in men at high risk of atherosclerosis due to high LDL cholesterol levels when LDL cholesterol is lowered by lifestyle modification and/or cholesterol-lowering medication. The benefit in outcome is directly related to the magnitude of LDL reduction (Lipid Research Clinics Coronary Prevention Trial, Helsinki Heart Study, Coronary Drug Project).

2. Coronary atherosclerosis ceases to progress and may reverse in patients with hypercholesterolemia who are treated for hyperlipidemia, even over a short duration (2.5 years) (Cholesterol Lowering Atherosclerosis Study, FATS Study).

3. Coronary artery disease events and mortality were decreased in men and women with a previous history of myocardial infarction over 5-year follow-up (Scandinavian Simvastatin Survival Study) when treated with simvastatin (HMG CoA reductase inhibitor) and diet vs. placebo and diet.

16. How should treatment goals be determined for the patient with hypercholesterolemia?

According to the NCEP Adult Treatment Panel II Recommendations, treatment of hypercholesterolemia is based on targeted LDL cholesterol levels determined by the presence of additional risk factors for coronary artery disease.

Positive risk factors
- Age: male > 45 years, female > 55 years or premature menopause without estrogen replacement
- Familial history of premature coronary artery disease (defined as myocardial infarction or sudden death before age 55 years in the father or other first-degree male relatives or before 65 years in the mother or other first-degree female relatives)

• Current cigarette smoking
• Hypertension (blood pressure > 140/90 mmHg or prescription of antihypertensive medication)
• Low HDL cholesterol (< 35 mg/dl)
• Diabetes mellitus

Negative risk factor
• High HDL cholesterol (> 60 md/dl)

Targeted LDL levels
• Without coronary artery disease and < 2 risk factors: 160 mg/dl
• Without coronary artery disease and ≥ 2 risk factors: < 130 mg/dl
• With coronary artery disease: < 100 mg/dl

17. Should hypertriglyceridemia (HTG) be aggressively treated?

The prevention of pancreatitis in patients at risk for severe HTG is a clear indication for lipid-lowering therapy. However, the relationship between HTG and atherosclerosis is much less clear. Because HTG is often accompanied by increases in cholesterol and diseases with risk factors for atherosclerosis, the question is less easily answered. In patients with familial HTG (and increased VLDL), no increased risk of atherosclerosis is found. In patients with familial combined hyperlipidemia or diabetes mellitus, HTG is a risk factor for cardiovascular disease. Evidence of benefit from lowering of triglycerides, however, is lacking.

18. What sequential recommendations for the treatment of hyperlipidemias should be followed by the primary care provider?

The following sequential recommendations may prevent the patient from appearing prematurely **DEAD** in the emergency department:

1. **D**iscontinue or reduce dosage of all drugs that may contribute to hyperlipidemia and treat any specific etiologies (e.g., thyroid disorder).

2. **E**xercise aerobically. Lipoproteins appear to be altered in proportion to the level of exercise; usually VLDL is decreased, HDL is increased, and LDL is not affected.

3. **A**bstain from excessive calories and from bad calories in the form of dietary saturated fats.

Disorder	Restriction
Chylomicronemia	Fat < 20% of calories; alcohol
Hyperlipidemia, obesity	Calories ± alcohol
Hypertriglyceridemia	± Alcohol
Hypercholesterolemia	Cholesterol, saturated fat (< 10% of calories)

4. **D**rugs may be used to treat specific lipid abnormalities; however, the anticipated outcome and known side effects must be carefully monitored.

19. What is the expected response to dietary management of hyperlipidemia?

1. For severe hypertriglyceridemia, dietary fat restriction leads to remission within days.

2. With weight reduction maintained over several months, triglycerides decrease and HDL cholesterol rises; LDL cholesterol is unaffected.

3. Dietary restriction of cholesterol (300 mg) accompanied by restriction of saturated fat (< 10% of calories) produces a maximal decrement in LDL cholesterol of 25%. However, the decrement is usually much less (5–10%).

20. Does increasing fiber in the diet reduce cholesterol?

Soluble fiber has a dose-dependent effect on lowering total and LDL cholesterol. However, the reduction is usually insignificant when cholesterol (< 300 mg) and saturated fat (< 10% of calories) are already restricted.

21. Why has gemfibrozil replaced clofibrate as the drug of choice to lower triglycerides?

Although both gemfibrozil and clofibrate lower triglycerides and increase HDL cholesterol, gemfibrozil has become the drug of choice because it does not lead to the major side effect seen with clofibrate: cholelithiasis. Whether both drugs cause an increase in cancer is still open to question. Fish oils also lower triglycerides, but they do not increase HDL cholesterol or lower LDL cholesterol, and high doses are associated with a fishy odor.

22. When is nicotinic acid the preferred drug for therapy?

Because nicotinic acid lowers VLDL apo-B synthesis, it is the drug of choice for familial combined hyperlipidemia. Its use is otherwise limited by its side effects and the need for careful monitoring: flushing, gastrointestinal symptoms, glucose intolerance, transaminasemia, and hyperuricemia. Only the rapidly absorbed form should be used, and patients with prior hyperuricemia should be pretreated. Other side effects may be diminished by slow escalation of dose and/or aspirin.

23. How is pharmacologic therapy of LDL cholesterol optimized?

An HMG CoA reductase inhibitor (e.g., lovastatin, 10 mg at night to 40 mg twice daily, or others, depending on cost) can lower LDL cholesterol by 35–40%. Transaminases are monitored every 3 months. A second lipid-lowering drug—usually a bile acid-binding resin (cholestyramine), which lowers LDL cholesterol by an additional 25%—may be instituted to reach target levels.

24. When should levels of creatine phosphokinase (CPK) be monitored in lipid therapy?

Patients taking an HMG CoA enzyme inhibitor and a second lipid-lowering drug (gemfibrozil, nicotinic acid) or cyclosporine are at risk for the development of myositis. Thus, a careful history and CPK determination should be regularly done.

25. What options are available for patients with homozygous familial hypercholesterolemia?

Patients with homozygous familial hypercholesterolemia respond poorly to pharmacologic management. The decision to treat more aggressively with plasmapheresis or liver transplantation is difficult and must be individualized.

26. What guidelines should be followed in treating dyslipidemia in the elderly?

Because no convincing evidence indicates that aggressive control in the elderly, among whom dyslipidemia is more common, will alter outcome, individualized therapy is warranted in addressing primary prevention. The principle of "do no harm" with drug toxicity, strenuous exercise, and overly restricted diets should be followed. Realistic goals and correction of secondary factors (e.g., smoking, obesity, hypertension) should be pursued.

BIBLIOGRAPHY

1. American College of Physicians: Guidelines for using serum cholesterol, high-density lipoprotein cholesterol, and triglyceride levels as screening tests for preventing coronary heart disease in adults. Ann Intern Med 124:515, 1996.
2. Criqui MH, et al: Plasma triglyceride level and mortality from coronary heart disease. N Engl J Med 328:1220, 1993.
3. Grundy SM, et al: The place of HDL in cholesterol management: A perspective from the National Cholesterol Education Program. Arch Intern Med 149:505, 1989.
4. Kjekshus J, Pedersen TR: Reducing the risk of coronary events: Evidence from the Scandinavian Simvastatin Survival Study (4S). Am J Cardiol 76:64C, 1995.
5. Kreisberg RA: Low high-density lipoprotein cholesterol: What does it mean, what can we do about it and what should we do about it? Am J Med 94:1, 1993.
6. Manninen V, et al: Joint effects of serum triglyceride and LDL cholesterol and HDL cholesterol concentrations on coronary heart disease risk in the Helsinki Heart Study: Implications for treatment. Circulation 85:37, 1992.
7. Report of the National Cholesterol Education Program Expert Panel on Detection, Evaluation, and Treatment of High Blood Cholesterol in Adults. The Expert Panel. Arch Intern Med 148:36, 1988.
8. Summary of the Second Report of the National Cholesterol Education Program (NCEP) Expert Panel on Detection, Evaluation, and Treatment of High Blood Cholesterol in Adults (Adult Treatment Panel II). JAMA 269:3015, 1993.

33. INFERTILITY

Julie Rifkin, M.D.

1. What defines an infertile couple?

Normal couples are generally able to conceive within 9 months. Failure to conceive after 1 year of unprotected intercourse is highly suggestive of a fertility problem. Infertility affects 10–15% of all couples in the United States. Unfortunately, 15% of such couples receive no diagnosis to explain their inability to conceive. Approximately 1 in 7 couples is infertile at age 30–34 years; 1 in 5 at age 35–39 years; and 1 in 4 at age 40–44 years. The risk of infertility is doubled for women aged 33–44 years compared with women aged 30–34 years. Up to 50% of infertile couples may conceive spontaneously in the second year of unprotected intercourse.

2. How can the history aid in uncovering clues to infertility?

It is critical to perform a history of sexual intercourse. Sometimes simple layman's terms are required. Both partners require a thorough medical history. Poorly controlled systemic disorders may contribute to lower fertility rates (e.g., hypothyroidism, diabetes mellitus, ulcerative colitis). The following questions provide important clues to diagnosing infertility:

1. Has the woman been pregnant before? If so, what was the outcome?
2. Has the man fathered children before?
3. Has the couple previously used any birth control methods?
4. How long has the couple been together?
5. How long have they attempted to conceive?
6. Has the woman ever menstruated?
7. Are the menstrual cycles regular? (Ovulatory dysfunction or anovulation is suggested by cycles shorter than 21 or longer than 35 days.)
8. Is there a recent onset of dysmenorrhea (which may suggest endometriosis)?
9. How often does the couple have intercourse?
10. Is there a history of an abnormal pelvic exam or Papanicolaou smear?
11. Is there a history of prior abdominal or pelvic surgery?
12. Is either partner taking medications? (Minor tranquilizers, phenothiazines, or antihypertensives may interfere with ovulatory function.)
13. Is there a history of excessive smoking, caffeine intake, or excessive alcohol consumption?
14. Is there a history of pelvic inflammatory disease (PID), septic abortion, use of intrauterine devices (IUDs), ruptured appendix, or ectopic pregnancy? (Positive history alerts physician to possible tubal damage.)

3. What are common medical causes of infertility?

1. Ovulatory dysfunction
2. Inadequate luteal phase
3. Subclinical hypoprolactinemia
4. Subclinical hypothyroidism
5. Asymptomatic genital infection
6. Antisperm antibodies

4. What is the first step in evaluating male infertility?

Carefully performed semen analysis is a useful first step. The specimen is best collected by masturbation. Three specimens should be evaluated at least 2 weeks apart. At least 2 specimens must contain 1 ml of semen and $> 20 \times 10^6$/total sperm concentration. At least 50% of the sperm must demonstrate normal morphology, and 60% must show progressive movement.

5. Can the postcoital test substitute for a semen analysis?

No. The postcoital test (PCT) may determine whether a specific interaction takes place between a patient's sperm and his partner's cervical mucus. Although most physicians recommend PCT as an important step in infertility evaluation, it is a poorly standardized, nonspecific, and insensitive test. The PCT should occur 1–2 days before ovulation and 8–12 hours after coitus. A sample of the vaginal pool and samples from the ectocervix are aspirated into syringes and placed on slides. Microscopic examination provides information about spinnbarkeit (stretchability of cervical mucus), ferning, amount of cervical mucus, cellularity, and viscosity. Normal mucus characteristics are indicative of ovulation. The number and movement of sperm are also recorded. Oligoasthenospermia or abnormal cervical mucus is suspected when less than 5 sperm/hpf are found.

6. What is the simplest way to assess the presence of ovulation in the majority of women?

Ovulation disorders account for 10–24% of female infertility. Thus assessment of ovulatory function is important; the simplest method is to obtain a menstrual history. A history of uterine bleeding at 21–36-day intervals, accompanied by midcycle mittelschmerz, premenstrual symptoms, and dysmenorrhea, indicates ovulation in 90% of women. Other methods include the following:

Basal body temperature. Charting of basal body temperature (BBT) is a noninvasive, inexpensive method to detect ovulation. The patient records her oral temperatures each morning while still in bed after 6–8 hours of uninterrupted sleep. The preovulatory phase averages 97.5°F, and the luteinizing hormone (LH) surge results in an increased temperature 2 days following the LH peak. A biphasic BBT indicates ovulation, although less frequently a monophasic BBT may also be normal.

Serum progesterone in mid luteal phase. A progesterone level of 5 ng/ml 4–7 days before the next predicted menstrual cycle is a reliable indicator of ovulation.

Transvaginal ultrasound. Although expensive and time-consuming, transvaginal ultrasound can track a follicle to pinpoint the time of ovulation.

7. How can a woman predict when ovulation will occur?

1. Basal body temperature, as described above.
2. Urine LH. Quick and reliable enzyme-linked immunosorbent assays that measure the LH surge are commercially available. Ovulation occurs approximately 32–38 hours after the onset of the LH surge.

8. When should a patient undergo an endometrial biopsy?

An endometrial biopsy performed in late luteal phase is the standard clinical test for diagnosing luteal phase defects. The corpus luteum must function normally for implantation to occur and persist. Thus, both infertility and recurrent abortion may result from defects in the luteal phase. Because endometrial biopsy is painful and expensive, infertility specialists may proceed directly to ovulation induction if this type of defect is suspected.

9. How does an inadequate luteal phase affect infertility? How is it treated?

The corpus luteum (ruptured follicle from the ovary) must function normally to allow implantation and to maintain early pregnancy. Infertility and recurrent abortion may be caused by luteal phase defects (inadequate amounts of progesterone produced by the corpus luteum). Serum progesterone levels drawn during the luteal phase are not useful in establishing defects. Endometrial biopsy in the late luteal phase is the standard clinical test for diagnosing luteal phase defects. Populations at infertility clinics demonstrate a 5–10% incidence of luteal phase dysfunction. It is usually an idiopathic disorder.

Treatment regimens that enhance folliculogenesis are helpful, including therapy with clomiphene, human menopausal gonadotropin (hMG), human gonadotropin (hCG), or progesterone vaginal suppositories.

10. When should a hysterosalpingogram and/or laparoscopy be considered?

Hysterosalpingography is useful in infertile patients with a history of PID, septic abortion, tubal surgery, or ectopic pregnancy. No history of tubal damage is obtained from about one-half of patients with an abnormal examination. Hysterosalpingography is performed to rule out uterine and/or tubal defects, usually before ovulation induction therapy. The test is performed by a radiologist who injects iodine-based contrast media into the external cervical os. Radiographs record the movement of the contrast liquid through the uterus and tubes. This examination does not detect endometriosis or periadnexal adhesions. The hysterosalpingogram is a screening procedure that provides the first clue to the possibility of a uterine anomaly.

11. What is the final diagnostic procedure of an infertility evaluation?

Laparoscopy is the final diagnostic procedure of an infertility work-up. It is useful in detecting pelvic adhesions and endometriosis. Such abnormalities may be treated through the laparoscope by lysis of the adhesions or fulguration of endometriosis implants.

12. Which tests should be ordered to evaluate amenorrhea and oligomenorrhea?

Beta chorionic gonadotropin (βCG)—to rule out pregnancy
Prolactin—to screen for pituitary adenoma
Thyroid-stimulating hormone (TSH)—to screen for hypothyroidism
Follicle-stimulating hormone (FSH)—to screen for primary ovarian failure

13. What is the purpose of a progesterone withdrawal test?

A progesterone withdrawal test is used to evaluate amenorrhea when the tests described above are normal. Withdrawal bleeding that occurs 4–14 days after 7–10 days of medroxyprogesterone (Provera) confirms an intact hypothalamic-pituitary-ovarian axis and patency of the reproductive tract. This test also confirms the adequacy of circulating estrogen to sustain a proliferative endometrium. In the absence of response, the patient is given estrogen (Premarin, 1.25 mg orally) for 25 days, followed by progesterone for 16–25 days; subsequent bleeding eliminates the uterus as a cause of amenorrhea.

14. When and how should ovulation be induced?

Ovulation induction may be used to treat infertile women with oligomenorrhea or amenorrhea without ovarian failure (i.e., the ovaries are able to produce estrogen). Clomiphene is the agent of choice to induce ovulation in most patients. By competing with endogenous estrogens for estradiol-binding sites in the hypothalamus, clomiphene blocks the normal negative estrogen feedback and leads to increased pulse frequency of gonadotropin-releasing hormone (Gn-RH). Ovulation is achieved in approximately 90% of patients; the overall pregnancy rate is roughly 50%.

15. What are the risks of stimulated ovulation?

Severe ovarian hyperstimulation is the most significant complication of gonadotropin therapy. The ovaries may become massively enlarged with development of ascites, hydrothorax, renal failure, and thromboembolic phenomenon. The exact pathogenesis of this syndrome is unknown.

16. How often does stimulated ovulation result in pregnancy when the cause of infertility is unknown?

Ovulation eventually can be induced in 99% of patients, with a 50% pregnancy rate. Multiple gestations result in 10% of patients.

17. Can women with pituitary or hypothalamic dysfunction become pregnant?

Yes. Gn-RH is the treatment of choice for amenorrhea secondary to pituitary or hypothalamic dysfunction. It is delivered subcutaneously by a pump in a pulsatile fashion. The pregnancy rate is 30–35% per treatment cycle. Repetitive treatment yields near-normal pregnancy rates. Referral to a specialist should not be denied to such patients.

18. What are assisted reproductive techniques (ARTs)?

1. **In vitro fertilization (IVF).** IVF allows conception in patients with surgically uncorrectable fallopian tube disease, endometriosis, or unexplained infertility. Pregnancy rates are highly variable. The 1990 pregnancy rate for IVF as reported by the American Fertility Society is 19% per retrieval.

2. **Gamete intrafallopian transfer (GIFT).** This method uses IVF protocols to obtain oocytes. The oocytes and spermatozoa are then placed directly into the fallopian tube via laparoscopy. GIFT pregnancy rates averaged 29% with 22% deliveries in 1990.

3. **Zygote intrafallopian transfer (ZIFT).** The technology and pregnancy rate are similar to IVF. The embryo is placed in the fallopian tube 24 hours after fertilization.

4. **Oocyte donation.** This procedure may be considered for women with ovarian failure whose endometrium is capable of responding to gonadal steroids. The patient's endometrium is prepared with an artificial steroid regimen. The donated oocytes are fertilized with the partner's sperm and placed into the patient's uterine cavity. One program has reported a live birth rate of nearly 50% per embryo transfer. Oocyte donation may be the most successful method of achieving pregnancy in older patients.

19. When is intracytoplasmic sperm injection (ICSI) used?

ICSI was introduced as a therapy for infertility in men with obstructive azoospermia or low sperm counts. Sperm are collected by surgical techniques from the epididymis or testicle. The sperm can be transferred into the oocyte for fertilization. The embryo is then introduced into the uterine cavity. ICSI has allowed men who have received chemotherapy or radiation to father children. These therapies, however, may cause permanent DNA breakages in the male germ line, with a theoretical increase of birth defects in the offspring.

20. What common psychological issues affect the infertile couple?

It is common for the affected partner to feel imperfect and for the unaffected partner to feel resentment. A grief reaction is set up by feelings of loss due to failed pregnancies and inability to experience a family. All stages of grief, including denial, isolation, anger, bargaining, and depression, are encountered. Financial stress is a major concern. Primary care providers can assist couples by providing information about local or national support groups and by encouraging the couple to use all available means of emotional support (clergy, family, close friends).

BIBLIOGRAPHY

1. Alexander NS, Sampson JH, Fulgram DL: Pregnancy rates in patients treated for antisperm antibodies with prednisone. Int J Fertil 28:63, 1983.
2. Bachmann GA, Ayers C: Psychosexual gynecology. Med Clin North Am 79:1299–1317, 1995.
3. Collins JA: Diagnostic assessment of the ovulating processes. Semin Reprod Endocrinol 8:145, 1990.
4. Corsan GH, Ghazi D, Kemmann E: Home urinary luteinizing hormone assays: Clinical applications. Fertil Steril 53:591, 1990.
5. Dodson WC, Hughes CL, Whitesides DB, Riley AG: The effect of leuprolide acetate on ovulation induction with human menopausal gonadotropins in polycystic ovary syndrome. J Clin Endocrinol Metab 65:95, 1987.
6. Kerin JF, Liu JH, Phillipai G, et al: Evidence for a hypothalamic site of action of clomiphene citrate in women. J Clin Endocrinol Metab 61:265, 1985.
7. Lobo RA: Unexplained infertility. J Reprod Med 38:241–249, 1993.
8. Martin MC: Infertility. In DeCherney AH, Pernoll ML (eds): Current Obstetric and Gynecologic Diagnosis and Treatment, 8th ed. East Norwalk, CT, Appleton & Lange, 1994, pp 996–1006.
9. Meldrum DR: Ovarian stimulation for assisted reproduction. Curr Opin Obstet Gynecol 8(3):166–170, 1996.
10. Morell V: Basic infertility assessment. Primary Care 24:195–204, 1997.
11. Palermo GD, et al: Evolution of pregnancies and initial follow-up of newborns delivered after intracytoplasmic sperm injection. JAMA 276:1893–1897, 1996.
12. Patrizio P: Intracytoplasmic sperm injection (ICSI): Potential genetic concerns. Hum Reprod 10:2520–2523, 1995.
13. Sauer MV, Paulson RJ: Human oocyte and pre-embryo donation: An evolving method for the treatment of female infertility. Am J Obstet Gynecol 163:1421, 1990.
14. Sauer MV, Paulson RJ, Lolo RA: A preliminary report on oocyte donation extending reproductive potential to women over forty. N Engl J Med 323:1157, 1990.
15. Seigal MS: The male infertility investigation and the role of the andrology laboratory. J Reprod Med 38:317–334, 1993.
16. Speroff L, Glass RH, Kase N: Female infertility. In Clinical Gynecologic Endocrinology and Infertility, 5th ed. Baltimore, Williams & Wilkins, 1994, pp 809–839.
17. Wong PC, Asch RH: Induction of follicular development with luteinizing hormone-releasing hormone. Semin Reprod Endocrinol 5:399, 1987.

34. THYROID DISEASE

Daniel H. Bessesen, M.D.

1. How is the secretion of thyroid hormone regulated?

As with a number of other endocrine systems, the hypothalamus works with the pituitary gland to regulate the production of bioavailable thyroid hormone. The hypothalamus secretes thyrotropin-releasing hormone (TRH) into the pituitary portal system. TRH stimulates the production of thyroid-stimulating hormone (TSH) by the anterior pituitary gland. In addition, dopamine and indirect effects of cortisol inhibit pituitary secretion of TSH. TSH, which is produced in a pulsatile manner with 2–3 peaks/day, stimulates the production of thyroid hormones (thyroxine [T_4] and triiodothyronine [T_3]) by thyroid follicular cells located in the thyroid gland. T_4 is in many respects a prohormone for the more potent T_3. About 10–15% of total peripheral T_3 comes from direct secretion from the thyroid gland; the remainder comes from the peripheral deiodination of T_4. Alternatively, T_4 may be peripherally deiodinated to form reverse T_3, which has no biologic activity. Ninety-eight percent of T_3 and 99.8% of T_4 are bound to plasma proteins, including thyroid-binding globulin, thyroid-binding prealbumin, and albumin. Circulating levels of T_4 and T_3 provide negative feedback for hypothalamic production of TRH and pituitary production of TSH. This system produces stable levels of T_4 and T_3 in healthy people.

2. Which tissues are affected by thyroid hormone?

Thyroid hormone has important effects on virtually every tissue of the body. These effects result from the interaction of thyroid hormone with its receptor. Some hormones act through cell membrane-associated receptors that are coupled to second messenger systems. Thyroid hormone is a member of a family of hormones that diffuse through the cell membrane of all cells and exerts its biologic actions through binding to an intranuclear receptor. Several isoforms of thyroid hormone receptors are present to different degrees in different tissues. These receptors interact with regulatory elements on thyroid-responsive genes as well as with a variety of other transcription factors to alter gene expression in a manner regulated by thyroid hormone. Thyroid hormone takes part in the regulation of metabolic rate, gastrointestinal motility, cardiac contractility, heart rate, body temperature, mood, body weight, and skin texture, among other parameters.

3. What is the most important laboratory test for evaluating the hypothalamic-pituitary-thyroid (HPT) axis?

Measurement of the serum TSH level is the most important test in evaluating the HPT axis. Because most thyroid disease results from the dysfunction of the thyroid gland rather than pituitary or hypothalamic disease, the TSH level is usually the first parameter to become abnormal during the development of thyroid disease. Older radioimmunoassays (RIAs) were relatively insensitive at low levels of TSH. As a result these assays were unable to distinguish between low and normal levels of TSH. Newer radioimmunometric assays (second-generation assays) and chemoluminescent assays (third-generation assays) are able to detect low levels of TSH and thus to diagnose glandular hypofunction (high TSH) and hyperfunction (low or suppressed TSH).

4. What must be considered in the interpretation of a serum T_4 level?

Various tests are available for assessing serum T_4 levels. The most commonly ordered test is a total serum T_4 level. However, because over 99% of circulating T_4 is protein-bound, this measure does not accurately reflect the level of free T_4. Therefore, if the total T_4 is measured, it is important also to assess the degree of protein binding through a test such as the T_3 resin uptake (T_3RU). If both T_4 and T_3RU are increased, hyperthyroidism is the likely diagnosis. T_3RU gives no direct information about the circulating level of thyroid hormones; it is an indirect test of available binding sites. Interpretation of these tests can be summarized as follows. If both T_4 and T_3RU are decreased, hypothyroidism is the likely diagnosis. However, if T_4 and T_3RU move in opposite directions, a protein-binding abnormality is the likely diagnosis. The laboratory often calculates a free thyroid hormone index (FTI) from the total T_4 and T_3RU to help in the interpretation of the two numbers. Alternatively, the level of free T_4 can be measured directly by either a radioimmunoassay or by equilibrium dialysis methods. Measuring free T_4 directly obviates the need for a T_3RU.

Assessment of Serum Levels

CONDITION	T_4	T_3RU	FTI	THYROID-BINDING PROTEINS
Hyperthyroidism	↑	↑	↑	NL
Hypothyroidism	↓	↓	↓	NL
Binding-protein excess	↑	↓	NL	↑
Binding-protein deficiency	↓	↑	NL	↓

FTI = free thyroxine index, NL = normal

5. What are the signs and symptoms of hypothyroidism?

Hypothyroidism may cause weight gain, fatigue, somnolence, depression, congestive heart failure, cold intolerance, constipation, and, in women, menstrual irregularities. Physical signs include periorbital puffiness; diastolic hypertension; cold, dry skin; delay in the relaxation phase of the reflexes; and bradycardia. Laboratory tests may reveal increased total and LDL cholesterol levels, anemia, CO_2 retention, and occasionally increased creatine phosphokinase (CPK). The diagnostic biochemical test is assessment of the serum TSH level, which is elevated in the presence of primary thryoid gland failure.

6. What causes hypothyroidism?

Most hypothyroidism is due to autoimmune destruction of the thyroid gland (primary hypothyroidism), which may be associated with increased circulating levels of antibodies directed against thyroid-specific antigens. The older test detected antimicrosomal and antithyroglobulin antibodies. The newer test detects antibodies directed against thyroid peroxidase, which is the microsomal enzyme detected by the older antimicrosomal antibody tests, and is more sensitive and specific. Previous neck irradiation for Hodgkin's disease or head and neck cancer also may cause thyroid gland destruction. Lithium therapy for manic depressive illness may unmask underlying hypothyroidism by reducing thryoid hormone secretion. Less commonly hypothyroidism is the result of destruction of the pituitary gland or the hypothalamus (secondary hypothyroidism) and loss of TSH. This scenario may result from a pituitary tumor, hemorrhage, or irradiation or from other neoplasms in the area, such as craniopharyngiomas.

7. Are special populations at high risk for hypothyroidism?

Biochemical hypothyroidism is present in as many as 8% of people over the age of 65 years. It is more common in people with diabetes, adrenal insufficiency, autoimmune hypogonadism, vitiligo, premature graying, and other autoimmune conditions.

8. How is hypothyroidism treated?

Many products are available for replacing thyroid hormone. Levothyroxine (LT_4) is the treatment of choice for hypothyroidism. The half-life of LT_4 in an euthyroid person is roughly 7 days. Thus, the clinician should wait 6 weeks after beginning a daily replacement dose before checking the TSH level to document adequacy of therapy. The goal of therapy is to normalize the TSH level. The physician needs to check only the TSH level when following a patient with primary hypothyroidism on hormone replacement therapy. The average dose required to achieve euthyroidism is 1.6 μg/kg ideal body weight. Levothyroxine requirements increase by an average of 45% during pregnancy; thus, the TSH should be monitored closely during pregnancy with an assumption that the dose probably will need to be increased. Several recent studies have shown that excessive thryoid hormone replacement (doses adequate to suppress TSH) is quite common. Overreplacement with LT$_4$ carries the risks of inducing osteoporosis and atrial arrhythmias and therefore should be avoided.

9. List the signs and symptoms of hyperthyroidism.

In the ambulatory setting, most patients with hyperthyroidism present with a single major complaint. Hyperthyroidism may develop gradually, and the person may not initially notice or complain of some of the symptoms. Deeper questioning, however, identifies a broadly positive review of systems.

Symptoms: heat intolerance, weight loss, nausea, hyperdefecation, amenorrhea, goiter, discomfort in the eyes, headache, psychic disturbances (e.g., anxiety, irritability, nervousness), tremulousness, sleep disturbances.

Physical signs: objective weight loss, tachycardia, widened pulse pressure (but not hypertension), atrial fibrillation, warm moist skin, stare, lid lag, onycholysis, goiter, tremor.

10. What is the most common cause of hyperthyroidism?

The most common cause of hyperthyroidism is Graves' disease, in which autoantibodies stimulate the TSH receptor and cause autonomous production of thyroid hormone by the thyroid gland. Graves' disease is associated with proptosis from retroorbital inflammatory infiltration and rarely with pretibial myxedema. The second most common cause of biochemical hyperthyroidism in most clinics is the use of thyroid-hormone medication. Less common causes of hyperthyroidism include an autonomously functioning thyroid nodule (hot nodule), toxic multinodular goiter, and thyroiditis.

11. Describe the most common varieties of thyroiditis.

The most common variety of thyroiditis is **subacute thyroiditis**, which usually follows a viral illness and presents with a painful, tender goiter and signs and symptoms of hyperthyroidism. **Painless thyroiditis** also follows a viral illness but is not associated with a painful, tender thyroid gland. **Postpartum thyroiditis** occurs 3–6 months after delivery and is usually painless and associated with mild enlargement of the thyroid gland; it tends to recur with subsequent pregnancies. **Hashitoxicosis** occurs in association with lymphocytic infiltration of the thyroid gland. The hyperthyroidism associated with thyroiditis is caused by injury to the thyroid gland and release of stored thyroid hormone. The hyperthyroid period, therefore, is short, lasting 2–3 months; it is followed by a hypothyroid period, which may last for 6–18 months. Approximately 50% of patients eventually become euthyroid.

12. Define apathetic hyperthyroidism.

Apathetic hyperthyroidism is an atypical presentation of hyperthyroidism in elderly patients. The placid or even depressed presentation may be more suggestive of hypothyroidism than hyperthyroidism. Weight loss is often a striking feature, as are cardiovascular manifestations such as atrial fibrillation and congestive heart failure. Many patients also manifest a proximal myopathy. The thyroid gland often is only minimally enlarged and may be multinodular. Eye findings typical of Graves' disease are minimal or absent.

13. How may the specific cause of hyperthyroidism be determined?

The physical examination often provides clues to the cause of hyperthyroidism. Graves' disease usually presents with a diffusely enlarged thyroid gland in association with proptosis. When autonomously functioning nodules are present within the thyroid gland, the remainder of the gland is usually suppressed (small or absent). A toxic multinodular goiter is usually palpable. Subacute thyroiditis is suggested when the thyroid gland is tender.

The most definitive method for determining the cause of hyperthyroidism, however, is the thyroid scan. In Graves' disease, the thyroid gland demonstrates diffuse, homogeneous increased uptake of radioactive iodine. An autonomously functioning nodule shows increased radioactive iodine uptake in the nodule, but the remainder of the gland shows no uptake. With a toxic multinodular goiter, multiple areas of autonomous uptake may be identified. With thyroiditis or hyperthyroidism caused by the ingestion of thyroid hormone medication, radioactive iodine uptake is suppressed or absent.

A number of laboratory tests also may be useful in confirming the diagnosis in confusing cases. The presence of thyroid-stimulating immunoglobulins in the serum suggests Graves' disease. Subacute thyroiditis usually is associated with a markedly elevated sedimentation rate. Hashitoxicosis is associated with high titers of thyroid peroxidase antibodies.

14. List the available treatments for Graves' disease.

Antithyroid medications, radioactive iodine, and surgery.

15. What medications can be used to treat Graves' disease?

Two classes of medications are used: those that provide symptomatic relief but do not alter the basic disease process and those that reduce the levels of thyroid hormone in the blood serum.

Symptomatic treatment. Beta blockers reduce the tremulousness and tachycardia associated with hyperthyroidism. Propranolol is the most widely advocated drug, but because of its relatively short half-life it should be given 3 or 4 times/day to be most effective. Metoprolol and atenolol may be used if compliance with more frequent dosing is a concern.

Antithyroid drugs. Two antithyroid drugs are commonly used: propylthiouracil (PTU) and methimazole. Both drugs are effective at inhibiting production of thyroid hormone. PTU has the added benefit of inhibiting peripheral conversion of T_4 to T_3 but the disadvantage of requiring administration 3 times/day. In addition to inhibiting production of thyroid hormone, these drugs may have an immunomodulating effect, reducing the levels of thryoid-stimulating immunoglobulins over time. Antithyroid drugs are effective in most patients with Graves' disease, if taken at a high enough dose, and work more rapidly than radioactive iodine. They also may be less likely to exacerbate Graves' ophthalmopathy than radioactive iodine. The downside of these medications is that many people require 4–12 pills/day to normalize thyroid hormone levels—in addition to the beta blockers that they may be taking for symptomatic relief.

Although expert opinion varies widely about the best form of treatment for Graves' disease, antithyroid medications are preferred as the initial treatment in (1) pregnant women, (2) elderly patients who are debilitated from hyperthyroidism, (3) very young patients, and (4) patients with relatively small thyroid glands and mild hyperthyroidism. In the first three groups, antithyroid medications are used to control the condition until more definitive treatment with radioactive iodine can be given. In the fourth group, antithyroid medications are given with the hope of inducing long-term remission. Estimates of the rates of remission that result from this approach vary widely in the literature. If antithyroid medications are given for 12–18 months, then tapered and discontinued, there is roughly a 30% chance of long-term remission. In the remaining 70%, radioactive iodine is needed for definitive treatment. Rare side effects include agranulocytosis and abnormal liver function tests.

16. What are the risks and benefits of radioactive iodine therapy for Graves' disease?

Radioactive iodine (I^{131}) is a highly effective and simple form of therapy for Graves' disease. In the United States it is the most commonly used form of treatment. A single dose successfully treats hyperthyroidism in 95% of patients. In 5% of patients a second dose is necessary to complete the treatment. Because one dose is the entire treatment compliance, a chronic medication regimen is not an issue as it is with PTU or methimazole therapy. The dose of I^{131} is adjusted in accordance with the size of the gland (the larger the gland, the higher the dose) and the avidity of the gland for the radionucleotide (the higher the uptake, the lower the dose necessary to deliver the same amount of radiation). Many patients may be concerned that treatment with I^{131} will increase their risk of developing cancer. This issue has been carefully studied, and no evidence indicates that I^{131} in the doses used to treat Graves' disease increases the risk of developing cancer. It is important to remind patients that anyone can develop cancer, whether or not they take radioactive iodine. Radioactive iodine does not protect against cancer, but neither does it increase the risk of developing cancer.

Several problems, however, are associated with the use of I^{131} to treat Graves' disease. First, this form of treatment takes on average 2 months to work. It is slower than medical therapy, which usually begins to work within 2 weeks. Second, more than 90% of patients eventually become hypothyroid after treatment, most within the first year and a half. They then need to take thyroid hormone supplementation for the rest of their lives. A third problem associated with the use of I^{131} is the potential for transient worsening of the hyperthyroid state before improvement because of radiation-induced thyroiditis in as many as 20% of patients. For this reason it is advisable not to use I^{131} in patients who have active or unstable ischemic cardiac disease or are severely malnourished and debilitated from Graves' disease.

If I^{131} is administered to a woman of reproductive age, the clinician must be certain that she is not pregnant. The most effective approach is to administer I^{131} within 10 days of the last menstrual period and to document a negative sputum pregnancy test on the day of administration. I^{131} is excreted in the urine, and because of the proximity of the bladder to the uterus there is concern over the teratogenic effects in pregnant women. In addition, I^{131} has the potential of being taken up by the thyroid gland of the fetus and destroying it. Studies, however, have shown that the fetus does not develop a thyroid gland until week 12–15 of gestation. In fact, the risk to the fetus if I^{131} is administered in the first trimester is quite small. However, it is prudent to be aggressive in ensuring that I^{131} is not given to pregnant women. In addition, it is important to counsel women of reproductive age to use a reliable form of contraception if they are sexually active and receiving I^{131} treatment. Many affected women have independently found that they are infertile and may not be using contraception. They may not realize that the infertility was due to the hyperthyroid state and that, once treated, they will become fertile again. Furthermore, in the 6–12-month period after the administration of I^{131}, thyroid hormone levels change on a regular and ongoing basis. This hormonal instability adds unnecessary risk and complication to pregnancy. Therefore, women of reproductive age should use contraception until thyroid hormone levels are normal and stable for at least 3 months.

17. When is surgery indicated to treat Graves' disease?

Surgery is rarely used to treat Graves' disease because other treatment options are highly effective and associated with less risk. In addition, because few surgeons have adequate ongoing experience in operating on patients with Graves' disease, complications, including hypoparathyroidism and recurrent laryngeal nerve palsy, are unacceptably high. The situations in which surgery may be considered include severe Graves' disease in a pregnant woman who is unable to take antithyroid medications, persistent or recurrent Graves' disease unresponsive to multiple doses of radioactive iodine, and the rare patient who simply refuses antithyroid drug and I^{131}.

18. When should a patient with Graves' disease be hospitalized?

The indications for hospitalization include altered mental status, fever, congestive heart failure, new atrial fibrillation, and intractable nausea and vomiting. Patients with atrial fibrillation associated with Graves' disease should be anticoagulated and treated with beta blockade for rate control. Digoxin usually is not effective in slowing ventricular response rate in hyperthyroid patients with atrial fibrillation. Despite the lack of good controlled data, it appears that the rate of systemic embolization is quite high in atrial fibrillation caused by Graves' disease. Efforts at cardioversion probably should be postponed until thyroid hormone levels are normal and adequate anticoagulation has been achieved.

19. How should Graves' disease be evaluated and managed?

Graves' disease is associated with inflammatory infiltration of the extraocular muscles, which usually causes mild proptosis and a sensation of dry eyes. If a patient has obvious eye changes associated with Graves' disease, visual acuity should be checked at each visit, along with assessment of visual fields by confrontation, extraocular movements, and degree of proptosis. Proptosis can be assessed objectively by measuring the perpendicular distance from the lateral orbital rim to the anterior surface of the cornea. This distance should be less than 19–20 mm in normal people. Graves' eye disease occasionally is markedly asymmetric. However, one should consider getting an orbital CT scan to rule out other serious retroorbital pathology when unilateral proptosis is the presenting finding. The patient should lubricate the eyes with eyedrops (daytime) or lubricating ointment (nighttime) and wear sunglasses. If the eyes remain open during sleep, corneal ulceration may result; thus, some patients may benefit from taping the eyes shut at night. Elevating the head of the bed and taking low doses of a thiazide diuretic also may help. Rare patients may experience a serious complication from Graves' eye disease, such as diplopia; decreased visual acuity, including restricted visual fields; or intractable, severe proptosis causing corneal ulceration. In these situations, aggressive treatment must be considered, such as use of oral steroids (prednisone, 60 mg/day, followed by a long, slow taper), retroorbital irradiation, or surgical decompression (removing the medial or inferior wall of the orbit). These treatments carry the risks of serious side effects. Therefore, if one of these signs develops, the patient should be referred to an ophthalmologist or endocrinologist with experience in managing Graves' eye disease.

20. Do any drugs cause abnormalities in thyroid hormone levels?

Amiodarone has been used in the United States since 1985 for treatment of serious ventricular and atrial arrhythmias. Roughly 35% of the mass of amiodarone is organic iodine. Patients treated with amiodarone may develop hyperthyroidism, hypothyroidism, or goiters. It is difficult to treat the hyperthyroidism caused by amiodarone because discontinuing the drug is often not a viable option; even if the drug is discontinued, hyperthyroidism may persist for several months. The most effective treatment for amiodarone-induced thyrotoxicosis is usually antithyroid drugs. The hypothyroidism associated with amiodarone should be treated with levothyroxine supplementation. Goiters associated with amiodarone use also may respond to levothyroxine. Patients treated with amiodarone should be screened periodically for thyroid dysfunction by measuring a serum TSH level. A number of medications interfere with absorption of levothyroxine, including aluminum hydroxide antacids, sucralfate, ferrous sulfate, cholestyramine, and activated charcoal. If one of these medications is added to a patient's medication regimen, the TSH should be monitored to ensure ongoing adequacy of levothyroxine therapy.

21. How common are thyroid nodules?

The prevalence of thyroid nodules is a function of the method used for their identification. In several series in which thyroid glands were palpated by experienced endocrinologists, 4–7% of normal adults were found to harbor thyroid nodules. In studies in which ultrasound of the neck was performed on normal adults, nodules were seen in 19–67%. Studies in which thyroid glands were examined at autopsy identified nodules in 3–60% of cadavers. Most nodules found incidentally after imaging studies are not palpable.

22. Which nodules are likely to be benign?

Nodules with autonomous functions (i.e., nodules that take up I^{131} independently of TSH) are virtually never malignant. Simple, thin-walled cysts are also unlikely to be cancerous. Nonpalpable nodules, if malignant, are less likely to have metastasized than large palpable nodules.

23. How should a solitary thyroid nodule be evaluated?

Thyroid cancer usually presents initially as a solitary thyroid nodule. However, only 3–5% of palpable thyroid nodules are malignant. The goal of the evaluation is to identify and remove the subset of nodules that are likely to be malignant. The first step is measurement of the serum level of TSH to determine whether the patient is biochemically euthyroid. If the TSH is normal, the usual second step is fine-needle aspiration (FNA), a safe, well-tolerated procedure performed with a 23–25-gauge needle. Five to 10% of FNA biopsies do not provide adequate tissue for a firm conclusion. If another attempt at FNA is made, adequate tissue is obtained 50% of the time. If there is adequate cellularity on FNA, 60–70% of nodules are found to be benign, and surgery can be avoided. In 5–10% of cases, the FNA suggests malignancy, and the nodule should be removed by a surgeon experienced in operating on patients with thyroid cancer. In 20–30% of cases, the FNA is suspicious for follicular cancer or follicular neoplasm, and a thyroid scan should be performed because an autonomous nodule may look like cancer on FNA. If the nodule is cold on scan and the FNA is worrisome, the risk of cancer is roughly 20–30%; as a result, most experts suggest that such nodules be removed. If the scan looks warm, indicating the possibility of autonomy, the patient may be placed on levothyroxine at a dose adequate to suppress TSH to an undetectable level. Then the scan can be repeated with levothyroxine. If the nodule takes up I^{131} on this suppression scan, it should be considered autonomous, and surgery is not necessary.

An alternative approach to this algorithm is to perform an initial thyroid scan on all patients with thyroid nodules. If the nodule demonstrates autonomous uptake, an FNA is unnecessary. Most thyroid nodules, however, are cold on scan and benign on biopsy. Therefore, if this approach is used, most patients with nodules will have both a scan and an FNA, which will increase the cost but not alter the ultimate diagnosis. Therefore, the most cost-effective approach is to perform the FNA first and to perform scans only on patients with abnormal FNA results.

If the FNA is either suspicious or suggests malignancy, the patient should be referred for surgical excision. If the nodule is hot or autonomous, thyroid function tests should be obtained every 6–12 months because such nodules tend to grow and eventually may cause overt hyperthyroidism. A hot nodule that causes hyperthyroidism may be treated with either I^{131} or surgical excision.

CONTROVERSIES

24. How should a benign thyroid nodule be managed?

If an FNA suggests that a nodule is a benign adenoma, reasonable treatment options include a dose of levothyroxine designed to lower the TSH level with a goal of suppressing or shrinking the nodule, oral iodine supplementation for the same purpose, or simple clinical observation. The standard approach in the past has been to administer suppressive doses of levothyroxine with the hope that reduction in TSH concentration will shrink the nodule and prevent malignant conversion. However, several recent randomized, controlled clinical trials suggest that suppressive therapy has no consistent effect on the size of solitary nodules. It does, however, shrink the normal surrounding thryoid tissue, giving the appearance by inspection and palpation that the nodule has shrunk. In addition, suppressive therapy with levothyroxine may predispose to osteoporosis, especially in postmenopausal women not taking estrogen replacement therapy. A reasonable middle course of action is to place the patient on levothyroxine with a goal of suppressing the level of TSH to 0.1–0.5 mU/L. If the nodule does not shrink within 6–12 months, therapy should be discontinued to minimize risks to the patient, including anxiety, atrial arrhythmias, and osteoporosis. The size of the nodule should then be measured periodically and FNA repeated if the nodule grows significantly.

25. What is the approach to the treatment of the patient with an elevated level of TSH but a normal level of T_4?

The patient with an increased level of TSH but a normal T_4 level presents a special problem. This condition is called **subclinical hypothyroidism**. Some clinicians suggest that because the T_4 level is normal, the patient requires no treatment. Others say that the increase in TSH suggests that the patient has mild hypothyroidism. Treatment with levothyroxine may be advocated for two reasons. The first is that patients with subclinical hypothyroidism may eventually become frankly hypothyroid. A number of prospective studies have demonstrated, however, that only a minority of patients progress to overt hypothyroidism; such patients have high titers of antimicrosomal antibodies (>1:1000) and higher values for TSH (> 15) at baseline compared with patients who do not progress. The second reason is to treat subtle clinical consequences of mild hypothyroidism, including depression, heart failure, weight gain, constipation, cold intolerance, abnormal menses, hyperlipidemia, or diastolic hypertension. Randomized, prospective clinical trials report subjective or objective improvement in approximately 60% of patients with subclinical hypothyroidism after treatment with levothyroxine. In practice it is reasonable to decide what clinical features provide justification for treating and then to place the patient on a dose of levothyroxine that normalizes

TSH for 6–12 months while monitoring the patient for objective or subjective improvement. If no improvement occurs and if the initial TSH was less than 15 and the titer of thyroid peroxidase is low, therapy may be discontinued and the patient followed clinically.

26. What is the approach to the treatment of a patient with a reduced level of TSH but a normal level of T_4?

This presentation is called **subclinical hyperthyroidism**. Treatment is again somewhat controversial. Like other anterior pituitary hormones, TSH is secreted in a pulsatile manner. A single value that is lower than the lower limits of normal for the assay (0.1–0.5) usually does not warrant intervention. In such patients the TSH should be remeasured periodically to make sure that overt hyperthyroidism does not develop. In patients with a TSH level < 0.03, treatment should be considered. As in subclinical hypothyroidism, a careful clinical evaluation should be conducted to look for subtle signs and symptoms of hyperthyroidism, including anxiety, osteoporosis, tachycardia, atrial fibrillation, weight loss, tremor, abnormal menses, or sleeplessness. A trial of antithyroid medications may be undertaken with a goal of normalizing the TSH for a period of 3–6 months. At the end of that time the clinician and patient can decide whether more definitive therapy with I^{131} would be beneficial. If the patient refuses therapy for subclinical hyperthyroidism, periodic assessment of bone density should be considered to ensure that osteoporosis does not develop.

27. Is the use of generic levothyroxine acceptable in the treatment of hypothyroidism?

Some alternative practitioners advocate the use of desiccated animal thyroid in the treatment of hypothyroidism. This approach is not acceptable because such preparations have been shown to contain doses of T_3 that are high enough to cause T_3 toxicosis and adverse clinical events when prescribed in usual doses. Historically, generic levothyroxine preparations had poor levels of bioavailability and were not recommended. More recently, however, a number of generic levothyroxine preparations were compared with brand-name versions and, by the standards used by the Food and Drug Administration to determine equivalence, were found to be interchangeable. However, many experts in thyroid disease believe that the standards used to determine equivalence were too low and that differences in the products are clinically meaningful. It is clear that the generic products performed better in recent tests than in older comparison studies. In practice it is important to be sure that the prescribed drug has been tested and found to be of good quality. Good quality is ensured if the product is a brand name. However, the brand-name products are a bit more expensive than the generics.

BIBLIOGRAPHY

1. Bartalena L, Marcocci C, Bogazzi F, et al: Relation between therapy for hyperthyroidism and the course of Graves' ophthalmopathy. N Engl J Med 338:73–78, 1998.
2. Blum M: Why do clinicians continue to debate the use of levothyroxine in the diagnosis and management of thyroid nodules? Ann Intern Med 122:63–64, 1995.
3. Dong BJ, Hauck WW, Gambertoglio JG, et al: Bioequivalence of generic and brand name levothyroxine products in the treatment of hypothyroidism. JAMA 277:1205–1213, 1997.
4. Figge H, Leinung M, Goodman AD, et al: The clinical evaluation of patients with subclinical hyperthyroidism and free T3 toxicosis. Am J Med 96:229–234, 1994.
5. Gharib H: Changing concepts in the diagnosis and management of thyroid nodules. Endocrinol Metab Clin North Am 26:777–800, 1997.
6. Harjai KJ, Licata AA: Effects of amiodarone on thyroid function. Ann Intern Med 126:63–73, 1997.
7. Klee GG, Hay ID: Biochemical thyroid function testing. Endocrinol Metab Clin North Am 26:763–776, 1997.
8. Klein I, Becker DV, Levey GS: Treatment of hyperthyroid disease. Ann Intern Med 121:281–288, 1994.
9. La Rosa GL, Lupo L, Giuffrida D, et al: Levothyroxine and potassium iodide are both effective in treating benign solitary solid cold nodules of the thyroid. Ann Intern Med 122:1–8, 1995.
10. Liel Y, Sperber AD, Shany S: Nonspecific intestinal adsorption of levothyroxine by aluminum hydroxide. Am J Med 97:363–365, 1994.
11. Mandel SJ, Brent GA, Larsen PR: Levothyroxine therapy in patients with thyroid disease. Ann Intern Med 119:492–502, 1993.

12. Ridgway EC: Modern concepts of primary thyroid gland failure. Clin Chem 42:179–182, 1996.
13. Surks MI, Ocampo E: Subclinical thyroid disease. Am J Med 100:217–223, 1996.
14. Tan GH, Gharib H: Thyroid incidentalomas: Management approaches to nonpalpable nodules discovered incidentally on thyroid imaging. Ann Intern Med 126:226–231, 1997.
15. Uzzan B, Campos J, Cucherat M, et al: Effects on bone mass of long term treatment with thyroid hormones: A meta-analysis. J Clin Endocrinol Metab 81:4278–4289, 1996.

35. OSTEOPOROSIS

Philip S. Mehler, M.D., and Fred D. Hofeldt, M.D.

1. Why is osteoporosis a major public health problem?

Osteoporosis affects 25 million Americans. It is responsible for 1.5 million fractures annually. The total health care expenditures for osteoporosis are more than $13 billion annually. Currently, it is estimated to be the twelfth leading cause of death in adults because around 20% of patients who sustain a hip fracture die from medical complications within 1 year after the fracture. Therefore, primary care physicians must intervene to prevent the progression of osteoporosis.

2. What is osteoporosis?

Osteoporosis is a systemic metabolic skeletal disease characterized by low bone mass and microarchitectural deterioration of bone tissue, which results in increased bone fragility and fracture susceptibility. This process may involve loss of both cortical and trabecular bone. **Type I osteoporosis** is postmenopausal and usually presents with type A fractures (i.e., fractures of trabecular bone, which is found in vertebrae and the wrist). **Type II osteoporosis** is senile osteoporosis that involves loss of cortical and trabecular bone and presents with type B fractures (hip). Type II occurs primarily in men and women over the age of 75. Osteoporosis may be due to high or low turnover states.

3. What leads to osteomalacia?

Osteomalacia is abnormal bone mineralization, frequently due to defects in substrate availability (i.e., calcium and/or phosphate). It also may be due to alterations in vitamin D metabolism or certain drugs that cause abnormal mineralization, such as sodium fluoride or bisphosphonates.

4. What does osteopenia mean in a radiologist's report?

Osteopenia is a descriptive radiologic diagnosis suggesting that the bone mass is reduced by standard radiographic techniques. This interpretation usually is based on radiographs of the chest and/or lumbar spine. When bone loss is evident radiographically, approximately 30–40% of the skeleton has demineralized.

5. When are bone density measurements medically indicated?

The appropriate use of bone densitometry is somewhat controversial. Currently mass screening for osteoporosis in all postmenopausal women by densitometry is not recommended. Instead, bone densitometry is useful to screen patients at high risk for osteoporosis. For example, densitometry may be useful in patients who require initiation of chronic steroid therapy. More commonly, a postmenopausal woman, hesitant to begin estrogen replacement, may be encouraged to do so by a bone density study that suggests she is at risk for osteoporosis. Repeat densitometry is also useful for assessing the efficacy of osteoporosis therapy and the need for more aggressive treatment programs. Dual-energy x-ray absorptiometry (DEXA) is the preferred screening tool. Results are expressed as a T-score, which is the difference between the patient's bone density and the mean value for young adults. **Osteopenia** is defined as a T-score between –1 and –2.5; **osteoporosis** is defined as a T-score below –2.5.

6. What are the most common causes of osteoporosis?

Idiopathic age-related osteoporosis (most common)

1. Juvenile
2. Young adults
3. Postmenopausal (type I)
4. Senile (type II)

Osteoporosis secondary to disease states

1. Metabolic conditions
   - Calcium deficiency
   - Vitamin D-deficient states
   - Malnutrition
   - Idiopathic hypercalciuria
   - Renal tubular acidosis and other systemic acidosis
   - Scurvy
2. Endocrine conditions
   - Thyrotoxicosis
   - Cushing's syndrome
   - Male and female hypogonadal states
   - Hypoamenorrheic female runners
   - Prolactinoma
   - Hyperparathyroidism
3. Renal disease
4. Gastrointestinal-liver disease
5. Hereditary connective tissue disease
   - Osteogenesis imperfecta
   - Homocystinuria
   - Ehlers-Danlos syndrome
   - Marfan syndrome
6. Bone marrow infiltrations
   - Multiple myeloma
   - Lymphoma
   - Leukemia
7. Drugs
   - Diphenylhydantoin
   - Phenobarbital
   - Thyroid hormone
   - Corticosteroids
   - Chronic heparin therapy
8. Lifestyle
   - Nutrition
   - Alcohol
   - Smoking
   - Inactivity
   - Immobilization
   - Excessive caffeine
   - Excessive phosphate intake (e.g., soft drinks, red meat)
9. Miscellaneous
   - Rheumatoid arteritis
   - Systemic mastocytosis

7. What risk factors need to be assessed in osteoporotic patients?

Risk factors for osteoporosis include positive family history; life-long history of poor dietary calcium intake, particularly during adolescent years; physical inactivity or immobilization; smoking; malnutrition; hypogonadal state; and ingestion of substances of high phosphate intake, such as soft drinks or large portions of red meat. Coffee is a calciuric substance. Because fat cells can act as an endocrine organ and convert adrenal androgens to estrogens, lean body mass is a risk factor for osteoporosis, especially in Asian or Caucasian females. Steroids, anticonvulsant therapy with either phenytoin or phenobarbital, long-term heparin use, and alcohol abuse also are predisposing factors.

8. What laboratory tests help to evaluate an osteopenic patient?

The initial tests are a complete blood count with sedimentation rate and routine chemistry panel that includes assessment of electrolytes, calcium, phosphate, and alkaline phosphatase as well as liver and renal function tests. A 24-hour urine collection is analyzed for calcium, phosphate, and creatinine. Calcium and phosphate measurements help to assess calcium-phosphate balance. In osteopenic patients with anemia and elevated sedimentation rate, multiple myeloma should be considered, and serum protein electrophoresis and/or urine protein electrophoresis should be performed.

Abnormalities of liver and kidney function define secondary causes of osteopenia. Electrolytes are helpful in identifying patients with renal tubular acidosis. Serum alkaline phosphatase is a marker of bone osteoblast function and helps to identify patients with high-turnover osteoporosis or osteomalacia. A 24-hour urine collection for measurement of calcium excretion identifies patients with renal hypercalciuria (i.e., urinary calcium greater than 4 mg calcium/kg body weight) or hypocalciuria, which suggests a calcium-deficient state. An extremely low urine phosphate value may identify a patient who is phosphate-depleted, consuming phosphate-binding antacids, or vegetarian.

Other more specific but expensive laboratory tests may be selectively indicated, including measurement of parathyroid hormone, serum osteocalcin, vitamin D metabolites [25(OH)D$_3$ and 1,25(OH)$_2$D$_3$], urinary hydroxyproline, pyridinoline, or n-telopeptide. Osteocalcin is a marker of osteoblast function, whereas urinary hydroxyproline, pyridinoline, and n-telopeptide reflect osteoclast function. These tests are generally reserved for patients followed by specialists in a metabolic bone clinic.

9. How can a bone biopsy help to evaluate patients with metabolic bone disease?

The bone biopsy is useful in evaluating high- and low-turnover osteoporosis, osteomalacia, primary and secondary hyperparathyroidism, osteogenesis imperfecta, and aluminum toxicity.

10. Is a bone biopsy similar to a bone marrow biopsy?

No. A bone biopsy is performed after administration of tetracycline, 250 mg 3 times/day for 3 days, followed by 10 days without medication and readministration of tetracycline, 250 mg 3 times/day for an additional 3 days. Three days after tetracycline labeling, an iliac crest bone biopsy may be performed. The biopsy shows the amount of trabecular bone volume, supporting the diagnosis of osteopenia. The amount of unmineralized matrix is measured and expressed as osteoid surface and osteoid seam thickness. The amount of tetracycline-labeled surface defines the amount of active mineralization by osteoblasts and determines rates of bone formation. Specific stains determine osteoclast counts and aluminum toxicity.

11. What preventive measures should be recommended to patients at risk for osteoporosis?

An adequate calcium intake of at least 1,000–1,500 mg of elemental calcium/day can be ingested in food substances; however, because of hypercholesterolemic issues and the recommendation to avoid foods high in saturated fats, patients may need calcium supplements. If calcium supplements are prescribed, they are best taken with meals. Because peak bone mass is the primary determinant of fracture risk, simple dietary interventions must be encouraged in adolescents and adults in their twenties and thirties. Outdoor activities should be encouraged; minimal erythremic sunlight exposure provides 400–1,200 units of vitamin D from synthesis in the skin. The recommended daily allowance of vitamin D is 400 units, which is contained in a multivitamin capsule. Weight-bearing exercises stimulate bone remodeling and inhibit osteolysis. Risk factor modification is important, including cessation of smoking and alcohol abuse as well as participation in a regular exercise program.

12. What are the drug treatment protocols for osteoporosis?

It is best to divide treatment protocols into primary prevention and therapy for established osteoporosis. A daily dose of 0.625 mg conjugated estrogen prevents postmenopausal bone loss through its antiresorptive effect. A smaller dose of 0.3 mg may also be effective. It is the current first-line therapy for prevention of osteoporosis along with adequate calcium and vitamin D. The transdermal patch is also effective. Addition of a progestational agent to prevent endometrial carcinoma does not impair the skeletal response to estrogen. The nasal formulation of calcitonin has reemerged as a substitute for osteoporosis prevention in postmenopausal women not able to receive estrogen replacement therapy. It is sprayed in an alternate nostril once a day (200 IU per activation), has no significant side effects, and works by inhibiting osteoclastic resorption. Alendronate, 5 mg daily, also has been approved recently by the Food and Drug Administration for prevention of osteoporosis in high-risk patients (see below).

The treatment of established postmenopausal osteoporosis also involves estrogen and calcitonin in the same doses used to prevent postmenopausal bone loss. Adjunctive calcium supplements play an ancillary role in a dose of 1500 mg of elemental calcium/day. Bisphosphonates, which are also antiresorptive agents, are the newest class of drugs approved in the United States for the treatment of established postmenopausal osteoporosis. Because of its favorable effects on bone—namely, an increase in the density of the lumbar spine and a 50% reduction in fractures—alendronate is now the first alternative to estrogen replacement therapy in women with postmenopausal osteoporosis. Serious esophageal disease (stricture, ulceration) has been reported in patients taking alendronate. Careful attention to dosing directions is imperative to avoid untoward events. The 10-mg daily dose is considered optimal. Sodium fluoride is the only therapeutic agent that actually stimulates osteoblastic activity. Because of concerns about increased fracture rates, it is still considered experimental.

13. How is glucocorticoid-induced osteoporosis prevented?

Prednisone therapy at doses of 7.5 mg/day or more for 6 months or longer often causes rapid bone loss. Glucocorticoids cause osteoporosis through a number of different mechanisms. Calcium and vitamin D_3 have been shown to be effective for preventing bone loss in patients treated with corticosteroids. Hormone replacement therapy (HRT) is also indicated for some patients. If a patient cannot take HRT, a bisphosphonate or calcitonin is recommended. Follow-up bone density studies are indicated to monitor the skeletal response to any of these therapeutic interventions.

14. When is the optimal time for initiating estrogen replacement therapy?

Based on the rapid bone loss observed at menopause, the usual recommendation is to begin estrogen therapy at the time of menopause and continue for life. Recent data suggest that estrogen begun even after age 60 years is beneficial for the maintenance of high bone density.

15. How should young amenorrheic female athletes or patients with anorexia nervosa be treated to prevent osteoporosis?

Because peak bone density is a major predictor of subsequent fracture risk, the amenorrhea associated with competitive female athletes and patients with anorexia nervosa can have profoundly deleterious effects on osteoporosis risk. Although restoration of weight and resumption of normal eating habits are the mainstays of treatment, vigilant attention to calcium and vitamin D intake, together with HRT and alendronate, may be needed to prevent further bone loss.

BIBLIOGRAPHY

1. Delmas PD: Bisphosphonates in the treatment of bone diseases. N Engl J Med 335:1836–1837, 1996.
2. Hofeldt PD: Proximal femoral fractures. Clin Orthop Rel Res 218:12–18, 1987.
3. Isenbarger DW: Osteoporosis. Postgrad Med 101:129–141, 1997.
4. Jackson RD, et al: Forestalling fracture in osteoporosis. Hosp Pract Feb:77–108, 1997.
5. Khosla S, et al: Treatment options for osteoporosis. Mayo Clin Proc 70:978–982, 1995.
6. Liberman UA, et al: Effect of oral alendronate on bone mineral density and the incidence of fractures in postmenopausal osteoporosis. N Engl J Med 333:1437–1443, 1995.
7. Mehler PS: Bone density in amenorrheic athletes and in anorexia nervosa. JAMA 276:1384–1385, 1996.
8. Ross PD: Osteoporosis. Arch Intern Med 156:1399–1411, 1996.
9. Schneider DL, et al: Timing of postmenopausal estrogen for optimal bone mineral density. JAMA 277:543–547, 1997.
10. Scott JC: Epidemiology of osteoporosis. J Clin Rheum 3:9–13, 1997.

VI. Problems of the Gastrointestinal Tract

36. HEARTBURN AND DYSPHAGIA

Stephen E. Steinberg, M.D.

1. What are the symptoms of gastroesophageal reflux disease (GERD)?

GERD is the spectrum of signs and symptoms related to the reflux of acid or alkaline secretions from the stomach into the esophagus. Common symptoms include heartburn (pyrosis) and noncardiac chest pain. Physicians also should suspect GERD when patients complain of dysphagia, recurrent nausea, nocturnal wheezing, atypical chest pain, chronic cough or sore throat, or hoarseness. Bleeding may result from chronic injury leading to inflammation and ulceration (erosive esophagitis). Symptoms often occur in the absence of even histologic evidence of inflammation; conversely, even severe esophagitis and its complications may be present without associated symptoms.

2. What is waterbrash?

It is the spontaneous and abrupt onset of salivary secretions followed by a bitter or acid taste in the mouth. This symptom is believed to be initiated by esophageal acid and therefore may represent a symptom of GERD.

3. What impact does GERD have on the health of the population?

Over one-third of healthy Americans experience heartburn at least once a month, and an estimated 7% experience heartburn daily. Two to three billion dollars are spent each year on over-the-counter and prescription medications to treat symptoms of acid reflux. Furthermore, reflux esophagitis may lead to complications, such as strictures, bleeding, ulceration, and perforation, which require hospitalization and/or invasive interventions.

4. How are diagnostic tools useful in the evaluation of patients with GERD?

For the majority of cases, the history combined with response to an antireflux regimen is sufficient to establish the diagnosis of GERD. In instances where the symptoms are unusual or do not respond as expected, additional tests may be helpful:

1. **Esophagoscopy** is the gold standard for evaluating esophageal mucosal and structural abnormalities that result from GERD. Upper endoscopy can demonstrate obvious evidence of acid injury to the esophagus (e.g., erosions, ulceration). Biopsies are taken at the esophagogastric (EG) junction to look for microscopic evidence of inflammation. Endoscopy cannot, however, quantitate the frequency or duration of esophageal reflux.

2. A **barium esophagogram** is useful in defining intraluminal lesions that may result as complications and acid reflux. It is poor overall in evaluating mucosal inflammation and, like endoscopy, does not aid in the quantitation of reflux episodes. Reflux demonstrated at esophagram does not correlate well with symptoms of GERD.

3. **Esophageal manometry** is helpful in evaluating the resting pressure of the lower esophageal sphincter and esophageal peristalsis (acid clearing) but provides little information about the actual extent of reflux. It is helpful as a preoperative evaluation to confirm that a procedure to tighten the lower esophageal sphincter (e.g., Nissen fundoplication) is likely to be helpful and that peristalsis is adequate to overcome the surgically increased pressures. It is also useful in evaluating noncardiac chest pain, which is occasionally related to motility abnormalities.

4. **Twenty-four-hour esophageal pH testing** is the gold standard for documenting and quantitating the number and extent of reflux episodes. It also helps to define which episodes are symptomatic. A probe is passed through the nose and positioned in the esophagus. The pH of the esophagus is measured over 24 hours and any symptoms noted (much like a Holter monitor for cardiac events). The patient's symptom diary may be correlated to the esophageal pH data. In patients whose symptoms do not respond to empiric therapy and in whom endoscopy does not demonstrate evidence of inflammation, it is the best test to confirm that reflux is indeed present and that symptoms are associated. It is particularly helpful for patients with atypical chest pain, and asthma that may be related to GERD.

5. The **acid perfusion test**, also known as the Bernstein test, involves dripping 0.1N solution of hydrochloric acid alternated (unknown to the patient) with normal saline into the distal esophagus. A positive test reproduces the patient's symptoms with the acid infusion phase of the test. This qualitative test is rarely used today.

5. What pathophysiologic factors influence GERD?
- Decreased resting amplitude of the lower esophageal sphincter results in reflux of gastric contents, including acid, into the esophagus.
- Impaired esophageal luminal clearance of acid caused by ineffective peristaltic activity (low-amplitude, aperistaltic, retrograde, or spastic esophageal contractions) allows a greater period of exposure to acid for any given episode of reflux.
- Decreased salivation (a source of bicarbonate) rarely may contribute to impaired acid neutralization.
- A decrease in the mucosal protective mechanisms, such as the unstirred mucus layer and epithelial bicarbonate secretion, often occurs.
- Increased pain sensitivity of the esophageal mucosal receptors to acid may cause some patients more symptoms than others for the same degree of acid exposure.

6. How is the patient with GERD managed?
When patients have symptoms of reflux more than 3 times/week, medical intervention is warranted. Mechanical measures should be implemented first, along with histamine (H_2) blockers. Because gravity is one of the most important factors in the reduction of esophageal reflux, elevating the head of the bed 4–6 inches is especially useful for patients with nocturnal reflux symptoms. It has been shown that the efficacy of this maneuver alone is equivalent to H_2 blockers. Other mechanical measures include the avoidance of tight-fitting clothing and weight loss for the obese. Dietary alterations also should be implemented. Avoiding offending foods or medications when possible may decrease the frequency and duration of reflux episodes.

If a patient does not respond to initial measures in 6–8 weeks, acid suppression therapy with a proton pump inhibitor is indicated. Increased doses may be required. Finally, in patients who are refractory to the above measures or who may require extended pharmacologic therapy (such as young patients), aggressive evaluation by a gastroenterologist and antireflux surgery should be considered.

7. What are the risks of prolonged therapy with proton pump inhibitors (PPI)?
Early data (omeprazole in rodents) suggested the possibility of increased risk of gastrinomas with prolonged PPI ingestion. Subsequent studies have demonstrated no increased risk, and these agents now have FDA approval for prolonged treatment regimens.

8. What foods and medications may contribute to GERD?
The following foods and medications have been shown to increase esophageal reflux by diminishing lower esophageal sphincter pressure or diminishing peristaltic activity.

Foods	Medications
Fatty foods	Xanthines (including caffeine)
Oils (including peppermint, onion, and garlic)	Beta-adrenergic antagonists
Chocolate, alcohol, and nicotine	Calcium channel blockers
	Anticholinergics

9. Which esophageal disorders are associated with an increased incidence of cancer?

1. **Barrett's esophagus**, also known as intestinal metaplasia of the mucosa. Columnar epithelium replaces the normal squamous epithelium, possibly as a result of continuous irritation and inflammation. Because 10–15% of patients with Barrett's epithelium may develop adenocarcinoma of the esophagus, frequent endoscopic surveillance with mucosal biopsy and brushings is warranted.

2. **Plummer-Vinson syndrome**. This syndrome, which consists of intermittent solid food dysphagia (from a cervical esophageal web) and iron deficiency anemia, may be associated with glossitis, stomatitis, and achlorhydria as well as an increased incidence of squamous cell carcinoma of the esophagus.

3. **Caustic ingestion**. In addition to the immediate injury and subsequent complications resulting from alkaline and acid substances, the risk of malignancy is significantly increased in subsequent years.

4. **Achalasia and a history of oral cancer** also increase the risk for the development of esophageal carcinoma.

10. List the major types of dysphagia and their common causes.

Dysphagia is the subjective sensation of impairment in the transit of a food bolus through the esophagus. A history of greater impairment to solids than to liquids generally implies a mechanical obstruction such as a stricture, whereas equal impairment or impairment to liquids implies a functional abnormality. Dysphagia can be subdivided into three categories:

1. **Oropharyngeal disorders of the neuromuscular components** of the proximal esophagus and distal pharynx may be caused by cerebrovascular accidents, multiple sclerosis, amyotropic lateral sclerosis, and Parkinson's disease.

2. **Mechanical obstruction** is caused by a structural abnormality that results in obstruction of food bolus transport. It may occur with strictures (benign and malignant), rings, webs, and Zenker's diverticulum.

3. **Esophageal motility disorder** is caused by motor dysfunction of the peristaltic mechanism of the esophagus. Etiologies include achalasia, scleroderma, diabetic neuropathy, amyloidosis, and various medications.

11. What causes the "steakhouse" syndrome?

Meat impaction of the lower tubular esophagus caused by a distal esophageal mucosal ring (B ring) or Schatzky's ring is referred to as steakhouse syndrome. Symptomatic dysphagia occurs when the diameter of the ring is 13 mm or less; mucosal rings are often asymptomatic until challenged with a large bolus of food. Rings are usually amenable to dilation treatment.

12. A patient presents to the emergency department with symptoms consistent with esophageal food impaction. The patient is unable to handle secretions and is drooling. What should or should not be done to resolve the impaction?

Medications that may help to relax the esophageal obstruction and thus relieve the impaction may be administered, including intravenous glucagon, sublingual nitroglycerin, or a calcium channel blocker, such as nifedipine. Meat tenderizers such as papain should be avoided, because they may injure the esophageal wall. Endoscopy should be used if conservative measures fail. Endoscopy is both diagnostic and therapeutic; the offending object may be removed and the type of esophageal obstruction identified. A barium swallow should be avoided because it provides no therapy; pulmonary aspiration of barium may result, and barium mixed with food and secretions in the esophagus makes subsequent endoscopy more difficult.

13. What diagnosis should be considered in a patient who complains of halitosis associated with dysphagia and regurgitation of undigested food?

Zenker's diverticulum is a mucosal herniation formed by the protrusion of the posterior hypopharyngeal mucosa between the oblique fibers of the inferior pharyngeal constrictor and the transverse fibers of the cricopharyngeus. Zenker's diverticulum is proximal to the esophagus and is not a true diverticulum because it has no muscular wall. The typical history includes dysphagia and occasional regurgitation of undigested food. It is often associated with bad breath from putrefaction of food remaining in the pouch. An upper GI series (cine swallow) is the best way to establish the diagnosis. Surgical resection, the definitive treatment, is usually reserved for markedly symptomatic cases.

14. On chest radiograph, a patient experiencing progressive dysphagia and weight loss over 1 year is found to have an air-fluid level midway up the esophagus. What is the most likely diagnosis?

Achalasia is a disorder of the esophagus in which peristalsis is absent and the sphincter between the esophagus and the stomach fails to relax in response to a swallow. As a result, food is not propelled down the esophagus through the sphincter and into the stomach. The chest radiograph often shows a dilated esophagus with an air-fluid level. Patients find that remaining upright allows gravity to assist in emptying the esophagus.

15. What swallowing problems do patients with scleroderma or CREST syndrome experience?

Progressive systemic sclerosis (scleroderma) and **CREST** syndrome (subcutaneous calcinosis, **R**aynaud's phenomenon, **e**sophageal dysmotility, **s**clerodactyly, and **t**elangiectasia) are associated with impaired or absent lower esophageal sphincter function and esophageal peristalsis due to involvement of esophageal smooth muscle. The result is often free reflux of acid into the esophagus, the effect of which is worsened by the inability to clear the acid (absent peristalsis). Reflux symptoms are often severe, and complications such as Barrett's esophagus, ulcerative esophagitis, and strictures are frequent.

16. What options are available for palliation of dysphagia related to malignant obstruction of the esophagus?

Options include surgical excision and bypass, laser and alcohol ablation of tumor, and placement of esophageal stents. Surgery has been shown to be effective palliation for cancers of the distal esophagus. Tumor ablation, which requires multiple sessions and follow-ups, had been the mainstay of endoscopic management, because repeated dilatation is generally ineffective in malignant disease. It has largely been replaced by the use of expandable metal stents. The stents are placed across a narrowing, after which their self-expanding property dilates the stricture. This outpatient procedure provides good palliation and may replace surgery.

17. Do all complaints of dysphagia warrant evaluation?

Single episodes of dysphagia may be followed if the event is minor (such as having a pill stuck in the esophagus); all others should be explained. Weight loss is the most significant associated finding. The following tests can be used to evaluate the cause of dysphagia, each with its own diagnostic and therapeutic strengths and weaknesses:

1. **Endoscopy** is the gold standard for evaluating esophageal lesions such as rings, webs, strictures, masses, and esophagitis. Biopsy can be performed to establish benignity of the lesion. Dilation of the obstruction with balloon dilators or esophageal bougienage also may be performed.

2. The **cine-esophagogram** is useful in investigating the swallowing mechanism and evaluating patients with oropharyngeal dysphagia. A tailored barium study also may be performed, in which barium "foods" with various consistencies are administered to evaluate the patient's ability to initiate swallowing.

3. An **esophageal motility** study helps to determine the general contraction profile of the esophagus. It provides amplitude and duration of the esophageal contraction wave and sphincter pressure.

18. What is the most common cause of dysphagia or odynophagia in patients with AIDS?

Candidal esophagitis is the most frequent cause of difficult or painful swallowing in patients with AIDS. Thus, an appropriate anticandidal agent should be initiated empirically early in the course of symptoms. Common agents include nystatin, ketoconazole, and fluconazole.

Ketoconazole, however, needs an acid environment for optimal absorption. Many patients with AIDS are achlorhydric or take acid-suppressing medications that may reduce the effectiveness of ketoconazole. Anticandidal therapy relieves symptoms in more than 50% of patients. However, if the patient's symptoms persist or progress after several days of anticandidal therapy, endoscopy with biopsy and brushing should be performed to evaluate the esophagus for lesions from cytomegalovirus, herpes simplex virus, or idiopathic ulceration due to human immunodeficiency virus (HIV). Barium studies miss a significant number of lesions, and definitive diagnosis is difficult to obtain from esophageal contrast studies.

BIBLIOGRAPHY

1. Kahrilas PJ: Gastroesophageal reflux disease [review]. JAMA 276:983–988, 1996.
2. Katz PO, Castell DO: Current medical treatment and indications for surgical referral for gastroesophageal reflux disease ("GERD") [review]. Semin Thorac Cardiovasc Surg 9:169–172, 1997.
3. Hogan WJ: Spectrum of supraesophageal complications of gastroesophageal reflux disease [review]. Am J Med 103(5A):77S–83S, 1997.
4. Orlando RC: The pathogenesis of gastroesophageal reflux disease: The relationship between epithelial defense, dysmotility, and acid exposure [review]. Am J Gastroenterol 92(4 Suppl):3S–5S; discussion, 5S–7S, 1997.
5. Reynolds JC: Influence of pathophysiology, severity, and cost in the medical management of gastroesophageal reflux disease [review]. Am J Health-Sys Pharm 53(22 Suppl 3):S5–S12, 1996.
6. Richter JE: Long-term management of gastroesophageal reflux disease and its complications [review]. Am J Gastroenterol 92(4 Suppl):30S–34S; discussion, 34S–35S, 1997.
7. Spechler SJ: Barrett's esophagus [review]. Semin Gastrointest Dis 7:51–60, 1996.
8. Wilcox CM: Esophageal disease in the acquired immunodeficiency syndrome: Etiology, diagnosis, and management. Am J Med 92:412–421, 1992.
9. Wilcox CM, Schwartz DA, Clark WS: Esophageal ulceration in human immunodeficiency virus infection. Causes, response to therapy, and long-term outcome. Ann Intern Med 123:143–149, 1995.

37. DYSPEPSIA AND PEPTIC ULCER DISEASE

Thomas E. Trouillot, M.D., and Stephen E. Steinberg, M.D.

1. What is dyspepsia? How is it treated?

Dyspepsia is a vague constellation of upper GI or biliary tract symptoms that may include epigastric discomfort or pain, nausea, vomiting, heartburn, bloating, belching, and dysphasia. Dyspepsia may represent organic disease, such as peptic ulcers, gastritis, or esophagitis. The more common condition is nonulcer dyspepsia, which refers to the above constellation of findings in the absence of peptic ulcers or other mucosal pathology (i.e., after a negative endoscopy). When mucosal lesions are present, treatment is directed at their etiology. There is no specific treatment for the "waste basket" diagnosis, "nonulcer dyspepsia."

2. What symptoms do patients with peptic ulcer disease (PUD) commonly exhibit?

Abdominal pain, primarily in the epigastrium, that radiates to the back is suggestive of PUD. Although the pain is not continuous, it usually occurs on a daily basis. Ingestion of food (an excellent antacid) or antacids may relieve the pain of patients with duodenal ulcers, although it may recur 1–3 hours after meals; it often awakens patients at night. PUD may be asymptomatic in 15–44% of cases, especially in the elderly, and the presence or absence of symptoms does not correlate with the risk of complications.

3. How is the diagnosis of PUD best made?

Endoscopy provides a safe means of diagnosis as well as an opportunity to obtain mucosal biopsies to confirm or eliminate the presence of *Helicobacter pylori* or malignancy. Endoscopic inspection of the mucosa also identifies esophagitis, gastritis, or duodenitis, which often are missed radiographically. In cases complicated by acute bleeding, endoscopy provides therapeutic intervention by various modalities that may result in hemostasis. The major complications from endoscopy, although rare (0.001–0.01), include perforation, bleeding, aspiration, and complications associated with the anesthetics used for conscious sedation. Compared with endoscopy, an upper GI series has lower morbidity, is less expensive, and, with an air contrast study, may have a sensitivity approaching 80–90%. However, direct comparisons between an upper GI series and endoscopy reveal a sensitivity of 54% vs. 92%, respectively, when other gastroduodenal lesions are included.

4. What is the role of *H. pylori* in PUD?

H. pylori has been associated with antral (type B) gastritis, duodenal ulcers (> 85%), and, to a lesser degree, gastric ulcers (> 65%). It should now be considered the most common cause of nonrelated peptic ulcers.

5. What tests are available for *H. pylori*? When is each used?

The presence of *H. pylori* can be confirmed either histologically from an antral biopsy or by the cod liver oil (CLO) test, which detects the urease enzyme contained in the organism.

6. What are the risk factors for *H. pylori*?

Risk factors for *H. pylori* include low socioeconomic status, geographic location, and ethnic background. There is a higher incidence of *H. pylori* infection in Third World countries compared to the United States and Europe. In developed countries, the annual infection rate of *H. pylori* increases at a rate of 1% per year.

7. What other diseases may be related to *H. pylori*?

H. pylori is associated with adenocarcinoma of the antrum and body of the stomach. There is also evidence that *H. pylori* is associated with an unusual non-Hodgkin's lymphoma of the stomach, mucosa-associated lymphoid tissue (MALT) lymphoma.

8. What pertinent history should be obtained from a patient with PUD?

1. Does the patient have a history of previous peptic ulcer disease? Previous PUD that has not been adequately treated (i.e., eradication of *H. pylori*) has a high recurrence rate.

2. Does the patient use aspirin or nonsteroidal antiinflammatory drugs (NSAIDs)? These agents interfere with normal mucosal defense mechanisms, which utilize prostaglandins. NSAIDs also may cause a topical irritation that directly damages the mucosa. Symptoms correlate poorly with NSAID-induced ulceration.

3. Does the patient smoke cigarettes? Smokers have an increased incidence of ulcer recurrence as well as impaired healing and require higher doses of histamine (H_2) blockers to achieve the same degree of acid suppression.

4. Are other risk factors present? Although the evidence is controversial, psychological stress, alcohol consumption, and caffeine have been implicated in ulcer formation and/or impaired healing.

9. Describe the relationship between upper GI bleeding and PUD.

Significant bleeding occurs in approximately 25% of patients with PUD. Patients may present acutely with orthostatic hypotension, hematemesis, and melena. When the bleeding is sudden, the hematocrit may be normal and the indices normocytic. Chronic blood loss from PUD may present more subtly with minimal peptic symptoms and microcytic anemia that, on further evaluation, is found to be related to iron deficiency and associated with hemoccult positive stools.

10. Why is careful observation necessary after an upper GI bleed?

Careful observation is necessary because the rebleed rate in the first 48 hours may be as high as 50%, depending on the endoscopic findings.

11. What complications other than GI bleeding may occur with PUD?

Scarring may result in obstruction, most often at the pylorus or in the duodenal bulb, that usually is associated with recurrent vomiting and weight loss. Severe esophagitis may result from impaired emptying of gastric contents. Perforation of an ulcer into the peritoneal cavity or penetration of the ulcer into adjacent structures, most commonly the pancreas, also may occur. In either instance, pain often is accompanied with an elevated level of amylase or lipase. Surgical repair is recommended when such complications occur.

12. How can benign and malignant ulcers be distinguished?

A benign-appearing ulcer has a smooth, regular rim with a smooth, flat base when evaluated endoscopically or radiologically. Folds radiating from the edge of the ulcer crater are usually symmetrical. In contrast, the malignant ulcer may have an irregular raised margin surrounded by clubbed gastric folds that suggest local tumor invasion. Large (> 2 cm), recurrent, or malignant-appearing gastric ulcers should be biopsied and brushed for cytologic evaluation to rule out cancer. Follow-up endoscopy may be required after 4–6 weeks.

13. What are the pharmacologic options in treating PUD?

First, medications or habits that impair ulcer healing, including aspirin, NSAIDs, cigarettes, and alcohol, should be discontinued. H_2 antagonists, the mainstay in PUD treatment before recognition of the role of *H. pylori*, bind to histamine receptors on the basolateral membrane of parietal cells and thus diminish gastric acid secretion. Proton pump inhibitors (omeprazole and lansoprazole) can essentially eliminate acid secretion by inhibiting the hydrogen-potassium adenosine triphosphatase pump on the luminal surface of parietal cells. Compared with H_2 antagonists, omeprazole shortens the healing rates of duodenal ulcers, although it is more costly when used longer than 8 weeks. Sucralfate provides local cytoprotection by enhancing mucosal defenses and has healing rates similar to those of H_2 blockers, although the relapse rate was lower in one study. Misoprostol inhibits acid secretion by blocking histamine stimulated cyclic adenosine monophosphate in the parietal cell. Misoprostol and H_2 antagonists are the only agents with proved efficacy in preventing NSAID-induced mucosal injury.

14. How does treatment affect the natural history of duodenal ulcer disease?

Although the complete healing rates for antacids (> 80%), H_2 blockers (85–90%), and omeprazole (> 90%) are high, each has a high recurrence rate once therapy is discontinued (> 50% in the first year). Studies have shown that eradication of *H. pylori* appears to alter the natural history and markedly reduces the relapse rate.

15. What are the indications for surgical management of PUD?

The primary indication for surgery is an ulcer that fails to heal, although with currently available agents this indication is uncommon. Recurrent disease is a more common indication, particularly when the cost of long-term medical management is considered. Ulcer disease complicated by bleeding, perforation, penetration, and gastric outlet obstruction is usually managed surgically. Lastly, giant duodenal ulcers (> 5 cm) are often resected because of the high complication rate.

16. What are the surgical options for treatment of PUD?

Vagotomy is the basis of all peptic ulcer operations. Proximal gastric vagotomy (highly selective vagotomy, parietal cell vagotomy) has become the most popular routine surgical procedure for the management of duodenal ulcer disease. The operation is designed to denervate the parietal (acid-secreting) cells in the stomach while preserving vagal innervation to the antropyloric region to allow near-normal gastric emptying of solids. The recurrence rate is 5–20%. Truncal vagotomy/antrectomy is the best operation in terms of ulcer recurrence (10–20%); however, the incidence of postoperative problems is greater.

17. What is the difference between a Billroth I and a Billroth II operation?

In a Billroth I operation, after resection of a portion of the stomach and the duodenal bulb, the cut ends are reanastomosed. After a similar resection, a Billroth II operation is completed by oversewing the duodenal remnant and anastomosing the cut edge of the stomach to the jejunum.

18. What problems result from ulcer surgery?

Virtually all ulcer operations result in the more rapid emptying of liquids from the stomach or gastric remnant and delayed emptying of solids. This delay may be so severe as to result in formation of a bezoar, a mass of fiber and food material that does not leave the stomach. The rapid movement of hypertonic liquid nutrients from the stomach into the small intestine may result in large volumes of intestinal fluid secretion (at the expense of blood volume) as well as elevation of various hormones (e.g., serotonin, bradykinin, substance P, vasoactive intestinal peptide). The patient may experience flushing, light-headedness, diaphoresis, tachycardia, and postural hypotension as well as cramping and diarrhea. This constellation is referred to as "dumping syndrome." Other problems include alkaline gastritis, when bile refluxes into the stomach and injures the gastric mucosa; ulcers at the gastrointestinal anastomosis; weight loss; and iron deficiency, particularly with Billroth II anatomy, in which blood loss at the anastomosis (small ulcers) is common.

19. In a patient with recurrent peptic ulcers, routine screening tests reveal an elevated level of serum calcium. In addition, the patient reveals a family history of pituitary tumor. What is the suspected etiology of her PUD?

Zollinger-Ellison syndrome is due to an endocrine tumor that secrets gastrin, which results in gastric acid hypersecretion. Such gastrinomas result in recurrent PUD that is refractory to conventional therapy. Gastrinomas, which are usually found in the duodenum or pancreas, are diagnosed most specifically by an elevated gastrin level, which paradoxically increases after an infusion of secretin. Approximately 25% of patients with gastrinomas have the multiple endocrine neoplasia (MEN I) syndrome, like the above patient. MEN I syndrome includes gastrinoma, hyperparathyroidism, and pituitary gland hyperplasia or tumor. The gastrinomas are often difficult to identify when they are solitary and rarely resectable when associated with the MEN I syndrome, because such tumors are frequently multifocal.

BIBLIOGRAPHY

1. Damianos AJ, McGarrity TJ: Treatment strategies for *Helicobacter pylori* infection [review] Am Fam Physician 55:2765–2774, 2784–2786, 1997.
2. Deltenre MA: Economics of *Helicobacter pylori* eradication therapy [review]. Eur J Gastroenterol Hepatol 1(Suppl 9):S23–S26; discussion, S27–S29, 1997.
3. Falk GW: *H. pylori* 1997: Testing and treatment options [review]. Cleve Clin J Med 64:187–192, 1997.
4. Graham DY: Nonsteroidal anti-inflammatory drugs, *Helicobacter pylori*, and ulcers: Where we stand (see comments) [review]. Am J Gastroenterol 91:2080–2086, 1996.
5. Hunt RH: Peptic ulcer disease: Defining the treatment strategies in the era of *Helicobacter pylori* [review]. Am J Gastroenterol 92(Suppl 4):36S–40S; discussion, 40S–43S, 1997.
6. Kuipers EJ: *Helicobacter pylori* and the risk and management of associated diseases: Gastritis, ulcer disease, atrophic gastritis and gastric cancer [review]. Aliment Pharmacol Ther 1(Suppl 11):71–88, 1997.
7. Lee J, O'Morain C: Who should be treated for *Helicobacter pylori* infection? A review of consensus conferences and guidelines [review]. Gastroenterology 113(Suppl 6):S99–S106, 1997.
8. National Institute of Health: *Helicobacter pylori* in peptic ulcer disease. NIH Consensus Statement 12(1):1–22, 1994.
9. Reed PI, Johnston BJ: Treatment of *Helicobacter pylori* infection [review]. Biomed Pharmacother 51(1):13–21, 1997.
10. Smalley WE, Griffin MR: The risks and costs of upper gastrointestinal disease attributable to NSAIDs [review]. Gastroenterol Clin North Am 25:373–396, 1996.
11. Wilcox CM: Relationship between nonsteroidal anti-inflammatory drug use, *Helicobacter pylori*, and gastroduodenal mucosal injury [review]. Gastroenterology 113(Suppl 6):S85–S89, 1997.

38. ABDOMINAL PAIN

Stephen E. Steinberg, M.D.

1. Distinguish between visceral (splanchnic) and parietal pain.

Visceral pain is associated with tension or stretching of a hollow viscus such as the intestine. Pain is diffuse and tends to be poorly localized. It is frequently associated with autonomic responses such as vomiting, tachycardia, bradycardia, diarrhea, hypotension, and muscle rigidity. Uncomplicated small bowel obstruction is an example of visceral pain.

Parietal pain results from irritation or inflammation of a parietal surface. As a result, the pain is sharp and more localized. It is associated with voluntary muscular rigidity called guarding. Parietal pain also may be associated with cutaneous hypesthesia. Severe acute appendicitis and peritonitis, in which parietal surfaces are inflamed and irritated, provide examples of parietal pain.

2. What is the difference between rebound and referred pain?

Both types of pain are due to irritation of serosal surface. **Rebound tenderness** occurs when the palpating hand pushes into the abdomen and is rapidly withdrawn. The inflamed surfaces of the peritoneum rub against each other, and the patient experiences sharp pain. The presence of rebound pain supports the diagnosis of disorders falling under the category of "surgical abdomen."

Referred pain occurs at a site distant from the location of the inciting process. Irritation of the diaphragm resulting from pancreatitis; subphrenic abscess following splenectomy; or a bile leak after laparoscopic cholecystectomy result in pain referred to the shoulder. The pain is referred to the shoulder as a result of irritation of a branch of the phrenic nerve in the diaphragm.

3. What is the significance of involuntary guarding?

Guarding is said to be present when the abdominal musculature becomes tense or rigid as a result of peritoneal irritation. It is one of the most important indicators of a surgical abdomen.

4. What physical exam maneuvers are helpful in assessing the retroperitoneal area?

1. The **psoas sign** is right or left lower quadrant pain resulting from psoas muscle irritation. To evaluate the right psoas, the patient lies on the left side and the right leg is passively extended at the hip. The test is positive if extension produces pain, suggesting a focal inflammatory process on the psoas muscle. The sign is frequently positive in retroperitoneal (psoas muscle) abscesses, which usually occur on the right side and are related to Crohn's disease; it may be positive with acute appendicitis, particularly when the appendix is in the retrocecal location.

2. The **obturator test** involves passive internal rotation of a flexed thigh with the patient in the supine position. A positive obturator sign indicates irritation at that site, often related to an abscess.

3. **Percussion of the paravertebral areas** may elicit pain in patients with renal inflammation, in particular pyelonephritis or perinephric abscess.

5. List the medical and surgical differential diagnosis of acute abdominal pain.

Surgical	Medical
Perforated viscus (stomach, duodenum, colon)	Biliary disease
Ruptured spleen	Pancreatitis pseudocyst
Dissecting or ruptured abdominal aortic aneurysm	Crohn's disease
Bowel obstruction	Intermittent small bowel obstruction
Appendicitis	Endometriosis
Ischemic bowel disease	Mesenteric lymphadenitis
Volvulus	Vasculitis

Surgical	Nongastrointestinal causes
Ruptured ovarian cyst	Pneumonia
Strangulated hernia	Diabetic ketoacidosis
Acute cholecystitis	Sickle cell crisis
Ruptured pancreatic pseudocyst	Porphyria
Ectopic pregnancy	
Ovarian tumor	

6. What is postcholecystectomy syndrome?

Ten to 15% of cholecystectomy patients continue to experience the same pain for which they underwent the operation. It is then referred to as the postcholecystectomy syndrome. Some patients have biliary tract disease (e.g., retained common duct stones) or sphincter of Oddi dysfunction (the muscle at the opening of the bile and pancreatic ducts into the small intestine is found to be hypertensive). Such patients usually have intermittently elevations of liver function tests and/or amylase, which may be associated with progressive dilation of the bile duct. Other patients with this syndrome have irritable bowel, esophagitis, or peptic ulcer disease. For many, no explanation will be uncovered. Most patients with postcholecystectomy syndrome had a cholecystectomy for symptoms not originating with the gallbladder.

7. Does the chest radiograph have value in the assessment of patients with acute abdominal pain?

The technique used for a chest radiograph may be helpful in the identification of free air under the diaphragm, which is not as easily seen with an abdominal series. Occasionally, pleural effusions may be associated with subdiaphragmatic processes such as pancreatitis. Lastly, pneumococcal pneumonia may present as abdominal pain in the absence of abdominal pathology.

8. What is a sentinel loop?

In the setting of a localized inflammatory process such as pancreatitis, a loop of bowel adjacent to the lesion may become distended with gas, thus becoming more apparent on radiographs. It occurs most often with small bowel and is described as a sentinel loop because it heralds an underlying process.

9. What is McBurney's point?

The pain of acute appendicitis typically originates as poorly localized periumbilical visceral pain; it then changes to a more localized right lower quadrant (RLQ) parietal pain that is frequently associated with guarding and rebound. The location in the RLQ midway between the symphysis pubis and the iliac crest where the pain settles is referred to as McBurney's point. Tenderness at McBurney's point is said to be pathognomonic of appendicitis; however, it may occur with inflammation related to Crohn's disease, Meckel's diverticulum, or the right ovary.

10. How may the location of abdominal pain be helpful?

Visceral pain tends to be poorly localized and diffuse. When visceral pain originates from the upper GI tract, it tends to occur above the umbilicus, whereas pain of colonic origin is more likely to be suprapubic. Pain produced by irritation of parietal peritoneum is confined to the area involved by the disease. Pain resulting from biliary tract disease, duodenal ulcers, or pancreatic disease is often described as radiating to the back.

11. How does the duration of abdominal pain help in the assessment of etiology?

Pain that lasts 6 hours or longer suggests a surgical problem.

12. Why is biliary colic a misnomer?

Whereas colicky pain usually means intermittent crampy pain, biliary colic is most often constant, lasting from a few minutes to several hours. Of note, it is impossible to distinguish gallbladder pain from stones that intermittently obstruct the common bile duct.

13. Which is more dangerous, ischemic disease of the colon or small intestines?

Because of its blood supply (the superior mesenteric artery), small bowel ischemia frequently involves the entire bowel from the ligament of Treitz (proximal jejunum) to the caecum, with dire consequences. In contrast, the collateral circulation to the large bowel usually means that vascular compromise resulting in ischemic colitis with pain and bloody diarrhea is usually self-limited. It does not often progress to full-thickness injury and perforation, although strictures may ultimately occur.

14. When should ischemic small bowel be considered a cause of abdominal pain?

Mesenteric ischemia is one of the most difficult and dangerous entities to be considered in patients with acute abdominal pain. It is most difficult because the clinical and laboratory findings often do not reflect the significance of the problem. The abdomen may be tender and bowel signs diminished, but early in the process the examination is not impressive. Likewise, the radiographs show a nonspecific bowel gas pattern. Only when injury has progressed to bowel necrosis and the likelihood of patient survival is markedly diminished does the seriousness of the situation become apparent. Ischemic bowel should be considered when prolonged mid or migratory abdominal pain occurs in a patient with risk factors, such as previous embolic events, atrial fibrillation, atherosclerotic cardiovascular disease, or diabetes. Nonthrombotic (vasospastic) mesenteric ischemia is even more difficult to diagnose because it may occur in patients with few, if any, risk factors. An elevated white blood cell count or acidosis may be clues that a significant process is involved. When mesenteric ischemia is suspected, an angiogram should be performed. Even when mesenteric ischemia is diagnosed early, mortality exceeds 60%.

15. What test proves that chronic pancreatitis is the cause of a patient's abdominal pain?

No proof is possible. Such patients frequently have exacerbation with no change in amylase or lipase and no evidence of acute disease activity by radiographic studies. This difficulty frequently results in the labeling of patients as "drug-seeking."

16. How does abstinence from alcohol affect the pain of chronic pancreatitis?

Abstinence from alcohol may diminish acute exacerbations in patients with chronic pancreatitis. Unfortunately, chronic pancreatitis is a process that, once initiated by chronic alcohol ingestion, progresses even in the absence of continued alcohol intake.

17. Describe the treatment options for the pain of chronic pancreatitis.

1. An empirical trial of pancreatic enzyme supplementation is usually the first option. An early study suggested that it may be effective, and there are few if any side effects. However, results are often disappointing.

2. Patients frequently require narcotic analgesics; regimens are best managed in the setting of a formal pain clinic.

3. Percutaneous or endoscopic celiac axis block may be beneficial and, in addition, may predict a favorable response to surgical ablation of the celiac axis.

4. Endoscopic retrograde cholangiopancreatography (ERCP) may be helpful in identifying a mechanical lesion (stone or stricture) that can be managed endoscopically or surgically.

5. The most radical step, surgical pancreatectomy, improves pain in 70–90% of patients.

6. Lastly, the pain of chronic pancreatitis burns out in many patients over years.

18. How should the patient with chronic undefined abdominal pain be managed?

Serious and/or identifiable processes are eliminated by negative endoscopic, radiographic, and laboratory studies, absence of constitutional findings (especially weight loss), and passage of time (the most important test). Patients should not be told that nothing is wrong or that they are not having pain; rather, they should be advised that by the means available today, it is not possible to identify the cause of their pain. They should be reassured that under such circumstances an undiscovered serious problem is unlikely. Attention should be turned to addressing quality-of-life issues. Patients may be better managed by referral to a pain clinic.

BIBLIOGRAPHY

1. Abdu RA, Zakhour BJ, Dallis DJ: Mesenteric venous thrombosis 1911 to 1984. Surgery 101:383–388, 1987.
2. Kaleya RN, Boley SJ: Acute mesenteric ischemia. Crit Care Clin 11:479–511, 1995.
3. Malfertheiner P, Buchler M: Indications for endoscopic or surgical therapy in chronic pancreatitis. Endoscopy 23:185–190, 1991.
4. Rolny P, Geenen JE, Hogan WJ: Post-cholecystectomy patients with objective signs of partial bile outflow obstruction: Clinical characteristics, sphincter of oddimanometry findings and results of therapy. Gastrointest Endosc 39:778–780, 1993.
5. Toskes PP: Medical therapy of chronic pancreatitis. Semin Gastrointest Dis 2:188, 1991.
6. Yamada T, et al: Textbook of Gastroenterology, 2nd ed. Philadelphia, J.B. Lippincott, 1995.
7. Vozkurt T, Orth KH: Long-term clinical outcome of post-cholecystectomy patients with biliary-type pain: Results of manometry, non-invasive techniques and endoscopic sphineterotomy. Eur J Gastroenterol Hepatol 8:245–249, 1996.

39. CONSTIPATION

James Goff, M.D., *and Stephen E. Steinberg,* M.D.

1. How does the caregiver determine whether the patient is constipated?

Constipation is diagnosed by the patient, not the physician; it is a subjective symptom, particularly in American culture. Most surveys suggest that a daily stool is common in healthy populations, but the frequency is quite variable and related to dietary intake. Of healthy persons, 5% report two or fewer stools per week. Consistency is also an aspect of constipation; hard, pelletlike stools, even if daily, often are considered to represent constipation. It is often best to use the patient's baseline pattern and to consider a decrease in frequency and/or an increase in hardness as constipation.

2. Can any test objectively assess constipation?

In addition to the history and a rectal examination that provides information about stool consistency, a test of colonic transit time may be helpful. The patient ingests radiopaque markers ("sitzmarks"), and daily flat plates are used to evaluate transit through the colon. This technique provides an objective test for a symptom that is often highly subjective. In normal people without a diet excessively high in fiber, stool transit time is about 3 days with a great deal of variability.

3. Is constipation more common with increasing age?

Depending on the definition, the prevalence of constipation is 5–20%. With increasing age, 3–5 times more women than men have complaints of constipation. Although the elderly often complain of constipation (23% in one study), one-half of the same individuals report daily bowel movements, and over 90% report at least 3 bowel movements per week.

4. What is the most common gastrointestinal (GI) condition that causes patients to visit a health care provider?

Irritable bowel syndrome (IBS) is characterized by bowel habits alternating between constipation and diarrhea, accompanied by abdominal pain. It is the most common GI condition for which help is sought. It appears to be a motor disorder that is affected by stress and food intake. Concomitant psychiatric illness is more common in patients with IBS.

5. How are patients with IBS managed?

The management of IBS usually consists of eliminating other significant pathology (chronicity with absence of weight loss, fever, other constitutional signs); high-fiber diet or supplements;

identification of specific dietary intolerances; antispasmodic, antidiarrheal, antiflatulent, and analgesic medications; and attention to contributing psychological factors.

6. What mechanical problems should be considered with new-onset constipation?
- Strictures related to tumors, inflammation (e.g., diverticulitis, ischemic colitis), or surgery
- Perianal disease (e.g., fissures, abscesses)
- Volvulus
- Hernias

7. Which metabolic and endocrine disorders may be associated with constipation?
- Diabetes (acidosis, neuropathy)
- Hypokalemia
- Hypothyroidism
- Pheochromocytoma
- Uremia
- Hypercalcemia (of any etiology)
- Panhypopituitarism

8. List the classes of drugs that may be associated with constipation.

• Analgesics	• Barium sulfate	• Antihypertensives
• Anesthetic agents	• Bismuth	• Laxative addiction
• Antacids (calcium, aluminum)	• Diuretics	• Monoamine oxidase inhibitors
• Anticholinergics	• Antiparkinsonian agents	• Heavy metals
• Anticonvulsants	• Ganglionic blockers	• Opiates
• Antidepressants	• Iron	• Psychotropic agents

9. How is constipation managed?
After eliminating mechanical, metabolic, endocrine, systemic, and drug etiologies, attention is turned to symptomatic management. Deficiency of dietary bulk is probably the most common cause of constipation in Western countries. This problem is addressed by an increase in dietary fiber (wheat bran, oatmeal, fruits, root vegetables) and supplementation with psyllium-containing compounds. Behavioral modification to varying degrees may be helpful in patients who frequently suppress the urge to defecate because of busy lifestyle or lack of facilities. Exercise also appears to enhance colonic motility. Often reassurance is the most important therapy.

10. What disorder should be considered in young adults with a history of chronic constipation and a dilated sigmoid on flat-plate radiography of the abdomen?
In addition to considering the above factors, the patient should be evaluated for Hirschsprung's disease, which in the absence of neurons in the diseased segment of the internal anal sphincter results in failure of reflex relaxation during defecation. The result is chronic constipation. Although more common in children, it is occasionally seen in young adults. Anal manometry documenting the sphincter disorder and biopsies showing the absence of neurons suggest the need for surgical correction.

11. What other neurologic problems are associated with constipation?
Peripheral: autonomic neuropathies; various disorders that affect the ganglions. **Central:** medulla and cord lesions and injuries (e.g., cauda equina tumor, tabes dorsalis, multiple sclerosis); cerebral lesions such as cerebrovascular accidents, parkinsonism, and tumors.

12. Describe the six different types of laxatives.
1. **Bulk-forming agents** are high in fiber (natural foods, psyllium). They increase stool volume by absorbing water and require water ingestion (without water, obstruction has been reported).

2. **Emollient laxatives** (dioctyl potassium sulfosuccinate) are surfactants that may increase water secretion into the gut and facilitate the mixture of water and fatty substances into the stool, thus softening it.

3. The most common **lubricant laxative** is mineral oil, which decreases the colonic removal of water from the stool and lubricates it for easier passage.

4. **Magnesium, sulfate, phosphate, and citrate-based laxatives** exert an osmotic effect to draw water into the colon; they also promote motility.

5. **Stimulant laxatives** (anthraquinone derivatives such as cascara and phenolphthalein) enhance motility by neurologic stimulation and may alter fluid secretion and absorption as well.

6. **Hyperosmotic laxatives** include glycerin and lactulose.

13. When should laxative abuse be suspected?

The patient may complain of abdominal pain, nausea, vomiting, weight loss, muscle weakness, and lassitude. Hypokalemia and abnormalities on barium enema and rectal biopsy may be noted. Diagnosis of laxative abuse may be supported by the finding of alkalization of the stool (and urine) or a change in the color of phenolphthalein from colorless (pH < 8.5) to pink or red (pH > 9.0).

14. Are there potential risks for patients who experience chronic constipation?

Yes. The frequency of urinary tract infections appears to increase in women with constipation. Several controlled studies have also shown a link between colorectal cancer and constipation, particularly in women. This association may be related to low dietary fiber intake, which leads to smaller stool volumes and slower colonic transit time. Potential carcinogens may spend more time in contact with the colonic mucosa.

BIBLIOGRAPHY

1. Abyad A, Mourad F: "Constipation": Common-sense care of the older patient [review]. Geriatrics 51:28–34, 36, 1996.
2. Dalton CB, Drossman DA: Diagnosis and treatment of irritable bowel syndrome [review]. Am Fam Phys 55:875–880, 883–885, 1997.
3. Mellgren A: Diagnosis and treatment of constipation. Eur J Surg 161:623–634, 1995.
4. Mollen RM, Claasen AT, Kuijpars JH: Evaluation and treatment of constipation. Scand J Gastrol 223(Suppl):8–17, 1997.
5. Read NW, Celik AF, Katsinelos P: Constipation and incontinence in the elderly. J Clin Gastrol 20:61–70, 1995.
6. Romero Y, Evans JM, Fleming KC, Phillips SF: Constipation and fecal incontinence in the elderly population. Mayo Clin Proc 71:81–92, 1996.
7. Velio P, Bassotti G: Chronic idiopathic constipation: Pathophysiology and treatment. J Clin Gastrol 22:190–196, 1996.
8. Verne GN, Cerda JJ: Irritable bowel syndrome: Streamlining the diagnosis [review]. Postgrad Med 102:197–198, 201–204, 207–208, 1997.

40. DIARRHEA

Terry Linn, D.O., and Stephen E. Steinberg, M.D.

1. Is diarrhea defined by the frequency of bowel movements?

No. Diarrhea is defined as daily stool weight > 200 gm, regardless of the consistency or frequency of the stool. It is important to make this distinction, because many patients complain of diarrhea when they experience loose stools, increased frequency of small amounts of stool, fecal incontinence, or urgency (tenesmus), all of which have distinct differential diagnoses. It should be differentiated from incontinence, which is the involuntary release of rectal contents often caused by abnormal neuromuscular function or pelvic problems.

2. What 10 elements should be included in the history of patients with diarrhea?
- Character of the stool
- Past medical and surgical history
- Weight loss
- Travel history
- Timing of bowel movements
- Fever
- Medications
- Relationship of diarrhea to food
- Duration of symptoms

3. What is the significance of nocturnal diarrhea?
Nocturnal occurrence suggests that the diarrhea is likely to have an identifiable pathologic etiology. For example, patients with irritable bowel syndrome frequently complain of diarrhea, but it occurs most often early in the morning and rarely awakens the patient from sleep. On the other hand, patients with diarrhea associated with diabetes frequently are awakened from sleep. The absence of nocturnal occurrence, however, does not exclude an organic cause, and is even typical of diarrhea related to malabsorption.

4. What food history is helpful in the evaluation of diarrhea?
Diarrhea may be caused by milk (lactose deficiency), soft drinks (sucrose intolerance), food allergies, or gluten-containing foods (celiac sprue). In addition, heavy alcohol consumption, through its effect on the intestinal mucosa, may lead to episodes of diarrhea.

5. How does the duration of diarrheal symptoms effect the evaluation and management?
The differential diagnosis for diarrhea varies by the duration of symptoms. Acute diarrhea, with a typical duration less than 2 weeks, is most commonly caused by infections. Chronic diarrhea, with a duration of more than 2–3 weeks, is more difficult to characterize and may be caused by either structural or functional diseases.

6. How does the symptom of weight loss help with the differential diagnosis of diarrhea?
Not all patients with diarrhea have weight loss. When present, weight loss is suggestive of malabsorption, inflammation (enteritis or colitis), hyperthyroidism, or malignancy.

7. Which historical features suggest that a patient may be at increased risk for infectious diarrhea?
- Recent travel (developing nations, camping, Peace Corps)
- Ingestion of unusual food (e.g., seafood, raw foods, picnics)
- Institutional care (hospitals, nursing homes, day care centers)
- Homosexual behavior (male)
- Prostitution
- Injection drug use

8. What is the most important consideration in managing patients with acute diarrhea?
The cardinal principle in the management of acute diarrhea is the assessment of the degree of dehydration and replacement of fluid and electrolyte deficits. For patients who have had symptoms less than 3 days and are not toxic, symptomatic therapies (i.e., anxiolytics, antiemetics; anti-motility agents are not recommended) and oral hydration are usually sufficient. In general, antibiotics are not appropriate.

For patients who are toxic and cannot tolerate oral intake, IV hydration, stool studies and antibiotic therapy are indicated. In patients who have persistent symptoms for more than 3 days, stool specimen for leukocytes, culture, and sensitivity may be considered along with empiric antibiotic therapy (e.g., quinolones). Flexible sigmoidoscopy is indicated if symptoms persist, stool studies are negative, or therapeutic trial of antibiotics fails.

9. What can patients do to prevent travelers' diarrhea?
Travelers' diarrhea generally occurs in people who have traveled from an industrialized to a developing country. Most cases of travelers' diarrhea are caused by bacterial pathogens, most

commonly enterotoxigenic *Escherichia coli*. Prevention can be attempted in two ways. First, travelers should avoid eating and drinking risky foods such as unpeeled fruits, tap water, and salads. Second, pharmacologic agents may be taken when the risk is high to reduce the incidence of travelers' diarrhea, although the risk of adverse side effects, the potential emergence of drug resistance, and the relative cost should be recognized. In immunosuppressed patients (e.g., HIV/AIDS, elderly patients) antibiotic prophylaxis is generally recommended. Appropriate antimicrobial agents include bismuth subsalicylate, trimethoprim-sulfamethoxazole, trimethoprim alone, mecillinam, norfloxacin, and ciprofloxacin. Protective efficacy is variable, correlating with site of travel, length of stay, and choice of antimicrobial agent.

10. What is the significance of bloody diarrhea? What is the most common cause in an otherwise healthy patient?

Bloody diarrhea indicates mucosal damage or invasion. It may be caused by infections (dysentery), inflammatory bowel disease (IBD), ischemic colitis, or malignancy (colon cancer with tissue necrosis and postobstructive diarrhea). Aggressive work-up is indicated. In an otherwise healthy person, the most common cause is infection by *Campylobacter jejuni*. In most cases, the disease is self-limited, and no treatment is required.

11. What does the symptom of tenesmus indicate?

Tenesmus is the sensation of incomplete rectal emptying. Tenesmus indicates rectal involvement in the pathologic process. Examples include proctitis from IBD or infections, anorectal fissures, and anorectal cancer.

12. Name six noninfectious causes of hospital-acquired diarrhea.
1. Fecal impaction (postobstructive diarrhea)
2. Medications (e.g., omeprazole, magnesium-containing antacids)
3. Radiographic studies using Gastrografin
4. Elixirs (high content of sorbitol)
5. Enteral feedings
6. Cancer treatment (chemotherapy, radiation-induced colitis)

13. What are the causes of noninfectious chronic diarrhea?

The causes are usually divided into four categories, based on their predominant underlying pathophysiology:
1. Osmotic
   Malabsorption
      Pancreatic insufficiency
      Sprue
      Lactose/fructose intolerance
   Bacterial overgrowth
   Dumping syndrome (i.e., after Billroth I or II, Roux-en-Y gastroenterostomy)
   Laxatives (magnesium-containing)
2. Secretory
   Diabetes mellitus
   Tumors (carcinoid syndrome, gastrinoma, glucagonoma, VIPoma, villous adenoma)
   Bile acid diarrhea (post partial ileal resection)
   Systemic mastocytosis
   Laxatives (Na_2SO_4, Na_2PO_4)
3. Inflammatory
   Inflammatory bowel disease (IBD)
   Microscopic and collagenous colitis
   Eosinophilic gastroenteritis
   Radiation colitis

4. Functional
   Irritable bowel syndrome (IBS)
   Causes may overlap (i.e., Billroth II may cause dumping and bacterial growth).

14. What clinical clues may help to distinguish functional from organic causes of chronic diarrhea?

Symptoms and signs suggestive of functional disease include diarrhea that occurs only during the day, absence of substantial weight loss, alternating constipation, and a long history of bowel problems dating back to adolescence or childhood.

15. What routine examinations should be done in the evaluation of diarrhea?

Unless the cause of diarrhea is obvious, stool should be examined for white blood cells and blood (occult or gross), which suggest inflammatory disease (usually colonic). Further evaluation for stool malabsorption may be useful. For example, a positive stool clinitest suggests carbohydrate malabsorption (usually related to proximal small bowel injury), as does a stool pH ~ 5.5. A sample of stool for assessment of fat content may suggest fat malabsorption. Most patients with chronic diarrhea also should undergo flexible sigmoidoscopy for evidence of colitis or tumors. Biopsies should be considered for histologic changes (i.e., microscopic, collagenous colitis) even if the mucosa appears normal on endoscopic examination.

16. What parasites are most likely to cause diarrhea?

Amebiasis and giardiasis. Three separate fresh stool specimens should be examined for ova and parasites, but examination for giardia cysts or trophozoites may be positive in only 50% of cases. Examination of small bowel fluid or small bowel biopsy may be necessary for diagnosis of giardiasis. Microscopic examination of the stool for amoebae has a higher yield (approximately 90%). Serology for antibody titer may be done to evaluate the possibility of amebiasis. These illnesses frequently occur after camping.

17. How is the diagnosis of pseudomembranous colitis established?

Pseudomembranous colitis is caused by a toxin produced by *Clostridium difficile*, which overgrows in the bowel after a patient has been treated with antibiotics or, occasionally, chemotherapy. Definitive diagnosis can be established by the use of endoscopy (sigmoidoscopy or colonoscopy) or by identification of *C. difficile* toxin in the stool. The distal colon is involved in most cases of pseudomembranous colitis, but up to one-third of patients have findings limited to the right colon and thus require colonoscopy for diagnosis. Typical lesions seen at endoscopy are multiple elevated yellowish-white plaques of varying sizes; adjacent mucosa either are normal or exhibit hyperemia and edema.

18. Name 11 pathogens associated with AIDS diarrhea.

- Parasitic infections: *Cryptosporidium* sp., *Microsporidians* sp., and *Isospora belli*
- Viral infections: Cytomegalovirus, herpes simplex virus, and adenovirus
- Bacterial infection: *Mycobacterium avium* complex, *Salmonella* sp., *Shigella flexneri*, *Campylobacter jejuni*, and *C. difficile*

19. Which viral pathogens most commonly cause diarrhea?

Rotavirus Norwalk agents and enteric adenovirus.

20. When do symptoms of food poisoning occur in relationship to ingestion?

Food poisoning is most often related to staphylococci or coliform contamination. Staphylococci grow in poorly refrigerated foods, producing an exotoxin. The exotoxin (rather than the bacteria itself) produces symptoms. Patients become ill shortly after ingestion (1–2 hours), and spread is said to be horizontal. In contrast, coliforms produce symptoms through actual invasion of the host by endotoxins as well as some exotoxins. This process involves live bacteria and requires an incubation time of 24–48 hours; spread is vertical.

BIBLIOGRAPHY

1. Blaser MJ: Epidemiologic and clinical features of *Campylobacter jejuni* infections [review]. J Infect Dis 176(Suppl 2):S103–S105, 1997.
2. Camilleri M: Gastrointestinal problems in diabetes [review]. Endocrinol Metab Clin North Am 25:361–378, 1996.
3. Donowitz M, Kokke FT, Saidi R: Evaluation of patients with chronic diarrhea [review]. N Engl J Med 332:725–729, 1995.
4. DuPont DL: Guidelines on acute infectious diarrhea in adults. The Practice Parameters Committee of the American College of Gastroenterology [review]. Am J Gastroenterol 92:1962–1975, 1997.
5. Farthing M, Feldman R, Finch R, et al: The management of infective gastroenteritis in adults. A consensus statement by an expert panel convened by the British Society for the Study of Infection [review]. J Infect 33:143–152, 1996.
6. Fekety R: Guidelines for the diagnosis and management of *Clostridium difficile*-associated diarrhea and colitis. American College of Gastroenterology, Practice Parameters Committee [review]. Am J Gastroenterol 92:739–750, 1997.
7. Framm SR, Soave R: Agents of diarrhea [review]. Med Clin North Am 81:427–447, 1997.
8. Kroser JA, Metz DC: Evaluation of the adult patient with diarrhea [review]. Primary Care 23:629–647, 1996.
9. Larson SC: Travelers' diarrhea [review]. Emerg Med Clin North Am 15:179–189, 1997.
10. Lew EA, Poles MA, Dieterich DT: Diarrheal diseases associated with HIV infection [review]. Gastroenterol Clin North Am 26:259–290, 1997.
11. Marousis CG, Cerda JJ: Malabsorption: A clinical update [review]. Comprehens Ther 23:672–678, 1997.
12. Nataro JP, Kaper JB: Diarrheagenic *Escherichia coli* [review]. Clin Microbiol Rev 11:142–201, 1998.
13. Neild RJ, Nelson MR: Management of HIV-related diarrhoea [review]. Int J STD AIDS 8:286–296, 1997.
14. Wolfe MS: Protection of travelers [review]. Clin Infect Dis 25:177–184, 1997.

41. ANORECTAL DISEASES

Iqbal S. Sandhu, M.D., and Stephen E. Steinberg, M.D.

1. What is the difference between internal and external hemorrhoids?

Internal hemorrhoids, which arise from the superior hemorrhoidal cushion above (internal to) the dentate line and occur in the right anterior, right posterior, and left lateral positions, are lined with columnar rectal mucosa. External hemorrhoids, which occur below (external to) the dentate line and arise from the inferior hemorrhoidal venous plexus, are lined by perianal squamous epithelium. Because of the many pain receptors in the squamous epithelium, thrombosis of external hemorrhoids causes a significant amount of pain.

2. Are hemorrhoids more common in patients with portal hypertension?

The incidence of hemorrhoids is not increased in patients with portal hypertension. Hemorrhoidal bleeding may be a significant problem in patients with liver disease because of accompanying thrombocytopenia and coagulopathy. Hemorrhoids and anorectal varices, however, are separate entities. Hemorrhoids have no connection to the portal system; although the distinction may be difficult, anorectal varices span the dentate line and may bleed from either the squamous or rectal side.

3. What are the usual presenting complaints of internal hemorrhoids?

Internal hemorrhoids may be associated with discomfort, pruritus, prolapse, fecal soiling, and, most commonly, hematochezia. Bright red blood usually is seen on toilet paper or dripping into toilet water at the end of defecation. Blood may coat the stool.

4. When is it appropriate to attribute occult bleeding to hemorrhoids?

Hemorrhoids should not be presumed to be the source of bright red or occult bleeding until flexible sigmoidoscopy or colonoscopy has excluded other, more significant sources.

5. What are the choices in the treatment of internal hemorrhoids?

Treatment is based on the severity of the hemorrhoids. Internal hemorrhoids are classified by the degree of protrusion. First-degree hemorrhoids bulge into the rectal lumen but not out of the anus; second-degree hemorrhoids protrude into the anal canal with straining but reduce easily; third-degree hemorrhoids require manual reduction; and fourth-degree hemorrhoids are not reducible and are at risk to strangulate. Treatment of first- and second-degree hemorrhoids is usually conservative, consisting of high fiber diet, sitz baths, and anal hygiene. Definitive therapies, which result in thrombosis of the hemorrhoidal vessels, include photocoagulation, electrocoagulation, rubber band ligation, and cryosurgery. For third- and fourth-degree hemorrhoids the treatment of choice is hemorrhoidectomy, in which both the vessel and redundant tissue are removed.

6. What triad of findings occurs with anal fissures?

Anal fissures are linear ulcers in the anal canal that cause pain and bleeding. The classic triad of a chronic anal fissure includes the fissure, a proximal hypertrophic anal papilla, and the sentinel pile, a fibrotic piece of skin just distal to the fissure.

7. When should a search for a secondary cause of anal fissures by undertaken?

Ninety percent of anal fissures are located in the posterior midline. If a fissure is found in the lateral position, a search for a secondary cause, such as Crohn's disease, tuberculosis, carcinoma, or syphilis, should be undertaken. A history of anal intercourse also should be sought.

8. How are anorectal abscesses related to the development of anorectal fistula?

The anal glands arise from the anal canal at the level of the crypts of Morgagni. Both anorectal abscesses and fistulas appear to begin with an infection in an occluded gland. Acutely infected anal glands result in anorectal abscess, whereas chronically infected glands give rise to anorectal fistulas. Approximately two-thirds of perirectal abscesses evolve into anal fistulas or recurrent abscesses.

9. Which patients should avoid surgical treatment for rectal fistulae?

In the majority of patients without underlying problems, fistulas should be managed surgically. However, the fistulas that develop in patients with Crohn's disease present a difficult problem. A rectal ulcer may give rise to fistulas that open into the perianal skin, scrotum, vulva, or groin. The management of such fistulas requires optimal treatment of the underlying Crohn's disease. Asymptomatic fistulas do not require treatment. A commonly used medical regimen is metronidazole, 20 mg/kg/day. Partial and complete healing is seen in up to 68% of patients, but therapy with metronidazole is hampered by a high rate of paresthesias with prolonged use and recurrence of fistulas after discontinuation of the antibiotic. Surgical management is considered only after medical treatments have failed.

10. Who is at risk for rectal prolapse?

Rectal prolapse is more common in women than men and is associated with straining at stool, fecal incontinence, poor pelvic muscle tone, and pelvic trauma (including childbirth). The three types of rectal prolapse are complete, occult, and mucosal. Complete rectal prolapse occurs when all layers of the rectum descend through the anal canal. Clinically one sees red concentric folds that protrude with double thickness with straining. In occult rectal prolapse no protrusion is visible; the intussusception occurs internally and is best seen with defecography. Mucosal rectal prolapse occurs when a short segment of rectum, not circumferential, protrudes through the anus. Instead of concentric rings, as in complete rectal prolapse, one sees radial folds.

11. What causes pruritus?

Pruritus ani (chronic perianal itching) most often occurs without obvious explanation. Toilet papers with perfumes, dyes, or cleansing agents may be identified as the irritant. Patients are advised to cleanse the area fastidiously with water only and to use absorbent cotton or plain white facial tissue for wipes.

12. What is the differential diagnosis of anorectal pain?

The various causes of anorectal pain include acute proctitis, tumor (e.g., cauda equina and pelvic tumors), anal fissure, intersphincteric abscess, prostatitis, endometriosis, trauma or arthritis of the coccyx, and idiopathic factors such as proctalgia fugax and levator syndrome. Proctalgia fugax is characterized by severe, short-lived (less than 1 minute) attacks of rectal pain that occur infrequently. Most patients do not seek medical attention. Although the cause is unknown, it appears to be associated with the irritable bowel syndrome. Levator syndrome is a chronic aching pain of the levator ani muscles, usually precipitated by defecation or prolonged sitting. Rectal exam reveals tenderness and spasm of the levator ani muscles, usually left-sided, as the examining finger sweeps forward from the coccyx.

13. What is the differential diagnosis of acute proctitis (rectal pain, discharge) in immunocompetent gay men?

The differential diagnosis includes four major etiologies: *Neisseria gonorrhoeae*, *Chlamydia trachomatis*, herpes simplex virus (HSV), and *Treponema pallidum*. The symptoms of gonorrhea include rectal discharge, bleeding, and anal dyspareunia. Asymptomatic infections are quite common. Constipation is more common than diarrhea. Acute chlamydial infection may cause bloody diarrhea, tenesmus, discharge, and, on rare occasions, fistula formation. It is associated with tender, enlarged inguinal lymph nodes that harbor the intracellular organism. Infection with HSV causes anal pain, constipation, urinary symptoms (e.g., retention), sacral paresthesias, and buttock and thigh pain. Many patients have no visible mucocutaneous lesions. Finally, anorectal syphilis may be associated with pain, discharge, and tenesmus. The chancre of primary syphilis is present on the squamous epithelium of the anal canal, and inguinal adenopathy is often present.

14. What are the risk factors for the development of anal carcinoma?

Anal carcinoma is associated with male homosexual behavior and a history of genital warts, which suggests a role for human papillomavirus as a causal agent. Other factors associated with increased risk include smoking, other sexually transmitted diseases, Crohn's disease, and renal transplantation. Recent studies suggest that radiation therapy and combination chemotherapy provide improved results over wide surgical excision for noninfiltrating anal carcinoma. Tumor regression occurs in most cases, and normal anal function is retained.

BIBLIOGRAPHY

1. Barnett JL, Raper SE: Anorectal diseases. In Yamada T (ed): Textbook of Gastroenterology. Philadelphia, J.B. Lippincott, 1995, pp 2027–2050.
2. Daling JR, Weiss NS, Hislop TG, et al: Sexual practices, sexually transmitted diseases, and the incidence of anal cancer. N Engl J Med 317:973–977, 1987.
3. Fazio VW, Tjandra JJ: Management of perianal diseases. Adv Surg 29:59–78, 1996.
4. Hyman NH: Anorectal disease: How to relieve pain and improve other symptoms. Rev Geriatr 52(4):75–76, 85–88, 91, 1997.
5. Goldstein ET: Outcomes of anorectal disease in a health maintenance organization setting. The need for colorectal surgeons. Dis Colon Rectum 39(11):1193–1198, 1996.
6. Metcalf A: Anorectal disorders. Five common causes of pain, itching, and bleeding [review]. Postgrad Med 98(5):81–84, 87–89, 92–94, 1995.
7. Nagle D, Rolandelli RH: Primary care office management of perianal and anal disease [review]. Primary Care 23:609–620, 1996.
8. Nelson RL, Abcarian H, Davis FG, Persky V: Prevalence of benign anorectal disease in a randomly selected population. Dis Colon Rectum 38(4):341–344, 1995.

9. Pfenninger JL, Surrell J: Nonsurgical treatment options for internal "hemorrhoids" [review]. Am Fam Physician 52:821–834, 839–841, 1996 [published erratum appears in Am Fam Physician 53:866, 1996.
10. Polglase AL: Hemorrhoids: A clinical update [review]. Med J Aust 167(2):85–88, 1997.

42. ACUTE LIVER DISEASE

Bahri Bilir, M.D., and Stephen E. Steinberg, M.D.

1. What are the causes of yellow skin discoloration aside from hyperbilirubinemia?

Yellow skin discoloration may be caused by ingestion of foods rich in carotene and lycopene (e.g., carrots and tomatoes) or use of antimalarial drugs (e.g., quinacrine, chloroquine), busulfan, or dinitrophenol.

2. How is the ratio of the hepatic transaminases AST to ALT useful in differentiating alcoholic hepatitis from viral and stone-related liver disease?

Alcohol represses the synthesis of alanine aminotransferase (ALT) more than the synthesis of aspartate aminotransferase (AST). With hepatic injury (alcoholic hepatitis), the released enzymes reflect this effect. Thus, a serum AST/ALT ratio > 2 is characteristic of acute alcoholic hepatitis. Elevations in AST are modest, rarely exceeding 300 IU/L, regardless of the severity of hepatic injury. In contrast, patients with acute common duct obstruction (e.g., gallstones) may have a transient (sharp) increase in transaminases, occasionally to very high levels and usually with associated elevation of alkaline phosphatase. However, the AST/ALT ratio is less than 1. In acute viral or drug-induced hepatitis, enzymes typically exceed 1,000 if the injury is moderate or severe; the AST/ALT ratio is again less than 1.

3. What problems are associated with cholestasis of pregnancy?

Premature birth, increased fetal distress, and a high perinatal mortality rate.

4. Which serologic tests are useful in evaluating acute hepatitis of possible viral etiology?

IgM antibodies to hepatitis A virus are the best test for diagnosing acute hepatitis A. For acute hepatitis B the appropriate tests are hepatitis B surface antigen (HbsAg), hepatitis B surface antibody, and IgM-antibody to hepatitis B core antigen. For hepatitis C, the first screening test is the enzyme-linked immunosorbent assay (ELISA) for the hepatitis C antibody. In the acute phase (and occasionally in the chronic phase) of hepatitis C infection, the antibody may not be positive despite active viral infection. In this case, detection of hepatitis C virus RNA by polymerase chain reaction (PCR) is the most sensitive test.

5. What is the range of incubation periods for hepatitis A, B, and C viruses?

It is easiest to remember the incubation periods by the "2 to 6" rule: hepatitis A, 2–6 weeks; hepatitis B, 2–6 months; and hepatitis C, 2 weeks –6 months.

6. Which hepatitis viruses are spread by sexual contact?

Hepatitis B can be transmitted by sexual contact, whereas this route has not been clearly established for hepatitis C virus. Hepatitis A and E viruses are spread by the fecal-oral route. Hepatitis B, C, and D viruses are spread by serum. Hepatitis G virus is a recently described virus transmitted parenterally. It may, however, not be a pathogen. In addition, another non–A-G hepatitis virus appears to be transmitted by the fecal-oral route.

7. What is the mode of transmission of hepatitis C?

Of 50 million persons worldwide believed to be infected with hepatitis C, only 25% give a history of blood transfusion, and in 40% the mode of infection is uncertain. Likewise, the route of infection in community-acquired cases is unknown. Body secretions from patients who test positive for RNA of the hepatitis C virus seem to contain the virus; thus, both dentists and oral surgeons appear to be at increased risk of infection. The virus may be passed in blood product concentrates, but this method of transmission can be prevented by vapor heating. All studies indicate that sexual transmission is not likely.

8. What recommendations should you give to persons traveling to areas endemic for hepatitis?

For **hepatitis A:** strict sanitation (handwashing, avoiding local water, peeling fruit); avoiding known vectors (e.g., oysters). Immunoglobulin (there is no "hyperimmune" globulin), and vaccination are indicated when prolonged stays are planned.

For **hepatitis B:** vaccination and avoidance of high-risk activities (any activity that provides exposure to blood or body fluids). Endemic areas include Southeast Asia.

For **hepatitis C:** no current recommendations.

9. What advice should you give to casual, household, and sexual contacts of patients with hepatitis A, B, and C?

HEPATITIS TYPE	CASUAL/HOUSEHOLD CONTACTS	SEXUAL CONTACTS
A	Strict sanitation practice Immunoglobulin is preferred	Strict sanitation practice Immunoglobulin is preferred
B	Avoid contact with blood and body secretions; vaccination	Hepatitis B immunoglobulin is preferred; vaccination
C	Simple hygiene principles (transmission rate is very low)	Controversial

10. How risky is hepatitis B vaccination?

Fewer than 0.1% of 43,618 persons immunized for hepatitis B experienced an adverse reaction other than transient fever or sore arm. Serious reactions (e.g., Guillain-Barré syndrome) did not occur, nor did transmission of the human immunodeficiency virus (HIV). All health care workers, family members, and sexual contacts of HbsAg-positive people, prison guards, and other persons with likelihood of exposure should be vaccinated.

11. Who should receive hyperimmune globulin to prevent hepatitis?

Hyperimmune globulin is used only in the prophylaxis of hepatitis B infection. It should be given in the following situations:

1. After homosexual or heterosexual contact with an HBsAg-positive partner

2. After a percutaneous puncture (e.g., in health care workers or drug abusers sharing needles)

3. In neonates who are born to HBsAg-positive mothers. Such offspring (except neonates) also should be started on hepatitis B vaccine.

4. Patients with cirrhosis due to HBV received after transplantation

12. Can patients be reinfected with hepatitis viruses?

It is extremely unlikely for HAV and HBV. Patients with chronic hepatitis C often have exacerbations that should not be confused with reinfection. However infection with different genotypes of HCV is possible.

13. Which patients with viral hepatitis should be considered for treatment with interferon?

Interferon does not have a proven role in the treatment of acute viral hepatitis. Chronic hepatitis due to B, C, or D viruses may be treated with interferon. Preliminary results from the treatment of acute hepatitis C exposure (e.g., needlesticks) with interferon are encouraging.

14. When should a patient with acute viral hepatitis be hospitalized?

Patients who are severely debilitated and, in particular, unable to maintain adequate oral intake should be hospitalized. In addition, any patient whose clinical features suggest the possible development of acute liver failure (encephalopathy and coagulopathy) should be hospitalized immediately.

15. What syndromes other than liver disease are associated with viral hepatitis?

Atypical manifestations of **hepatitis A** include immune complex deposition, which causes leukocytoclastic vasculitis; cryoglobulinemia; arthritis; and acute oliguric renal failure. All resolve spontaneously. An acute illness that resembles serum sickness—with symptoms of fever, rash, urticaria, arthralgias, and, on occasion, acute arthritis—occurs in 10–20% of patients during the incubation period of **hepatitis B**. HBsAg-HBs complexes apparently play a role in the pathogenesis. With persistent hepatitis B infection, immune complex glomerulonephritis may occur, and 30–50% of patients with polyarteritis nodosa have evidence of hepatitis B infections. **Hepatitis C** appears to be causal in some cases of aplastic anemia. Viral antibodies are highly prevalent in the serum and cryoprecipitate of patients with essential mixed cryoglobulinemia. Hepatitis C also has been associated with Sjögren's syndrome and glomerulonephritis.

16. What is the clinical course of acute liver failure?

Initially, nonspecific symptoms such as malaise and nausea develop in a previously healthy person; jaundice develops shortly thereafter, followed by the rapid onset and progression of altered mental status (hepatic encephalopathy) and coagulopathy. Death occurs within 2–10 weeks in 80% of patients unless they undergo orthotopic liver transplantation.

17. How often is acute liver failure of viral etiology?

Viral hepatitis accounts for about 40–70% of all cases, including hepatitis A (rare), B (most commonly identified virus), C (rare), D (common with B), and E (rare) but occurs in epidemics with a high incidence of fulminant hepatitis, particularly in pregnant women). Cytomegalovirus, Epstein-Barr virus, and herpes viruses are occasionally implicated; herpes viruses affect immunosuppressed patients and at times pregnant women. The remaining cases are accounted for by (1) drugs and toxins, including fluorinated hydrocarbons (trichloroethylene and tetrachloroethane), *Amanita phalloides* (death-cap mushroom), and acetaminophen; (2) vascular causes (low flow states); and (3) various other disorders, including Wilson's disease, acute fatty liver of pregnancy, and Reye's syndrome. In 40% of all cases of acute liver failure, the etiology is unclear and attributed to an unknown hepatitis virus (non-A, non-B, non-C).

18. What is the significance of a "flap" in acute liver disease?

A flap, or asterixis, is a manifestation of progressive hepatic encephalopathy, but it is not specific to liver disease. It also may be seen with other instances of metabolic toxicity, such as uremia and carbon dioxide narcosis, as well as after cerebrovascular events. Evaluation for a flap consists of having the patient extend the arms and pronate the hands (with fingers spread and extended). Patients with asterixis are unable to maintain tonic extension. The sudden relaxation results in a quick drop of the hand and slower restoration to the extended position.

19. What causes death in fulminant liver failure?

Cerebral edema is the usual cause of death. Less commonly, sepsis and metabolic complications, including hypoglycemia and multiorgan failure, are responsible.

20. What is the treatment of fulminant liver failure?

The most effective treatment is liver transplantation. Although some patients with acute liver failure recover spontaneously with supportive therapy, the mortality rate without transplantation approaches 80%. A progressive increase in prothrombin time, development of encephalopathy, and progressive renal failure are indications for transplantation. Such patients are best cared for in an intensive care setting by specialists with access to liver transplantation. Because the transport of patients with advancing encephalopathy is hazardous, consideration should be given to early transfer of any patient with altered mentation; bleeding, decrease in liver size, or precipitous fall in transaminases predicts a poor prognosis.

21. What is the success rate of orthotopic liver transplantation in acute liver failure?
The 1-year survival rate exceeds 60%.

BIBLIOGRAPHY

1. Bernstein D, Tripodi J: Fulminant hepatic failure. Crit Care Clin 14:181–197, 1998.
2. Carre G, Schiff ER: Viral, bacterial, and parasitic causes of liver disease. Curr Opin Gastroenterol 9:349, 1993.
3. Huber RR, Sebestr C, Bauer K: Detection of hepatitis C virus subtypes with a third generation enzyme immunoassay. Hepatology 24:471–473, 1996.
4. Muraca M, Fevery T, Blancheart N: Analytical aspects and clinical interpretation of serum bilirubin. Semin Liver Dis 137:138, 1988.
5. O'Grady JG, Alexander GJM, Hugler KM, Williams R: Early indicators of prognosis in fulminant liver failure. Gastroenterology 97:439, 1989.
6. Reichling O, Kaplan MM: Clinical use of serum enzymes in liver disease. Dig Dis Sci 31:1601–1633, 1988.
7. Schafer DF, Sorrell MF: Power failure, liver failure. N Engl J Med 336:1173–1174, 1997.
8. Sherlock S: Viral hepatitis C. Curr Opin Gastroenterol 9:341–349, 1993.
9. Stolz A, Kaplowitz N: Approach to the patient with cholestatic jaundice. N Engl J Med 308:1515–1518, 1983.
10. William R: Classification etiology and considerations of outcome in acute liver failure. Semin Livers Dis 16:343–348, 1996.

43. CHRONIC LIVER DISEASE

Bahri Bilir, M.D., and Stephen E. Steinberg, M.D.

1. At what point should a patient be evaluated for chronic hepatitis?
Chronic hepatitis is defined as persistence of elevated transaminases for at least 6 months. Because enzyme levels may fluctuate (particularly with hepatitis C), occasional normal values do not exclude the diagnosis of chronic hepatitis.

2. What disorders should be considered in patients with chronic hepatitis?
The differential diagnosis includes viral hepatitis (B, C, and D), drug-induced hepatitis, autoimmune hepatitis, Wilson's disease, and alpha$_1$ antitrypsin deficiency. Alcoholic hepatitis, nonalcoholic steatohepatitis (NASH), and primary biliary cirrhosis also should be considered.

3. Describe the proper use and interpretation of hepatitis B serology.
Of the widely available serologic tests, hepatitis B surface antigen is the most useful marker of chronic infection and/or carrier state. Antibody to surface antigen is found in patients who have cleared the infection or who have been immunized. Core antibody can be useful in identifying early hepatitis B infections (before tests for surface antigen become positive). Because it is long-lived, core antibody is also useful in epidemiologic studies to identify people infected with hepatitis B in the past. HBV DNA test, like hepatitis B early antigen (HBcAg) is indicative of a high replicative, highly infectious state.

4. Describe the test for chronic hepatitis C.
Hepatitis C antibody identifies patients whose chronic hepatitis may be due to C virus. The third-generation ELISA is over 95% sensitive and specific, decreasing the need to use the RIBA

II antibody test. Because of the 5–10% false-negative rate, antibody-negative patients may be evaluated by the more sensitive RIBA assay. Identification of hepatitis C virus RNA by polymerase chain reaction (PCR) is highly sensitive but has a longer turn-around time.

5. When is it appropriate to test for hepatitis A and D viruses and cytomegalovirus (CMV) as causes of chronic hepatitis?

Hepatitis A virus does not cause chronic hepatitis. The hepatitis D virus is incomplete and requires the presence of the hepatitis B virus for infectivity; therefore, the test for delta antigen should be performed only in patients with B infections. CMV cultures should be considered in immunocompromised patients.

6. What is the likelihood of chronicity for hepatitis B and C?

Of acute hepatitis B infections, 10–15% ultimately progress to chronicity; for hepatitis C infections, the rate is at least 50%.

7. What tests should be ordered to screen for hemochromatosis?

Transferrin saturation (greater than 61%) and serum ferritin level are the primary screening tests for hemochromatosis. The gold standard for the diagnosis of hemochromatosis is quantitation of iron in the liver biopsy specimen. Magnetic resonance imaging and computed tomography may be suggestive but are not diagnostic of hemochromatosis. Family members of affected people should be screened. A genetic screening test will likely become available in the near future.

8. When should Wilson's disease be considered?

Wilson's disease should be considered in children or young adults with chronic elevation of transaminases. The disease is almost always diagnosed before the age of 30 years. Patients with classic Wilson's disease show both liver and neurologic involvement and a positive family history; often, however, only one organ is affected initially. Initial tests include serum copper (high), 24-hour urine copper (high), ophthalmologic examination (for Kayser-Fleischer rings), and ceruloplasmin levels (low). If the screening tests are abnormal, the diagnosis is established by quantitation of copper in liver biopsy specimen. Recent cloning of the Wilson's gene suggests the availability of a genetics screening test in the near future.

9. How are patients screened for alpha$_1$ antitrypsin deficiency?

Alpha$_1$ antitrypsin is a protease inhibitor synthesized by the liver. People who are homozygous for a variant of the normal protein are predisposed to the early onset of chronic active hepatitis, liver cirrhosis, and emphysema. Screening for the alpha$_1$ peak on serum protein electrophoresis helps to rule out alpha$_1$ antitrypsin deficiency. The diagnosis is established by measuring the serum alpha$_1$ antitrypsin level and phenotyping. Because expression is variable, some patients with the deficiency may not develop hepatitis or may do so only with additional insults (alcohol, hepatitis C).

10. Which patients are at risk for the development of hepatocellular carcinoma?

Chronic hepatitis that results in cirrhosis is a significant risk factor for the development of hepatoma; chronic hepatitis B and C infection confers an additional risk, independent of cirrhosis. Hepatic ultrasonography and alpha-fetoprotein have been used as screening modalities in high-risk patients.

11. What three laboratory findings suggest the diagnosis of primary biliary cirrhosis?

Increased levels of alkaline phosphatase, gammaglobulins (mostly IgM type), and antimitochondrial antibody titers are highly suggestive of primary biliary cirrhosis. Bilirubin is elevated late in the disease, which occurs with greatest frequency in middle-aged women.

12. List five findings in the extremities that are associated with chronic liver disease.

Palmar erythema   Dupuytren's contracture (most often seen in alcoholic cirrhosis)
Spider angiomata   Thenar and hypothenar atrophy
White nails

13. When is a caput medusae seen?

Caput medusae is the name given to engorged veins surrounding the umbilicus; normally venous filling is away from the umbilicus. This physical finding is most commonly seen in portal hypertension due to cirrhosis, but it may occur with thrombosis of the inferior or superior vena cava.

14. Should asymptomatic esophageal varices be treated prophylactically to prevent bleeding?

Prophylactic eradication of incidentally discovered varices by sclerotherapy or variceal ligation banding is not indicated. Sclerotherapy has proved ineffective, and ligation has not yet been evaluated. However, recent data suggest that one can delay the time to initial bleeding by treating nonbleeding varices with beta-adrenergic blockage and nitrates.

15. What is the role of endoscopy in the initial management of acute variceal hemorrhage?

After resuscitation, patients should undergo endoscopic evaluation with sclerosis or banding of varices. This approach controls the initial bleeding in more than 90% of patients.

16. Why should acetaminophen be avoided in patients with alcoholic liver disease?

Chronic alcohol intake increases the activity of the cytochrome P450 system, normally a minor pathway of acetaminophen metabolism. In this setting, a larger fraction of the acetaminophen is metabolized through the P450 system, resulting in increased amounts of toxic metabolites that need to be detoxified by glutathione. Alcoholics also have low amounts of glutathione in the liver because of concomitant poor nutrition. As a result, the increased levels of toxic metabolites cannot be detoxified, and hepatocyte necrosis results, occasionally even with modest amounts of acetaminophen (3–6 gm/day).

17. Describe the management of the patient with moderate ascites.

Most patients with mild ascites can be managed with salt restriction (< 2 gm/day). Moderate ascites (visible but not tense) usually requires a potassium-sparing diuretic (spironolactone or amiloride), occasionally in combination with a loop diuretic (furosemide or bumetanide). The combination is synergistic in patients with liver disease. If ascites is still refractory, large-volume paracentesis, placement of a LeVeen shunt, or transjugular portosystemic shunt (TIPS) may provide alternatives.

BIBLIOGRAPHY

 1. Berg PS, Klein R, Lindenborn-Fotmos T: Antimitochondrial antibodies in primary biliary cirrhosis. J Hepatol 2:123, 1986.
 2. Edwards CQ, Kushner JP: Screening for hemochromatosis. N Engl J Med 328:1616–1620, 1993.
 3. Hollinger FB, Lemon SM, Margolis HS: Viral hepatitis and liver disease. In Proceedings of the Seventh International Symposium. Baltimore, Williams & Wilkins, 1991.
 4. Madden WC: Chronic hepatitis. Dis Month 2:53–126, 1993.
 5. McIntyre N: Symptoms and Signs of Liver Disease. Oxford Textbook of Clinical Hepatology, vol. 1. Oxford, Oxford University Press, 1991.
 6. Rowdley KV, Smanik EJ, Tavill AS: Metabolic liver diseases. Curr Opin Gastroenterol 2:466–473, 1992.
 7. Runyon BA: Care of the patient with ascites. N Engl J Med 330:337–342, 1994.
 8. Runyon BA: Bacterial infection in patients with cirrhosis. J Hepatol 18:271–272, 1993.
 9. Wong F, Blendi LM: Ascites and porto-systemic encephalopathy as complications of cirrhosis. Curr Opin Gastroenterol 9:391–395, 1993.
10. Bula ZJ, Griffen LM, Jorde LB, et al: Clinical and biochemical abnormalities in people heterozygous for hemacromatosis. N Engl J Med 335:1799–1805, 1996.

44. BILIARY TRACT DISEASE

Stephen E. Steinberg, M.D.

1. Is fatty food intolerance related to gallstone disease?

It is commonly believed that fatty foods cause increased biliary pain; however, studies using test meals in a blinded fashion have shown no correlation between fat content and symptoms. In addition, gallbladder contractility does not change significantly when fatty or nonfatty foods are ingested. Symptoms such as belching, bloating, and fatty food intolerance are not statistically related to gallstones.

2. A 49-year-old obese woman on estrogen replacement therapy has gallstones. What is the most likely composition of the stones?

In the United States 80% of gallstones are composed of cholesterol. Cholesterol stones are extremely common and occur more frequently in women and with advancing age. By age 75 years, 20% of men and 35% of women have gallstones.

3. List the risk factors for cholesterol gallstones.

Age: 50 years and over	Obesity: > 20% above ideal body
Gender: female	Ethnic group: American Indian
Diet: high fat	Pregnancy
Drugs: Clofibrate, oral estrogens	Rapid weight loss
Genetics: siblings	Total parenteral nutrition

4. What is the risk of cholelithiasis during pregnancy?

The risk is related to both number and frequency of pregnancies. For example, a woman who has four pregnancies before age 25 has a 4–12-fold increased risk of cholesterol cholelithiasis. Certain changes in hepatobiliary physiology during pregnancy promote gallstone formation. This period is characterized by stimulation of cholesterol synthesis, decreased secretion of the bile acids, and hypomotility of the gallbladder.

5. A 30-year-old African-American man with sickle cell anemia has gallstones. What type of gallstone is the patient most likely to have?

The patient most likely has pigment stones, which are formed in the presence of unconjugated bilirubin and precipitate with calcium to form calcium bilirubinate stones. Amounts of unconjugated bilirubin are increased in hemolytic anemia and cirrhosis. Pigment stones come in two varieties: brown and black. Black stones are radiopaque and hard, whereas brown stones are soft and radiolucent. Brown stones are common in Asia as a result of infection by bacteria and parasites that deconjugate bilirubin.

6. What is biliary sludge?

Biochemically, sludge is composed of calcium bilirubinate and cholesterol monohydrate crystals embedded within a mucous gel. It has been called by many names—bile gravel, microcrystal disease, microlithes, and bile sand. Sludge is best diagnosed by microscopic examination of a fresh sample of gallbladder bile; it can be seen ultrasonographically as echogenic material that layers in the dependent portion of the gallbladder. In certain conditions, sludge is a risk factor for the subsequent development of cholelithiasis. It is quite common in patients receiving prolonged total parenteral nutrition (TPN). By 4–6 weeks, 50% of TPN recipients usually have sludge, and after 6 weeks its appearance is universal. Significantly, the reinstitution of oral feedings results in sludge resolution. Ceftriaxone also may contribute to sludge formation because it precipitates as a calcium salt.

7. **What is the current recommendation for patients with an incidental finding of gallstones?**

Most patients with gallstones (60–80%) are asymptomatic. Several studies have followed patients with initially asymptomatic stones and recorded the incidence of symptoms or complications. In a study of 123 faculty members of the University of Michigan who were followed for 24 years, the rate of development of biliary pain was 1.3% per year. At 20 years of follow-up only 18% were symptomatic. Other studies have confirmed the development of symptoms at 1–2% per year. These studies show that most patients with gallstones have a benign course; therefore, prophylactic therapy is not warranted. In certain subsets of patients, it may be prudent to make exceptions, including children with gallstones, patients with sickle cell disease and gallstones, and morbidly obese patients. In the last group, cholecystectomy is recommended at the time of other abdominal surgery if indicated.

8. **Once symptoms develop, does the natural history of gallstones change?**

Once a patient develops biliary pain, recurrent attacks are likely, although up to 30% of patients have no further episodes. The rate of recurrence may be as high as 30–50% per year in the first few years. Acute complications in patients who present with biliary pain occur at a rate of approximately 1–1.5% per year.

9. **What is the appropriate treatment for gallstones in diabetic patients?**

Early autopsy studies purported to show an increased risk for gallstones in diabetic patients, but the studies were not controlled for confounding risk factors such as obesity and hyperlipidemia, disorders that are common in the diabetic population. Studies that controlled for these factors have not shown an increased risk of gallstone formation. In addition, previous studies appeared to show significantly greater morbidity and mortality for cholecystectomy in diabetic patients than in the general population. More recent data indicate that biliary surgery in diabetic patients is not associated with increased morbidity and mortality. Therefore, diabetic patients should be managed no differently from other patients.

10. **What radiologic studies are useful in the diagnosis of patients with suspected gallstones?**

Ultrasonography has high specificity and sensitivity for the diagnosis of gallstones and is usually the first test. The false-negative rate is approximately 5%. Ultrasound is also useful in detecting thickening of the gallbladder wall (chronic cholecystitis), fluid around the gallbladder (acute cholecystitis), and dilation of the biliary tree (choledocholithiasis). However, it is not helpful in excluding stones in the common bile duct; the false-negative rate is high unless the bile duct is markedly dilated. Oral cholecystography may identify stones that are not picked up by ultrasonography.

11. **What is the best test to order when acute cholecystitis is suspected?**

When the clinical findings are not definitive, hepatobiliary scintigraphy (HIDA scan) is useful in the diagnosis of acute cholecystitis. After a 2-hour fast the patient is given a radiolabeled agent, which is taken up by the liver and excreted into the biliary system. Images of the gallbladder, common bile duct, and small bowel should appear within 45 minutes. Failure to image the gallbladder by 90 minutes is strongly suggestive of cystic duct obstruction. False-positive scans may result from prolonged fasting or in the presence of TPN. The false-negative rate of this test is less than 5%.

12. **Can cholecystitis develop without gallbladder stones?**

Acalculus cholecystitis accounts for 5–10% of the patients presenting with acute cholecystitis. It usually occurs in the setting of major surgery, critical illness, intensive trauma, or burn-related injury. Hypotension and sympathetic vasoconstriction may predispose the patient to ischemic injury. The patients are predominantly male and older than 50 years. Many are on TPN. The pathogenesis probably involves a combination of stasis, chemical inflammation, and ischemia. Acalculus cholecystitis is a more fulminant disorder than calculus cholecystitis, possibly because the patients are older and sicker.

13. Which procedure is associated with more complications—laparoscopic or open cholecystectomy?

Laparoscopic cholecystectomy. Open cholecystectomy is one of the safest surgical procedures with mortality rates of less than 1%, although the rate increases with age and for urgent procedures. The incidence of bile duct injury is 0.1–0.2%. Recovery time after open cholecystectomy may take months because of the extensive abdominal incision. Laparoscopic cholecystectomy has gained popularity since its introduction in 1989. The advantages include minimal incisions, decreased postoperative pain, improved recovery time with discharge from the hospital in 1–2 days, and unrestricted activity at 8 days. The disadvantages of laparoscopic cholecystectomy include longer anesthesia time and an increased rate of complications, which is likely to improve as experience with the procedure increases. The rate of bile duct injury is approximately 0.5%; 5% of patients require conversion to open cholecystectomy.

14. What are the contraindications to the performance of laparoscopic cholecystectomy?

Contraindications to laparoscopic cholecystectomy include generalized peritonitis, severe acute pancreatitis, cirrhosis with portal hypertension, unresponsive coagulopathy, and carcinoma of the gallbladder. Pregnancy in the third trimester is a contraindication because of potential injury to the uterus. Patients with chronic obstructive pulmonary disease need to be monitored carefully because the CO_2 used to insufflate the abdominal cavity may cause hypercarbia and acidosis. Obesity is generally not a problem unless the abdominal wall is so large that the instruments cannot reach the gallbladder.

15. What are alternatives to surgery for acute and chronic cholecystitis?

Patients with acute cholecystitis who are high risk for surgery can often be managed initially by percutaneous drainage, usually under ultrasound guidance. For patients in need of a longer-term solution, cannulation of the cystic duct at endoscopic retrograde cholangiopancreatography (ERCP) can be done fairly predictably, and stents or nasobiliary tubes can be passed into the gallbladder with resolution of cholecystitis in most cases. This procedure is indicated in high-risk patients in whom an operation is to be avoided (e.g., before liver transplantation). Elective dissolution of gallbladder stones with a nasobiliary tube also has received limited application.

16. Distinguish among cholelithiasis, choledocholithiasis, and biliary colic.

Cholelithiasis and choledocholithiasis are simply the descriptions for stones in the gallbladder and bile duct, respectively. Both often occur without symptoms. Biliary colic, however, is the term used to refer to pain caused by stones or other abnormalities of the gallbladder. In reality, biliary pain is not colicky but rather a steady (not fluctuating) pain localized to the epigastrium or the right upper quadrant. It may last from 1–6 hours and often occurs at random with no relation to meals. Pain frequently radiates to the right scapula or shoulder or into the back. Because it is related to obstruction rather than infection, it usually occurs without constitutional signs (e.g., fever, chills). The biliary colic of a typical "gallbladder attack" is indistinguishable from that of transient obstruction of the bile duct with a stone.

17. Which tests provide the strongest clues to a common duct stone?

Serial liver function tests, including assessment of direct bilirubin, transaminases, and alkaline phosphatase, provide the strongest evidence for or against the diagnosis of choledocholithiasis. When a stone obstructs the duct, the transaminases rise abruptly, occasionally to very high levels. Within a few hours they begin to fall (even if the obstruction persists), and the levels of direct bilirubin and alkaline phosphatase rise at a moderate pace. When the obstruction is alleviated (by passage, movement of the stone back into the duct, or removal), all abnormalities rapidly return toward normal. Cholecystitis is associated with only minimal changes in liver function tests. In hepatitis the liver may be tender, but pain is not a common feature and liver function tests do not fluctuate dramatically. Although the finding of a dilated common duct on ultrasound or computed tomographic (CT) scan suggest biliary pathology, both modalities often fail to find common duct stones, especially when the duct is of normal caliber. Neither test is required to make or act on the diagnosis of common bile duct stone. If the clinical features and liver function tests suggest biliary obstruction, ERCP should be performed for diagnosis and treatment.

18. What is Charcot's triad? Reynold's pentad?

Stones within the common bile duct are usually associated with infected bile, and cholangitis results if obstruction occurs. **Charcot's triad** consists of upper abdominal pain, fever secondary to bacteremia, and jaundice from extrahepatic obstruction. **Reynold's pentad** is the addition of hypotension and mental confusion in more severe suppurative cases. The most common organisms include *Escherichia coli*, *Klebsiella* sp., *Pseudomonas* sp., enterococci, and anaerobes.

19. What is the most common cause of pancreatitis in nondrinkers?

Gallstone-related (biliary) pancreatitis is the most frequent type in nondrinkers. It typically occurs in patients with smaller rather than larger stones, presumably because small stones are able to migrate to the end of the bile duct at its junction with the pancreatic duct. The mechanisms by which the stones cause pancreatitis are unclear. Biliary sludge and crystals are also associated with pancreatitis. Biliary sludge occurs when cholesterol or calcium bilirubinate precipitates in bile and may be a precursor to gallstone formation. Studies have shown that after gallstones and alcohol, biliary sludge is the third most common cause of acute pancreatitis. Sphincter of Oddi dysfunction, pancreas divisum, and unsuspected stones are less common causes of pancreatitis. Ceftriaxone, a third-generation cephalosporin, has been implicated as a cause of biliary sludge; it may precipitate with calcium to form crystals and sludge. The crystals and sludge dissolve when the drug is discontinued; thus, symptoms rarely require surgical intervention.

20. What percentage of patients with pancreatitis secondary to gallstones will pass the gallstone?

It is postulated that the lodging of a gallstone at the duodenal papilla is the precipitant of an attack of acute gallstone pancreatitis. In approximately 80–90% of patients with gallstone pancreatitis, the stone will pass without intervention.

21. What is the role of ERCP in acute gallstone pancreatitis?

A recent study found that ERCP with papillotomy performed within 24 hours of the onset of symptoms resulted in a decrease in incidence of biliary sepsis. There was no change in mortality or other complications, such as pseudocyst. ERCP is indicated in episodes of gallstone pancreatitis that are deemed to be severe, that do not resolve with conservative measures, or that are associated with possible acute cholangitis.

22. What are the causes of acute cholecystitis in immunocompromised patients?

Cytomegalovirus and cryptosporidia can infect the biliary system and produce symptoms in patients with AIDS or after bone marrow transplantation.

23. What are the manifestations of the bile duct injury?

Bile duct injury leads to two clinical manifestations: bile leakage into the peritoneum, with resulting bile peritonitis and abdominal pain, and biliary obstruction due to partial or complete hepatic or common duct ligation or to late-onset stricture. Patients may present 3–7 days after surgery with fever, abdominal pain, anorexia, nausea, jaundice ileus, and ascites. Cholescintography with 99m Tc-1DA may be used to diagnose bile leakage and may show activity in the right paracolic gutter. ERCP can be used for diagnosis as well as treatment (stricture dilation, stent placement). Surgical repair may be necessary in some patients.

24. What is the role of magnetic resonance cholangiopancreatography (MRCP)?

MRCP represents a noninvasive method of obtaining cholangiography and pancreatography. It is based on imaging capabilities of MR combined with powerful computers, which can subtract unwanted portions of the image and reconstruct them in three dimensions. It can be performed without administration of contrast agents and with any degree of obstruction. There are several disadvantages, however: MRCP cannot currently distinguish stones from tissues, and there is no potential for interventions such as biopsy or brushings.

A number of studies have compared MRCP with ERCP. In general, the correlation of findings has been high. However, in most cases MRCP ultimately was an additional procedure and did not replace ERCP, resulting in additional cost rather than more efficient evaluation.

25. What is the association between gallstones and gallbladder carcinoma?

The incidence of gallbladder cancer in the United States is low. Despite a definite association with gallstones (70–90% of patients with gallbladder cancer have gallstones), the incidence of gallbladder cancer in patients with gallstones is low (0.5–3%). A causal role has not been proved. In general, cholecystectomy is not recommended for the prevention of gallbladder carcinoma, with the possible exception of very large stones (> 3 cm).

BIBLIOGRAPHY

1. Aucott JN, Cooper GS, Bloom AD, et al: Management of gallstones in diabetic patients. Arch Intern Med 153:1053–1058, 1993.
2. Borum ML: Hepatobiliary diseases in women [review]. Med Clin North Am 82:51–75, 1998.
3. Fan ST, Lai ECS, Mok FPT, et al: Early treatment of acute biliary pancreatitis by endoscopic papillotomy. N Engl J Med 328:228–232, 1993.
4. Fenster LF, Lonborg R, Thirlby RC, Traverso LW: What symptoms does cholecystectomy cure? Insights from an outcomes measurement project and review of the literature [review]. Am J Surg 169:533–538, 1995.
5. Ghumman E, Barry M, Grace PA: Management of gallstones in pregnancy [review]. Br J Surg 84:1646–1650, 1997.
6. Lai ECS, Mok FPT, Tan ESY, et al: Endoscopic biliary drainage for severe acute cholangitis. N Engl J Med 326:1582–1586, 1992.
7. Nash JA, Cohen SA: Gallbladder and biliary tract disease in AIDS [review]. Gastroenterol Clin North Am 26:323–335, 1997.
8. Siegel JH, Kasmin FE: Biliary tract diseases in the elderly: Management and outcomes [review]. Gut 41:433–435, 1997.
9. Schwesinger WH, Diehl AK: Changing indications for laparoscopic cholecystectomy. Stones without symptoms and symptoms without stones [review]. Surg Clin North Am 76:493–504, 1996.
10. Soto JA, et al: Magnetic resonance cholangiography comparison with endoscopic retrograde cholangiopancreatography. Gastroenterology 110:589–597, 1996.
11. Tait N, Little JM: The treatment of gall stones [review]. BMJ 311:99–105, 1995.

45. ENDOSCOPY: INDICATIONS AND OUTCOMES

Terry Linn, D.O., and Stephen E. Steinberg, M.D.

1. When should colonoscopy be performed instead of a double-contrast barium enema?

Colonoscopy is the preferred method for evaluation of symptoms of hematochezia, surveillance after resection of colon cancer or polyps, and surveillance of inflammatory bowel disease. For these indications, the ability to perform hemostasis therapy, to obtain biopsies, and to remove polyps during colonoscopy outweighs the cost savings of the purely diagnostic double-contrast barium enema. Double-contrast barium enema, combined with flexible sigmoidoscopy, represents an effective strategy for colon cancer screening.

2. What is the recommended surveillance interval after colonoscopic removal of a few benign adenomatous polyps?

According to data from the National Polyps Study, after an initial high-quality colonoscopy during which all synchronous adenomas were removed, a follow-up colonoscopy should be performed in 3 years. The purpose of this surveillance is to check for adenomas that may have been missed on the first colonoscopy (synchronous lesions) or that may have formed in the interim (metachronous lesions). If the examination at the 3-year interval is unremarkable, the subsequent intervals may be extended to 5 years. Because it takes 3–6 years for a polyp to grow to visibility and another 4–6 years for the small proportion that will become malignant to do so, a long screening window is possible.

3. What is the current recommendation for colorectal cancer screening in asymptomatic patients at average risk (i.e., no family history of colorectal cancer or history of polyps)?

For patients who are age 50 or older, the recommendation is to have fecal occult blood test (FOBT) annually and flexible sigmoidoscopy every 3–5 years. With the above combination screening tests, one can achieve 50% risk reduction in preventing cancer development. If the FOBT is positive or adenomatous polyps are found on sigmoidoscopy, a colonoscopy is recommended to assess the proximal colon. The test should then be repeated every 3–5 years, depending on number and/or size of polyp(s). Screening tests should be continued until patients reach age 80. After age 80, further screening is not cost-effective.

4. What is the diagnostic accuracy of colonoscopy?

The sensitivity of colonoscopy varies with the size of the lesion. Colonoscopy has a detection rate greater than 95% for lesions larger than 1.0 cm, 85–90% for lesions between 0.5–1.0 cm, and 70–80% for lesions less than 0.5 cm in diameter.

5. What are the usual indications for esophagogastroduodenoscopy (EGD)?

An EGD is usually indicated to evaluate upper abdominal symptoms that have not responded to an appropriate trial of therapy or that are associated with anorexia and weight loss, complaints of dysphagia or odynophagia, or persistent nausea and vomiting. Additionally, EGD is indicated to biopsy lesions detected by radiographs, to treat upper gastrointestinal (GI) bleeding, and to assess mucosal injury after ingestion of a corrosive agent.

6. How effective is endoscopic therapy of bleeding peptic ulcers?

Endoscopic therapy with thermal probe, bipolar electrical probe, or epinephrine injection induces acute hemostasis in an actively bleeding peptic ulcer in approximately 90% of patients. Compared with conservative medical therapy, endoscopic hemostasis significantly reduces the cost of hospitalization, need for transfusions, and requirement for emergency surgery.

7. What are the advantages of early upper endoscopy for acute gastrointestinal bleeding?

In addition to controlling hemorrhage in many situations, early endoscopy can be used to assess the risk of ongoing or additional bleeding. This assessment may allow a decision for early discharge in patients with a Mallory-Weiss tear (low risk of rebleed), esophagitis, or low-risk ulcer disease; it also affects decisions about which patients need monitoring in an intensive care setting and for how long.

8. When should EGD be performed for a complaint of bright red blood per rectum (BRBPR)?

Melena, or black, tarry stools and "coffee grounds," results from bleeding in the stomach or proximal small bowel. In patients with massive upper GI bleeding, there may not be enough time (or acid) for the conversion to melena because of rapid intestinal transit. Any patient who is hemodynamically unstable or who has an uncertain source of BRBPR should undergo upper endoscopy. A nasogastric tube, even if it returns bile, does not exclude an upper GI source.

9. Why is EGD essential in the evaluation of patients who may have swallowed a corrosive substance?

An EGD offers a better assessment of the extent and severity of the chemical burn than the history and physical examination or an upper GI barium radiograph, and thus allows better therapeutic decisions. Minor mucosal burns may be managed conservatively. Severe mucosal burns should prompt consideration of urgent surgical resection before perforation develops. Small-caliber, flexible endoscopes do not increase the risk of perforation.

10. What are the usual indications for endoscopic retrograde cholangiopancreatography (ERCP)?

ERCP is usually indicated to evaluate and treat symptoms that suggest disorders of the biliary system and pancreas. Examples include jaundice that is possibly obstructive; cholangitis; acute or recurrent pancreatitis; recurrent upper abdominal pain associated with transient liver function test abnormalities; and, less commonly, steatorrhea. Specific disorders that may be diagnosed and treated by ERCP include choledocholithiasis, benign or malignant bile duct stricture, bile duct leak, pancreatic pseudocyst, and pancreatic duct disruption.

11. What is the role of ERCP in suspected acute cholangitis?

Acute cholangitis is caused by infection in the setting of biliary obstruction from a gallstone or, less often, a stricture. When severe, it is associated with a high mortality rate (> 30%), whether managed conservatively or surgically. Endoscopic drainage is safe and reduces mortality. It should be used as early as possible in the course of the disease.

12. What is the role of ERCP in the evaluation of recurrent acute pancreatitis?

In approximately 30% of patients with recurrent pancreatitis of uncertain etiology, ERCP yields an explanation. Findings include previously unsuspected common duct stones; anatomic abnormalities (pancreas divisum, choledochocele); sphincter of Oddi dysfunction; and, rarely, pancreatic malignancy.

13. What are the indications for placement of a percutaneous endoscopic gastrostomy tube (PEG)?

A PEG should be considered when a patient with a functional GI tract is not expected to ingest orally for 3 or more weeks. Examples include patients with altered mental status after neurologic injury or trauma, oropharyngeal dysphagia due to neurologic injury, and oropharyngeal and esophageal obstruction during treatment of oropharyngeal and esophageal tumors. In addition, a PEG provides effective decompression for patients with chronic bowel obstruction due to peritoneal carcinomatosis.

14. Describe the management of suspected esophageal foreign body impactions.

If the suspected foreign body is radiopaque, it is helpful to search for it with a plain radiograph of the neck and chest. Endoscopy is the primary modality for evaluation and removal. The prior performance of a barium study makes endoscopy more difficult and is contraindicated. Meat tenderizer may be harmful to the esophagus and should be avoided. For sharp objects (chicken/fish bones) lodged near the cricopharangeus, rigid endoscopy under general anesthesia is often the safest option.

15. When is an endoscopic ultrasound (EUS) helpful?

EUS detects mediastinal lymph node involvement with an accuracy of 70–80%, whereas CT detects only 20–50% of such lesions. In addition, EUS is more sensitive than CT for detecting malignant invasion into the diaphragm, aorta, and pericardium. Mounting data suggest that an EUS examination should be performed on all candidates for curative resection of esophageal carcinoma and that it is the most sensitive staging test for primary lung cancers.

16. How may endoscopy help palliate an unresectable esophageal cancer?

When surgical resection is not possible, several options are available, most of which require endoscopic manipulation. A list of potential options includes the following:

- Metal stent placement
- Chemical injection (i.e., ethanol polidocanol, sodium morrhuate)
- Laser treatment (Nd:YAG)
- Esophageal dilation
- Photodynamic therapy
- Intracavitary irradiation
- Thermal/bipolar electrocoagulation

17. How does endoscopic management of obstructive biliary tract lesions compare with surgical or percutaneous palliation?

The endoscopic placement of biliary stents is safer and more effective than percutaneous placement of similar stents and allows shorter hospital stays than surgical decompression. Surgery has been preferred when the tumor threatens to obstruct the bowel, although endoscopic techniques are now available to stent bowel lesions as well.

18. What are the alternatives for the management of pseudocysts?

Endoscopic pseudocysts drainage has been shown to be as effective as traditionally preferred surgical drainages (i.e., cystogastrostomy, cystoduodenostomy, cystojejunostomy) and has, in general, mild complications. When the pseudocyst is immediately adjacent to the stomach or duodenum and bulges into the lumen or communicates with pancreatic duct, endoscopic drainage can be performed by placing stent(s) into the pseudocyst to drain cystic fluid into GI tract. The limiting factor is the favorable anatomic relationship.

19. What is the primary indication for small bowel enteroscopy?

When a patient has recurrent bleeding of obscure origin (i.e., failure to identify the source of bleeding by both EGD and colonoscopy), push enteroscopy may be indicated. The 240-cm endoscope can reach as far as 40–60 cm beyond the ligament of Treitz. It has a success rate of up to 50% in identifying the source of bleeding. Most cases result from ateriovenous malformations.

BIBLIOGRAPHY

1. Bond JH: Colonoscopy and neoplastic disorders of the colon. Gastrointest Endosc Clin North Am 3:585–776, 1993.
2. Bond JH: Polyp guideline: Diagnosis, treatment, and surveillance for patients with nonfamilial colorectal polyps. Ann Intern Med 119:836–848, 1993.
3. Jensen DM: Severe nonvariceal upper GI hemorrhage. Gastrointest Endosc Clin North Am 1:209–433, 1991.
4. Kozarek RA: Endoscopic approach to biliary stones. Gastrointest Endosc Clin North Am 1:208, 1991.
5. Tytgat GN (ed): Precancerous Conditions and Endoscopic Screening. Gastrointest Endosc Clin North Am 7(1), 1997.
6. Yamada T (ed): Textbook of Gastroenterology, 2nd ed. Philadelphia, J.B. Lippincott, 1995.

VII. Gender-Specific Care

46. BREAST MASSES AND PAIN

Julie Rifkin, M.D.

1. How good is the physician at determining the presence of a breast mass?
Determining whether an actual mass is present in the breast can be difficult. Discrete and dominant describe a mass that needs to be biopsied. Suspicious masses are three-dimensional, distinct from surrounding tissues, and generally asymmetrical in relation to the other breast. Only 10–20% of breast masses are initially discovered by the physician; therefore, an area that the patient feels is abnormal must be evaluated thoroughly. The examining physician must always err on the side of caution.

2. What aspects of the history are important in the evaluation of a breast mass?
Duration of the mass
Related and referred pain
Change in physical characteristics with menstrual cycle variations
Preexisting breast cancer risk factors (menstrual and family history, previous breast disease)

3. What characteristics of a breast mass are suggestive of cancer?
Masses that are firm, nontender, irregular with indistinct borders, immobile, and fixed due to skin or deep fascial attachments are suggestive of cancer. Skin dimpling and nipple retraction are also suspicious for carcinoma. Bloody nipple discharge and palpably enlarged lymph nodes are other worrisome findings.

4. What is the likely diagnosis in an adolescent with a discrete breast mass?
The mass is most likely a fibroadenoma, which rarely grows to more than 1 or 2 cm. The fibroadenoma is a benign and self-limited condition in most patients. A patient under age 25 can be safely observed. Fibroadenomas that are 5 cm or larger in women under 25 do not usually regress, and surgical excision is warranted. Fibroadenomas in women over 25 are usually surgically removed.

5. What causes breast pain or tenderness?
Up to 70% of women have some form of premenstrual breast tenderness or pain. One-third of such women seek medical advice for their symptoms. The use of mammography in women with cyclic mastalgia who are under the age of 35 and at low risk for breast cancer should be minimized. However, other more serious causes of breast pain include mastitis, breast abscess, and inflammatory breast carcinoma.

6. What is meant by fibrocystic changes of the breast?
This term has replaced fibrocystic breast disease. All women develop some degree of fibrocystic breast change. During the mature reproductive years, cyclic pain and nodularity are usual features. Fibrocystic changes clinically manifest as diffuse firmness, fine granularity, coarse granularity, irregular patterns of firmness, or a single nodule. Microcysts and macrocysts are common after age 35. Rarely, a thin discharge (clear, opaque, or colored) can be expressed from ectatic ducts.

7. Do fibrocystic breast changes place a woman at increased risk for breast cancer?

Most fibrocystic changes are benign. Women with diffuse fibrocystic changes are routinely biopsied. A dominant mass or nodule, however, should be histologically evaluated. Certain histologic diagnoses (atypical epithelial hyperplasia, atypical lobular hyperplasia, and diffuse papillomatosis with atypia) are potential premalignant findings. Atypical lobular hyperplasia increases the risk of breast cancer six-fold, especially in women under 45. Women with a family history of breast cancer and atypia in the setting of fibrocystic change have a 20% chance of developing breast cancer over 15 years. The presence of atypia without a positive family history reduces the risk to 8%.

8. What types of treatment are useful in relieving breast pain associated with cyclic mastalgia?

Firm brassiere support	Tamoxifen
Local heat application	Danazol
Aspirin, ibuprofen, acetaminophen	Bromocriptine
Evening primrose oil	Abstinence from nicotine, coffee, caffeinated sodas,
Oral contraceptives	chocolate, nuts, wine, avocados, and cheese

9. What causes mastitis? How is it treated?

Mastitis most commonly occurs in the lactating breast. Staphylococci and anaerobic organisms (peptostreptococci) are the usual pathogens. It is important for women to continue to empty the breast completely even though it is painful. A breast pump may be helpful. Improvement should be noted in 24–48 hours after starting an oral penicillin derivative. If symptoms worsen, a breast abscess, which requires incision and drainage, should be suspected.

10. What clue suggests inflammatory breast carcinoma as opposed to infection?

Erythema completely surrounding the areola suggests malignancy until proved otherwise. This finding is virtually absent in breast infection.

11. What role does mammography play in the evaluation of a woman with a palpable breast mass?

It is absolutely critical to place mammography in its proper perspective. The purpose of mammography is not to characterize mass but to evaluate the breasts for clinically occult lesions. A normal mammogram adds no information to the evaluation of a palpable breast mass. An abnormal mammogram may or may not be of value; even when a suspicious lesion is seen on a mammogram, it may not coincide with a palpable mass. Therapeutic decisions should not be based on a negative mammogram in women with a palpable breast mass.

12. Are mammograms necessary in evaluating a woman with a palpable breast mass?

Mammography is part of the examination of a woman with a breast mass but its limitations must be kept in mind. One study reported that when both palpation and mammography suggest that a mass is benign, the error rate is 3.7%—far too high to be acceptable to patients and physicians.

13. What are the sensitivity and specificity of mammography, physical examination, and a combination of both?

	SENSITIVITY (%)	SPECIFICITY (%)	OVERALL ACCURACY
Combination mammography and physical examination	95	—	77
Mammography alone	94	55	73
Physical examination alone	88	71	81

From Van Dam PA, Van Goethem MLA, Kersschot E, et al: Palpable solid breast masses: Retrospective single and multimodality evaluation of 201 lesions. Radiology 166:435–439, 1988.

14. What is the role of fine-needle aspiration (FNA) in the evaluation of a solid breast mass?

Fine-needle aspiration can be both diagnostic and therapeutic, but it is not necessarily a substitute for open biopsy. The use of FNA has reduced the need for open surgical biopsy for lesions that ultimately turn out to be benign. An ultrasound may be needed to confirm whether the lesion is cystic or solid. The false-negative rate varies with the cytopathologist and ranges from 1–35%. This false-negative rate is the Achilles' heel of FNA; therefore, a negative FNA in the presence of a suspicious mass does not exclude cancer. The combination of physical examination, mammography, and FNA has a diagnostic accuracy approaching 100%. The use of FNA in the diagnosis of cancer and subsequent determination of surgical therapy is controversial. However, an excisional biopsy can be done immediately before the operation to confirm a positive FNA.

15. Can FNA be performed before obtaining a mammogram?

Yes. For patient convenience an FNA can be performed on the same day as the office visit. The FNA may produce a hematoma, but mammography can be accurately read when done 2 weeks later.

16. What is a triple negative diagnostic test?

"Triple negative" refers to the combination of a "not suspicious" physical examination, a normal mammogram, and fine-needle aspiration cytology that is not suspicious for cancer. When all three tests are negative, the chance that the lesion is cancerous is reduced to less than 1%. This reduction from the higher false-negative rate of FNA alone is important to justify the use of aspiration cytology. In a combined positive diagnostic test, the physical exam, mammogram, and FNA are suspicious for breast cancer.

17. What is the modified triple test?

The modified triple test substitutes ultrasound for mammography. It is comparable to the standard triple test in women under age 40 but has not been well studied in older women. The ultrasound machine is easily maintained in a physician's office and can distinguish whether the area in question is indeed a mass and whether the mass is solid or cystic.

18. What should be done with the fluid from a cyst aspiration?

The fluid may be discarded if it is not bloody, if the mass disappears, and if the mammogram is normal. Cytologic analysis of cyst fluid is recommended if the fluid is bloody or aspirated from a cyst in a postmenopausal woman. A follow-up mammogram is important to visualize tissue surrounding the collapsed cyst. If a residual mass remains, either FNA or biopsy is recommended.

19. What should be done with a cyst that reappears after the first aspiration?

A cyst may be aspirated one or two times after the initial aspiration. With each repeat aspiration, the physician must review whether the mammogram is normal and whether the mass completely disappears. Statistically, less than 20% of cysts require repeat aspirations, and less than 9% reappear after two or three aspirations.

20. What is the role of stereotactic-guided core needle biopsy in a woman with a palpable breast mass?

Once again, the management of a palpable mass must not be confused with the management of a mammographic lesion. A palpable mass can be evaluated without stereotactic or other radiologic guidance. If a mammographic lesion is present in the same breast, one must be careful to ensure that the mammographic lesion is coincident with the palpable mass.

21. Can a woman under the age of 30 years develop breast cancer?

Yes. A substantial number of women under the age of 30 years develop breast cancer; however, the chance that a breast mass is malignant in women less than 25 years of age is essentially zero.

22. List four pitfalls in the management of palpable breast masses.

1. Assuming that mammography is diagnostic. Mammography seldom defines a mass well enough to avoid further diagnostic evaluation (FNA or excisional biopsy). Thus the value of mammography in managing a palpable breast mass is minimal (detection of occult or multifocal disease).

2. Assuming that the radiographic lesion seen on mammography is the same as the palpable lesion. If there is any question about this correlation, further evaluation is essential. A follow-up mammogram should be obtained 3 or 4 months after biopsy of all mammographically diagnosed lesions to determine that the suspicious mass was actually excised. The follow-up mammogram also serves as a new baseline, showing the changes after biopsy.

3. Letting a negative or nonsuspicious mammogram influence the judgment of whether a palpable mass needs to be biopsied. The decision to biopsy or aspirate should be made on physical examination criteria.

4. Assuming that a benign aspiration cytology is definitive.

BIBLIOGRAPHY

1. Adler DN, Browne MW: Prevalence and impact of cyclic mastalgia in a United States clinic-based sample. Am J Obstet Gynecol 177:126–132, 1997.
2. Bland KI, Copeland B, Copeland EM III (eds): The Breast: Comprehensive Management of Benign and Malignant Diseases. Philadelphia, W.B. Saunders, 1991.
3. Donegan WL: Evaluation of a palpable breast mass. N Engl J Med 327:937–942, 1992.
4. Donegan WL, Spratt JS: Cancer of the Breast. Philadelphia, W.B. Saunders, 1995.
5. Drukker BH: The breast. In Seltzer VL, Pearse WH (eds): Women's Primary Health Care. New York, McGraw-Hill, 1995.
6. Hindle WH, Chen EC: Accuracy of mammographic appearances after breast fine-needle aspiration. Am J Obstet Gynecol 176:1286–1292, 1997.
7. Layfield LF, Glasgow BJ, Cramer H: Fine-needle aspiration in the management of breast masses. Pathol Annu 24(Pt 2):23–62, 1989.
8. Page DL, Dupont WD: Histologic indicators of breast cancer risk. Am Coll Surg Bull 76:16–23, 1991.
9. Van Dam PA, Van Goethem MLA, Kersschot E, et al: Palpable solid breast masses: Retrospective single and multimodality evaluations of 201 lesions. Radiology 166:435–439, 1988.
10. Vetto JT, Rodney FP, et al: Diagnosis of palpable breast lesions in younger women by the modified triple test is accurate and cost-effective. Arch Surg 131:967–974, 1996.
11. Zitarelle J, Burkhart LL, Weiss SM: False negative breast biopsy for palpable mass. J Surg Oncol 52:61–63, 1993.

47. DYSFUNCTIONAL UTERINE BLEEDING

Julie Rifkin, M.D.

1. Define dysfunctional uterine bleeding.

Loss of the coordinated cyclic hormonal changes that govern the normal menstrual cycle leads to abnormal uterine bleeding. Abnormal uterine bleeding is the most common complaint presented to a gynecologist. Most causes of dysfunctional uterine bleeding fall into the following categories:

1. Dysfunctional bleeding, with no evidence of organic lesions
2. Pregnancy
3. Pelvic lesions—benign or malignant
4. Extragenital problems: coagulopathies, endocrinopathies

2. What is a normal menstrual cycle?

The normal menstrual cycle ranges from 25–35 days. Day one of the cycle is the first day of bleeding. The average amount of blood lost is 30 ml per cycle; less than 80 ml is considered normal. Many women flow for as few as 2 days or as many as 8 days.

3. What hormonal abnormalities are associated with dysfunctional uterine bleeding?

The endometrium is stimulated by estrogen. Without estrogen, the endometrium becomes atrophic. Persistently low levels of estrogen are associated with intermittent spotting and light bleeding. High levels of estrogen for prolonged periods are associated with intervals of amenorrhea followed by heavy bleeding.

4. What causes amenorrhea or irregular menses in women of reproductive age?

Anovulation causes irregular menses or amenorrhea. Ovulation must occur for progesterone to be produced by the corpus luteum. Without progesterone, the endometrium becomes abnormally thick and vascular. Eventually the endometrium outgrows its hormonal support and becomes friable and sloughs. Women of reproductive age without identifiable medical problems or genital pathology who do not menstruate normally generally have one of the following:

1. Anovulatory cycles (most common). Of women with heavy bleeding and irregular cycles or amenorrhea, 75% have polycystic ovarian syndrome. Other common causes include obesity (androstenedione is converted to estrogen by adipose tissue) and psychological or physical stress (peripheral conversion of adrenal C19 androgenic precursors to estrogen).

2. Ovarian failure. Usually these genetic disorders present with secondary amenorrhea and elevated gonadotropins; however, evaluation for autoimmune disorders is warranted.

3. Central failure. This condition may be caused by a pituitary tumor, the empty sella syndrome, severe weight loss, anorexia nervosa, and bulimia.

5. What may cause mid-cycle spotting?

Mid-cycle (ovulatory) spotting may occur because ovarian estrogen production is inhibited by the high levels of luteinizing hormone (estrogen withdrawal bleeding).

6. Define these 10 terms that refer to abnormal bleeding patterns.

Amenorrhea	Absent menstrual flow of more than 90 days
Hypermenorrhea	Excessive uterine bleeding occurring during a *regular* menstrual duration
Hypomenorrhea	Decreased menstrual flow, usually with a decrease in duration
Menometrorrhagia	Irregular intermenstrual bleeding with prolongation of menstrual flow
Menorrhagia	Excessive bleeding during a menstrual period either in number of days, amount of blood, or both
Metrorrhagia	Irregular bleeding between menstrual cycles
Oligomenorrhea	Menstrual bleeding at intervals greater than 35 days
Polymenorrhea	Menstrual cycles of less than 22 days' duration
Postmenopausal bleeding	Bleeding that occurs 12 months after the cessation of menses
Premenstrual spotting	A frequent variant of metrorrhagia limited to the few days before the beginning of menses

7. What are the common causes of genital bleeding in a young girl?

Menses before the age of 9 years is abnormal. The patient and family should be questioned about maternal use of diethylstilbestrol during pregnancy, possible patient ingestion of birth control pills, and family history of bleeding problems or sexual precocity.

Sexual molestation is the most tragic cause of genital bleeding in a young girl. Known or suspected cases of sexual trauma must be reported to appropriate child protection authorities. Abdominal perforation or rectal entry should be ruled out with examination under anesthesia. All significant hematomas should be followed for enlargement.

Urethral prolapse may cause bleeding as a result of congenital weakness or external trauma. Genital neoplasms are rare in young girls but should be considered. Benign growths include vaginal or cervical polyps and genital hemangiomas. Malignant tumors include sarcoma botryoides, ovarian tumors, and adenocarcinoma of the cervix or vagina.

8. What causes abnormal perimenarcheal bleeding?

The most common cause of abnormal bleeding in perimenarcheal girls is anovulatory cycles. An immature hypothalamic-pituitary-ovarian axis is usually a factor. Most girls enter menarche at 12–13 years of age. During the first year, 80% of the menstrual cycles are anovulatory. When menorrhagia is present, a coagulation defect is the cause in up to 20% of patients. Pregnancy and genitourinary infections (chlamydia and gonorrhea) should be ruled out.

9. Describe the management of abnormal perimenarcheal bleeding.

If the history, physical examination, and pertinent laboratory data reveal no underlying pathology, the treatment of choice is oral contraceptives. With each successive cycle of the pill, the menses become lighter. After several cycles the pill can be stopped, and the patient may be observed for onset of regular menses. Oral medroxyprogesterone, 10 mg/day for 7–10 days, also may be used. The withdrawal bleeding is heavy. The patient must be advised that withdrawal bleeding does not represent treatment failure. Intravenous Premarin, 25 mg intravenously every 4 hours for up to 3 doses, may be required for the patient with profuse, persistent bleeding. After the bleeding stops, oral contraceptives or progesterone is started immediately. Failure to control bleeding with intravenous Premarin calls for further investigation and may require curettage.

10. What causes dysfunctional uterine bleeding in a woman of reproductive age?

The most common cause of abnormal uterine bleeding in women ages 18–40 years is pregnancy and its complications. Beta-human chorionic gondadotropin (β-hCG) is assessed (serum pregnancy test). If the test is positive, the differential diagnoses include threatened, incomplete, or missed abortion; ectopic pregnancy; or gestational trophoblastic disease. If the β-hCG test is negative, then anovulation, uterine leiomyomas, and pelvic inflammatory disease are likely causes. Anovulation with metromenorrhagia may be seen more frequently in women who undergo rapid weight changes and is more common in very thin or obese women.

11. What type of menstrual flow is abnormal for the perimenopausal or postmenopausal woman?

Any bleeding occurring 12 months after the cessation of regular menstrual flow is defined as postmenopausal bleeding. Perimenopausal women often have irregular anovulatory bleeding that may make it difficult to determine when the menopause actually started. The older the patient, the higher the likelihood that the bleeding is related to malignancy. Endometrial carcinoma causes approximately 5% of perimenopausal and 20% of postmenopausal abnormal bleeding. Thus, the differential diagnosis of abnormal bleeding in women 50 years or older is malignancy until proved otherwise. Anovulatory bleeding, atrophic endometrium, and benign etiologies are diagnoses of exclusion.

12. When should a work-up for primary amenorrhea be initiated?

A 16-year-old girl without pubic or axillary hair (adrenarche) and without breast development (thelarche) requires evaluation. Failure to begin menstruation by age 18 years is considered delayed menarche. Primary amenorrhea is uncommon. Abnormal fetal development of the müllerian and wolffian systems or external genitalia accounts for two-thirds of cases. Pituitary-hypothalamic disorders and insensitive follicles account for most of the remaining cases.

The physical examination includes the patient's stature (a height of 60 in suggests gonadal dysgenesis), breast development, hair distribution, inguinal or labial masses, and cutaneous lesions (multiple pigmented nevi, gonadal dysgenesis, acanthosis nigricans, sclerotic ovary syndrome). If the patient appears to have definite pubertal development, a serum pregnancy test should be obtained before any evaluation. Management of primary amenorrhea is guided by the correct diagnosis. Initial evaluation includes measurement of pituitary gonadotropins (follicle-stimulating hormone and luteinizing hormone) and serum prolactin. Further assessment with estrogen and progesterone withdrawal, along with anatomic and chromosomal assessment, may then be undertaken.

13. How is secondary amenorrhea evaluated?

Secondary amenorrhea is defined as the loss of regular menstrual cycles for 3 months. The evaluation includes a serum pregnancy test. If the test is negative, the levels of prolactin and thyroid-stimulating hormone (TSH) are assessed. If the levels are normal, the next step is a progestational challenge. If withdrawal bleeding is noted, anovulation is confirmed. If withdrawal bleeding does not occur, the patient is challenged with oral estrogen on days 1–25 and progesterone on days 16–25. Absence of bleeding indicates a defect in the endometrium or uterine outflow tract. Destruction of the endometrium, referred to as Asherman's syndrome, is generally caused by overzealous postpartum curettage. Multiple synechiae are found on hysterogram. Dilatation and curettage may break up the adhesions.

14. What is the most common presentation of patients with polycystic ovarian disease?

Over 50% of patients with polycystic ovarian disease present with secondary amenorrhea. The diagnosis is strongly supported by the onset of symptoms in adolescence (irregular menses and varying degrees of hirsutism). Serum free testosterone, adrostenedione and LH are usually somewhat elevated; however, the levels overlap considerably with normal values. In many cases the ovaries are not palpably enlarged. Ovarian ultrasound or biopsy is not indicated. Anovulatory amenorrhea may be treated with oral contraceptives or monthly progesterone if the patient does not desire fertility.

15. When should patients with dysmenorrhea be referred to a gynecologist?

Dysmenorrhea, or "difficult monthly flow," is characterized by crampy lower abdominal or pelvic pain that may radiate to the back and thighs. Associated symptoms often include nausea, vomiting, diarrhea, bloating, weakness, fatigue, headaches, and, rarely, syncope. Such symptoms may occur before and during menstruation.

Primary dysmenorrhea begins shortly after menarche and is not caused by pelvic pathology. It affects 50–60% of all women in some form. Secondary dysmenorrhea begins later in life. Causes of secondary dysmenorrhea include endometriosis, pelvic inflammatory disease, postsurgical adhesions, myomas, polyps, and use of an intrauterine device. Because secondary dysmenorrhea is usually associated with pelvic pathology, referral to a gynecologist is appropriate.

16. Describe the management of dysmenorrhea.

High levels of endometrial prostaglandins are the most likely causes of dysmenorrhea. The pain may be related to prostaglandin-mediated, high-intensity uterine contractions or prostaglandin-induced sensitivity of nerve terminals.

Nonsteroidal antiinflammatory drugs (NSAIDs) are the treatment of choice for primary dysmenorrhea. The following medications are approved for use:

• Motrin, Advil, Nuprin, Rufen: 400–600 mg 4 times daily
• Naprosyn (naproxen): 250 mg 4 times daily
• Anaprox (naproxen sodium): 275 mg 4 times daily
• Ponstel (mefenamic acid): 250 mg 4 times daily to 500 mg 3 times daily.

There is no advantage to beginning treatment before the onset of menses unless symptoms begin premenstrually. Gastrointestinal upset is a common side effect of NSAIDs. A patient may require a trial of two or more medications to find the one that gives the best pain relief. Most women have good pain relief with NSAIDs.

An alternative regimen for the woman not desiring pregnancy is an oral contraceptive. Because of the inhibition of ovulation, oral contraceptives prevent the development of a lush endometrium and the associated high levels of prostaglandin. If both NSAIDs and oral contraceptives fail, nifedipine (a calcium channel blocker), 10 mg 3 times daily, may be helpful. Oral nifedipine may cause headaches, facial flushing, palpitations, and moderate increases in heart rate. Failure to respond to any treatment modality suggests secondary dysmenorrhea, and the patient should be referred to a gynecologist.

BIBLIOGRAPHY

1. Awwad JT, Togh TL, Schiff I: Abnormal uterine bleeding in the perimenopause. Int J Fertil 38:261–269, 1993.
2. Barnes R: Pathophysiology of ovarian steroid secretion in polycystic ovary syndrome. Semin Reprod Endocrinol 15:159–168, 1997.
3. Bayer S, De Cherney AH: Clinical manifestations and treatment of dysfunctional uterine bleeding. JAMA 269:1823–1828, 1993.
4. Carlson KJ, Nichols DH, Schiff I: Indications for hysterectomy. N Engl J Med 328:856–860, 1993.
5. Duncan KM: Nonsteroidal anti-inflammatory drugs in menorrhagia. Ann Pharmacother 27:1353–1354, 1993.
6. Emanuel MH, Verdel MJ, Wamsteker K, et al: A prospective comparison of transvaginal and diagnostic hysteroscopy in the evaluation of patients with abnormal uterine bleeding: Clinical implications. Am J Obstet Gynecol 172:547–552, 1995.
7. Farquhas C: Management of dysfunctional uterine bleeding. Drugs 44:578–584, 1992.
8. Jennings JC: Abnormal uterine bleeding. Med Clin North Am 79:1357–1376, 1995.
9. Thorneycroft IH: Medical management of abnormal uterine bleeding in the patient in her 40s. Obstet Gynecol Clin North Am 20:333–336, 1993.
10. van Eijkeren MA, Christians GCML, Scholten PC, et al: Menorrhagia: Current drug treatment concepts. Drugs 43:201–209, 1992.

48. MENOPAUSE AND ITS COMPLICATIONS

Julie Rifkin, M.D.

1. What is the climacteric?

The climacteric is the period in which a woman's ovarian function gradually fails. With each menstrual cycle fewer follicles are recruited in the estrogen-producing phase of folliculogenesis. Circulating estrogen begins to decrease. Variations in the menstrual cycle may begin to occur after age 35 but usually not until age 45 years. Menstrual irregularity lasts roughly 2–8 years before the onset of menopause. Women may experience oligomenorrhea and/or hypermenorrhea. Fertility during this time is unpredictable, because not all cycles are ovulatory.

2. What causes hot flashes?

Vasomotor symptoms (hot flush or flash) may occur during the perimenopausal years. The flush may occur sporadically or recur every 10–30 minutes. It is rare for a flush to last an hour. Hot flashes seem to be worse at night. Generalized vasodilation occurs throughout the body and skin temperature rises. Pulsatile release of gonadotropin-releasing hormone (GNRH) from the hypothalamus is responsible for the flush. Stimuli that trigger hot flashes include caffeine, alcohol, spicy foods, hot weather, warm rooms, and emotional distress.

3. What other symptoms may occur as a result of the normal changes associated with the climacteric?

A variety of other estrogen-dependent changes also occur. The vaginal and vulvar epithelium thins. Dyspareunia, pruritus, and abacterial urethritis or cystitis may occur. Other bothersome symptoms during the climacteric include anxiety, tension, depression, irritability, headaches, insomnia, myalgias, and libido changes.

4. What therapies are useful to treat climacteric symptoms?

Vasomotor symptoms can be alleviated by wearing cool comfortable clothes and avoiding warm rooms and caffeine. In addition, 400 IU of vitamin E daily may be useful. If necessary, 0.3 mg of Premarin daily may be tried. Monthly synthetic or natural progestins ease mood changes and heavy menstrual bleeding due to progesterone deficiency (luteal phase defect). A cyclic, continuous, combined hormone replacement regimen also may be used, but it does not provide contraceptive protection. Low-dose birth control pills are safe for nonsmoking, healthy, peri-menopausal women.

5. What is menopause?

Menopause is the absence of menses for 6–12 months. A level of serum follicle-stimulating hormone (FSH) above 40 IU/L is diagnostic of ovarian failure. Levels of estradiol and luteinizing hormone (LH) are not routinely used to diagnose menopause. No one can predict which menstrual period will be the last.

6. What causes premature menopause?

The average age of menopause is 50 years with a range of 48–55 years. Menopause before the age of 40 is considered premature. Patients with rheumatoid arthritis or diabetes may experience premature menopause. Previous abdominal hysterectomy is also associated with early menopause. This association is believed to be due to compromise of the ovarian vasculature.

7. How is hormone replacement therapy (HRT) used?

HRT is used to treat women with any stigmata of hormone deprivation. Most authorities advocate HRT as prophylaxis against osteoporosis and cardiovascular disease. The decision to use estrogen belongs to the patient once the risks and benefits have been explained. HRT may be used for as long as the patient desires. Vasomotor symptoms that begin before the cessation of menstrual bleeding may be treated with estrogen. If the patient has not had a hysterectomy, a progestational agent is added to prevent endometrial hyperplasia.

8. What type of evaluation is performed before HRT is used?

After a definitive reason to use HRT is established and discussed with the patient, the following evaluation is generally performed:

1. Examination and laboratory tests
   - A complete physical, including breast and pelvic examinations
   - Stool guaiac analysis
   - Papanicolaou smear
   - Mammogram
   - Fasting lipid profile
   - Fasting glucose level
   - Liver function tests (with past history of liver disease)
2. Conditions that contribute to the development of osteoporosis are evaluated in each patient (see chapter 25). Patients unsure about estrogen therapy may be better able to reach a decision if there is evidence of or high risk for osteoporosis. HRT can be prescribed when causes of secondary osteoporosis have been excluded.

9. How do the various regimens of HRT differ, especially for women who have not had a hysterectomy?

Commonly used estrogen-progesterone combinations are described below. Each regimen affords benefit for vasomotor symptoms and osteoporosis. The usual dose of conjugated estrogen is much lower than the dose of synthetic estrogen (ethinyl estradiol) commonly used in oral contraceptives. The usual dose of conjugated estrogen (Premarin) is 0.625 mg. Oral contraceptives usually contain 30–50 µg of ethinyl estradiol.

$$5 \text{ mg of conjugated estrogen} = 50 \text{ µg of ethinyl estradiol}$$

HRT Regimens

1. Women who have had a hysterectomy are treated with estrogen alone.
   - The usual dose of conjugated estrogen (Premarin, Ogen, Estratab) is 0.625 mg–1.25 mg/day orally.

- The estrogen patch (Estraderm) is prescribed as 0.05–0.1 mg patches that are applied twice weekly.
- Injectable estrogen is not recommended for routine use. The peak estrogen level, which is often supraphysiologic, is reached days to weeks after injection. The level then declines over several more weeks. Such patients are most prone to marked fluctuations of estrogen and may seek frequent injections.

2. Women who have **not** had a hysterectomy require a progestin in addition to the estrogen.
- Oral conjugated estrogen, 0.625 mg–1.25 mg, may be given daily, with the addition of Provera, 5–10 mg orally on days 1–12 of each month. Withdrawal bleeding usually occurs after the Provera is finished.
- Both conjugated estrogen, 0.625 mg–1.25 mg, and Provera, 2.5–5.0 mg orally, may be used daily. This regimen is associated with irregular bleeding during the first 4–6 months. After 6 months nearly all patients are amenorrheic.
- All of the above regimens may be used with the estrogen patch instead of oral estrogen. Pills and patches containing both hormones may be available in the future.

10. What are the side effects of HRT?

Patients usually note breast tenderness and on occasion breast enlargement. Estrogen increases the risk for developing gallbladder disease that requires cholecystectomy. Less common problems include headache, nausea, fluid retention, weight gain, and chloasma. These symptoms are related to estrogen. The progestin component also contributes to breast tenderness and fluid retention and, less commonly, may produce some degree of depression. Unscheduled breakthrough bleeding is the most serious side effect. Prompt investigation (endometrial biopsy) is performed to rule out endometrial cancer.

11. When is HRT contraindicated?

Absolute contraindications:
- Pregnancy
- Undiagnosed dysfunctional uterine bleeding
- Active thrombophlebitis or thromboemboli disorders
- Suspected breast or uterine cancer
- Active liver disease

A history of venous thrombosis is **not** an absolute contraindication to estrogen replacement. Caution is recommended for the following patients:
- Patients who are obese and/or have diabetes are at increased risk for endometrial cancer.
- Patients with a history of migraine headaches may not be able to tolerate HRT.
- Patients with uterine myomata or gallbladder disease may experience worsening of these conditions.
- There is no clear consensus regarding HRT for women with a past history of breast cancer who have been disease-free for several years.

12. What is the association between HRT and endometrial cancer?

The use of estrogen alone in a woman who has not had a hysterectomy significantly increases the risk of developing endometrial cancer. Endometrial hyperplasia, which is believed to be a precursor to endometrial cancer, occurs in 20–40% of women taking unopposed estrogens. Endometrial hyperplasia may be prevented by the addition of a progestin. Currently available studies suggest that the addition of a progestin prevents the increased risk of endometrial cancer associated with the use of estrogen alone.

13. Is an endometrial biopsy required before HRT is prescribed?

A baseline endometrial biopsy is not required before prescribing an estrogen-progestin regimen. The exceptions are patients without evaluation of dysfunctional perimenopausal bleeding and postmenopausal patients with vaginal bleeding. Routine surveillance endometrial biopsies are not required. Unscheduled breakthrough bleeding, however, must be promptly evaluated.

14. What is the currently perceived relationship between estrogen replacement therapy and breast cancer?

Data suggest that estrogen levels most likely influence the risk of developing breast cancer in postmenopausal women. The risk of breast cancer is increased in women with early menarche, late menopause, and obesity. The following statements reflect current information regarding the association of estrogen use and breast cancer risk:

• Women currently using estrogen may have an increased incidence of breast cancer, but the relationship to mortality is unknown.

• Long-term estrogen use (> 10 years) may lead to a small increase in risk of breast cancer.

The small increased risk among current and long-term estrogen users may be misleading. Such patients must see a physician regularly to renew their prescriptions and are therefore screened for breast cancer on a regular basis. Withholding estrogen therapy because of fear of increasing the risk of breast cancer is not well justified.

The risk for breast cancer among estrogen users is not influenced by the dose, the addition of a progestin, or the type of menopause (surgical vs. natural). In addition, the risk of breast cancer is not influenced by a family history of breast cancer or a personal history of benign breast disease.

15. Does HRT reduce a woman's risk of coronary heart disease?

Current data suggest a significant decrease in coronary heart disease among postmenopausal women who use estrogen. Beneficial effects of oral conjugated estrogen on libido are seen: it lowers serum levels of low-density lipoprotein cholesterol about 10–15% and increases serum levels of high-density lipoprotein cholesterol about 10–15%. Triglyceride levels may increase with oral estrogen. The transdermal estrogen patch decreases total cholesterol and LDL cholesterol but does not increase triglycerides. The addition of medroxyprogesterone acetate does not abolish estrogen's beneficial effects on lipoproteins.

The addition of a progestin to estrogen replacement therapy may attenuate estrogen's beneficial effects on lipoproteins. Few good studies are available to analyze the results. Recent studies, however, indicate that users of a combined estrogen-progestin regimen have favorable lipid profiles and receive cardiovascular protection. It is currently suggested that women who use an estrogen-progestin regimen have a lower risk of coronary heart disease compared with women who do not take estrogen.

16. When should HRT be prescribed to prevent or treat postmenopausal osteoporosis?

Any time, but the sooner the better. The benefit of estrogen increases with duration of therapy. The optimal benefit of HRT is seen when estrogen is prescribed within 3 years of menopause. However, estrogen therapy may be prescribed at any time after menopause to prevent additional bone loss. Benefit has been demonstrated even for older women with established osteoporosis.

17. How may vasomotor symptoms be treated if the patient cannot use estrogen?

Several agents may provide relief from vasomotor symptoms in patients who are unable to use estrogen. The therapy should be determined by the severity of the symptoms. Possible therapies include the following:

• **Progestins alone**

Depomedroxyprogesterone acetate (DMPA), 150 mg intramuscularly each month

• **Alpha-2 adrenergic agonists**

Clonidine, 0.1 mg orally twice daily

Methyldopa, 250–500 mg orally twice daily

• **Bellergal-S** (contains 40 mg of phenobarbital, 0.6 mg of ergotamine tartrate, and 0.2 mg of bellafoline alkaloids of belladonna)

• **Natural remedies**

B vitamin supplements	Vitamin E	Bee pollen
Vitamin C	Licorice root	Fenugreek
Zinc	Ginseng tea	Sarsaparilla

• **Avoidance of stimuli that trigger vasomotor symptoms**

Caffeine	Hot weather
Alcohol	Warm rooms
Spicy foods	Emotional distress

18. How does menopause affect sexual function and libido?

Most menopausal women have normal sexual responses and frequently report improved sexual function. Dyspareunia secondary to urogenital atrophy can be alleviated with estrogen replacement. Decreased libido is more often caused by relationship difficulties, depression, and medication than low testosterone levels. The exception is surgical menopause, because ovarian production of androgen is abruptly lost.

19. When should women on cyclic HRT and continuous combined HRT expect withdrawal bleeding?

For women using cyclic HRT (daily estrogen plus progesterone on days 1–12), withdrawal bleeding can be expected on or after the tenth day of the month. The flow is usually mild to moderate. Women using a continuous combined regimen can have unpredictable irregular spotting for the first 4–6 months. Unexpected or excessive bleeding must be investigated.

BIBLIOGRAPHY

1. Belchetz PE: Hormonal treatment of postmenopausal women. N Engl J Med 330:1062–1071, 1994.
2. Colditz GA, Hankinson SE, Hunter DL, et al: The use of estrogen and progestins and the risk of breast cancer in postmenopausal women. N Engl J Med 332:1473–1480, 1995.
3. Gorsky RD, Koplan JP, Peterson HB, et al: Relative risks and benefits of long-term estrogen replacement therapy: A decision analysis. Obstet Gynecol 83:161–166, 1994.
4. Hargrove JT, Eisenberg E: Menopause. Med Clin North Am 79:1337–1356, 1995.
5. Lobo RA, Pickar JH, Wild RA, et al: Metabolic impact of adding medroxyprogesterone to conjugated estrogen therapy in postmenopausal women. Obstet Gynecol 84:987–995, 1994.
6. Oldenhave A: Pathogenesis of climacteric complaints: Ready for a change? Lancet 343:649, 1994.
7. Report of the U.S. Preventive Services Task Force: Postmenopausal Hormone Prophylaxis—Guide to Clinical Preventive Services, 2nd ed. Baltimore, Williams & Wilkins, 1996, pp 829–843.
8. Schneider DL, et al: Postmenopausal hormone therapy after age 60. JAMA 277:543–547, 1997.
9. Thacker HL: Current update in menopausal hormonal replacement therapy. Cleve Clin J Med 63:979–982, 1996.
10. Udoff L, Langenberg P, Adashi EY: Combined continuous hormone replacement therapy: A critical review. Obstet Gynecol 86:306–316, 1995.
11. Writing Group for the PEPI Trial: Effects of estrogen/progestin regimens on heart disease risk factors in postmenopausal women. The Postmenopausal Estrogen/Progestin Interventions (PEPI) trial. JAMA 273:199–208, 1995.

49. CONTRACEPTION

Julie Rifkin, M.D.

1. What contraceptive methods are available to women in the United States?

Currently women in the U.S. have several contraceptive methods from which to choose. Concern for efficacy and safety as well as the user's age, general health, and future childbearing plans influence the choice.

Hormonal contraceptives are available as a synthetic estrogen combined with one of several C-19 progestational steroids or as a progestational agent alone. Barrier methods include the diaphragm, cervical cap, spermicide, and condoms. Hormone-impregnated intrauterine devices

(IUDs) use both biochemical and barrier protection. Fertility awareness (rhythm, basal body temperature, cervical mucus method) and coitus interruptus are not predictably effective. Surgical contraception may be achieved with tubal ligation or vasectomy.

2. How effective are the various contraceptive methods?
The table below lists the first-year failure rates of contraceptive methods per 100 users in 1 year of use.

METHOD	% OF WOMEN EXPERIENCING AN ACCIDENTAL PREGNANCY WITHIN THE FIRST YEAR OF USE		% OF WOMEN CONTINUING USE AT ONE YEAR
	TYPICAL USE	PERFECT USE	
Chance	85	85	
Spermicides	21	6	43
Periodic abstinence	20		67
Calendar		9	
Ovulation method		3	
Symptothermal		2	
Postovulation		1	
Withdrawal	19	4	
Cap			
Parous women	36	26	45
Nulliparous women	18	9	58
Diaphragm	18	6	58
Condom	12	3	63
Pill	3		72
Progestin only		0.5	
Combined		0.1	
IUD			
Progestasert	2.0	1.5	81
Copper T 380A	0.8	0.6	78
LNg 20	0.1	0.1	81
Depo-Provera	0.3	0.3	70
Norplant (6 capsules)	0.09	0.09	85
Female sterilization	0.4	0.4	100
Male sterilization	0.15	0.10	100

3. How do oral contraceptives work?
Oral contraceptives contain a synthetic estrogen plus a synthetic progestin or a synthetic progestin alone. Oral contraceptives prevent ovulation by suppressing pituitary and hypothalamic hormones and by altering the endometrial lining.

4. Are users of oral combined contraceptives at a higher risk for future development of cancer?
No convincing evidence links oral contraceptives with increased risk of breast cancer. Women who have taken an oral contraceptive for more than 5 years have a small increase in the risk of squamous carcinoma of the cervix. This type of neoplasm, however, is also associated with a woman's level of sexual activity. There appears to be no increase in the risk of cervical cancer for users of oral contraceptives once difference in sexual activity is accounted for. Women taking oral contraceptives have a small risk of developing hepatocellular carcinoma after 8 years of use. Hepatitis B infection is also strongly linked with hepatocellular carcinoma. Oral contraceptives protect against uterine and endometrial cancers.

5. What complications are associated with the use of oral contraceptives?

Severe complications are rare. They are usually related to the cardiovascular system. Adverse reactions include thrombophlebitis, pelvic vein thrombosis, pulmonary embolism, cerebrovascular accidents, myocardial infarction, hepatic adenoma, hypertension, gallbladder disease, retinal vein thrombosis, vascular headache, and depression. Other side effects include nausea, weight gain, fluid retention, breast tenderness or fullness, and menstrual irregularities.

6. What group is at greatest risk of cardiovascular complications from oral contraceptives?

Contraceptive users over the age of 35 who smoke are at highest risk for cardiovascular morbidity and mortality. The five danger signs are summarized by the mnemonic **ACHES**.

A = **A**bdominal pain
C = **C**hest pain or shortness of breath
H = **H**eadaches
E = **E**ye problems (blurred vision, flashing lights, blindness)
S = **S**evere leg pain

7. Are oral contraceptives safe for adolescents?

Oral contraceptives can be safely prescribed for adolescents. Because oral contraceptives offer no protection against acquired immunodeficiency syndrome (AIDS), regular use of a condom **in addition to the pill** is advised until a long-term relationship with one partner is established. The estimated risk of death from oral contraceptive use is 1.3 per 100,000 adolescent users. The estimated risk of death in childbirth is 11.1 per 100,000 adolescent pregnancies.

8. How does the prescription of oral contraceptives differ if the patient is over age 35 years of age?

Women who do not smoke and have no associated risks for premature cardiovascular disease may use oral contraceptives into the fourth and fifth decades. Women over 35 years of age should be prescribed an oral contraceptive containing 35 μg of estrogen or less and a low-potency progestin.

9. Do oral contraceptive users need to be concerned about efficacy when other medications are prescribed?

Yes. Many medications may reduce the efficacy of oral contraceptives. A partial list includes rifampin, dilantin, phenobarbitol, and possibly ampicillin and tetracyclines. Oral contraceptives may alter the activity of the other drugs. A thorough medication list must be obtained before prescribing oral contraceptives. Likewise, careful thought must be given to prescribing additional medications for oral contraceptive users.

10. Is a woman's infertility altered after discontinuing oral contraceptives?

About 25% of women have some delay in establishing ovulatory cycles after stopping oral contraceptives. Most women, however, immediately resume ovulation. Three months after discontinuing oral contraceptives the conception rate returns to normal. The pregnancy rate for oral contraceptive users and users of other methods is the same after 42 months.

11. Why may a care provider recommend that a patient use a nonhormonal contraceptive method after discontinuing oral contraceptives?

Many care providers recommend using a nonhormonal contraceptive method for at least 2 or 3 cycles before attempting to conceive. This advice allows a woman's natural cycle to reestablish itself, thereby providing more accurate pregnancy dates. No evidence suggests an increased risk of spontaneous abortion or birth defects in women who have used oral contraceptives. Any woman who has not resumed menstrual function after 12 months should be evaluated for secondary amenorrhea.

12. Are oral contraceptives safe for nursing mothers to use?

No. Contraceptive steroids have been identified in small amounts in breast milk. In rare instances, jaundice and breast enlargement may occur in infants consuming such milk. The quantity and quality of breast milk is altered by oral contraceptives. Nonhormonal contraceptives are recommended for nursing mothers until the child is weaned.

13. What types of oral contraceptives are available?

Combinations, biphasic, triphasic, and progestin-only oral contraceptives are available. Combination oral contraceptives use fixed doses of estrogen and progestin. In biphasic and triphasic oral contraceptives the progestin dose is varied to resemble more closely the natural menstrual cycle. Progestin-only oral contraceptives (mini-pills) are taken continuously and contain no estrogen. The progestin dose in most combination oral contraceptives is 1 mg or less. Progestin-only preparations contain 0.075–0.35 mg of progestin. The estrogen dose does not need to exceed 50 µg.

There is no difference in failure rates among oral contraceptives using 20, 30, 35, or 50 µg of estrogen. The failure rate with a progestin-only pill is somewhat higher (up to 1.1%) than that of combination preparations.

14. What is the "morning-after" pill?

After unprotected intercourse, two tablets of Ovral (ethinyl estradiol and norgestrel) may be taken within 72 and preferably 24 hours. Two more tablets are taken 12 hours after the first dose. Postcoital treatment reduces the pregnancy rate to 1–2%. A pregnancy test is mandatory if menses do not begin within 21 days.

15. What is Norplant?

The Norplant system consists of six Silastic capsules that are placed under the skin of the upper arm. Each capsule contains 36 µg of levonorgestrel. The progestin prevents conception by suppressing ovulation and thickening the cervical mucus to inhibit sperm penetration. Approximately one-third of women have prolonged and irregular bleeding with Norplant, whereas 10% may become amenorrheic. Most women resume regular menses after 6–12 months.

The typical first-year pregnancy rate with Norplant is 0.09%. The 5-year cumulative pregnancy rate is 3.9%. Norplant is not acceptably effective after 5 years. The average cost of Norplant is $450–$750. Fertility returns almost immediately when the system is discontinued. Norplant is an excellent contraception system for women who have chronic disease and/or require teratogenic medications. It is also safe for women over the age of 35 who smoke. Antiseizure medications and rifampin may reduce levels of serum levonorgestrel and decrease the efficacy of the system.

16. List the absolute contraindications for Norplant.

Known or suspected pregnancy
Benign or malignant liver tumors
Active thrombophlebitis or thromboembolic disease
Undiagnosed vaginal bleeding
Known or suspected breast cancer

17. What is the current status of the IUD?

The Dalkon Shield (manufactured by A. H. Robins Company) was removed from the market in 1975 because of its association with high rates of pelvic inflammatory disease and an increased incidence of septic abortion. A large settlement was paid to over 100,000 women who had claims of problems related to the shield. Several companies removed IUDs from the market, because they were no longer a profitable item. Less than 1% of women in the U.S. choose the IUD for contraception.

Two modern IUDs are more effective than oral contraceptives and all of the barrier methods: the copper T 380A (ParaGard) and the progesterone-releasing IUD (Progestasert). The copper T 380A is effective for 8 years. The Progestasert is replaced annually and is not quite as effective (especially in preventing ectopic pregnancies). Medically, an IUD is not a good contraceptive choice for a nulliparous woman. If the patient is unable to conceive after its removal, she may blame the device.

The IUD's mechanism of action is still poorly understood. It prevents fertilization by several mechanisms. The patient needs to know that the IUD is **not** an abortifacient. Side effects of IUDs include spotting, bleeding, anemia, cramping, and pain. A woman with more than one sexual partner is not a good candidate for the IUD because she is at increased risk for sexually transmitted diseases (STDs).

18. How effective are barrier methods?

All barrier methods are comparable for efficacy. The first-year failure rate ranges between 18 and 22%. Barrier methods include condoms, the cervical cap, the contraceptive sponge, spermicides, and the diaphragm. All barrier methods provide significant protection from STDs. Barrier methods are associated with a decreased risk of developing cervical dysplasia.

Synthetic condoms have been available since the 1840s. Condoms for men should be made of latex to protect against STDs. They must not be used with petroleum-based lubricants, and they must be applied before any genital-to-genital contact. Morning-after hormone treatment should be offered to couples who use condoms.

The **female condom** was approved for use in May 1993. The condom is manufactured as a prelubricated polyurethane sheath. One end is open, and the other is closed. Both ends are fitted with flexible rings. The upper ring aids as an insertion guide and an anchor during use. The outer ring remains outside of the vagina and fits over the labia.

The **cervical cap** is a soft thimble-shaped cup that fits over the cervix and is held in place by suction. The cap is partially filled with spermicide before application. The cap with spermicide provides contraception protection for 48 hours, no matter how many times intercourse occurs.

Nearly two million women use the **diaphragm**, which was first described in 1880. Diaphragms are prescribed in various sizes and are used with a spermicide. The diaphragm is a dome-shaped rubber cup with a flexible rim that is inserted into the vagina. The rubber dome covers the cervix and the rim (flat coil, or arching spring) tucks behind the symphysis pubis and fits snugly in the posterior vaginal fornix. The diaphragm must be left in place at least 6 hours after intercourse but should not be left in place for more than 24 hours.

Spermicides kill sperm after immobilizing them. They are available as foam, gels, or creams and contain octoxynol or nonoxynol 9.

Allergic reactions to latex and spermicides may occur. For the woman recurrent cystitis and vaginal discharge also may be troublesome. Toxic shock syndrome may occur if a barrier method is left in place longer than the recommended time.

19. What is fertility awareness?

Fertility awareness requires a woman to chart the most likely days during which she may conceive. Charting involves use of a calendar, recording basal body temperature, and following changes in the cervical mucus. Intercourse is avoided during the periovulatory days. The life span of an ovum is estimated to be 72 hours. Sperm are viable in the female reproductive tract for 2–7 days. The span of fertility may be from 7 days before ovulation to 3 days after ovulation. Approximately 20% of users experience failure during the first year. The most effective way to use fertility awareness is to postpone intercourse until after ovulation has been clearly documented.

20. What is the most commonly used form of birth control in the United States?

Sterilization is the treatment of choice for more than 16 million couples. The failure rate for tubal ligation is 0.2–0.4% in the first year. The failure rate for vasectomy is similar to that for tubal ligation. Vasectomy is simpler, safer, and less expensive than tubal ligation.

21. What is mifepristone?

Mifepristone (RU 486) is a progestin antagonist. Mifepristone may be used as a postcoital contraceptive within 72 hours of unprotected intercourse. The drug is given as a single oral dose of 600 mg. It is highly effective in preventing pregnancy. Mifepristone (600 mg orally) given with a prostaglandin 48 hours later results in a complete abortion rate approaching 100%. The combination is highly effective in women with pregnancy-induced amenorrhea for up to 9 weeks. Side effects are uncommon but may include heavy bleeding, nausea, vomiting, abdominal pain, and fatigue.

22. How effective is the female condom?

The female condom (Reality) was released in 1993. It provides a physical barrier for both the vagina and part of the perineum. It is made from polyurethane, which offers protection against HIV (unlike Latex) and is not susceptible to oil-based products. The pregnancy rate reported in several small studies is unfortunately as high as 15 pregnancies per 100 women.

23. How is Depo-Provera prescribed? How does it work?

Depo-Provera acts by inhibiting ovulation. A 150-mg injection is given every 3 months. Therapy is initiated within 5 days of the onset of menses. Women who are more than 2 weeks late for a shot should have a pregnancy test before proceeding. Unpredictable, irregular bleeding and spotting lasting 7 days or more are common during the first few months of use. Nearly one-half of women using Depo-Provera for more than 1 year become amenorrheic. Menstrual irregularity is the most frequent reason cited for discontinuation. Depo-Provera does not increase the risk of breast, endometrial, ovarian, or cervical cancer.

BIBLIOGRAPHY

1. American College of Obstetricians and Gynecologists: Hormonal contraception. ACOPG Technical Bulletin 48, 1995.
2. Colditz G: Oral contraceptive use and mortality during 12 years of follow-up: The Nurses' Health Study. Ann Intern Med 120:821–826, 1994.
3. Creinin MD, et al: Methotrexate and misoprostol for early abortion: A multicenter trial. I: Safety and efficacy. Contraception 53:321–327, 1996.
4. d'Or LC, Parazzini F: Barrier methods of contraception, spermicides, and sexually transmitted diseases: A review. Genitourin Med 70:410–417, 1994.
5. Farr G, Gabelnick H, Sturgen K, et al: Contraceptive efficacy and acceptability of the female condom. Am J Public Health 84:1960–1964, 1994.
6. Hatcher RA, Stewart F, et al: Contraceptive Technology, 16th ed. Manchester, NH, Irvington Publishers, 1994.
7. Kaunitz AM: Long-acting injectable contraception with depot medorxyprogesterone acetate. Am J Obstet Gynecol 170:1543, 1994.
8. Mauk C, et al: Lea's Shield: A study of the safety and efficacy of a new vaginal barrier contraceptive used with and without spermicide. Contraception 53:325–329, 1996.
9. Report of the U.S. Preventive Services Task Force: Counseling to Prevent Unintended Pregnancy—Guide to Clinical Preventive Services, 2nd ed. Baltimore, Williams & Wilkins, 1996, pp 739–753.
10. Schlesselman J: Net effect of oral contraceptive use on the risk of cancer in women in the United States. Obstet Gynecol 85:793–801, 1995.
11. Shoupe D: Contraception in the 1990s. Curr Opin Obstet Gynecol 8:211–215, 1996.

50. VAGINAL DISCHARGE AND PELVIC INFLAMMATORY DISEASE

Kavita Nanda, M.D., M.H.S., and Susan J. Diem, M.D., M.P.H.

1. Characterize the normal and abnormal vaginal discharge.

Some degree of vaginal discharge is normal. **Normal discharge** consists of desquamated vaginal epithelial cells and secretions from cervical glands, sebaceous glands, sweat glands, Bartholin's glands, and Skene's glands. Transudate through the vaginal wall also contributes to the composition of a normal discharge. Normal secretions are usually clear or white, odorless, and viscous. Polymorphonuclear leukocytes are rare. The amount of discharge varies with the menstrual cycle, age, sexual arousal, pregnancy, and use of oral contraceptives. An **abnormal discharge** is usually accompanied by a change in odor, a change in color, or an increase in the amount of discharge. In addition, patient may note pruritis, dysuria, or staining of underwear.

2. What causes an abnormal vaginal discharge?

1. Infections of the vagina, vulva, cervix, or upper genital tract

2. Atrophic vaginitis due to estrogen deficiency, which causes thinning and fragility of the vaginal and vulvar epithelium. Hence the epithelium is more vulnerable to injury and inflammation, producing desquamation of cells and stimulation of glandular secretions from the cervical area. In addition, such changes may elevate the pH in the vagina and thus result in a change in the bacteria.

3. Foreign bodies, such as tampons or diaphragms, if left in the vagina for a prolonged period

4. Irritation from frequent douching

5. Neoplasms of the cervix and uterus

3. List the five common infectious causes of a vaginal discharge.

Bacterial vaginosis   Chlamydial cervicitis and pelvic inflammatory disease
Trichomonal vaginosis   Gonococcal cervicitis and pelvic inflammatory disease
Candidal vulvovaginitis

4. Which of the infectious causes of a vaginal discharge are sexually transmitted?

Trichomoniasis, chlamydial infection, and gonococcal infection are sexually transmitted. Bacterial vaginosis and candidal vulvovaginitis are not generally thought to be sexually transmitted, although occasionally treatment of sexual partners is considered for persistent or recurrent infections.

5. What is bacterial vaginosis (BV)?

Also known as nonspecific vaginitis, BV is the most common cause of vaginal discharge. Although its etiology has been debated for years, it is believed to represent an alteration in the microbial flora of the vagina, with an increase in anaerobes and gram-negative bacilli and a decrease in the endogenous *Lactobacillus* flora. The presence of *Gardnerella vaginalis* also has been implicated in the pathogenesis of BV, but its role is not clearly elucidated. It is cultured commonly in patients with BV but may be found in up to 50% of healthy, asymptomatic women. Most authors believe that *G. vaginalis* may be necessary but not sufficient alone to cause BV. Patients with BV often present with a vaginal discharge associated with a change in odor, described as musty or fishy. The odor is due to the production of aromatic amines by the bacteria. The discharge is usually thin, white-yellow, homogeneous, and moderately increased in volume over the patient's normal discharge.

6. How is the diagnosis of BV made?

The diagnosis of BV requires three of the following four findings:

1. The pH of the vaginal discharge should be greater than 4.5. The normal pH of vaginal secretions, ranging from 3.8–4.4, is raised by the production of aromatic amines in the altered microbial environment.

2. "Clue" cells are seen on wet mount. Clue cells are epithelial cells with a granulated surface due to adherence of bacteria. They can be seen under high-dry magnification after a drop of the discharge is mixed with a drop of saline.

3. The "whiff" test is positive. A fishy odor is often produced when a drop of discharge is mixed with 10% potassium hydroxide. The alkalinization is thought to volatize amines, producing the characteristic fishy odor.

4. The discharge is consistent with BV.

7. Is BV associated with serious complications?

Yes. BV has been associated with several complications of pregnancy, including preterm delivery, premature rupture of membranes, amnionitis, chorioamnionitis, and postpartum endometritis. For this reason, it is important to treat BV in pregnant patients. It has also been associated with pelvic inflammatory disease (PID) and posthysterectomy vaginal cuff cellulitis.

8. Describe the treatment of BV.

Metronidazole is the drug of choice for the treatment of BV. The standard regimens include 500 mg twice daily for 7 days or 250 mg 3 times/day. Patients should be warned to avoid alcohol because of a disulfiram-like reaction. Other options include intravaginal clindamycin cream, metronidazole vaginal gel, and oral clindamycin at a dose of 300 mg twice daily for 7 days. Patients in the first trimester of pregnancy should be treated with one of the alternatives because of potential risks of teratogenicity from metronidazole. Clindamycin, either as intravaginal cream or as an oral dose of 300 mg twice daily for 7 days, is an effective option. After the first trimester, oral or topical therapy with metronidazole is an acceptable alternative.

9. Why is it important to diagnose and treat trichomonal vaginitis?

Trichomonal vaginitis is caused by *Trichomonas vaginalis*, a protozoan usually transmitted by sexual contact. Infection with *T. vaginalis* is associated with an abnormal discharge that ranges in color from white to yellow, gray, or green. Other manifestations may include vaginal itching, dysuria, and dyspareunia. As many as 50% of infected women are asymptomatic, as are the majority of infected men. Microscopic examination of a drop of the vaginal discharge mixed with saline reveals motile flagellated trichomonads that are approximately twice the size of WBCs. The sensitivity of this procedure in symptomatic women is approximately 50–75%, and the specificity approaches 100%. Cultures for *T. vaginalis* have a sensitivity of approximately 90%. In addition, monoclonal antibody tests are available with sensitivities and specificities that approach those of culture. The standard treatment for trichomoniasis is a single dose of 2 gm of metronidazole. Partners also should be treated. Other dosing regimens may be tried for treatment failures. Topical metronidazole is not effective.

10. What infection is suggested by a "strawberry cervix"?

Cervicitis due to *T. vaginalis*, although rare, is characterized by a strawberry cervix.

11. What infection is suggested by a white, cheesy discharge?

Candidal vulvovaginitis is caused by *Candida* species of fungi, most commonly *C. albicans*. Candidal infection may cause vulvar and vaginal irritation and inflammation, resulting in burning, itching, dyspareunia, and dysuria. Many women have an abnormal discharge, often thick and clumpy. These fungi also are found as part of the normal flora in approximately 30% of women. The diagnosis is made by examining the discharge with a Gram stain or 10% potassium hydroxide solution for the fungal forms. Culture is a more sensitive method for detecting the yeast, but because many women without symptoms have positive yeast cultures, routine cultures are not recommended. Culture for *Candida* sp. is indicated for chronic or recurrent infections to identify resistant strains.

12. What factors predispose to candidal vaginitis?

Predisposing factors for candidiasis include diabetes, acquired immunodeficiency syndrome, recent antibiotic use, pregnancy, corticosteroids, and immunosuppressants.

13. What is the role of oral agents in the treatment of candidal vaginitis?

Candidiasis can be treated with several topical agents, including miconazole or clotrimazole; all have cure rates of 85% or higher. Oral agents include fluconazole, ketoconazole, and itraconazole. The risk of side effects of oral agents restricts their use to resistant or recurrent candidal vulvovaginitis. They do not appear to be significantly more effective than topical treatments.

14. What is chlamydial cervicitis? How is it treated?

One common cause of cervicitis, *Chlamydia trachomatis*, is transmitted through sexual contact. Symptoms include a mucopurulent discharge, lower abdominal discomfort, fever, and dysuria. However, many patients infected with *C. trachomatis* are asymptomatic. On examination the cervix is red, edematous, and friable. The diagnosis can be made by culture, a technique that is expensive and technically difficult. Fluorescent antibody testing and enzyme-linked immunoassays are easier to perform and have good sensitivity and specificity. Newer techniques include the polymerase chain reaction (PCR) or ligase chain reaction (LCR).

The mainstay of treatment for chlamydial infection is doxycycline, 100 mg twice daily for 7 days, or azithromycin, 1 gm orally in a single dose. Alternatives include ofloxacin, 300 mg orally twice daily for 7 days, or erythromycin base, 500 mg orally 4 times/day for 7 days. Erythromycin or azithromycin should be used in pregnant patients, and ofloxacin should not be used in adolescents under 18. Erythromycin is not as effective, and a test of cure is recommended 2–3 weeks after treatment. Partners also should be referred for treatment.

15. When else should patients be treated for chlamydial infection? Why?

Patients should be treated for presumed chlamydial infection in the presence of gonococcal cervicitis. Up to 40% of patients with gonorrhea are also infected with chlamydia.

16. What infection is caused by *Neisseria gonorrhoeae*?

Infection with *N. gonorrhoeae* causes gonorrhea, a sexually transmitted disease. Gynecologic manifestations include a purulent vaginal discharge due to cervicitis and PID. The discharge may be accompanied by pruritus, dyspareunia, dysuria, and lower abdominal discomfort. The diagnosis of gonococcal cervicitis is made by Gram stain of the discharge demonstrating gram-negative intracellular diplococci. Cultures of Thayer-Martin medium are used to confirm the diagnosis. PCR may also be used.

First-line treatment of gonococcal cervicitis consists of ceftriaxone, 125 mg intramuscularly (IM) in a single dose, or cefixime, 400 mg orally, followed by a 7 day course of doxycycline, 100 mg twice daily, or azithromycin, 1 gm orally, to treat undiagnosed coexistent chlamydial infection. Ciprofloxacin, 500 mg orally, or ofloxacin, 400 mg orally, may be used for patients allergic to cephalosporins. Partners also should be treated.

17. Describe the approach to a patient with a vaginal discharge.

History, physical examination, and a few simple laboratory tests identify the cause of many cases of vaginal discharge. The history should focus on the nature of the discharge, associated symptoms, sexual and contraceptive history, and other medical conditions. The physical examination should include inspection of the vulva, vagina, and cervix, noting any erythema, edema, atrophy, abnormal lesions, trauma, or foreign bodies. Characteristics of the discharge, such as color and consistency, also should be noted. A bimanual examination should be performed to evaluate cervical motion tenderness, adnexal masses, and uterine masses or tenderness.

Laboratory studies should include a saline wet-mount preparation to look for clue cells and trichomonads. A 10% solution of potassium hydroxide added to a sample of discharge facilitates identification of *Candida* sp. A Gram stain of the discharge should be performed if gonococcal infection is suspected. In addition, pH testing of the discharge may be helpful. Cultures of the discharge for *N. gonorrhoeae* should be performed if mucopurulent cervicitis is seen on physical examination. Infection with *C. trachomatis* can be evaluated with direct immunofluorescent testing or cultures. Other tests to consider include a urinalysis, particularly if dysuria is present, and a complete blood count if PID is a diagnostic consideration.

18. Define PID.

PID is an infection of the upper genital tract in women and may include salpingitis, tuboovarian abscess, endometritis, and pelvic peritonitis. An estimated 1 million American women per year are diagnosed with PID; the direct and indirect costs of the disease and its complications are estimated to be over $5.5 billion annually.

19. Which organisms are responsible for PID?

PID is caused by a variety of bacteria, most importantly *N. gonorrhoeae* and *C. trachomatis*, both of which are sexually transmitted. Other organisms that may play a role either in the initial development of PID or as secondary pathogens include aerobes, such as *Streptococcus* sp., *Escherichia coli*, and *Hemophilus influenzae*, and anaerobes, such as *Bacteroides* sp., *Prevotella* sp., *Peptostreptococcus* sp., and *Peptococcus* sp. *Actinomyces israelii*, a gram-positive anaerobic organism, is seen in PID related to the use of intrauterine devices.

20. Describe the pathogenesis of PID.

C. trachomatis and *N. gonorrhoeae* initially affect the endocervical canal and cause cervicitis. The infection ascends the cervix and spreads into the uterus and fallopian tubes and then to the ovaries and peritoneal cavity. Factors that promote ascension include damage to the endocervical canal by the bacteria, extension of the endocervical columnar epithelium beyond the endocervix, and hormonal changes during the menstrual cycle that affect characteristics of the cervical mucus.

21. List risk factors for PID.
- Young age
- Multiple sex partners
- Vaginal douching
- Bacterial vaginosis
- Intrauterine device
- Previous PID

22. How is the diagnosis of PID made?

The minimal criteria for diagnosis of PID are cervical motion tenderness, lower abdominal tenderness, and adnexal tenderness. Additional criteria used to increase the specificity of the diagnosis include fever > 100.9 F, abnormal cervical or vaginal discharge, elevated erythrocyte sedimentation rate, elevated C-reactive protein, or laboratory confirmation of infection with *N. gonorrhoeae* or *C. trachomatis*. Further testing is warranted if the diagnosis remains in question. Pregnancy should be excluded, and a pelvic ultrasound may help to evaluate a palpable pelvic mass. The gold standard for the diagnosis of PID is laparoscopy. Laparoscopy should be considered if the diagnosis is unclear, if the patient fails to respond to conventional treatment, or if an unexplained pelvic mass is present.

23. What should be considered in the differential diagnoses of PID?
- Acute appendicitis
- Endometriosis
- Ruptured ovarian cyst
- Ectopic pregnancy
- Inflammatory bowel disease
- Spontaneous abortion

24. What are the three principal complications of PID?
(1) Infertility due to tubal occlusion, which occurs in 8–40% of patients after PID; (2) chronic pelvic pain, which develops in up to 18% of women after acute PID; and (3) ectopic pregnancy, which occurs in approximately 9% of women who have had PID.

25. What is Fitz-Hugh–Curtis syndrome?
Fitz-Hugh–Curtis syndrome is the acute perihepatitis seen with the spread of *N. gonorrhoeae* or *C. trachomatis* from the fallopian tube through the peritoneal cavity to the liver capsule. Patients usually present with right upper quadrant pain and often have clinical evidence of PID.

26. What is the recommended treatment for PID? When should patients with PID be hospitalized?
Empirical broad-spectrum treatment is essential. The Centers for Disease Control (CDC) recommends outpatient treatment for mild PID with ceftriaxone, 250 mg IM along with doxycycline, 100 mg orally twice daily for 14 days. An alternative regimen is ofloxacin, 400 mg/day orally for 14 days, and either clindamycin, 450 mg orally 4 times/day, or metronidazole, 500 mg orally twice daily for 14 days. If the diagnosis is uncertain; if a pelvic abscess is suspected; or if the patient is severely ill, cannot take oral medications, or is pregnant, hospitalization should be considered. Hospitalization is also recommended for HIV-positive, nulliparous, or adolescent patients and patients who cannot return for follow-up. Treatments recommended for severe PID include intravenous cefoxitin, 2 gm every 6 hours, along with doxycycline, 100 mg orally or intravenously twice daily. An alternative regimen is clindamycin, 900 mg intravenously every 8 hours, accompanied by gentamicin intravenously. Intravenous treatment should be continued for at least 48 hours after the patient shows clinical improvement. If the patient does not improve in 72 hours, surgical intervention should be considered.

BIBLIOGRAPHY

1. American College of Obstetrics and Gynecologists: Vaginitis. ACOG Technical Bulletin 226, 1996.
2. Centers for Disease Control and Prevention: 1998 Guidelines for treatment of sexually transmitted diseases. MMWR 198:74(No. RR-1):1–111.
3. Goode MA, Grauer K, Gums JG: Infectious vaginitis: Selecting therapy and preventing recurrence. Postgrad Med 96(6):85–88, 1994.
4. Hillis SD, Wasserheit JN: Screening for chlamydia—a key to the prevention of pelvic inflammatory disease. N Engl J Med 334:1399–1401, 1996.
5. McCormack WM: Current concepts: Pelvic inflammatory disease. N Engl J Med 330:115–119, 1994.
6. McCoy MC, Katz VL, Kuller JA, et al: Bacterial vaginosis in pregnancy: An approach for the 1990s. Obstet Gynecol Surv 50:482–488, 1995.
7. Reed BD, Eyler A: Vaginal infections: Diagnosis and management. Am Fam Physician 47:1805–1818, 1993.
8. Sweet RL: Role of bacterial vaginosis in pelvic inflammatory disease. Clin Infect Dis 20(Suppl 2): S271–275, 1995.

51. PROSTATE DISEASE

Norman E. Peterson, M.D.

1. What are the most common disorders affecting the prostate?
Prostatitis, benign prostatic hypertrophy (BPH), and prostatic cancer.

2. What are the typical clinical manifestations of BPH?
BPH is manifested by any combination of the following symptoms: slowing of the size and force of the urinary stream, urinary frequency or urgency, sensation of incomplete bladder

emptying, and nocturia. Usually symptoms are gradually progressive and therefore may be tolerated until severe. Examination may reveal varying levels of residual urine. Digital rectal examination (DRE) typically discloses homogeneous, symmetric enlargement of the prostate. Urodynamic evaluation may demonstrate uninhibited detrusor contractions, which may be relieved by anticholinergic medication or corrected by surgical means. Symptoms of prostate obstruction (prostatism) may be exaggerated by coexisting urinary infection or disorders that deleteriously influence bladder function, such as diabetes or chronic vesicle overdistention.

3. List the complications of BPH.

Obstruction may culminate in acute urinary retention that requires catheter relief. Less common complications include urinary incontinence, infection, stone formation, and hematuria.

4. Can patients present with prostatism and a gland of normal size?

Younger patients (early 50s) presenting with prostatism frequently demonstrate an unenlarged, clinically benign gland. Incongruously severe voiding dysfunction is produced by a small fibrous prostate, or median bar hypertrophy of the posterior vesicle neck. Management is similar to that for BPH, although less likely to respond to medical management, warranting surgical incision rather than resection.

5. What is the recommended approach to the patient with BPH?

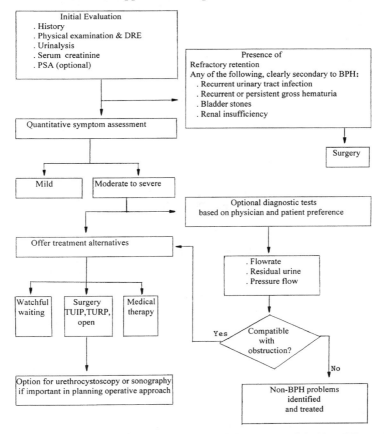

Decision diagram for benign prostatic hypertrophy. (From U.S. Department of Health and Human Services: Clinical Practice Guideline: Benign Prostatic Hyperplasia, 1994.)

6. What is the most common operative option for treatment of BPH?

Transurethral prostatectomy (TURP) is appropriate for most patients because it limits hospitalization and convalescence. "Prostatectomy" for BPH is in reality adenomectomy of the obstructing hypertrophied periurethral tissue, leaving the prostate gland largely undisturbed. Perineal prostatectomy is rarely performed for benign disease and is generally limited to the patient who is vulnerable to pulmonary or other complications associated with alternative surgical approaches. Suprapubic and retropubic approaches are similar open procedures and are often used for larger glands; blood loss and fluid absorption are considerably less than what may occur with prolonged transurethral resection.

Treatment alternatives currently under investigation include transurethral incision (TUIP) rather than resection of smaller obstructive prostates, permanent dilating prostatic urethral stents, and tissue removal by laser and hyperthermic applications. Advantages of nonresection procedures are basically paraoperative and are offset by postoperative disadvantages largely avoided by TURP, which remains the overall gold standard.

7. What is the spectrum of pharmacologic options available for the treatment of BPH?

AGENT	PRIMARY SITE OF ACTION
Androgen suppressors	Inhibition of LH secretion $\rightarrow$ T $\downarrow$ + DHT $\downarrow$
Diethylstilbestrol	Desensitization of LHRH receptors in the pituitary $\rightarrow$ inhibition
LHRH agonists	of LH secretion $\rightarrow$ T $\downarrow$ + DHT $\downarrow$
Nafarelin	
Buserelin	
Goserelin	
Leuprolide	
Cyproterone acetate	Androgen receptor inhibition
	Inhibition of LH secretion $\rightarrow$ T $\downarrow$ + DHT $\downarrow$
Flutamide	Androgen receptor inhibition through competitive blockade of T +
	DHT binding to androgen receptors
Progestins	Inhibition of LH secretion $\rightarrow$ T $\downarrow$ + DHT $\downarrow$
Megestrol acetate	Androgen receptor inhibition
Hydroxyprogesterone caproate	
Medrogestone	
Finasteride	5-Alpha reductase inhibitor $\rightarrow$ T $\rightarrow$ DHT
Ketoconazole	Antifungal imidazole derivative and potent inhibitor of gonadal steroid biosynthesis through inhibition of 17 alpha-hydroxylase and 17,20-desmolase activity
	Aromatase inhibition
Spironolactone	Aldosterone antagonist with anti-androgenic action through competitive inhibition of androgen receptors, and inhibition of androgen biosynthesis by inhibiting 17 alpha-hydroxylase and 17,20-desmolase activity
H_2-receptor antagonist	
Cimetidine	H_2-receptor antagonist with antiandrogenic action
Aromatase inhibitors	
Nonsteroidal	Converts 4-androstenedion to estrone
Ketoconazole	Testosterone to estradiol
Miconazole	
Clotrimazole	
Steroidal	
1-methyl-1,4-androstatriene-3,17-dione	
1,4,6-androstatriene-3,-17-dione	
Testolactone	

(Table continued on following page.)

AGENT	PRIMARY SITE OF ACTION
Alpha-adrenergic receptor antagonists	
Nonselective	Blockade of both alpha$_1$ and alpha$_2$ adrenoreceptors
Phenoxybenzamine	
Thymoxamine	
Selective	Blockade of alpha$_1$ adrenoreceptors only
Prazosin	
Alfuzosin	
Doxazosin	
YM 617	
Nicergoline	

LH = luteinizing hormone, LHRH = luteinizing hormone-releasing hormone, DHT = dehydrotestosterone.

8. Describe the clinical utility of the three most frequently used hormonal therapies for reducing prostatic volume.

1. Agonists of luteinizing hormone-releasing hormone (LHRH), which include leuprolide and nafarelin acetate, produce significant benefits but require permanent uninterrupted therapy. Side effects include decreased libido, impotence, gynecomastia, hot flushes, and decreased levels of serum prostate-specific antigen (PSA). Therapy, therefore, is ideally restricted to impotent patients. An additional disadvantage is the requirement for intramuscular or subcutaneous administration. Depot forms permit administration every 3 months.

2. Antiandrogen medication is dominated by flutamide, which has advantages similar to LHRH agonists but also alters PSA levels. Side effects include gastrointestinal upset and gynecomastia or nipple tenderness. Sustained serum testosterone levels produce the advantage of undiminished libido, potency, and ejaculation. Flutamide is administered orally but may require up to 6 months to achieve maximal benefit. Uninterrupted maintenance therapy is necessary. Observance for hepatotoxicity is advised.

3. Inhibition of 5-alpha reductase (finasteride/Proscar) is a once-daily medication that has no significant side effects and may reduce prostatic volume and modestly improve symptoms in 30–50% of patients. Up to 6 months may be required for maximal benefit, and permanent maintenance therapy is required. PSA levels typically fall by 50%, and this effect must be considered during monitoring for prostate cancer. An added advantage is the potential for halting disease progression due to suppressed androgen stimulation of the prostate.

All three agents appear equally effective in reducing prostatic volume by approximately 25% and improving obstructive symptoms and urinary flow rate. However, adrenergic inhibition is commonly preferred as initial therapy.

9. What medical therapy is available for outlet obstruction that results from BPH?

Selective alpha$_1$ antagonists relax smooth muscle fibers at the vesicle outlet, thus reducing outlet resistance and improving urinary flow. Nonselective alpha antagonists (phenoxybenzamine/Dibenzyline) may reduce voiding symptoms but also have adverse side effects. Selective alpha$_1$ antagonists include prazosin (Minipress), terazosin (Hytrin), and doxazosin (Cardura). Minipress requires twice daily dosage, whereas Hytrin and Cardura are administered at bedtime. No clinical advantage favors Cardura over Hytrin. Brief transitory lightheadedness, dizziness, and fatigue may occur with initiation of therapy; it is advisable to administer the first several doses under conditions that minimize the risk of complications. Dosage options are 1, 2, 5, and 10 mg, and dosage is titrated for effect. A newly released agent, tamsulosin (Flomax) is reputed to convey equal benefit with fewer side effects.

10. What is the preferred management of acute injury retention?

The obvious answer is catheter decompression of the bladder. Decisions about removal or maintenance of catheter drainage relate to the level of bladder overdistention. Retained volumes exceeding 500 cc are probably best treated by two days of catheter decompression to permit recovery of detrusor tonus. Smaller volumes are usually amenable to immediate drainage, with prompt restoration of pre-retention voiding dynamics. When urethral catheterization is unsuccessful, urologic referral is advised.

11. When urethral catheterization cannot be performed and consultation with a urologist is unavailable, what can be done to relieve urethral obstruction?

Temporary relief is obtainable by suprapubic trocar cystostomy or suprapubic insertion of a large-bore needle into the bladder through which a polyethylene drainage tube is passed. Commercial products are available for these purposes. Suprapubic maneuvers require a distended bladder and the absence of previous surgical procedures that may jeopardize the small bowel and colon because of adhesions.

12. What is the recommended practice for improving early diagnosis of prostate cancer?

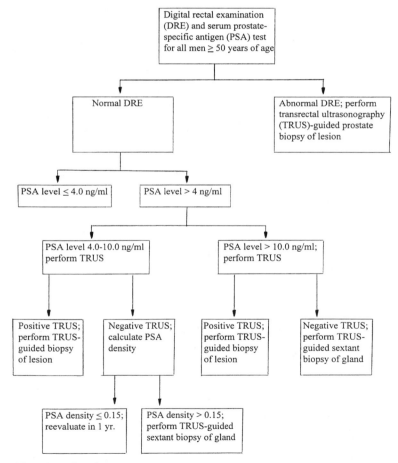

(Adapted from Oesterling JE: PSA leads the way for detecting and following prostate cancer. Contemporary Urology, pp 60–81, 1993.).

Screening for prostate cancer is recommended for all men aged 50–70. Earlier screening (age 40–45) is advised for African-American patients and patients with familial (father, brother, uncle) incidence of prostate cancer. PSA elevation without abnormalities at DRE or transrectal ultrasonography (TRUS) warrants referral for sextant needle biopsy. A PSA level less than 20 ng/ml is statistically unassociated with identifiable metastatic dissemination; metastasis is more likely as levels progressively exceed 20 ng/ml. Elevation of the serum prostatic acid phosphatase is associated in most cases with cancer that escapes the confines of the prostate gland.

13. What conditions other than prostatic carcinoma may elevate the PSA to intermediate levels?

Prostatitis, prostate infarction, large BPH, and trauma, including biopsy or surgery.

14. Describe the staging of prostatic cancer.

Staging Systems for Prostate Cancer

WHITMORE-JEWETT STAGE	DEFINITION
A1–A2	No palpable tumor; incidental finding in operative specimen; positive random biopsy
B1–B3	Palpable tumor confined to the gland or small nodule confined to one lobe
C1–C2	Extension beyond prostatic capsule with or without involvement of lateral sulci and/or seminal vesicles
D1–D2	Metastases to any site, often including elevated prostatic acid phosphatase

15. What are the contemporary options for management of prostate cancer?

- Watchful waiting   • Surgical extirpation
- External or interstitial (seed) radiotherapy
- Pharmacologic or surgical hormone suppression
- Chemotherapy   • Methods for pain control of bony metastases

Management may be directed by the patient's wishes or by clinical factors that limit options. Patients diagnosed at age 70 are likely to live out normal lives unaffected by nontreatment. Otherwise management is selected according to staging. **Stage A and B** lesions (confined to the prostate) are candidates for radical prostatectomy. Radiotherapy has produced improved results in many recent studies. Open or laparoscopic pelvic lymphadenectomy is necessary to ensure absence of latent dissemination. PSA levels < 20 ng/ml reduce the likelihood of understaging. **Stage C** disease (invasion of prostate capsule or seminal vesicle) is occasionally downstaged by androgen suppression, but such patients are otherwise maintained on suppression therapy until hormonal independence is manifested by rapidly escalating PSA or clinical complications. **Stage D** (dissemination to bone or lymphatics) is treated as stage C. Clinical manifestations of hormone resistance may benefit from radiotherapy, interruption of hormone suppression therapy, intravenous strontium, and various chemotherapy regimens.

16. List potential complications or side effects seen with therapy for prostatic carcinoma.

Surgery
Impotence
Incontinence
Anastomotic stricture
Rectal injury

External radiotherapy
Cystitis
Bladder contracture
Urethral stricture
Incontinence
Impotence

Estrogen therapy (rarely used)
Breast enlargement and tenderness
Increased incidence of cardiovascular events
Isolated leuprolide therapy
Testosterone flare (temporary increase in bone pain and other symptoms suppressible with antiandrogen therapy)
Testicular atrophy
Loss of libido
Impotence
Flutamide therapy
Gynecomastia
Nausea and vomiting

17. What is meant by prostatitis?

A misdiagnosis of prostatitis is often applied to nonspecific complaints of low back pain, perineal pain or discomfort, constipation, premature ejaculation, or vague voiding discomfort or dysfunction. Prostatitis or prostatic inflammation is subcategorized into acute bacterial prostatitis, chronic bacterial prostatitis, nonbacterial prostatitis, prostadynia, or granulomatous prostatitis (rare). Each requires specific diagnosis and treatment.

18. Describe the presentation and management of a patient with acute prostatitis.

Acute bacterial prostatitis presents as a florid clinical disorder characterized by toxic systemic symptoms, extreme dysuria with increased frequency, urgency and strangury, severely tender prostate, and rusty urine containing red blood cells, white blood cells, and bacteria. The prostatic barrier to antibiotic penetration is destroyed by the acute inflammatory process; therefore, any effective antibiotic suffices. Potentially severe local and systemic symptoms may necessitate hospitalization for parenteral antibiotics, fluid repletion, pain control, and urethral catheter drainage. Recovery is usually prompt.

19. Why should chronic bacterial prostatitis be distinguished from nonbacterial prostatitis?

Prolonged, uninterrupted antibacterial therapy is required for cure of chronic bacterial prostatitis. Diagnosis depends on culture positivity of prostatic secretions (after prostatic massage) or semen in the presence of sterile urine. Clinical manifestations are dominated by recurrent episodes of bacterial cystitis. Effective therapy is usually provided by trimethoprim-sulfamethoxazole (published cure rates of 30%) or quinolone (70%). Recommended duration of therapy is 6–8 weeks, thereby underscoring the importance of accurate diagnosis.

20. How is nonbacterial prostatitis managed?

Nonbacterial prostatitis is manifested as vague, nonspecific symptoms (see question 17). Prostatic secretions contain inflammatory cells but no bacteria or culture-positivity. Antibiotic therapy is, therefore, inappropriate. Symptoms dominate, and therapy is directed to symptomatic alleviation. Prostatic congestion may benefit from massage to express accumulated secretions. Other modalities include pharmacologic relaxation of the pelvic floor (diazepam), warm sitz baths, pyridium for urethral discomfort, and occasionally dilation of the anal sphincter.

21. Define prostadynia.

Prostadynia is a term intended to incorporate the nonspecific symptoms often misinterpreted as prostatitis. Prostatic secretions are devoid of inflammatory cells. Management is the same as for chronic nonbacterial prostatitis and focuses on symptom alleviation.

22. What is the significance of a diagnosis of prostatic abscess?

Prostatic abscess is uncommon. Contributing factors, therefore, should be considered, including diabetes, AIDS, and other immunosuppressive states. Specific bacterial diagnosis is warranted to identify atypical opportunistic infections. A prostatic abscess may present as either an acute systemic toxic event or as a chronic low-grade, nonspecific disorder. Urethral obstruction may result from the abscess mass. DRE reveals asymmetry and nonhomogeneity; the involved lobe may be bulging, fluctuant, and variably sensitive. Prostatic abscess frequently ruptures into the rectum or urethra with resolution of the acute clinical status. Interventional drainage may be accomplished by transurethral resection or transrectal needle aspiration.

BIBLIOGRAPHY

1. Beduschi MC, Oesterling JE: Percent free-PSA and the early diagnosis of prostate cancer. Urol Grand Rounds 2:1–8, 1997.
2. Berger RE: Prostatitis—so what? Clin Care Prost Dis 1:13–16, 1994.

3. Childs SJ: Ultrasound-guided laser-assisted transurethral resection of the prostate. Surg Techn Urol 7:2–8, 1994.
4. Evans DTP: Treatment of chronic abacterial prostatitis: A review. Int J STD AIDS 5:157–164, 1994.
5. Falagas ME, Gorbach SL: Practice guidelines: Prostatitis, epididymitis, and urethritis. Infect Dis Clin Pract 4:325–333, 1995.
6. Kabalin JN: Invasive therapies for BPH. Monogr Urol 18:17–47, 1997.
7. Kabalin JN: Transurethral laser prostatectomy. Infect Urol 1994, pp 71–84.
8. Keetch DW, Andriole GL: Prostate cancer screening. Monogr Urol 17:31–48, 1996.
9. Labrie F, Belenger A, Simard J, et al: Combination therapy for prostate cancer. Cancer 71:1059–1067, 1993.
10. Nixon RC, Brawer MK: PSA testing. Mediguide Urol 9:1–6, 1995.
11. Perez-Marrero R, Emerson LE: Expandable titanium prostatic urethral stent for the treatment of BPH. Infect Urol 1992, pp 183–188.
12. Peterson NE: Primary care treatment of prostatic disorders. Prim Care Rep 2:19–26, 1996.
13. Peterson NE: Urinary incontinence and retention. In Harwood-Nuss A, et al (eds): The Clinical Practice of Emergency Medicine, 2nd ed. Philadelphia, Lippincott-Raven, 1996, pp 258–263.
14. Raghavan D, Cooney G, Rosen M, et al: Management of hormone resistant prostate cancer. Semin Oncol 23:20–23, 1996.
15. Schellhammer PF: Radiation therapy for localized prostate cancer. Monogr Urol 15:77–92, 1994.
16. Shortliffe LD: Evaluation and management of prostatitis. Mediguide Urol 3:1–7, 1989.
17. Slawin KM, Ohori M, Dillioglugil O, Scardino PT: Screening for prostate cancer. Cancer J Clin 45:134–147, 1995.
18. Stamey TA: Prostate cancer: Who should be treated? Monogr Urol 16:1–16, 1995.

52. SCROTAL MASSES

Norman E. Peterson, M.D.

1. List the masses that may involve intrascrotal contents, and specify the presence or absence of pain as a distinguishing feature.

Scrotal Masses

Benign	PAIN	Inflammatory	PAIN
Hydrocele	−	Epididymitis	+
Varicocele	−	Orchitis	+
Spermatocele	−	Abscess	+
Inclusion cyst	−	Tuberculosis	−
Lipoma	−	**Malignant**	
Adenomatoid tumor	−	Seminoma	−
Hematocele	+	Embryonal carcinoma	−
Spermatic cord torsion	+	Teratocarcinoma	−
Torsion, testis appendage	+	Yolk sac carcinoma	−
		Choriocarcinoma	−

Hydrocele and varicocele may present with pain, but palpation discomfort is uncommon and symptoms may be exaggerated by anxiety and apprehension. Spermatocele may be painful only in its earliest and smallest manifestations. As the spermatocele enlarges, the fibers of its capsule separate, thereby relieving the pain of capsular distension. Testis tumors are characteristically painless, although intralesional hemorrhage (rare) may be painful. Chronic discomfort also may result from the weight and mass of larger lesions.

2. What is the recommended clinical reaction to discovery of an intrascrotal mass?

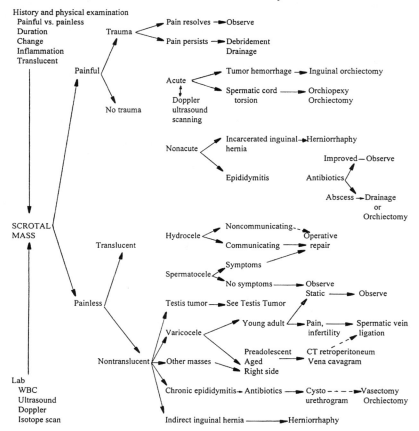

3. What is the significance of acute vs. chronic scrotal pain?

Scrotal pain of acute onset characterizes torsion of the spermatic cord or testicular appendages, and acute epididymitis. Acute pain also may result from hemorrhage into a tumor or traumatic rupture of the testicular capsule (tunica albuginea). Doppler ultrasound scanning is often effective in diagnosis, but contradictory studies impose the requirement for surgical exploration. **Chronic scrotal pain** may occur with any subacute inflammatory disorder, including epididymitis, orchitis, or abscess. It also may result from the weight and mass of larger testis tumors. Chronic testicular pain is often claimed with hydrocele, varicocele, and spermatocele but may result from anxiety. Chronic pain associated with testicular elevation may represent chronic cremaster muscle spasm, which is usually self-limited but requires operative intervention in extreme cases.

4. Why is orchiectomy maintained as a last resort for patients with chronic orchidynia?

Debilitating, incapacitating testicular pain resistant to myriad analgesic and psychogenic relief efforts is termed orchidynia or orchalgia. Postoperative complaints of ipsilateral or contralateral testis pain often follows removal of the symptomatic testis. Referral to pain management consultants or psychotherapy is advised.

5. What diagnostic adjuncts are available for evaluation of intrascrotal pathology?

- Urinalysis (to exclude infection)
- Color Doppler ultrasound (for blood flow)

- Isotope scintigraphy
- Plain radiographs (for evidence of calcification)
- Ultrasound scanning
- Serum tumor marker evaluation (human chorionic gonadotropin, alpha fetoprotein)
- Drainage cultures
- Surgical exploration

6. How may physical examination be implemented in patients with severe pain?

Pain resulting from epididymitis, spermatic cord torsion, or posttraumatic hematocele inhibits palpation. Injection of local anesthetic (1% lidocaine) into the spermatic cord above the testis provides instant relief, and examination may then proceed.

7. What clinical features are helpful for distinguishing spermatic cord torsion from epididymitis?

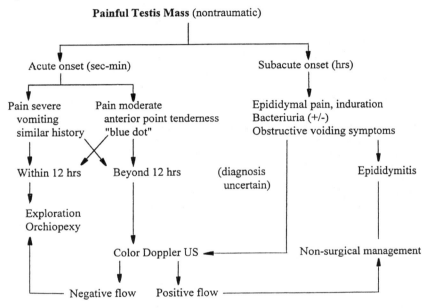

Clinical distinctions are reported to include transverse orientation of testis/epididymis, Prehn's sign (pain improvement with testis support or elevation), high-riding testis, and cutaneous erythema. The most reliable clinical feature is rate of onset of pain: instantaneous with torsion, over several hours with epididymitis. Emesis is frequent in pediatric patients. Diagnosis of epididymitis may be supported by pain and induration limited to the posterior aspect of the testis or to one pole.

8. Is spermatic cord torsion restricted to young patients?

Spermatic cord torsion is thought to be limited to boys under age 16 and epididymitis to adults. Neither statement is accurate. Acute severe testis pain is spermatic cord torsion until proved otherwise, regardless of age or other clinical features. Recurrent episodes with spontaneous resolution (derotation) is common in adults and may contribute to the diagnosis.

9. What is the recommended management of spermatic cord torsion?

Prompt detorsion is required. Successful manual derotation permits elective (nonemergency) scheduling for bilateral orchiopexy. Manual or spontaneous derotation is more frequent in adults, perhaps related to less fixation by fibrin exudate than in pediatric patients. Emergency operative scrotal exploration usually is required for derotation, appraisal of viability, orchiectomy or orchiopexy, and prophylactic fixation of the opposite uninvolved testis. When clinical diagnosis is uncertain or when excessive time has elapsed between onset and presentation (thereby questioning testicular viability), color Doppler ultrasound or isotope scintigraphy is recommended. Orchiectomy for definitive infarction may be deferred or omitted.

10. Describe the management of acute epididymitis.
Symptoms of acute epididymitis range from nominal polar tenderness to extreme indurated painful mass with systemic toxicity. Management, therefore, ranges from outpatient antibiotics and pain medication to hospitalization for fluid repletion, intravenous antibiotics, and perhaps therapeutic orchiectomy. Extreme pain can be alleviated by spermatic cord block.

11. What is the anticipated response to therapy for acute epididymitis?
Epididymitis that does not respond to therapy within 24–48 hours implies inappropriate antibiotic treatment, inaccurate diagnosis, or abscess formation. Abscess may be identified by ultrasound scanning, and orchiectomy should be considered.

12. What is the potential significance of an episode of epididymitis in a child?
Epididymitis is uncommon in children and, therefore, suggests the possibility of obstructive or fistulous urinary defects, usually identified by voiding cystourethrogram. Bacteriuria or history of urinary tract infections increases suspicion.

13. What is the potential significance of recurrent epididymitis in an adult?
Recurrent epididymitis suggests lower urinary tract obstruction. An alternative possibility in patients engaged in vigorous work or exercise is retrograde reflux of urine into the vas deferens with straining, producing a chemical epididymitis that tends to be recurrent.

14. What is the potential significance of varicocele to a child? To an adult?
Varicoceles usually become manifest in early or mid adolescence and often regress spontaneously during the fourth decade. Thus, the published incidence of varicocele among military inductees is 12–15% compared with a nominal incidence of varicocele among older men. Pathologic etiologies such as intraabdominal or retroperitoneal masses that produce venous obstruction and collateral venous drainage should be considered in preadolescent or presenile patients. Nonpathologic varicoceles in preadolescent boys are significant, because of possible deleterious influences on testicular growth and maturation. Therefore, varicocelectomy is recommended to reverse suppressive influences in a testis that is noticeably smaller than its mate. Semen analysis of infertile patients with varicocele may include reduced sperm motility and increased numbers of immature and abnormal forms. Semen characteristics and fertility potential may improve after varicocelectomy, although absolute sperm counts and densities are rarely improved.

15. What is the usual presentation of a testicular tumor?
Testicular tumors present as a painless mass. Lack of symptoms is reflected in the frequent delay of presentation until the size of the mass is several times normal.

16. Should needle aspiration of a painless testicular mass be undertaken for diagnosis?
No. The mainstay of diagnosis is inguinal orchiectomy for establishment of tumor histology. Needle aspiration is contraindicated, because tumor seeding and inaccurate histologic subtyping may result. Also needed are a chest radiograph and assessment of serum tumor markers (alpha fetoprotein and beta human chorionic gonadotropin) as an index of tumor volume, aggressiveness, and histology and later as a measure of response to therapy. Additional diagnostic maneuvers include computerized abdominal scanning and excretory urography.

17. Is testicular carcinoma curable?

Yes. Therapy is selected according to histology, volume, staging (degree of dissemination), status of tumor markers, and previous therapy. Seminoma is traditionally curable with small doses of radiotherapy; large-volume seminoma or extranodal disease often warrants chemotherapy. Nonseminomatous germ-cell carcinoma (embryonal carcinoma, teratocarcinoma, choriocarcinoma) requires platinum-based chemotherapy, with retroperitoneal lymph node dissection selected according to persisting nodal masses.

18. What should be considered in the management of indurated testicular enlargement in a neonate?

Intrauterine testicular torsion presents as an apparently painless, smooth, homogeneously enlarged testis that may appear blue through the scrotal integument and may be distinguished from hydrocele or other lesions by testicular ultrasound. Orchiectomy is usually not necessary.

19. What is the presentation and significance of torsion of a testicular appendage?

Torsion of a testicular appendage presents with symptoms of spermatic cord torsion, but they are much less intense. Vomiting is unlikely. Less extreme pain and swelling contribute to delayed presentation, which is provoked more often by chronicity than intensity of symptoms. Therefore, emergency operative intervention is avoided in favor of adjunctive diagnostic maneuvers (color Doppler ultrasound, isotope scanning). The natural history of a twisted appendage is symptomatic resolution and regression of the tender mass (which may appear blue through the skin, producing the "blue dot" sign). Such lesions may calcify and become separated, accounting for intrascrotal "foreign bodies" occasionally discovered at routine physical examination.

20. What is the significance of acute pain and testicular enlargement after scrotal trauma?

Acutely painful posttraumatic testicular enlargement reflects rupture of the testicular capsule (tunica albuginea) with parenchymal extrusion and hematoma formation (hematocele). Pain may be extreme, with pallor, sweating, and nausea. Diagnosis may be confirmed in equivocal circumstances by scrotal ultrasound scanning. Patients managed conservatively usually recover spontaneously after an extended symptomatic convalescence, whereas scrotal exploration, evacuation of hematoma and infarcted tissue, and surgical repair of the testicular capsule contribute to a rapid benign recovery.

BIBLIOGRAPHY

1. Berman JM, Beidle TR, Kunberger LE, Letourneau JG: Sonographic evaluation of acute intrascrotal pathology. AJR 166:857–861, 1996.
2. Brown JM, Hammers LW, Barton JW, et al: Quantitative Doppler assessment of acute scrotal inflammation. Radiology 197:427–431, 1995.
3. Chinegwundoh FL: The post-traumatic painful testis. Postgrad Med J 72:251–252, 1996.
4. Doherty AP, Bower M, Christmas TJ: The role of tumor markers in the diagnosis and treatment of testicular germ cell cancers. Br J Urol 79:247–252, 1997.
5. Donohue JP, Foster RS, Little JS Jr, et al: Biology of metastases and its clinical implications: Testicular germ-cell tumors. W J Urol 14:197–203, 1996.
6. Flores LG II, Shiba T, Hoshi H, et al: Scintigraphic evaluation of testicular torsion and acute epididymitis. Ann Nucl Med 10:89–92, 1996.
7. Hendrikx AJ, Dang CL, Vroegindeweij D, Korte JH: B-mode and colour-flow duplex ultrasonography: A useful adjunct in diagnosing scrotal diseases? Br J Urol 79:58–65, 1997.
8. Herbener TE: Ultrasound in the assessment of the acute scrotum. J Clin Ultrasound Med 24:405–421, 1996.
9. Herr HW, Sheinfeld J, Puc HS, et al: Surgery for a post-chemotherapy residual mass in seminoma. J Urol 157:860–862, 1997.
10. Lewis AG, Bukowski TP, Jarvis PD, et al: Evaluation of acute scrotum in the emergency department. J Pediatr Surg 30:277–281, 1995.
11. Middleton WD, Middleton MA, Dierks M, et al: Sonographic prediction of viability in testicular torsion: Preliminary observations. J Ultrasound Med 16:23–27, 1997.

12. Moul JW, Heidenreich A: Prognostic factors in low-stage nonseminomatous testicular cancer. Oncology 10:1359–1368, 1996.
13. Oliver RT: Testicular cancer. Curr Opin Oncol 8:252–258, 1996.
14. Peterson NE, Schwab R: Acute scrotal pain requires quick thinking and plan of action. Emerg Med Rep 13:11–18, 1992.
15. Rabinowitz R, Hulbert WC Jr: Acute scrotal swelling. Urol Clin North Am 22:101–105, 1995.
16. Schwaibold H, Fobbe F, Klan R, Dieckmann KP: Evaluation of acute scrotal pain by color-coded duplex sonography. Urol Int 56:96–99, 1996.

53. IMPOTENCE

Norman E. Peterson, M.D.

1. What is impotence?

Impotence is a diagnostic term indicating erectile dysfunction that interferes with the ability to obtain or maintain penile erection satisfactory for intercourse. Erectile dysfunction is distinct from infertility and also must be distinguished from unrealized ambitions of sexual potency.

2. How common is impotence in the United States?

The number of men with erectile dysfunction is estimated at 10–20 million. Annual estimates include 525,000 office visits and 30,000 hospital admissions for this disorder. Erectile dysfunction often may go undiagnosed because of embarrassment and reluctance to acknowledge symptoms and to pursue remedies.

3. What are the potential etiologies of erectile dysfunction?

Erectile dysfunction may be categorized into organic and nonorganic etiologies:

Organic causes

Trauma

Inflammatory disorder (prostatitis)

Neurogenic disorders: spinal cord injury, multiple sclerosis, temporal lobe epilepsy, cerebrovascular accident, autonomic neuropathy, peripheral neuropathy

Vasogenic disorders: arterial or venous

Endocrine (hormonal): hypogonadism, decreased testosterone, hyperprolactinemia

Systemic disorders: diabetes, hypertension, hyprcholesterolemia, hyperthyroidism

Pharmacologic impotence

Miscellaneous factors: cigarettes, priapism, Peyronie's disease, dialysis, alcoholism, zinc deficiency, angina, arthritis, chronic obstructive pulmonary disease, postoperative dysfunction (abdominoperineal resection, prostatectomy, renal transplantation)

Nonorganic causes

All etiologies not qualifying as organic and involving basically psychogenic factors

4. What traumatic injuries may result in erectile dysfunction?

Excluding trauma-induced emasculation, injuries involving the spinal cord below the L1–L2 level and pelvic fracture with cicatrix-related or direct injury to the pudendal and genital arterial supply are most likely.

5. What are clues to psychogenic impotence?

Clues to psychogenic impotence include descriptions of periodic erections or coitus, spontaneous nocturnal or early morning erections, or satisfactory potency in selected circumstances such as illicit romance or during drug or alcohol use. Psychogenic impotence typically involves patients in younger age groups and an absence of other potential pathologic influences. Psychogenic erectile dysfunction is equally deserving of every modality of care.

6. Can psychogenic erectile dysfunction be treated?

Therapeutic remedies for psychogenic erectile dysfunction include psychiatric counseling, which may be prolonged and of variable benefit, and initiation of therapy to induce erection artificially. Successful therapy is often associated with progressive independence from such methods.

7. List the indications for psychiatric counseling.
- Sex therapy
- Ambiguous impotence
- Psychiatric fitness for prosthesis
- Preexisting functional impotence
- Ethanol or drug abuse
- Personality disorder
- Hypochondriasis
- History of psychiatric disorder
- Situation impotence

8. Are objective means available for identifying or verifying nocturnal erections?

Erectile response to intracavernous injection of erection-inducing agents is satisfactory evidence of intact erectile physiology. Thus, referral to the urologist for this test may eliminate greater expense and help to direct therapy. Specific monitoring for nocturnal penile tumescence is largely abandoned as unimportant to the diagnosis.

9. What drugs or medications may deleteriously influence penile erection?

Diuretics
Hydrochlorothiazide
Chlorthalidone
Spironolactone
Hydroflumethiazide

Tranquilizers
Phenothiazines
Butyrophenones
Thioxanthines

Antiandrogens—flutamide

Addictive and abused substances
Alcohol
Opiates
Barbiturates
Nicotine
Cannabis

Alpha-adrenergic blockers
Phenoxybenzamine
Phentolamine
Prazosin
Terazosin

Beta-adrenergic blockers
Propranolol
Metoprolol

Anticholinergic agents
Atropine
Clinidium
Dicyclomine
Isopropamide

Antihypertensive agents
Hydralazine
Minoxidil
Clonidine
Methyldopa
Reserpine

Antispasmodic agents
Propantheline

Antiparkinsonian agents
Benztropine
Biperiden
Procyclidine
Trihexyphenidyl

Antihistamines

Muscle relaxants
Cyclobenzaprine
Orphenadrine

Miscellaneous drugs
Cimetidine
Clofibrate
Digoxin
Estrogens
Indomethacin
Lithium carbonate
Methysergide
Metoclopramide
Metronidazole
Phenytoin
Antineoplastic agents
Thiabendazole
Tolazoline

(Continued on next page.)

Antidepressants
Tricyclics
Monoamine oxidase (MAO)
    inhibitors
Antianxiety agents
Benzodiazepines
Meprobamate

Miscellaneous drugs
Ethionamide
Phentolamine
Dicyclomine
Diethylpropion
Phentermine

When it is suspected that an agent may be responsible for erectile dysfunction, discontinuation of the drug and rechallenge, if necessary, should be undertaken. The patient may also relate onset or exaggeration of erectile dysfunction with initiation of drug therapy.

10. What systemic disorders are associated with erectile dysfunction?

Diabetes may be the single most frequent cause of erectile dysfunction. Impotence occurs in 35–75% of diabetic men. Whereas many studies claim no correlation between impotence and duration and severity of diabetes, other reports assert that impotence affects 50% of male diabetics after 10 years. Impotence is often associated with peripheral and/or autonomic diabetic neuropathy. Patients with erectile dysfunction and poorly controlled hyperglycemia occasionally improve with careful medical management, but improvement is uncommon and limited. Artificial remedies are advised rather than a futile wait for spontaneous recovery.

11. Which hormone tests are important in evaluating patients with erectile dysfunction?

Normal serum testosterone values obviate the need for additional endocrine testing or exogenous testosterone therapy. The rare patient with hypogonadism characteristically presents with a serum testosterone level of 200 mg/dl or less, a small prostate, and small, soft testes (< 3.5 cm). Impotence occasionally results from hyperprolactinemia (> 15–20 mg/dl), which is typically associated with subnormal testosterone and diminished libido. Bromocriptine is specific therapy, but management depends on the specific etiology, which may be idiopathic or related to the following conditions:

Postoperative state
Postraumatic state
Primary hypothyroidism
Renal disease
Hypothalamic-pituitary disease
Craniopharyngioma
Sarcoid
Pituitary tumors

Drugs
Phenothiazines
Tricyclic antidepressants
Meprobamate
Haloperidol
Reserpine
Amphetamines

12. What medical therapy is available for erectile dysfunction?

Medical Therapy for Impotence

Oral agents		Intracavernous	
Yohimbine	6 mg 3 times/day	Papavarine HCl	30–90 mg
Intramuscular agents		Phentolamine	5 mg
Testosterone propionate	400 mg every 3 wk	Prostaglandin E$_1$	5–25 ng

Oral therapy was previously limited to yohimbine, 2–6 mg 3 times/day. Yohimbine is expensive and of no objective benefit, although some patients claim improvement; placebo effect may explain the claim. **Intramuscular testosterone** (either proprionate or ethionate, 400 mg every 3 weeks) is directed to patients with documented subnormal levels of serum testosterone. Some patients with normal serum testosterone claim benefit from such therapy, but placebo effect is likely. For men with normal testosterone levels, endocrine treatment is inappropriate. **Intracavernous therapy** of any combination of papaverine (30–90 mg), Regitine (5 mg), and/or prostaglandin E$_1$ (PGE$_1$; 5–25 ng) injected directly into one cavernous compartment usually induces erection within 10 minutes and maintains erection for 30–90 minutes. Smaller doses are required for neurogenic erectile dysfunction and for agents given in combination. Responsible patients can be educated to perform self-injection so that urologic evaluation and prescription refills are necessary only 3–4 times/year. Potential complications of therapy include cavernous scarring (papaverine), which requires discontinuance; local pain (PGE_1); priapism, which often is associated with injection of excessive volumes; and drop-out due to patient dissatisfaction with the procedure itself.

More recent remedies include alprostadil (PGE_1) in pellet form for intraurethral insertion and absorption, commercially available as Muse. Effective doses range between 500 and 1,000 μ. It is expensive and has not achieved commercial success. Sildenafil (Viagra), an oral phosphodiesterase blocker, is administered in doses between 50 and 100 μ. Sildenafil is clinically effective and has few and nominal side effects. Other remedies awaiting approval are oral phentolamine (Regitine, Vasomax), which has a shorter latency period than sildenafil, and sublingual apomorphin, which acts centrally.

13. What is a vacuum erection device?

The vacuum erection device is a plastic tube that fits over the penis. Air is ejected from the tube by an attached hand pump, resulting in attraction of blood into the cavernosal tissues by negative pressure. An elastic constriction applied to the penile base maintains an erection satisfactory for coitus. Such devices are effective for many patients and have a low incidence of side effects. Cost ranges between $250–400 and may be partially covered by insurance. Battery-energized pump devices are available as affordable options.

14. What role does penile/pelvic vascular surgery play in therapy for erectile dysfunction?

Penile vascular surgery is of uncertain value and may best be limited to investigational centers. Such therapy is traditionally indicated for younger patients with posttraumatic vascular obstructions amenable to repair. Surgery has a high failure rate; many early successes deteriorate later.

15. What are penile prostheses?

Penile prostheses are intracavernosal implants available to patients who fail or refuse other forms of treatment. Several models are available, including semirigid devices with malleability features for convenience and inflatable-deflatable hydraulic models. Semirigid devices are reliable and have a low failure rate. Improvements in materials and bioengineering have reduced the mechanical dysfunction of inflatable models, although cost remains significant.

16. Is there an effective treatment for premature ejaculation?

This variant of erectile dysfunction dominates clinical complaints of sexual inadequacy and deserves every therapeutic resource. Care traditionally has been reduced to reassurance and psychotherapy with disappointing results. Contemporary management favors methods developed for erectile failure, including intracavernous and intraurethral drugs and vacuum erectile devices. Benefit also has been described with low doses of selective serotonin uptake inhibitors, including fluoxetine (Prozac), 7.5–30 mg/day; sertraline (Zoloft), 50 mg/day, and clomipramine (Inapramil), 25–50 mg/day. Paradoxically, larger doses may increase sexual complaints.

BIBLIOGRAPHY

1. Borirakchanayavat S, Lue TF: Evaluation of impotence. Infect Urol 1997, pp 12–29.
2. Brock G, Lue TF: Impotence. Monogr Urol 13:99–110, 1992.
3. Broderick GA, Schwartz S: Sexual dysfunction in diabetes. Hosp Pract 1991, pp 85–97.
4. Fallon B, Grahem H: Sexual performance and satisfaction with penile prosthesis in impotence of various etiologies. Int J Impotence Res 2:35–42, 1990.
5. Gilbert HW, Gingell JC: Vacuum constriction devices: Second-line conservative treatment for impotence. Br J Urol 70:81–83, 1992.

6. Gupta R, Kirschen S, Barrow R, et al: Predictors of success and risk factors for attrition in the use of intracorporal injection therapy. J Urol 157:1681–1686, 1997.

7. Lewis RW: Long-term results of penile prostheses implants. Urol Clin North Am 22:847–856, 1995.

8. Linet OL, Ogrinc FG: Efficacy and safety of intracavernosal alprostadil in men with erectile dysfunction: The Alprostadil Study Group. N Engl J Med 334:873–877, 1996.

9. McLean RH, Barrett DM: Patient and partner satisfaction with the AMS 700 penile prosthesis. J Urol 147:62–65, 1992.

10. Morales A, Heaton JPW: The medical treatment of erectile dysfunction. Urol Int 1996, pp 9–11.

11. Montorsi F, Guazzoni G, Barbieri L: Recovery of spontaneous erectile function after nerve sparing radical prostatectomy with and without early intracavernous injections of prostaglandin E-1: Results of a prospective, randomized trial. J Urol 155(Suppl):468A, abstract 628, 1996.

12. Moreland RB, Traish A, Mc Millin MA: PGE-1 suppresses the synthesis by transforming growth factors β1 in human corpus cavernosum smooth muscle. J Urol 153:826–834, 1995.

13. Mulcahy JJ, Eid F, Fair WF, et al: Treatment options for erectile dysfunction in the post-prostatectomy patient. Contemp Urol 9(Suppl):3–22, 1997.

14. Padma-Nathan H: Corporal pharmaco-therapy for erectile dysfunction and priapism. Monogr Urol 17:51–64, 1997.

15. Padma-Nathan H, Auerbach SM, Barada JH: Multicenter, double-blind, placebo-controlled trial of transurethral alprostadil in men with chronic erectile dysfunction. J Urol 155(Suppl):496A, abstract 740, 1996.

16. Padma-Nathan H, Hellstrom WJG, Kaiser FE: Treatment of men with erectile dysfunction with transurethral alprostadil. N Engl J Med 336:1–7, 1997.

17. Porst H: The rationale for prostaglandin E-1 in erectile failure: A survey of worldwide experience. J Urol 155:802–815, 1996.

VIII. Common Disorders of the Renal and Urinary System

54. URINARY TRACT INFECTIONS

Randall R. Reves, M.D., MSc, and David W. Lehman, M.D., Ph.D.

1. Are urinalysis and urine culture always necessary to confirm the diagnosis of a urinary tract infection (UTI)?

No. By age 65 years up to one-third of women experience one or more episodes of cystitis, the great majority of which are uncomplicated. Factors that increase the risk of UTI include recent sexual intercourse, recent use of a diaphragm with spermicide, and a history of prior UTI. Such infections, which are usually due to *Escherichia coli* (80%) or *Staphylococcus saprophyticus* (5–15%), follow predictable susceptibility patterns and respond to a short course of antimicrobial agents. Thus, a young woman with typical symptoms and signs of uncomplicated cystitis and with pyuria documented with a positive urine dipstick test for leukocyte esterase may be treated without urine microscopy or culture. If the leukocyte esterase test is negative in such patients, microscopic examination of urine or a urine culture should be done.

2. How can one be certain that genitourinary symptoms in young women are due to cystitis?

Dysuria may be due to cystitis, urethritis, vulvovaginitis with or without urethritis, or noninfectious inflammatory processes such as chemical irritation. UTI is the cause of dysuria in about one-half of female patients. Among young women cystitis is characterized by the abrupt onset of rather severe symptoms of urgency, dysuria, and urinary frequency, often with suprapubic or low back pain. Women with urethritis or vaginitis are more likely to report gradual onset of symptoms, vaginal discharge, and a recent new sexual contact; examination often reveals cervicitis or vulvovaginitis. Significant pyuria is strongly associated with UTI.

3. Define "significant pyuria."

Most recent studies indicate that 8–10 leukocytes/mm^3 (as determined by cytometer) correlate with UTI. This level is probably similar to 10 cells per high power field on examinations of centrifuged urinary sediment.

4. What is the role of single-dose treatment of UTIs?

Uncomplicated cystitis in young women may be treated with a single dose of trimethoprim, trimethoprim/sulfamethoxazole, or a fluoroquinolone (which is far more expensive), but treatment failures are slightly higher than with 3-day courses of therapy. Beta-lactam drugs are less effective. Treatment for 7 days should be considered for women who are diabetic or pregnant, who have recently experienced a UTI or have had symptoms for over 1 week before treatment, or who use a diaphragm for contraception.

5. Should young women with repeated episodes of cystitis be evaluated differently?

Repeated episodes of cystitis usually are due to recurrent episodes of infection rather than relapses of chronic infection. At least one culture should be done for confirmation, but cultures during recurrent infections are not necessary. Frequent recurrences can be managed by daily or thrice-weekly prophylaxis or postcoital prophylaxis. Self-diagnosis with prompt single-dose or 3-day treatment is an effective alternative.

6. Can recurrent cystitis in women be prevented without antibiotics?

High fluid intake, postcoital voiding, drinking cranberry juice, and other practices have been widely recommended to decrease the frequency of cystitis in young women. Pathophysiologically, frequent irrigation of the urethra and drainage of the bladder, including postcoital voiding, seem to complement immune mechanisms in aborting an early infection, but data to support these recommendations are limited. A retrospective case-control study showed a lower relative risk for UTI in young women who reported postcoital voiding. In the same study, tampon use, oral contraceptive use, voiding before intercourse, and direction of wiping after a bowel movement did not correlate with UTI. A randomized, double-blind, placebo-controlled trial showed that consumption of 300 ml of cranberry juice decreased bacteriuria in elderly women. The previously proposed mechanism of urinary acidification was not supported by this study; the cranberry group had a higher median urinary pH (6.0) than controls (5.5). The beneficial effects of cranberry juice may be due to compounds that inhibit bacterial adhesion to mucosal surfaces.

7. Why is a colony count >10⁵/ml of urine no longer the single standard for defining UTI?

Colony counts $> 10^5$/ml of a single species of bacteria are found in about 80% of patients with pyelonephritis; this concentration also reliably distinguishes between true (significant) asymptomatic bacteriuria and low-level contamination that occurs during specimen collection (frequently with several species). The value of $> 10^5$ is not useful in defining significant bacteriuria among several other populations (see table below). Only 50% of young women with documented cystitis are correctly identified with such a definition.

Colony-forming Units (CFU)/ml of Urine Used to Define
Significant Bacteriuria among Different Populations

POPULATION	CFU/ml	COMMENTS
Patients with pyelonephritis	$> 10^5$	80% have $> 10^5$; most $> 10^6$
Asymptomatic patients	$> 10^5$	Repeat to confirm
Young women with cystitis	$> 10^2$	Pyuria/dysuria syndrome
Men with UTI	$> 10^3$	Contamination uncommon
Recently catheterized inpatients	$> 10^2$	CFUs usually rise; symptoms develop

8. How important is it to discriminate between upper and lower UTIs before considering a 3-day course of therapy?

Up to one-third of women with symptoms of cystitis have been shown to have occult pyelonephritis. Nonetheless, single-dose antibiotic therapy is 85–95% effective, and 3-day treatment is even less likely to fail. When symptoms and signs of upper tract involvement are present, however, urine culture should be obtained, and treatment for pyelonephritis should be given.

9. Should all patients with symptoms of pyelonephritis be admitted to the hospital?

Young women who have relatively mild symptoms without nausea and emesis that preclude oral therapy and for whom follow-up can be ensured may be treated as outpatients. Pyelonephritis during pregnancy should be treated in the hospital. Resistance to amoxicillin and first-generation cephalosporins is noted in 20–30% of bacteria causing community-acquired pyelonephritis. Treatment may be initiated with trimethoprim/sulfamethoxazole; if trimethoprim resistance is common in the community, a fluoroquinolone should be used. Two weeks of therapy appears adequate in most cases. Amoxicillin is less effective than trimethoprim/sulfamethoxazole, even for susceptible strains.

Blood cultures should be obtained from patients requiring hospitalization; up to 20% are positive. Options for initial empirical intravenous therapy include a third-generation cephalosporin such as ceftriaxone (1 gm/day), a fluoroquinolone, or gentamicin for the usual gram-negative organisms. Ampicillin is often given initially in combination with ceftriaxone or gentamicin for the possibility of enterococci. After several days of intravenous therapy, treatment often can be completed with an oral agent.

10. What is the value of a Gram stain of uncentrifuged urine?

The detection of one or more bacteria per oil-immersion field correlates with a colony count > 10^5/ml and identifies the organism in about 80% of cases of pyelonephritis. In addition, the detection of gram-positive cocci provides rapid indication of the possibility of enterococcus as the cause.

11. Should imaging procedures or urologic evaluations be used in all cases of pyelonephritis?

When fever and other symptoms fail to resolve after 72 hours of appropriate therapy, ultrasonography or computed tomography should be considered to look for obstruction, urologic abnormalities, or complications such as perinephric abscess.

12. When should a complicated UTI be suspected?

Complicated UTIs are defined as those due to organisms resistant to antibiotics or occurring among patients with urinary tract abnormalities. Complicated infections should be considered in patients who recently received antibiotics or acquired infection nosocomially or after urinary tract instrumentation during urinary tract catheterization. UTIs are more likely to be complicated in men, diabetics, pregnant women, and immunosuppressed individuals.

13. What is the recommended therapy for complicated UTIs?

Recommendations vary, depending on the severity of the illness and the known or anticipated drug-susceptibility patterns of the infecting organism. A greater frequency of *Proteus* sp. enterococci, and nosocomial pathogens such as *Pseudomonas aeruginosa* can be anticipated. Empiric therapy of the seriously ill patient should include coverage for *P. aeruginosa* and *Enterococcus* sp., pending culture results.

14. Should all men with a single UTI receive a urologic evaluation?

UTIs in men were previously considered to be complicated by definition, but later studies demonstrated that young men (18–50 yr) occasionally experience uncomplicated cystitis. Sexual partners of women with vaginal colonization with *E. coli* or homosexual men engaging in insertive anal intercourse appear to be at greater risk. A 7-day course of therapy with pre- and posttreatment cultures is recommended. If the infection responds promptly, urologic evaluation may be deferred. Recurrent infections, pyelonephritis, or other complicating factors warrant urologic evaluation. Male infants and boys should be evaluated for structural abnormalities with an intravenous pyelogram (IVP). Men > 50 years old should be assessed for clinical symptoms suggestive of urinary tract obstruction, usually due to benign prostatic hypertrophy (urgency, nocturia, and decreased flow rates). Men with symptoms of obstruction or recurrent infections should be evaluated with a serum creatinine and measurement of postvoid residual volume. IVP and cytoscopy are often required for further evaluation. Invasive procedures should be delayed until the acute infection has been treated.

15. What are the indications for repeat cultures after treatment of a UTI?

Routine posttreatment cultures of asymptomatic patients are not recommended except for patients with pyelonephritis, complicated UTIs, UTI associated with pregnancy, and infections in men. Follow-up cultures are usually obtained 2 weeks after treatment.

16. Who should be screened and treated for bacteriuria?

Only two patient groups are known to benefit from treatment of asymptomatic bacteriuria and to warrant screening with two separate urine cultures. Bacteriuria during pregnancy should be treated to prevent pyelonephritis and the risks of premature delivery. Patients with bacteriuria before urologic surgery should be treated to prevent infectious complications of surgery.

17. When should one consider treatment of a UTI for longer than 2 weeks?

Women with positive posttreatment cultures following pyelonephritis may have subclinical pyelonephritis and may require 4–6 weeks of antibiotics for a cure. Men with positive posttreatment cultures may have either an upper tract or prostatic source of infection and benefit from a 4–6-week course of therapy.

18. Should one treat patients with indwelling urinary catheters and positive urine cultures?
Bacteriuria in patients with chronic, indwelling urinary catheters should not be treated unless patients become symptomatic. Removal or replacement of catheters that have been in place for more than 2 weeks may be helpful. Bacteriuria in recently catheterized patients in the hospital frequently leads to clinically important UTI. Defining asymptomatic bacteriuria in a patient in the intensive care unit is often difficult.

19. What is the significance of staphylococcal isolates from urine cultures?
S. saprophyticus is a recognized cause of cystitis in young women. *Staphylococcus aureus* is an unusual cause of community-acquired UTI, and the diagnosis of staphylococcal bacteremia with or without a renal cortical abscess should be considered. Diabetes mellitus, hemodialysis, and intravenous drug use are predisposing factors for staphylococcal sepsis. Complications of pyelonephritis may lead to a perinephric abscess, usually due to *E. coli* or other enteric bacilli. Ultrasonography or computed tomography is usually required to diagnose either type of renal abscess.

20. What factors may alter the vaginal flora and increase the risk of UTI?
The use of spermicides with or without a diaphragm for contraception increases the frequency of both vaginal colonization with uropathogens and UTIs. Estrogen deficiency in postmenopausal women leads to a decrease in the frequency of vaginal colonization with *Lactobacillus* sp., a higher vaginal pH, and increased frequency of colonization with *E. coli*. Topical application of estriol has been shown to decrease the frequency of recurrent UTIs in postmenopausal women.

21. Describe the special considerations associated with UTIs in the elderly.
Factors that increase the rate of UTIs in the elderly include incomplete bladder emptying, decreased immune response, and the consequences of chronic disease, such as institutional living and more frequent hospital admissions. Bladder instrumentation is frequent, making the urinary tract the most common (40%) site of nosocomial infections. The presentation of UTI in the elderly may be atypical, lacking some or all of the classic symptoms and signs. Fever is not invariably present in elderly patients. The evaluation of elderly patients presenting with acute onset of confusion, lethargy, abdominal pain, and decline in functional status should include UTI in the differential diagnosis. Septic shock, a not infrequent complication of urosepsis in the elderly, causes a significant rate of mortality.

BIBLIOGRAPHY

1. Abrutyn E, Mossey J, Berlin JA, et al: Does asymptomatic bacteriuria predict mortality and does antimicrobial treatment reduce mortality in elderly ambulatory women? Ann Intern Med 120:827–833, 1994.
2. Avorn J, et al: Reduction of bacteriuria and pyuria after ingestion of cranberry juice. JAMA 271:751–754, 1994.
3. Fihn SD, Boyko EJ, Chen C-L, et al: Use of spermicide-coated condoms and other risk factors for urinary tract infection caused by staphylococcus saprophyticus. Arch Intern Med 158:281–287, 1998.
4. Gratacos E, Torres P-J, Vila J, et al: Screening and treatment of asymptomatic bacteriuria in pregnancy prevent pyelonephritis. J Infect Dis 169:1390–1392, 1994.
5. Hooten TM, Stamm WE: Management of acute uncomplicated urinary tract infection in adults. Med Clin North Am 75:339–357, 1991.
6. Hooton TM, Scholes D, Hughes JP, et al: A prospective study of risk factors for symptomatic urinary tract infection in young women. N Engl J Med 335:468–474, 1996.
7. Johnson CC: Definitions, classification, and clinical presentation of urinary tract infections. Med Clin North Am 75:241–252, 1991.
8. Kunin CM: Urinary tract infections in females. Clin Infect Dis 18:1–12, 1994.
9. Lipsky BA: Urinary tract infections in men. Ann Intern Med 110:138–150, 1989.
10. Raz R, Stamm WE: A controlled trial of intravaginal estriol in postmenopausal women with recurrent urinary tract infections. N Engl J Med 329:753–756, 1993.
11. Rubin RH: Infections of the urinary tract. Sci Am Med 7:1–12, 1997.
12. Stamm WE, Hooton TM: Management of urinary tract infections in adults. N Engl J Med 329:1328–1334, 1993.
13. Strom BL, et al: Sexual activity, contraceptive use, and other risk factors for symptomatic and asymptomatic bacteriuria. Ann Intern Med 107:816–823, 1987.

55. SEXUALLY TRANSMITTED DISEASES

Mary Ann De Groote, M.D.

1. Why should women be especially targeted for control of gonorrhea?

It is estimated that 600,000 new cases of infection due to *Neisseria gonorrhoeae* develop each year in the United States. While screening and treatment of all patients with gonorrhea is important, most men with new infection display symptoms and seek care. Many women are asymptomatic until complications such as pelvic inflammatory disease (PID), tubal scarring, or ectopic pregnancy occur. Undiagnosed chronic pelvic infections are considered the major cause of infertility.

2. Which nongenital infections and complications due to *N. gonorrhoeae* may occur in adult patients?

1. **Pharyngeal infection** may be asymptomatic. A pharyngeal culture should be obtained in patients with a history of orogenital contact. Occasionally, overt pharyngitis with cervical lymphadenitis may occur.

2. **Anorectal infection** occurs in women and homosexual men.

3. **Disseminated gonococcal infection** (DGI) occurs in up to 1% of patients. Patients present with fever, tenosynovitis, petechial or pustular skin lesions, and occasionally septic arthritis.

4. **Perihepatitis**, also known as Fitz-Hugh–Curtis syndrome, is most often caused by *Chlamydia trachomatis* but may be a rare complication of gonococcal infection.

5. **Tubo-ovarian abscess and pelvic peritonitis** may be serious complications of *N. gonorrhoeae* infection that require hospitalization.

6. **Long-term complications** of gonorrhea include tubal scarring, which leads to ectopic pregnancy, infertility, and chronic pelvic pain.

3. What anatomic sites may be involved in women with *C. trachomatis* infection of the genital tract?

1. The **endocervix** is the most frequent site of infection. Most patients present with a vaginal discharge. On examination of the cervix, a yellow or green mucus is often visible. Although not specific for *Chlamydia*, a swab obtained of the discharge reveals polymorphonuclear cells (PMNs) without gram-negative intracellular diplococci.

2. The **urethra** is also a common site of infection. In up to 65% of women with dysuria or urgency and a negative urine culture for bacteria, *C. trachomatis* is the etiologic agent.

3. Numerous studies have shown that chlamydial infection of the **endometrium** may be the most common cause of endometritis and PID.

4. Damage to the **fallopian tube**s leading to obstructive infertility and ectopic pregnancy has been linked to *C. trachomatis*.

4. How is chlamydial infection diagnosed?

The diagnosis begins with a careful history. Chlamydial infection is most common in younger women (≤ 24 years old), women with a new sexual partner, and women who do not use barrier contraceptives. The patient may present with no symptoms, abdominal or pelvic pain, or vaginal or urethral symptoms. In most women, the cervix is the initial site of infection. Vaginal discharge, vaginal bleeding, and postcoital spotting may occur. On examination the cervical discharge may be clear or purulent, and cervical bleeding after using a culture swab is common. Culture for *C. trachomatis*, the gold standard, is not always available. Culture is performed using a Dacron swab (after mucus has been removed from the endocervix) and must be sent on ice within 24 hours. Other diagnostic modalities include direct fluorescent antibody, enzyme-linked immunosorbent assay, DNA probe, and polymerase chain reaction (PCR). These techniques are more widely used than culture because of ease of collection, transport, and performance. They carry a sensitivity rate of 75–90% and a specificity rate of 95%. Empirical therapy while the patient is still in the clinic is often begun before the results are confirmed. The treatment of choice is doxycycline or tetracycline. If the patient is pregnant, erythromycin is the drug of choice.

5. Why is therapy recommended for both gonococcal and chlamydial infections?

Persons infected with *N. gonorrhoeae* are often also infected with *C. trachomatis*. In fact, chlamydial infection accompanies 20–40% of gonococcal infections. Chlamydial treatment is safe and inexpensive.

Treatment for **gonococcal infections** involves one of the following:
• Cefixime, 400 mg orally in a single dose
• Ceftriaxone, 125 mg intramuscularly as a single dose
• Ciprofloxacin, 500 mg as a single dose
• Ofloxacin, 400 mg as a single oral dose

There are sporadic reports of fluoroquinolone-resistant gonococci from around the world. This problem will continue to be monitored carefully; however, quinolones are still recommended at the time of this writing.

For **chlamydial infections** the following are effective:
• Doxycycline, 100 mg twice daily for 7 days
• Azithromycin, 1 gm orally as a single dose

6. Which organisms are thought to cause PID?

PID represents a spectrum of diseases of the upper genital tract in women and includes infection and inflammation of the endometrial tissue, tubes, and ovaries. It also may cause pelvic peritonitis. Symptoms include lower abdominal tenderness, adnexal tenderness, and cervical motion tenderness. PID may be caused by one or more organisms. The most common is *C. trachomatis*, but *N. gonorrhoeae* is also important. Polymicrobic infection, including facultative aerobic and anaerobic bacteria, also occurs. Laparoscopic cultures of fallopian tubes and culdocentesis from patients with PID often reveal a combination of aerobic and anaerobic organisms, such as *Bacteroides* sp., *H. influenzae*, *Escherichia coli*, group B streptococci, *Gardnerella vaginalis*, and other anaerobic cocci. In addition, *Mycoplasma hominis* and *Ureaplasma urealyticum* may be etiologic agents of PID. These organisms are frequently isolated in the presence of *N. gonorrhoeae* or *C. trachomatis* from endocervical cultures.

7. Discuss the evaluation of a man who presents with urethritis.

Although some men may be asymptomatic, a history of urethral discharge, dysuria, itching, or recent diagnosis of a sexually transmitted disease (STD) in a partner should be ascertained. A Gram stain of the urethral discharge typically reveals increased PMN cells. A first-void urine sediment also may be used for diagnosis using new nucleic acid amplification tests for *N. gonorrhoeae* and *C. trachomatis*. The presence of intracellular gram-negative diplococci is diagnostic of gonorrhea. Because the Gram stain may miss some cases, a urethral swab for *N. gonorrhoeae* culture also should be done. When no bacteria are detected in the presence of PMNs, the diagnosis of nongonococcal urethritis (NGU) is made. NGU is most frequently caused by *C. trachomatis* but *U. urealyticum, Trichomonas vaginalis,* and other organisms also may be responsible.

Treatment of NGU consists of doxycycline or azithromycin. Because the coisolation of *N. gonorrhoeae* and *C. trachomatis* is common, patients with evidence of gonorrhea should be treated for both.

8. Name the three most common causes of genital ulcers.

1. **Herpes simplex virus** (HSV). Although the incidence varies geographically in the U.S., HSV is the most common cause of genital ulcers and appears to be increasing.

2. **Syphilis.** The classic syphilitic ulcer is a painless, indurated chancre. Syphilis is a frequent cause of genital ulceration both in the United States and in developing nations.

3. **Chancroid.** This common cause of genital ulcers in the developing world is also gaining a foothold in the U.S. *Haemophilus ducreyi*, the etiologic agent, needs to be cultured on special media.

More than one pathogen may exist in a small number of lesions (3–10%). Less common causes are lymphogranuloma venereum and donovanosis (granuloma inguinale). The presence of a genital ulcer is a risk factor for transmission of the human immunodeficiency virus (HIV). All patients should be evaluated with syphilis serology. Other miscellaneous noninfectious causes include trauma, allergic reactions, Behçet syndrome, malignancy, and Stevens-Johnson syndrome. HIV serology should be done in patients with chancroid and syphilis and considered for patients with herpes simplex ulcers.

9. Describe the clinical stages and the consequences of untreated syphilis.

There are no pathognomonic presentations for each stage, and a high index of suspicion is needed to make the diagnosis. Syphilis is a systemic disease caused by the spirochete *Treponema pallidum*. Primary syphilis is manifested by a chancre that begins as a macule at the site of inoculation (usually on the genitals) and then becomes an indurated ulcer. Secondary syphilis, which usually appears 3–6 weeks after the initial chancre, includes a wide variety of signs and symptoms that reflect the systemic nature of the infection. The skin rash is a hallmark and characteristically appears on the palms and soles but may be highly variable. Lymphadenopathy, mucous membrane lesions, arthritis, hepatitis, nephrotic syndrome, meningitis, and cranial abnormalities may be seen with secondary syphilis. Syphilis is called the great masquerader because of the plethora of findings; most patients, however, display only one or a few of these findings.

If untreated, syphilis progresses to a latent stage with no evidence of disease, although serologic tests are positive. Early latent infection refers to a duration of less than 1 year. Patients who have been infected more than 1 year or for an unknown duration are considered to have late latent infection. In the preantibiotic era, approximately 25% of untreated patients with latent syphilis progressed to the tertiary stage, which includes gummas, granulomas of bones and soft tissues, cardiovascular symptoms, and neurosyphilis. Currently rates of complications of unrecognized latent syphilis are probably lower because of the likelihood of receiving antibiotics with antisyphilitic activity for unrelated reasons.

10. How can the laboratory assist the clinician in making the diagnosis of syphilis?

The definitive diagnosis of syphilis is made by demonstrating the presence of characteristic spirochetes on a darkfield examination of infected tissue. However, two types of serologic tests assist in diagnosis: nontreponemal and treponemal. The first consists of the rapid plasma reagin (RPR) and Venereal Disease Research Laboratory (VDRL) tests. The two specific treponemal tests are the fluorescent treponemal antibody-absorbed assay (FTA-ABS) and the microhemagglutination assay for antibody to *Treponema pallidum* (MHA-TP). The nontreponemal serologic tests may be quantitated and followed to assess response to therapy and to diagnose reinfection. The RPR and VDRL are associated with occasional false-positive results and must be confirmed with a specific treponemal test. Both abnormally high and low syphilis titers have been described in patients infected with HIV, but serologic tests remain reliable for the vast majority of patients. The diagnosis of neurosyphilis relies on serology of the cerebrospinal fluid as well as abnormalities of CSF cell counts and protein levels.

11. Does the treatment of syphilis depend on the stage of infection?

Yes. Although the drug of choice for all stages is penicillin, late latent, tertiary, and neurosyphilis require a longer duration of therapy. Careful follow-up includes history, physical examination, and serologic tests. Patients should be reexamined clinically and serologically at 6 and 12 months. Failure of nontreponemal test titers to decline fourfold by 6 months after therapy for primary or secondary syphilis may suggest the need to retreat. All patients should be tested for HIV.

STAGE	THERAPY*
Primary	Benzathine PCN G, 2.4 million units IM once
Secondary	Benzathine PCN G, 2.4 million units IM once
Latent (early)	Benzathine PCN G, 2.4 million units IM once
Latent (late or unknown)	Benzathine PCN G, 2.4 million units IM weekly for 3 weeks
Neurosyphilis	18–24 million units aqueous crystalline PCN G daily for 10–14 days or 2.4 million units procaine PCN IM + probenecid, 500 mg 4 times/day for 10–14 days

* For HIV infection, PCN allergy, and treatment of pregnant patients, see Centers for Disease Control: 1998 Guidelines for Treatment of Sexually Transmitted Diseases. MMWR 47(RR-1), 1998.

12. Genital warts are caused by the human papilloma virus (HPV). Which malignant lesions are also linked to the virus?

HPV has been linked to cervical and vulvar cancer in women and squamous cell cancer of the penis and anus in men. Genital warts are commonly caused by HPV types 6 or 11. Other types, including 16, 18, 31, 33, and 35, have been associated with dysplasia and cancer. External warts can be removed in a number of ways, including cryotherapy with liquid nitrogen, podophyllin, and trichloroacetic acid, but recurrences are common. As alternatives to these provider-applied treatments, patients can be instructed to apply podofilox gel or imiquimod. Laser treatment and surgery are reserved for extensive warts. Patients should be counseled about recurrences, use of condoms, and the importance of annual Papanicolaou smears.

13. Which STD is caused by a protozoan?

Trichomoniasis is caused by the protozoan *Trichomonas vaginalis*. Signs and symptoms include vaginal inflammation and malodorous discharge. Some women and most men are asymptomatic. Occasionally men have mild urethritis. Organisms can be demonstrated in 30–40% of sexual partners. Diagnosis can be made in the office by performing a microscopic evaluation of vaginal secretions and demonstrating typical motile organisms. Metronidazole is the only oral medication available in the United States for treatment of trichomoniasis. Sexual partners should be treated.

14. Differentiate between the clinical manifestations of primary and recurrent genital herpes infections.

The two serotypes of herpes simplex virus are HSV-1 and HSV-2. Most cases of genital herpes are caused by HSV-2. Although the course may vary, primary disease is usually more severe. The patient lacks specific antibodies at the time of the lesions. Mucosal lesions may be multiple. Urethritis, cervicitis, lymphadenopathy, fevers, headaches, and occasionally aseptic meningitis or sacral nerve symptoms (urinary retention or laxness of the anal sphincter) may complicate primary genital herpes infection. Primary disease is often treated with acyclovir to reduce the duration of symptoms, although therapy does not cure or prevent latent infection.

Recurrent disease tends to be milder. The small clusters of lesions usually crust over in a few days. Some patients have a prodromal tingling sensation, numbness, or paresthesias before the development of vesicles. Early treatment (i.e., on or before day one of lesions) can lessen the duration of lesions. In addition, daily therapy can suppress recurrences and is indicated if patients have frequent (e.g., > 6/year) recurrences. Options for suppression of recurrences or episodic treatment include acyclovir, famciclovir, and valacyclovir. Cost of treatment may be an important consideration. Patients with HIV may have prolonged or extensive disease.

15. Why are the diagnosis and treatment of genital herpes important? Describe each.

In addition to the morbidity associated with genital ulcers, the major serious sequela of genital HSV infection is transmission to the newborn infant at the time of delivery. The greatest risk occurs when the mother acquires a primary infection near the time of delivery. Viral cultures of the birth canal at delivery are helpful in guiding management of the neonate.

In nonpregnant patients with HSV, clinicians should perform a careful examination with culture of suspicious lesions. Sexual transmission of virus is most efficient in the presence of overt lesions. However, virus can be shed in the absence of obvious lesions, and many cases are thought to be transmitted during asymptomatic periods. Patients should be advised to refrain from sexual activity in the presence of overt lesions. Condoms are not foolproof but should be encouraged during all sexual exposures. Sexual partners benefit from evaluation and counseling, even if they are asymptomatic.

16. Do STDs pose special risks to travelers?

All general guidelines apply to STDs during travel, but a few points deserve special mention:

1. Frequently the incidence of STDs is much higher in developing countries than in most areas of the U.S. In addition to gonorrhea, chlamydia, and syphilis, two other important STDs—hepatitis B and HIV—are often more common. Hepatitis B antibody prevalence is well over 50% in some countries of Africa and Asia, and carriage of the surface antigen (HBsAg) may be as high as 25%. Unprotected sex in the developing world increases the risk of acquiring STDs that are uncommon in Western countries, such as chancroid, lymphogranuloma venereum, and granuloma inguinale.

2. HIV-1 and HIV-2 seroprevalence rates are high in certain areas of the world. The major route of transmission is heterosexual intercourse. Solid evidence suggests that the presence of an STD increases the risk of transmission of HIV.

3. Avoidance of high-risk sexual behavior is clearly the best course, but barrier contraception is also effective at decreasing the transmission of STDs.

BIBLIOGRAPHY

1. Ault KA, Faro S: Pelvic inflammatory disease: Current diagnostic criteria and treatment guidelines. Postgrad Med 93(2):85–91, 1993.
2. Centers for Disease Control and Prevention: 1998 Guidelines for Treatment of Sexually Transmitted Diseases. MMWR 47(RR-1), 1998.
3. Freund KM: Chlamydial disease in women. Hosp Pract 27(2):175–186, 1992.
4. Hansfield HH: Sex, science, and society: A look at sexually transmitted diseases. Postgrad Med 101: 268–278, 1997.
5. Hansfield HH: Recent developments in STDs. I: Bacterial diseases. Hosp Pract 26(7):47–56, 1991.
6. Hansfield HH: Recent developments in STDs. II: Viral and other syndromes. Hosp Pract 27(1):175–200, 1991.
7. Holmes KK, Mardh PA, Sparling PF, Wiesner PJ (eds): Sexually Transmitted Diseases, 2nd ed. New York, McGraw-Hill, 1990.
8. Jong EC, McMullen R (eds): The Travel and Tropical Medicine Manual, 2nd ed. Philadelphia, W.B. Saunders, 1995.
9. Mandell GL, Douglas RG, Bennett JE (eds): Principles and Practice of Infectious Diseases, 3rd ed. New York, Churchill Livingstone, 1990, pp 931–975.
10. Mogabgab WJ: Recent developments in the treatment of sexually transmitted diseases. Am J Med 91(Suppl 6A):140S–143S, 1991.
11. Parenti DM: Sexually transmitted diseases and travelers. Med Clin North Am 76:1449–1461, 1992.
12. Vinson RP, Epperly TD: Counseling patients on proper use of condoms. Am Fam Physician 43:2081–2085, 1991.
13. Woodridge WE: Syphilis: A new visit from an old enemy. Postgrad Med 89(1):193–202, 1991.

56. PROTEINURIA AND HEMATURIA

Katherine M. Fitting, M.D., and Arlene B. Chapman, M.D.

1. How should one prepare a urine specimen for analysis?

A fresh urine specimen voided at the beginning of the day gives the most concentrated and acidic urine, which preserves formed elements. Urine specimens should be reviewed within 30 minutes of collection to avoid disintegration of red cells and red cell casts. All samples should be collected in midstream; therefore, a moderately full bladder is required. At least 200 ml of urine should be voided before the specimen is collected. Contamination is avoided by foreskin retraction in men and good labial separation in women. Proper preparation includes gentle cleansing with cotton wool swabs moistened with saline. Even midstream urine collections in the majority of women demonstrate contamination unless cleaning instructions are clear. If it is impossible to obtain a good midstream urine specimen, as in patients with physical handicaps, a catheter specimen may be required.

2. What are the main components of urinalysis?

1. **Visual inspection.** The color and consistency of the urine should be assessed visually before centrifugation. Gross hematuria, marked pyuria, heavy crystalluria, and, occasionally, funguria can be detected by visual inspection. A layer of foam at the top of the specimen is indicative of heavy proteinuria.

2. **Dipstick or chemical analysis.** Commercially available dipsticks measure a number of different components, including pH, glucose, ketones, hemoglobin, protein, leukocyte esterase, and bilirubin. Dipsticks screen most accurately for the presence of proteinuria, whereas microscopic analysis is a more informative method for the evaluation of hematuria. Dipstick evaluation of protein involves a pad that contains tetrabromophenol, which changes from yellow to green to blue as increasing amounts of protein are available for binding. Dipstick evaluation of hematuria involves hemoglobin or myoglobin to catalyse a reaction between hydrogen peroxide and the chromogen O-toluidine. When hemoglobin or myoglobin is present in the urine, the test pad turns blue.

2. **Microscopic analysis.** Fresh urine samples are aliquoted into a 10-ml test tube and centrifuged at 2500–3000 rpm for 5 minutes. The supernatant is poured off, and after resuspension the sediment is poured onto a slide and placed under a coverslip. A bright-field microscope is commonly used for analysis of urinary sediment, although phase-contrast microscopy provides better vision of all elements. Microscopic analysis is commonly viewed without staining. This approach allows rapid preparation. Two magnifications are required, with the lower (100×) for a general overview and the higher (400×) for details and cell evaluation. The complete slide should be evaluated, which can take 10–15 minutes; most formed elements, however, adhere to the edges of the coverslip. Casts are reported as number per low power field and cells as number per high power field.

3. What is considered normal proteinuria?

Under physiologic conditions, urinary excretion of protein does not exceed 150–180 mg/day. The main proteins normally excreted are albumin, immunoglobulins, immunoglobulin light chains, and Tamm-Horsfall protein. In some conditions, excessive proteinuria is benign, including functional proteinuria in patients with fever or after exercise; idiopathic transient proteinuria, as in patients with congestive heart failure; and orthostatic proteinuria.

4. What conditions produce false-negative and false-positive results for proteinuria?

False-negative results for proteinuria occur when urine is extremely dilute or when Bence Jones protein (immunoglobulin light chains) is the predominant source of protein. Dipsticks are more sensitive to albumin. Sulfosalicylic acid should be added to determine whether immunoglobulin light chains are present.

False-positive results occur when urine is highly concentrated, when urine pH is greater than 8, when the dipstick has been immersed too long (> 30 seconds), and in the setting of gross hematuria when plasma proteins accompany blood.

5. What is proteinuria?

The three types of proteinuria are glomerular, tubular, or overproduction proteinuria. Proteinuria is most commonly of glomerular origin, and albumin is the major component of protein that leaks through an abnormal glomerular basement membrane. Tubular proteinuria is due to decreased tubular reabsorption of proteins contained in the glomerular filtrate, as in tubulointerstitial disorders. Overload proteinuria is secondary to increased production of immunoglobulin light chains, as in monoclonal gammopathies, or lysozyme, as in some forms of leukemia.

6. How does one evaluate a patient with proteinuria?

The first approach is to quantify the amount of protein in the urine by collecting a 24-hour urine specimen and determining rates of creatinine and protein excretion. Creatinine excretion rates are determined to assess the accuracy (total time) of urine collection. Men should excrete 15–25 mg/kg/day and women 12–20 mg/kg/day of urinary creatinine. Nephrotic range proteinuria is more than 3.5 gm/day. Protein/creatinine ratios have been found to be extremely useful in patients with established creatinine excretion rates, noncompliant patients, or patients for whom rapid diagnoses are sought. Ratios greater than 3.5 in a single voided sample represent more than 3.5 gm of proteinuria in 24 hours, and ratios less than 0.2 represent less than 0.2 gm of proteinuria in 24 hours.

After quantitation, qualitative analysis of proteinuria should be performed. Qualitative analysis of proteinuria is typically carried out by using electrophoresis on cellulose acetate or agarose after concentrating the urine specimen. This procedure reveals dense bands in β and γ regions. Immunoelectrophoresis is used to identify a monoclonal component.

7. What is considered normal hematuria?

Normal hematuria is defined simply as no red blood cells (RBCs). The dipstick method is extremely sensitive for detecting RBCs in the urine and is positive with as little as 3–5 RBC/hpf. Healthy people excrete as many as 1×10^6 RBCs every 24 hours. Therefore, occasional RBCs seen microscopically in urine sediment are normal. Approximately 10% of normal people excrete up to 10 RBC/hpf of centrifuged urine sediment. However, less than 3% of normal people excrete more than 3 RBC/hpf. When repeat urinalyses demonstrate 1–3 RBC/hpf, further investigation for a cause of hematuria is warranted.

8. Are the characteristics of hematuria clinically useful?

Yes. Increased excretion of erythrocytes is a nonspecific finding and may be associated with bleeding at any site in the urinary tract. Patterns of hematuria usually are determined by four parameters:
1. Color and appearance of urine (gross or macroscopic vs. covert or microscopic hematuria)
2. Timing of the hematuria (persistent or constant, intermittent or recurrent)
3. Presence or absence of symptoms
4. Isolated hematuria or evidence of proteinuria, leukocytopenia, or bacteriuria

9. What may cause false-positive hematuria?

A color of red or dark brown may be seen in conjunction with dyes in foods, including beets, paprika, and senna. Drugs such as rifampin, phenothiazines, and phenytoin (Dilantin) also may have this effect. Myoglobin also gives a red-brown color to the urine. After intravascular hemolysis, free hemoglobin may be excreted, giving a distinct red color to the urine. Both myoglobin and hemoglobin pigments cause the standard urinary dipstick to give a positive reaction in patients with microscopic hematuria, but the correct diagnosis of urinary RBCs is based on microscopic analysis of the same urine specimen. In female patients, menstrual blood occasionally finds it way into an improperly collected urine specimen. Such patients need to return when they are not having menstrual bleeding. Microscopically, yeast, calcium oxalate crystals, starch granules, and air bubbles have been mistaken for hematuria.

10. What are the causes of isolated hematuria?

Isolated hematuria is almost always due to an extrarenal source. The major causes of both gross and microscopic hematuria include acute and chronic prostatitis or urethritis, hemorrhagic cystitis, renal stones, and tumors of the kidney, renal pelvis, ureter, bladder, prostate, and urethra.

11. How does one approach a patient with isolated hematuria?

Patients need repeat urinalyses to demonstrate persistent hematuria. Examination of the prostate and external urethra in conjunction with a urine culture is the basic first step in evaluation. A three-glass urine test is helpful in diagnosing lower urinary tract hematuria. The patient voids into three different containers. Hematuria only in the initial void suggests urethral bleeding, whereas hematuria in the terminal void suggests a prostatic or bladder origin. Intravenous pyelography and renal ultrasonography are the next tests to be performed if more information is needed. Renal stones, cysts, or urinary tract tumors can be identified in this fashion. Cystoscopy or retrograde pyelography may be needed to identify the source of bleeding. If these studies are uninformative, renal biopsy should be considered.

12. What suggests that hematuria may be renal in origin?

Associated proteinuria almost always suggests a renal origin of hematuria. However, in renal diseases in which proteinuria alone predominates (e.g., diabetes mellitus), evaluation for extrarenal sources of hematuria should be done, such as cystoscopy to screen for transitional cell carcinoma of the bladder. When red cell casts (RBCs enmeshed in Tamm-Horsfall protein) are found, the hematuria is almost always glomerular in origin.

Glomerular hematuria also is suspected when abnormalities in size, shape, and membrane appearance of the RBCs are present (dysmorphic erythrocytes). Phase-contrast microscopy is necessary to identify such abnormalities. RBCs from a nonglomerular source have normal and regular morphology (isomorphic erythrocytes). More recently, automated blood-cell volume analysers have been proposed to distinguish glomerular from nonglomerular hematuria. Decreased cell volumes are more commonly found in glomerular bleeding.

13. What is the most common cause of hematuria?

Extrarenal sites are the most common source of isolated hematuria. Of a consecutive series of 1000 patients with gross hematuria, 67% demonstrated a lesion in the bladder or lower urinary tract. The most common causes of gross hematuria originating in the kidney are nephropathy and polycystic kidney disease. In 10–15% of patients, no cause for hematuria can be found.

14. Should hematuria in a patient taking anticoagulant therapy be worked up?

A normal urinary tract should not bleed spontaneously when a patient is taking anticoagulants. Up to 82% of such patients have a lesion somewhere in the urinary tract. Examples include renal cell carcinoma, vesicoureteral reflux, urethral strictures, cancer of the prostate or bladder, and stone disease.

15. What are the most common causes of idiopathic nephrotic syndrome and nephrotic syndrome secondary to another disease process?

Nephrotic syndrome, defined as proteinuria ≥ 3.5 gm/24 hr, edema, and hypoalbuminuria, may be the result of primary renal disease (idiopathic) or part of a systemic disease (secondary). The most common idiopathic diseases are focal segmental glomerulosclerosis (FSGS) (35%), membranous nephropathy (33%), and minimal change (mil) disease (15%). Systemic diseases frequently associated with nephrotic syndrome include diabetes, systemic lupus erythematosus, multiple myeloma/amyloid disease, and HIV nephropathy. Drugs and toxins also may cause nephrotic syndrome; most notably, NSAIDs, heroin, and heavy metals (including gold used therapeutically).

BIBLIOGRAPHY

1. Abuelo JC: Proteinuria: Diagnostic principles and procedures. Ann Intern Med 98:186–191, 1983.
2. Antolak SJ, Mellinger GT: Urologic evaluation of hematuria occurring during anticoagulant therapy. J Urol 101:111–113, 1969.
3. Ginsberg JM, Chung BS, Materese RA, Garella S: Use of single voided urine samples to estimate quantitative proteinuria. N Engl J Med 309:1543–1546, 1983.
4. Glassock RJ: Hematuria and pigmenturia. In Massry S, Glassock R (eds): Textbook of Nephrology, vol. 1. Baltimore, Williams & Wilkins, 1989, pp 4.14–4.22.
5. Haas M, Meehan SM, Karrison TG, Spargo BH: Changing etiologies of unexplained adult nephrotic syndrome. A comparison of renal biopsy findings from 1976–1979 and 1995–1997. Am J Kidney Dis 30: 621–631, 1997.
6. Kubota M, et al: Mechanisms of urinary erythrocyte deformity in patients with glomerular disease. Nephrology 48:338–339, 1988.
7. Larson TS: Evaluation of proteinuria. Mayo Clin Proc 69:1154–1158, 1994.
8. Raman VG, Peud L, Leu HA, Haskell R: A blind controlled trial of phase-contrast microscopy by two observers for evaluating the source of hematuria. Nephrology 44:304–308, 1986.
9. Sutton JM: Evaluation of hematuria in adults. JAMA 263:2475, 1990.

57. KIDNEY STONES

Jeffrey Pickard, M.D.

1. What is the likelihood that any individual will develop kidney stones during his or her lifetime?

About 5–15% of people develop kidney stones during their lifetime.

2. Will a person who has had one kidney stone later develop another one?

Although formerly it was believed that first-time stone formers usually would not develop another stone, the opposite is, in fact, true. Most stone formers develop other stones during their lifetime and should be evaluated for historical, physical, and laboratory findings that predispose them to developing stones.

3. List the five types of kidney stones.

Types of Kidney Stones

COMPOSITION OF STONE	CAUSES
1. Calcium oxalate	Primary hyperparathyroidism Idiopathic hypercalciuria Low urine citrate level Hyperoxaluria Hyperuricosuria
2. Calcium phosphate	Renal tubular acidosis
3. Uric acid	Low urine pH Hyperuricosuria
4. Struvite	Infection with bacteria that express urease
5. Cystine	Cystinuria

From Coe FL, Parks JH, Asplin JR: The pathogenesis and treatment of kidney stones. N Engl J Med 327:1141–1152, Copyright © 1992 Massachusetts Medical Society. All rights reserved.

4. What is the most common type of kidney stone?

Three-fourths of all kidney stones are made of calcium oxalate. In fact, in normal urine calcium oxalate is concentrated to 4 times its solubility (i.e., the urine is supersaturated). Nucleation (the nidus for crystal formation) occurs when the concentration reaches 7 times solubility. About 10–20% of kidney stones are struvite (magnesium ammonium phosphate); 5% are uric acid; 5% have mostly hydroxyapatite or brushite (calcium monohydrogen phosphate); and < 1% are cystine.

5. How does hypocitraturia contribute to the formation of calcium stones?

Citrate forms soluble complexes with calcium oxalate in the urine to keep the crystals from coalescing to form stones.

6. What causes calcium oxalate stones?

The most common cause of calcium oxalate stones is idiopathic hypercalciuria, which is responsible for > 50% of all calcium oxalate stones. Other causes include primary hyperparathyroidism, low urinary citrate level, hyperoxaluria, and hyperuricosuria.

7. What are the causes of hyperoxaluria?

The normal 24-hr urinary excretion of oxalate is ≤ 45 mg. Increase in dietary intake of foods that are rich in oxalate increases the concentration of oxalate in the urine (spinach, rhubarb, beets, peppers, cocoa, chocolate, wheat germ, peanuts, pecans, okra, lime peel). Small bowel malabsorption, as in regional enteritis, increases intestinal absorption of oxalate. Primary hyperoxaluria is a rare disorder, which is inherited in an autosomal recessive pattern. Kidney stones start forming in childhood, and analysis of the urine reveals a marked increase in the concentration of oxalate (135–270 mg/24 hr).

8. What laboratory evaluation should be done in a person who develops a kidney stone?

A spot urine should be collected for culture and pH testing. A 24-hr urine and corresponding blood sample should be collected. Calcium, magnesium, phosphorus, uric acid, and creatinine should be measured in both. In addition, it is important to measure serum sodium and potassium and to analyze the urine for oxalate, citrate, volume, and cystine.

9. How do you prevent recurring stones in a patient with idiopathic hypercalciuria?

The answer depends on the specific cause based on stone analysis. All patients with stones probably benefit from increasing fluid intake, which increases urine volume and decreases concentrations. Dietary manipulation may be helpful for patients with hyperoxaluria (decrease dietary intake) or hypocitraturia (supplement with citrate), but calcium restriction is not helpful, as discussed below. Patients with calcium stones benefit from thiazides, which decrease urinary calcium by increasing fractional reabsorption of calcium from the distal tubule. It appears that reabsorbed calcium is shunted directly into bone. However, thiazides must be used for 2 years before a beneficial effect on stone recurrence is seen.

10. What is the value of dietary calcium restriction in patients with calcium stones?

Dietary calcium restriction is not helpful for preventing the recurrence of calcium stones and, in fact, may be harmful. In patients with idiopathic hypercalciuria, bone mineral is unusually labile. Those who restrict dietary calcium appear to compensate by increasing calcium resorption from bone, although this effect may not be universal. Some patients given a low calcium diet manifest a reciprocal hyperoxaluria, which can maintain calcium oxalate stone-forming potential even in the face of decreased urinary calcium.

11. What analgesics are best for acute renal colic?

Narcotics have typically been first-line analgesics for controlling the pain of renal colic in both outpatient and inpatient settings. However, prospective trials using NSAIDs have shown them to be roughly equivalent in the ability to control pain, although the onset of pain relief from narcotics may be slightly faster. It appears that much of the pain is caused by the release of renal prostaglandins (primarily PGE_2) and localized inflammation, both of which may be counteracted by NSAIDs. It may be that combining narcotics (which act centrally) and NSAIDs (which act peripherally) may work better than either drug alone, but no studies have addressed this possibility.

12. What treatment should you recommend for an impacted stone?

Stones < 5 mm in diameter generally pass on their own, whereas stones > 7 mm generally do not. Stones in the distal ureter (i.e., below the pelvic brim) may be removed either ureteroscopically or by extracorporeal shock wave lithotripsy (ESWL). Although ESWL is less invasive than ureteroscopy, it is less effective in removing distal stones. Proximal stones ≤ 1 cm in diameter are best removed by ESWL. Stones ≥ 1 cm in the upper ureter may be treated by either of the above techniques or by percutaneous nephrolithotomy. Open surgery is done only if other modalities have failed or if the stones are unusually large or complex.

13. What beverages are best and worst for preventing recurrent stones?

This question was examined prospectively as part of the Health Professionals Follow-up Study, which included a cohort of 45,289 men 40–75 years of age with no history of kidney stones. Follow-up was for 6 years (242,100 person years). In addition, 81,093 women in the Nurses' Health Study were followed for 533,081 person years. After simultaneously adjusting for a variety of factors, the risk of stone formation was decreased for each 8-oz serving consumed daily of coffee, decaffeinated coffee, tea, beer, and wine. The risk was increased by apple juice and grapefruit juice. In contrast to a previously published report, these studies found no statistically significant effect for carbonated soft drinks.

14. How are struvite stones formed?

Struvite stones are caused by urine infected with urease-producing bacteria: *Proteus* sp., *Klebsiella* sp., *Pseudomonas* sp., and enterococci. *Escherichia coli* does not produce struvite stones.

BIBLIOGRAPHY

 1. Coe FL, Parks JH, Asplin JR: The pathogenesis and treatment of kidney stones. N Engl J Med 327:1141–1152, 1992.
 2. Coe FL, Parks Favus MJ: Diet and calcium: The end of an era? Ann Intern Med 126:553–555, 1997.
 3. Cordell WH, Larson TA, Lingeman JE, et al: Indomethacin suppositories versus intravenously titrated morphine for the treatment of ureteral colic. Ann Emerg Med 23:262–269, 1994.
 4. Curhan CG, Willet WC, Rimm EB, Stampfler MJ: A prospective study of dietary calcium and other nutrients and the risk of symptomatic kidney stones. N Engl J Med 328:833–838, 1993.
 5. Curhan CG, Willet WC, Rimm EB, et al: Prospective study of beverage use and the risk of kidney stones. Am J Epidemiol 143:240–247, 1996.
 6. Curhan CG, Willet WC, Speizer FE, Stampfler MJ: Beverage use and risk for kidney stones in women. Ann Intern Med 128:534–540, 1998.
 7. Curhan CG, Willett WC, Speizer FE, et al: Comparison of dietary with supplemental calcium and other nutrients as factors affecting the risk of kidney stones in women. Ann Intern Med 126:497–504, 1997.
 8. Gault MH, Longerich LL, Crane G, et al: Bacteriology of urinary tract stones. J Urol 153:1164–1170, 1995.
 9. Labrecque M, Dostaler LP, Rousselle R, et al: Efficacy of nonsteroidal anti-inflammatory drugs in the treatment of acute renal colic: A meta-analysis. Arch Intern Med 154:1381–1387, 1994.
10. Wrenn K: Emergency intravenous pyelography in the setting of possible renal colic: Is it indicated? Ann Emerg Med 26:304–307, 1995.

58. INCONTINENCE

Evelyn Hutt, M.D.

1. What percentage of community-dwelling elders are incontinent?

Prevalence of urinary incontinence varies by age and gender. Among the population aged 65–74 years, approximately 5–7% are incontinent. Over age 75 years, at least 10% of men and 15–20% of women living in the community are incontinent. About 10 million Americans suffer from urinary incontinence; annual costs are estimated at $10.3 billion.

2. What is the differential diagnosis of acute incontinence?

About 50% of incontinence is acute and therefore readily treatable. It may be the only presenting sign of a serious underlying disorder, such as delirium or spinal cord compression. A simple mnemonic, **DRIP**, helps to remember the differential diagnosis:

D = **D**elirium and **D**rugs. Any patient with new-onset incontinence should have formal mental status testing (e.g., Mini-Mental Status Exam) and a review of medications, including over-the-counter (OTC) preparations. Drugs that precipitate incontinence can be divided into three main groups: diuretics, sedatives, and anticholinergics. Alcohol is both a sedative and a diuretic. It is easy to miss the diagnosis of excessive alcohol intake in older women. Anticholinergics may precipitate acute urinary retention by direct action on bladder innervation and by central sedative effect; they are common in OTC cold preparations.

R = **R**estricted mobility and **R**etention. Many older people have impaired mobility, which limits their ability to get to the bathroom quickly. Retention of urine may be caused by drugs, as mentioned above; an enlarged, obstructing prostate; or neurologic damage from an acute spinal cord compression. New-onset incontinence in the setting of back pain is a medical emergency and should prompt an immediate work-up for spinal cord lesions.

I = **I**nfection, **I**nflammation, and **I**mpaction. Every patient with new-onset incontinence should have a urinalysis and rectal examination.

P = **P**olyuria, which serves as a reminder that diabetes and hypercalcemia may present in the elderly as incontinence.

3. What simple clinical test distinguishes between inability to retain urine and inability to empty the bladder?

Bladder catheterization to measure postvoid residual volume (PVR) determines whether or not the patient is retaining urine. A volume greater than 60 cc immediately after the patient voids freely is abnormal and suggests retention.

4. Is it useful in women to distinguish between stress and urge incontinence?

In reality, most incontinent women have a mixture of stress and urge symptoms and pathophysiology. Predominance of one type of symptom may suggest what treatment modality to start with.

5. What is detrusor instability? How is it treated?

Detrusor instability is defined as uninhibited bladder contraction sufficient to overcome urethral resistance. It is the most common cause of incontinence. Because bladder contraction is cholinergically mediated and urethral contraction is sympathetically mediated, one can either give an anticholinergic to block bladder contraction or an alpha-adrenergic agonist to increase urethral resistance. Alpha agonists are generally better tolerated than anticholinergics.

6. Define bedside cystometrics. When is it useful?

Bedside cystometrics is a series of maneuvers, described by Ouslander, Leach, and Staskin, that assess stress incontinence, detrusor instability, and bladder capacity. The patient is asked to come to the exam with a full bladder and to cough 3 times in the standing position, with a small pad over the urethral area. Then the patient voids privately. A 14-French straight catheter is inserted into the bladder with the patient supine to measure PVR. A 50-ml catheter tip syringe is attached to catheter, and the bladder is filled with room-temperature sterile water at 50-ml increments until the patient feels the urge to void and then at 25-ml increments until bladder capacity is reached. The catheter is removed, and the stress maneuvers are repeated. The patient voids again privately. Involuntary contractions visible as a rise in the meniscus of the syringe or urgency at relatively low volume (< 300 cc) suggests detrusor instability. The tests are useful in women for whom a drug trial is contraindicated (e.g., dementia) and in men with benign prostatic hypertrophy (BPH) who are contemplating transurethral prostatectomy to detect the presence of detrusor instability and to plan for the possible onset of worsening of incontinence postoperatively.

7. How effective are nonpharmacologic treatments for incontinence?

Nonpharmacologic treatment consists of either timed toileting techniques or pelvic floor muscle-strengthening techniques. In **timed toileting** the patient is taught to void on a schedule determined by the frequency of incontinent episodes as revealed by a diary. With or without biofeedback in several small trials, this technique achieved a 60–80% reduction in incontinent episodes. The technique is also effective in demented patients with conscientious caregivers. **Pelvic muscle (Kegel's) exercises** have been shown to be effective in stress incontinence. One study found them to be as effective as alpha agonist therapy. Their utility is limited, however, by the need for strong motivation and a clear sensorium.

8. What is the role of estrogen in the treatment of stress incontinence?

Estrogen has not been shown to affect pure stress incontinence, but it improves dysuria and urgency caused by atrophic vaginitis. Because most incontinent women have both stress and urge symptoms as well as atrophic vaginitis, a trial of estrogen is often beneficial. It is contraindicated, however, in women with breast cancer. For women reluctant to try hormone therapy, a 3-week trial of vaginal estrogen cream may help to assess its utility.

9. How effective are alpha agonists in the treatment of stress and urge incontinence?

Alpha agonists have been shown to be 60–80% effective in reducing episodes of wetness, but placebo-controlled trials are lacking. The side-effect profile of alpha agonists compares favorably with that of anticholinergics; therefore, alpha agonists should be tried first.

10. When should an incontinent woman with cystocele be referred for surgery?

Only a grade 3 cystocele, with extension to the back of the vaginal vault or through the introitus, is likely to cause incontinence. Such patients are unlikely to benefit from drug or behavioral therapy and should seek surgical attention. All other patients deserve a trial of conservative management.

11. How useful are alpha agonists in the treatment of urinary retention due to BPH?

Alpha antagonists may be of some benefit in the treatment of retention due to BPH. They are particularly useful in patients who are too frail for surgery or who have concomitant hypertension. Caution must be exercised to prevent syncope with the first dose, and the patient should be checked for orthostatic hypotension after initiation of therapy.

12. What is the role of finasteride in the treatment of retention due to BPH?

Finasteride is a 5-alpha-reductase inhibitor that may reduce prostate volume by approximately 25% and improve urine flow rates in 30% of patients. Side effects include decreased libido and a confounding of the prostate-specific antigen (PSA) values used to screen for prostate cancer. It is at least twice as expensive as an alpha antagonist. Combining finasteride with alpha antagonists provides no additional benefit.

13. When is an indwelling Foley catheter indicated in the management of chronic incontinence?
The clearest indication for long-term use of a Foley catheter is protection of skin in a patient who has or is at risk for pressure ulcers and who has failed condom catheterization. Patients with urinary retention who are difficult to catheterize intermittently or who are too frail for surgery also may benefit from an indwelling Foley catheter.

14. Is there a relationship between chronic incontinence and otherwise asymptomatic bacteriuria?
No. A recent study in nursing home patients showed no effect of eradicating bacteriuria on chronic incontinence.

BIBLIOGRAPHY

1. Fanti JA, Wyman JF, McClish DK, et al: Efficacy of bladder training in older women with urinary incontinence. JAMA 265:609–613, 1991.
2. Kane RL, Ouslander JG, Abras IB: Incontinence. In Essentials of Clinical Geriatrics, 2nd ed. New York, McGraw-Hill, 1989, pp 139–191.
3. Lepor H, Williford WO, Barry MJ, et al: The efficacy of terazosin, finasteride, or both in benign prostatic hypertrophy. N Engl J Med 335:533–539, 1996.
4. McConnell JD, Bruskewitz R, Walsh P, et al, for the Finasteride Long-term Efficacy and Safety Group: The effect of finasteride on the risk of acute urinary retention and the need for surgical treatment among men with benign prostatic hyperplasia. N Engl J Med 338:557–563, 1998.
5. Monda JM, Osterling JE: Medical treatment of benign prostatic hypertrophy: 5-Alpha-reductase inhibitors and alpha-adrenergic antagonists. Mayo Clin Proc 68:670–679, 1993.
6. Ouslander JG, Leach GE, Staskin DR: Simplified tests of lower urinary tract function in the evaluation of geriatric urinary incontinence. J Am Geriatr Soc 37:706–714, 1989.
7. Ouslander JG, Schnelle JF: Incontinence in the nursing home. Ann Intern Med 122:438–449, 1995.
8. Resnick NM, Ouslander JG: NIH Conference on Urinary Incontinence: Urinary incontinence—Where do we stand and where do we go from here? J Am Geriatr Soc 38:263–368, 1990.
9. Wells TJ, Brink CA, Diokno AC, et al: Pelvic muscle exercise for stress urinary incontinence in elderly women. J Am Geriatr Soc 39:785–791, 1991.

59. RENAL FAILURE

Katherine M. Fitting, M.D., Alan B. Cooper, M.D., and Arlene B. Chapman, M.D.

1. What is chronic renal failure?
Chronic renal failure is an irreversible loss of nephrons and is usually asymptomatic until 70–90% of the nephron population is destroyed. Renal disease progresses through various stages:
Decreased renal reserve: nephron loss without the loss of measured renal function.
Renal insufficiency: a measurable decline in renal function, usually associated with an impaired ability to concentrate the urine or a decreased maximal urinary osmolality that causes nocturia or polyuria and is often accompanied by hypertension.
Renal failure: a progressive decline in renal function to the point that homeostasis cannot be maintained; associated with worsening azotemia, anemia, hyperphosphatemia, hypocalcemia, and metabolic acidosis.
Uremia: a clinical syndrome with severe decline in renal function, associated with dysfunction of multiple organ systems potentially manifested as anorexia, taste change, nausea, epigastric pain, pruritus, chest pain (pericarditis), shortness of breath, fatigue, weakness, and depression.

2. How does one differentiate acute from chronic renal failure?
History, supported by medical records, is the most important way to differentiate acute from chronic renal failure. Often records are not available. Classically, hypocalcemia, hyperphosphatemia,

and anemia have been associated more often with chronic than acute renal failure. However, calcium, phosphorus, and acid-base derangements are often seen in patients with acute renal failure as early as 48–72 hours after the onset of illness. Anemia is also a nonspecific indicator. A more reliable indicator of chronic renal failure is the finding of small kidneys with a decrease or absence of renal cortex, as assessed by ultrasonography. Ultrasound is noninvasive with image resolutions of 0.5 cm and is highly effective in determining renal size and ruling out obstructive disease. A kidney length of less than 9 cm is abnormal and indicates chronic and significant renal disease. A difference of greater than 1.5 cm in renal length indicates unilateral or asymmetric renal disease. The echogenicity of the renal cortex is increased in chronic renal disease.

Another reliable indicator of chronic renal failure is the presence of renal osteodystrophy; osteitis fibrosa cystica, osteomalacia, and osteoporosis are present to varying degrees in all patients with chronic renal disease.

3. What conditions causing chronic renal failure are associated with normal to increased renal size?

Diabetic nephropathy	Polycystic kidneys
Hydronephrosis	Nephropathy associated with the human
Amyloidosis	immunodeficiency virus
Congenital malformations	Myeloma kidney

4. What evaluation should be done in patients with renal insufficiency?

In the evaluation of patients with renal disease, it is important to establish the degree of renal impairment and to identify reversible factors causing a decrease in renal function, such as infection, obstruction, volume depletion, nephrotoxic drugs, less than optimal cardiac output with or without hypertension, uncontrolled hypertension, hypercalcemia, and hyperuricemia. A thorough history and physical examination should be performed, including orthostatic blood pressure and pulse measurements. Besides the history and physical, the database should include urinalysis by dipstick and microscope; assessment of serum electrolytes, blood urea nitrogen (BUN), and creatinine; complete blood count; evaluation of postvoid residual; and ultrasonography.

5. How does urinalysis aid in the evaluation of renal failure?

The simplest, most cost-effective element of the evaluation of a patient with chronic renal failure is routine urinalysis. In chronic renal disease, one may see unconcentrated or isothenuric urine, as indicated by a specific gravity of 1.010 or less. Dipstick glucose may be seen in diabetes mellitus or in chronic renal failure as the ability of the proximal tubule to reabsorb glucose decreases with progression of disease. The urine pH in chronic renal failure is usually less than 7.0; if it is greater than 8.0, the question of infection with urease-splitting organisms should be raised. Proteinuria is the hallmark of intrinsic renal disease; nephrotic-range proteinuria is seen in glomerular lesions and 1–2 gm of protein excretion in interstitial diseases. If the dipstick is positive for blood but no red blood cells are seen microscopically, the question of myoglobinurias and rhabdomyolysis should be raised. Cellular or red blood cell casts indicate active renal disease of a glomerular or vascular etiology. White blood cells are usually seen in infections but may be present in allergic interstitial nephritis, renal tuberculosis, glomerulonephritis, or chlamydial infection. Hansel's stain for eosinophils helps to differentiate allergic interstitial nephritis from other conditions.

6. Aside from correcting reversible factors, what can be done to change the chronic progression of renal disease?

Relatively few renal diseases are responsive to therapy, and once the serum creatinine concentration is greater than 2.0 mg/dl, progression often occurs even if the initial insult completely resolves. However, control of blood pressure is paramount in slowing the progression of renal disease. Some antihypertensive agents also show promise of slowing the progression of renal disease independently of blood pressure control, particularly in diabetic nephropathy. Examples include angiotensin-converting enzyme (ACE) inhibitors, such as enalapril or captopril, and the nondihydropyridine calcium channel blockers, such as diltiazem or verapamil. The beneficial effects of the ACE inhibitors are secondary to their predominant actions on the glomerular efferent arteriole. Both groups of drugs demonstrate antiproteinuric effects, which are important because proteinuria is an independent risk factor for progressive loss of renal function.

Dietary modification may slow the progression of renal disease. Protein restriction (with attendant phosphorus restriction) has been demonstrated to decrease loss of renal function in animal studies and has been used for decades to prevent loss of renal function in humans. However, clinical trials demonstrate no clear benefit. Because of the risk of malnutrition, patients should not be placed on long-term severe protein restriction without careful monitoring. According to conservative recommendations, patients should ingest no more than 0.8–1 gm of protein/kg/day with dietetic counseling to ensure adequate nutritional intake. Three-day dietary recall and diet diaries are reliable ways to determine the level of protein intake.

7. Which antihypertensive agents are contraindicated in patients with chronic renal failure?
Contraindicated antihypertensives in patients with renal disease include the potassium-sparing diuretics, such as triamterene, spironolactone, and amiloride. Medications that cause large changes in systemic blood pressure or in potassium handling by the kidney (such as ACE inhibitors) require close monitoring in patients with chronic renal failure.

8. When do patients with renal failure have problems maintaining potassium balance?
Without renal tubular acidosis, patients with renal failure are able to maintain potassium balance on a regular diet until the glomerular filtration rate (GFR) is reduced to 5–10 ml/min/1.73 m^2. In chronic renal failure, total body stores of potassium are either normal or low; shifts of potassium from the intracellular to extracellular compartment predominate. The colon secretes potassium, but its contribution to potassium balance is negligible until chronic renal failure occurs, at which point stool potassium excretion increases to 35% of intake.

9. How should acute hyperkalemia be managed? When should hyperkalemia be treated in renal failure?
Patients with chronic renal failure may have chronically elevated concentrations of serum potassium; chronic hyperkalemia is often better tolerated by the cardiovascular system than acute hyperkalemia. The predominant effects of hyperkalemia are cardiac and require treatment when EKG changes are present. Peaked T waves (isosceles triangle) or widening of the PR interval, which may be followed by widening of the QRS complex and a sine wave complex and asystole, require emergent therapy. Intravenous calcium should be given to stabilize the cardiac membrane; the effect of this treatment lasts for approximately 20 minutes. Insulin, glucose, and bicarbonate are given to increase cellular uptake of potassium. Depending on the severity of the EKG changes, bolus therapy (10 U regular insulin, 1 ampule D50, 50 cc $NaHCO_3$) or continuous infusion (10 U regular insulin in 250 cc D10W with 50 cc $NaHCO_3$ running at 75–100 cc/hr) may be used. Beta agonists such as albuterol have been shown to potentiate the potassium-lowering effects of insulin and may be used as a prolonged nebulizer treatment. This technique provides a small but measurable effect. The effects of this regimen last as long as the treatment continues, but some method of potassium removal must be provided—either Kayexelate (sodium polystyrene exonate (30–50 gm with 20% sorbitol) or dialysis. Intracellular shifts of potassium should be avoided during hemodialysis, because they prevent effective removal of potassium. Continued monitoring of serum potassium is required to avoid severe hypokalemia during dialysis.

10. What indications are used for treatment of chronic metabolic acidosis in renal failure?
Exogenous alkali treatment should be used in symptomatic patients with renal failure. Symptoms include dyspnea (from respiratory compensation) and persistent hyperkalemia. Treatment of milder asymptomatic metabolic acidosis minimizes the loss of skeletal calcium with resultant

osteodystrophy. In addition, acidemia interferes with protein metabolism and may lead to muscle wasting and cardiac dysfunction. Treatment of metabolic acidosis secondary to uremia is recommended when serum bicarbonate levels reach 15 mg/dl.

11. Which agents are available to provide exogenous alkali in chronic renal failure?

The most commonly used agents are sodium bicarbonate or citrate. The sodium content may worsen blood pressure control or contribute to volume overload; citrate should be used with caution when patients are also taking albumin as a phosphate binder (e.g., Amphojel, Basaljel). Citrate increases aluminum absorption and may lead to toxic aluminum levels, which are associated with dementia in patients with renal failure. Calcium carbonate has been advocated as the buffering agent, but it is not as effective as the others in restoring neutral pH, because large doses (more than 1500 mg/day) are required. This dosage may increase the calcium-phosphorus product, resulting in metastatic calcium deposition, and predispose patients to calcium oxalate stone formation.

12. When is renal failure predominantly polyuric?

Renal failure caused by certain conditions may present with advanced renal insufficiency (elevated BUN, creatinine) yet be polyuric, hypokalemic, and salt-wasting. This condition is most commonly seen in obstructive nephropathy (vesicoureteral reflux) and hypokalemic nephropathy (caused by prolonged, severe potassium depletion—often associated with eating disorders). Such patients require both sodium and potassium supplementation and need to be encouraged to increase fluid intake to avoid dehydration.

13. Are patients with renal failure at increased risk for depression?

Many believe that depression is the most common psychiatric disorder in patients with renal disease. However, the true incidence is unknown, because the data are scarce. Presenting symptoms of depression in renal failure may mimic a primary depressive illness (e.g., anhedonia, sense of helplessness, depressed mood) or may involve more subtle findings. Such findings include increased irritability, bad dreams, or somatic complaints that cannot be explained after careful diagnostic evaluation. Treatment of depression should be strongly considered in patients with chronic renal failure. Because tricyclic antidepressants are predominantly metabolized by the liver and are not dialyzable, no dosage adjustments need be made. Some investigators have found that patients with renal failure respond better to certain antidepressants, such as imipramine or sertraline.

14. What bleeding diathesis is associated with renal failure?

A qualitative platelet defect is present and manifested only by an increased bleeding time. The platelet count is normal, whereas platelet aggregation and adhesion are normal. Treatment, directed at increasing release of von Willebrand's factor from vascular endothelium, consists of administration of 1-deamino-8-D-arginine vasopressin (DDAVP) at 3 µl/kg. This treatment, which is effective for 4–6 hours after administration, is accompanied by tachyphylaxis. Cryoprecipitate rapidly corrects the diathesis and is effective for 24–36 hours but carries the risk of blood-borne viruses. Estrogens (25 mg orally or 3 mg/kg divided over 5 doses intravenously) have been shown to be effective for as long as 3–10 days. Maintaining the patient's hematocrit at greater than 30% is also beneficial. Dialysis improves platelet function without normalizing the bleeding time and should be considered as an adjunctive therapy for life-threatening hemorrhage that is attributed to uremia.

15. How common is upper gastrointestinal (GI) bleeding in patients with renal failure?

Upper GI bleeding is a major complication in patients with renal failure and accounts for 3–7% of deaths. Superficial mucosal abnormalities are more common than ulcerative disease. Duodenitis and gastritis have been reported in 10–60% of patients with moderate-to-severe renal failure. The incidence of angiodysplasia is also increased in renal failure and is believed to be the source of bleeding in 23% of patients. Therapy for upper GI bleeding in renal failure is the same as for patients without renal disease, except that H_2 receptor antagonists, such as cimetidine, should be given at reduced dosages because they are cleared by the kidney.

16. List five indications for acute hemodialysis.

1. Medically unresponsive hyperkalemia with EKG changes
2. Profound metabolic acidosis causing cardiovascular compromise and hypotension
3. Medically unresponsive pulmonary edema with hypoxemia
4. Drug ingestions (lithium, theophylline, salicylates, methanol, or glycols)
5. Uremic encephalopathy

17. When is hemodialysis contraindicated?

Most contraindications to hemodialysis are relative and depend on the individual patient. However, in acute hemorrhage involving the central nervous system, hemodialysis should be deferred, because rapid fluid shifts between the arachnoid and subarachnoid space may worsen the injury. Peritoneal dialysis is the modality of choice.

18. What therapeutic options are available for patients with end-stage renal disease?

The three forms of renal replacement are hemodialysis, peritoneal dialysis, and transplantation. Chronic hemodialysis is performed for 2.5–4 hours 3 times/week based on patient characteristics and may be provided at home or in a dialysis center. Peritoneal dialysis, which allows patients more freedom and control of therapy, is either continuous over a 24-hour period or performed at night for approximately 8 hours on a cycler machine. The cycler machine allows the patient to hang the dialysate before going to bed; the cycler performs the exchanges throughout the night. Renal transplantation can be performed using either a living or cadaveric donor; good outcomes are expected with either source. The life expectancy for patients on dialysis is 6–7 years for those less than age 60 years and 2–3 years for those who are older than 60 years or diabetic. Survival after renal transplantation is 90% at 3 years with cadaveric transplantation and approximately 95% with living related donations.

BIBLIOGRAPHY

1. Giovannetti S, Cupisti A, Barsotti G: The metabolic acidosis of chronic renal failure: Pathophysiology and treatment. Contrib Nephrol 100:48–57, 1992.
2. Khan S: New insights into the consequences and mechanisms of renal impairment in obstructive nephropathy. Am J Kidney Dis 18:689–699, 1991.
3. Kupin WL, Narins RG: The hypokalemia of renal failure: Pathophysiology, diagnosis and therapy. Contrib Nephrol 102:1–22, 1993.
4. Malluche HH, Monier-Faugere MC: Uremic bone disease: Current knowledge, controversial issues, and new horizons. Miner Electrolyte Metab 17:281–296, 1991.
5. Murphey MD, Sartoris DJ, Quale JL, et al: Musculoskeletal manifestations of chronic renal insufficiency. Radiographics 13:357–379, 1993.
6. Oldrizzi L, Rugiu C, De Biase V, Maschio G: The place of hypertension among the risk factors for renal function in chronic renal failure. Am J Kidney Dis 5(Suppl 2):119–123, 1993.
7. Peterson JC, Tisher CC, Wilcox CS (eds):
8. Procci WR, Massry SG, Glassock RL (eds): Textbook of Nephrology. Baltimore, Williams & Wilkins, chapter 66 (Pt 1), 1980.
9. Remuzzi G: Bleeding in renal failure. Lancet i:1205–1208, 1988.
10. Sevy N, Snape WJ, Massry SG, Glassock RJ (eds): Textbook of Nephrology. Baltimore, Williams & Wilkins, chapter 70 (Pt 1), 1989.
11. United States Renal Data System: 1997 Annual data report: Patient mortality and survival. Am J Kidney Dis 30(2-1):S86–S106, 1997.

IX. Common Problems of the Blood and Lymph System

---

60. ASYMPTOMATIC FINDINGS ON THE HEMOGRAM

Jeanette Mladenovic, M.D.

---

1. What value on the complete blood count (CBC) is helpful when the mean corpuscular volume (MCV) is disproportionately low in comparison with the mildly low hemoglobin (Hb)?

The major consideration is whether the low MCV results from iron deficiency or an abnormality of globin chain synthesis (thalassemia). Clues that suggest thalassemia trait rather than iron deficiency may be provided by the following: a red cell count higher than expected for the hemoglobin; a near-normal mean corpuscular hemoglobin count (MCHC), and a red cell distribution width (RDW) within normal range. Microcytosis, when due to iron deficiency, usually is accompanied by a low red cell count, low MCHC, and high RDW.

	HEMOGLOBIN (gm/dl)	MCV	RDW
Iron deficiency	8	74	> 15.3%
Chronic disease	10	86	Variable
Thalassemia syndromes	12	68	< 14%

2. What causes an elevated platelet count?

Thrombocytosis may result from primary or secondary causes. In primary thrombocytopenia, an intrinsic defect in the stem cell leads to abnormally increased platelets, often irregular in size with variable granularity. Diseases such as polycythemia vera, chronic myelogenous leukemia, and essential thrombocythemia fall into this category. Secondary thrombocytosis is seen in patients with chronic inflammatory states, hemolysis, iron deficiency, gastrointestinal bleeding, and postsplenectomy syndrome. Chronic inflammatory states include malignancies in addition to conditions that result in a cellular immune response, such as chronic infections and autoimmune disease. Patients with primary thrombocytosis may be at risk from bleeding or clotting with platelet counts higher than 1 million, whereas patients with secondary thrombocytosis rarely develop such high counts.

3. Besides infection, what causes leukocytosis?

Leukocytosis may be secondary or due to primary bone marrow abnormalities. Secondary leukocytosis may be due to demargination, accelerated release of cells from the marrow, increased production of white cells, or even decreased removal. Demargination may be seen with sepsis or any stress-mediated response, such as hypotension or hypoxia. Increased release and production, indicative of infection, also may be seen with inflammation (such as blood in a closed space) or even with tumors that produce stimulatory factors (lung carcinoma). Primary leukocytosis occurs with leukemia. If the differential white blood cell count shows young white blood cells in circulation (blasts or cells of earlier differentiation than metamyelocytes), a primary marrow disorder (leukemia) is more likely.

4. Define lymphocytosis. With what disorders is it associated?

Lymphocytosis is defined as an absolute lymphocyte count $> 3.5 \times 10^9$/L. Lymphocytosis or a lymphoid leukemoid reaction may be seen in viral infections, such as infectious mononucleosis, cytomegalovirus (CMV), measles, and pertussis (in children). Lymphocytes may be atypical in appearance, variable in size, and reactive. In an adult without evidence of infection, a persistent lymphocytosis $> 5 \times 10^9$/L suggests the diagnosis of chronic lymphocytic leukemia. Typing to determine that all lymphocytes are B-lymphocytes confirms the diagnosis.

5. What is significant leukopenia?

Leukopenia is defined as a white blood cell count $< 4 \times 10^9$/L. Usually, as the count falls, cells of the neutrophil series are most affected. The percentage of the white blood cell count of granulocytic lineage (bands and mature cells) determines the absolute neutrophil cell count and the risk of life-threatening infection. Patients with granulocyte counts $< 1 \times 10^9$/L are at risk of sepsis. Fever $> 38.3°$ should be evaluated aggressively to determine the cause and treated empirically with broad-spectrum antibiotics that cover gram-negative (including *Pseudomonas* sp.) and gram-positive (including staphylococci) organisms. As the absolute count falls, the association of fever with bacteremia increases.

6. What test should be ordered first to determine the cause of a prolonged prothrombin time (PT) and/or partial thromboplastin time (PTT)?

The first test that should be requested is a 1:1 mix, in which normal plasma is mixed with the patient's plasma and both PT and PTT are repeated. Complete correction suggests that prolongation is due to factor deficiency. Failure to correct suggests the presence of inhibitors in the patient's plasma. Patients with liver disease often have two defects; thus, correction is incomplete. Alternatively, a prolonged PTT with evidence of inhibition is consistent with a lupus inhibitor.

7. What is the appropriate response when the hematocrit is elevated above normal?

An increased hematocrit may be due to decreased plasma volume (relative erythrocytosis) or a true increase in the red cell mass (primary polycythemia vera or secondary erythrocytosis). At a hematocrit of 55%, the odds of a true increase are only 50/50, whereas at a hematocrit of 60%, the red cell mass almost certainly is increased. Thus, at levels in the 52–58% range, the red cell mass should be determined to evaluate a persistently elevated hematocrit. Patients with elevated hematocrits should not undergo surgery or dye loads without evaluation because of the risk of thrombosis.

8. With automated counters, which abnormalities may cause a false change in CBC values?

Erythrocytosis: lipids

Pseudoanemia: cold agglutinins

Pseudothrombocytosis: red cell fragments or microcytic red cells

Pseudothrombocytopenia: clumped platelets

Pseudoleukocytosis: giant platelets

Pseudoleukopenia: leukoagglutination

Thus, unexpected values should be evaluated visually and usually are flagged for further laboratory analysis.

9. What is the significance of polychromatophilia and nucleated red blood cells on the peripheral blood smear?

Such findings suggest early release of cells from the marrow in response to erythropoietin or secondary to displacement of the marrow with other elements (myelophthisis). A reticulocyte count is required to determine which process caused the increase in early circulating red cells.

10. Define significant eosinophilia and significant basophilia.

Mild eosinophilia (0.2–1.5×10^9 cells/L) may be seen with mild skin disease, atopy, and allergic reactions. Marked eosinophilia occasionally is seen in patients with asthma (especially in the presence of *Aspergillus* sp.) or angioneurotic edema. Extremely high or progressively increasing numbers of eosinophils also may suggest tissue helminthic infection or eosinophilic syndromes related to any organ of the body or secondary to malignancies. Prolonged, marked elevation of eosinophils may lead to tissue damage due to the eosinophils themselves. Eosinophilic leukemia is exceedingly rare.

Basophilia ($> 0.1 \times 10^9$) is seen in myeloproliferative diseases of all types. In the presence of leukocytosis or thrombocytosis, basophilia of any degree supports a diagnosis of primary myeloproliferative disease. Mild transient basophilia also is seen with ulcerative colitis and allergic systemic or skin diseases.

BIBLIOGRAPHY

1. Diagnostic hematology. Hematol Oncol Clin North Am 8:1–34, 1994.
2. Jandl JH: Blood: Textbook of Hematology, 2nd ed. Boston, Little, Brown, 1996.
3. Lee GR, Bithell TC, Foerster J, et al (eds): Wintrobe's Clinical Hematology, 9th ed. Philadelphia, Lea & Febiger, 1993.

61. ANEMIA

Jeanette Mladenovic, M.D.

1. Define anemia.

Normal hemoglobin levels are influenced by age, sex, ethnic group, and altitude. Normal values were calculated to a 95% reference range for a large population, thus providing the laboratory reference. Values for men are higher than for women, a finding attributed to testosterone. For children, the lower hemoglobin level at age 2 years (10.7 gm/dl) rises gradually until normal limits are reached by age 15 and 18 for girls and boys, respectively. Values for African-Americans are approximately 0.5–0.6 gm lower than for Caucasian Americans. In men older than 65 years, hemoglobin tends to decline; if the value of 12 gm/dl is used as the norm, 25% of patients may be abnormal, but the anemia has no pathologic etiology. It is also important to compare the patient's hemoglobin values over time, thus determining when deviation from the norm occurs. Mild anemia may be important primarily as a barometer of the patient's overall health and as an early clue to disease.

2. What are the most common causes of anemia?

Iron deficiency	25%
Blood loss	25%
Anemia of chronic disease	25%
Megaloblastic anemias	10%
Hemolysis	10%
Other bone marrow failure	5%

3. Can anemia be diagnosed by the physical exam?

Often physical examination is diagnostic only indirectly when anemia is severe: by resting tachycardia, wide pulse pressure, hyperdynamic precordium, or evidence of high-output heart failure. Pallor is highly subjective and influenced by vascular tone and intrinsic skin hue. Even absence of palmar creases in severe anemia is currently in question. When a patient appears pale in the face, conjunctiva, and mucous membranes, the physician is likely to order a complete blood count (CBC) to evaluate systemic illness. In most other instances, anemia is diagnosed asymptomatically or during the evaluation of other complaints.

4. How does the mean corpuscular volume (MCV) help in the differential diagnosis of anemia?

Classification of anemia has traditionally relied on the size of red blood cells (RBCs), as determined by the RBC volume. The normal MCV is 80–95 fl; values above and below this range define macrocytic and microcytic anemias, respectively. However, because the value represents the arithmetic mean of all RBCs, a mixed population of cells may contribute to the overall value. Furthermore, in several instances a single deficiency may be masked by a combined deficiency. Thus, low or high values of the MCV are useful in directing the diagnosis, but a normal MCV does not exclude any of the causes that may contribute to the etiology of anemia. The table below outlines the classification of anemia based on the MCV in conjunction with the reticulocyte count.

Practical Evaluation of Anemia

RETICULOCYTE	HALLMARK ON SMEAR	LABORATORY TESTS
Reticulocytes < 2%		
MCV low	*Microcytosis*	
Iron deficiency	—	Ferritin < 12 μg/L or ↓Fe/↑TIBC = Sat < 16%
		↓Fe/↑TIBC = Sat < 16%
Chronic disease	—	↓Fe/↑TIBC = Sat < 20%
		Ferritin low or may be > 100 μg/L
Thalassemia (αα–, β-minor, or HbE)	—	Hemoglobin electrophoresis normal, ↑A$_2$ or E
MCV high	*Macrocytosis*	
Vitamin B$_{12}$ deficiency	Multilobed neutrophils	B$_{12}$ level
Folate deficiency	Multilobed neutrophils	Serum/RBC folate
Myelodysplasia or other stem cell defect	—	Bone marrow aspiration and biopsy
MCV normal		
Early iron deficiency or chronic disease	Normal	As above
Renal or endocrine disease	Normal	As indicated
Marrow replacement or stem-cell diseases	Abnormal cells from the marrow; teardrops or nucleated red cells	Bone marrow biopsy
Mixed defects	Large and small cells, or normal	As needed from clinical suspicion
Corrected reticulocytes > 2%		**Tests for RBC breakdown**
Extravascular hemolysis	Spherocytes	Direct Coombs' test
Intravascular hemolysis	Abnormal RBC shapes and sizes	Tests for free hemoglobin, DIC evaluation
Intrinsic RBC defects	Clues: shapes, Heinz bodies	Evaluation for defect in RBC membrane, hemoglobinopathy, enzyme

MCV = mean corpuscular volume, TIBC = total iron-binding capacity, Sat = saturation, HbE = hemoglobin E, RBC = red blood cell, DIC = disseminated intravascular coagulation.

5. When is a reticulocyte count helpful?

The reticulocyte count is the only available measure of daily marrow production. As such, it is the most important test for determining whether anemia is due to increased RBC destruction or inadequate marrow production. Normal production of RBCs is 1–2% per day. Thus, any number less than 2% in the patient with anemia is considered inadequate production, which may be due to hematinic deficiencies (iron, vitamin B$_{12}$, folate); chronic inflammatory, endocrine, or renal disease; or infiltrating marrow diseases, such as tumor or primary stem-cell failure.

However, when the reticulocyte count is greater than 2%, further analysis is required to determine whether chronic stimulated marrow production due to increased destruction of RBCs is truly present. Because the reticulocyte count is expressed as a percentage of RBCs, measurement of daily production of RBCs requires correction of this percentage when the absolute RBC count is decreased (as in anemia). The following equation may be used for the correction:

Corrected reticulocyte = observed hematocrit/45 (used as the normal hematocrit)
                          × measured reticulocyte count

Alternatively, an absolute reticulocyte count $> 90 \times 10^9$ is considered increased. In reality, the severity of the increased destruction (hemolysis) tends to be reflected in the measured reticulocytes. More importantly, correction of the reticulocytes is a helpful reminder of underlying pathophysiology in the following circumstances: mild reticulocytosis with intramedullary hemolysis in B_{12} or folate deficiency when the underlying problem is hypoproliferative; after a single episode of acute hemorrhage with an appropriate marrow response; and in the instance of hemolytic disease, when it is necessary to determine whether the marrow is adequately responding (i.e., is the amount of iron or folate sufficient to maintain the marrow production needed for the increased destruction, or is the patient entering an aplastic crisis?).

6. When may the red blood cell volume distribution (RDW) be useful?

The RDW reflects the degree of homogeneity or heterogeneity in size among the RBCs. This measurement is meant to detect the degree of anisocytosis on a peripheral blood smear. A wide RDW may be the first clue to iron deficiency; a manifestation of dual populations of cells; or a sign of anisocytosis due to RBC fragments. The RDW may be highly sensitive for early iron deficiency, but it is not specific. A normal value is helpful in distinguishing thalassemia minor from iron deficiency as a cause of microcytosis.

7. When should the clinician evaluate the peripheral blood smear?

Ideally the smear should be evaluated in all patients with anemia or even leukocytosis, but this often becomes practically unfeasible and does not change the primary care provider's evaluation. Thus, it is important to determine when the smear should be further evaluated—a heretical but realistic approach. Often the smear needs to be viewed to confirm abnormalities detected by automated procedure before further work-up is pursued. Automated values require review of the smear in the following circumstances:

- Abnormal types of circulating cells; for example, blasts or lymphocytes
- Confirmation and evaluation of extremely high or low values of blood counts (especially platelets and neutrophils)
- RBC fragments of any type (teardrops, schistocytes, sickle cells)
- Perplexing hypoproliferative anemia to look for clues of rouleaux (paraprotein) or mixed populations of cells (large and small)
- Anemia with reticulocytosis to search for spherocytes or other clues, such as shape abnormalities in hereditary membrane disease

8. What are the indications for a bone marrow aspirate and/or biopsy?

The provider should obtain consultation for the purpose of a bone marrow analysis under the following circumstances:

1. Pancytopenia or bicytopenias
2. A peripheral blood smear that shows abnormal early cells (i.e., blast, myelocytes) or evidence of myelophthisis (teardrops)
3. For rare causes of anemia, such as sideroblastic anemia and pure RBC aplasia, which must be suspected because of unique clinical situations or in patients in whom the anemia is unexplained
4. Severe thrombocytopenias
5. Severe leukopenia
6. Monoclonal serum protein
7. Culture for granulomatous diseases in unique situations

A biopsy is not always indicated; however, when evaluation of cellularity or a search for tumor cells or other infiltrating disease is required, a biopsy is necessary along with the aspirate. Although bone marrow examination has traditionally been advocated for the evaluation of iron stores, the diagnosis of iron deficiency is made by other means.

9. Which single test most frequently yields a diagnosis of iron deficiency anemia?

Two laboratory tests are in common use to detect iron deficiency: the ferritin level, a measure of iron stores, and the serum iron saturation (serum iron/total iron-binding capacity [TIBC] = iron saturation; a value less than 16% in the presence of normal-to-high TIBC reflects iron deficiency). In uncomplicated cases of iron deficiency, the ferritin level most often leads to the diagnosis (level less than 12 µg/L). However, this test lacks sensitivity. A normal value does not exclude iron deficiency, but a value greater than 100 µg/L is inconsistent with iron deficiency. Both tests are not necessary in the initial evaluation; on occasion, however, both may prove helpful.

10. When is the ferritin level likely to be falsely elevated?

Ferritin reflects true iron overload at values greater than 100 µg/ml (hemochromatosis; hemosiderosis from blood cell dyscrasias). However, both inflammation and liver disease with destruction of hepatocytes increase ferritin to values ranging from 100 to > 1000 µg/ml.

11. What are the hallmarks of the anemia of chronic disease?

1. Nonprogressive anemia that usually does not fall below a hematocrit of 25% and parallels the severity of the underlying inflammatory disease. In this instance, inflammation is a broad term that includes systemic diseases accompanied by a major cellular response. An elevated sedimentation rate often correlates with the presence of chronic disease.

2. MCV that is not increased and usually is mildly decreased

3. Low reticulocyte count (less than 2%)

4. Low serum iron. The pathophysiologic problem appears to be tissue avidity for iron and failure to release iron to the serum; thus, although ferritin may be above normal, serum iron is characteristically low. This defect may be seen immediately in infectious processes, even before the 1–2 months required for the development of anemia with chronic inflammation. Low serum iron, often with a low TIBC, results in low iron saturation, which characterizes the anemia of chronic disease.

12. What further evaluation is required for the diagnosis of iron deficiency?

The etiology of the iron deficiency must be evaluated. A chronic loss of 3–4 cc of blood per day (1–2 mg of iron) leads to iron deficiency. Although gastrointestinal (GI) blood loss may occur with common entities, including use of nonsteroidal antiinflammatory drugs, aspirin, and anticoagulants, hemorrhoids, and various acid peptic entities (ulcers, esophagitis), they should not be assumed to be the etiology. Chronic loss of iron from the lower GI tract as an initial manifestation of malignancy must always be considered.

Another common cause of iron deficiency is menses. The history may provide clues to excessive menstrual loss; menses greater than 7 days in duration; passage of clots greater than 2 cm in size; and inability to control flow with tampons. In the absence of such manifestations, excessive menstrual flow is poorly assessed by the history.

Urinary blood loss is not a cause of iron deficiency, unless excessive gross hematuria is chronically present or unless intravascular hemolysis is persistent (as in the presence of a cardiac valve that causes hemolysis or in rare blood disorders, such as paroxysmal nocturnal hemoglobinemia).

The above observations have led to the practical clinical recommendations that men with GI blood loss and women over the age of 35–40 years require evaluation of iron deficiency anemia to exclude sources of occult GI blood loss due to malignant or premalignant lesions.

13. What is runner's anemia?

Iron deficiency has been seen in up to one-half of long-distance competitive runners. The cause of the iron loss appears to be chronic and multifactorial: low-grade intravascular hemolysis; low-grade hematuria; and low-grade GI loss. However, this diagnosis remains one of exclusion in populations at risk.

14. Can a patient have both iron deficiency and chronic disease?

Yes. Iron deficiency is particularly common in patients with rheumatoid arthritis, although it may be seen in other conditions. Clues to iron deficiency include a fall in the usually low hematocrit of chronic disease; ferritin < 100 µg/L; and a very low (5–10%) iron saturation. Oral iron supplementation may be given on a trial basis, with an anticipated increase in the hematocrit or hemoglobin to low plateau levels consistent with the inflammatory state.

Iron deficiency also may occur with a defect in folate or vitamin B_{12} and initially high iron studies. Thus normal iron studies in the presence of or at the initiation of treatment for folate or B_{12} deficiencies are not helpful in excluding iron deficiency. A more accurate reflection of iron stores is obtained when normal marrow maturation has resumed after replacement of B_{12} or folate.

15. How should iron deficiency be treated?

Multiple preparations are available to treat iron deficiency, with variable amounts of iron available for absorption. Overall, lower amounts of iron are better tolerated. Thus, ferrous gluconate or slow-release preparations may be better tolerated than traditional ferrous sulfate, 300 mg 3 times/day. However, the required rate of correction determines the choice of preparation. In any case, iron supplementation must be continued for 3–6 months beyond correction of the anemia.

Failure to correct iron deficiency is due to poor compliance, inadequate absorption, continued blood loss that exceeds supplementation, or incorrect diagnosis. Absorption may be enhanced by changing preparations or mode of administration. Systemic iron should be reserved for patients at extreme risk of malabsorption (inflammatory bowel disease).

16. When is evaluation of the folate level useful?

Evaluation of folate level is rarely useful in the usual patients at risk, such as nutritionally deficient patients who consume alcohol or the nutritionally replete patient who consumes alcohol but has a mildly elevated MCV. It is much more important to eliminate B_{12} deficiency as the cause of macrocytosis than to evaluate the serum folate level, which is easily and rapidly corrected by alcohol cessation or food intake. If the B_{12} level is normal, folate deficiency may likely be treated with multivitamin and folate supplements. If the B_{12} level is low, further evaluation is necessary, because spuriously low levels may be seen in folate deficiency. Although the evaluation of multiple levels, including folate, B_{12}, red blood cell folate, and iron, is common in the shotgun evaluation of anemia, the cost-effectiveness of this approach is suspect. As a marker of malabsorption in high-risk patients or in the evaluation of a difficult-to-diagnose anemia with megaloblastosis, evaluation of levels of serum and erythrocyte folate is clearly useful.

17. When should levels of vitamin B_{12} be measured?

In addition to the evaluation of megaloblastic anemia, certain conditions lead predictably to B_{12} deficiency or result from B_{12} deficiency in the absence of hematologic defects:

1. Gastrectomy, ileal resection, or malabsorption. Because stores of B_{12} are large, deficiency is not suspected until years later. The average time to deficiency after gastrectomy is 5 years (2–12-year range).

2. Neurologic complaints, especially with a peripheral neuropathy manifested by numbness and tingling, dementia, or evidence of posterior column disease, should prompt a search for vitamin B deficiency.

3. Associated immune disease, including the following:
   - Patients, usually young, who have combined variable immune deficiency or selective IgA deficiency.
   - Patients with autoimmune endocrinopathies, including Hashimoto's thyroiditis, Addison's disease, Graves' disease, and non–insulin-dependent diabetes.
   - Patients with other autoimmune disease: vitiligo, myasthenia gravis, primary ovarian failure.

18. What regulates the red blood cell mass?

RBC mass is maintained within well-defined limits through a feedback mechanism regulated by the hormone erythropoietin. Tissue oxygenation, as sensed within the kidney, governs the amount of hormone released from renal peritubular cells. Erythropoietin stimulates early marrow cells to undergo differentiation, proliferation, and maturation. Production and destruction of

RBCs in the spleen are carefully matched to tissue oxygen demands. Thus, maintenance of hemoglobin also depends on bone marrow that can respond adequately to external demands.

19. When is measurement of the erythropoietin level helpful?

In the presence of anemia, erythropoietin should be appropriately elevated for the level of hematocrit and is especially high with bone marrow failure. Measurement of erythropoietin is most useful for distinguishing high from normal values. The hormone level also is useful in distinguishing causes of erythrocytosis: high levels indicate secondary causes of erythropoietin secretion, whereas low levels indicate primary marrow-induced polycythemia. Measurement is helpful in considering the use of erythropoietin therapy for patients with malignancy or those diseases that may result in a blunted erythropoietin response to anemia. In patients with AIDS, an erythropoietin level > 500 IU/ml suggests that erythropoietin therapy will not be effective.

20. Which patients are candidates for therapy with erythropoietin?

1. Patients with chronic renal failure, undergoing dialysis or predialysis.

2. Patients with AIDS (on zidovudine therapy) who require transfusions. If the erythropoietin level is > 500 IU/ml, hormone therapy is not likely to be effective.

3. Patients with malignancy or undergoing treatment for cancer, in whom anemia is severe enough to result in transfusions and is likely to respond to erythropoietin. Treatment with erythropoietin may improve the anemia without exposing patients to the potential immunomodulating effect of transfusions.

4. Patients scheduled to undergo preoperative autologous blood donation in noncardiac, nonvascular surgery. A cost-effective approach may be to target patients whose initial hematocrit ranges between 33–39% and who are scheduled to undergo surgery in which blood loss is expected to be between 1000–3000 ml (e.g., hip replacement).

21. When may anemia be attributable to chronic renal failure?

The anemia of chronic renal failure, which is due to deficient production of erythropoietin, is not likely to become manifest clinically until the creatinine clearance is < 40 ml/min. There is a rough correlation between creatinine and anemia, although this correlation cannot be extrapolated to the individual patient. With polycystic kidney disease, the erythropoietin level appears to be maintained; patients become anemic much later (if at all) in the natural course of the disease. With progressive renal failure, additional causes of anemia must be considered, especially iron deficiency and volume expansion.

22. What laboratory tests support the diagnosis of hemolysis or increased RBC destruction?
Measures of cellular breakdown of RBCs

• *Bilirubin.* A slightly elevated bilirubin may be a clue to underlying RBC destruction in the absence of a hepatic explanation. However, the liver can compensate tremendously for increased bilirubin production. Thus, values over 4 mg/dl are likely to reflect liver disease as well as excessive RBC breakdown.

• *Lactate dehydrogenase (LDH).* Although nonspecific for red cells or hemolysis, the presence of an elevated LDH is consistent with the diagnosis of hemolysis.

Evidence of free hemoglobin

• *Low haptoglobin.* This protein, one of the measurable carriers of free hemoglobin, falls to undetectable levels as it is catabolized when it is bound to free hemoglobin. Thus haptoglobin may not be low in patients who have decreased RBC survival that is localized to the spleen (extravascular). Because haptoglobin may be elevated in inflammatory disease, the absolute value is not helpful clinically. However, an undetectable or very low level is consistent with hemolysis.

• *Free serum hemoglobin.* When overwhelming hemolysis is present, as in a mismatched transfusion reaction, free hemoglobin results in pink serum. Otherwise, hemoglobin is cleared and degraded quite rapidly.

- *Urine hemoglobin.* When haptoglobin is saturated, free hemoglobin dissociates into molecules that pass freely through the glomerulus and thus are detected in the urine when the tubular reabsorption threshold is exceeded. Therefore, urine hemoglobin is also a measure of hemolysis due to excessive RBC breakdown, if other mechanisms cannot clear serum hemoglobin.
- *Urine hemosiderin.* With excessive free serum hemoglobin, free heme pigment may precipitate in the distal tubular cells. Hemoglobin iron in the renal epithelial cell is rapidly stored as hemosiderin or ferritin. As the tubular cell sloughs, hemosiderin and iron can be measured in the urine. Thus, urine hemosiderin is a good measure of chronic intravascular hemolysis. After a single episode of hemolysis, measurement of urine hemosiderin may not be positive for 2–3 days, but it may then persist for up to 14 days. Thus it is a useful clue for an earlier event.

23. What classic disease results in extravascular hemolysis?

Autoimmune hemolytic anemia results in shortened RBC survival due to complement and/or antibody detection on the RBC membrane by the splenic macrophage. Hallmarks of the disease are the spherocyte and the direct Coombs'-positive antibody test in the presence of reticulocytosis. A spleen tip is palpable in one-half of patients. The majority of all other hemolysis is due to intravascular causes (including RBC mechanical or fibrinous breakdown in the vascular space) or intrinsic RBC defects.

24. What considerations should be given to optimizing hemoglobin concentration in patients with chronic anemia?

Although patients with chronic anemia appear to tolerate low hemoglobin better than patients with acute anemia, consideration should be given to optimizing oxygen-carrying capacity (by transfusion, erythropoietin, or autologous transfusion) in certain circumstances:

1. Patients with underlying symptomatic coronary artery disease
2. Patients with poor exercise and temperature tolerance who wish to be more physically active (including patients with cancer or chronic inflammatory disease)
3. Elderly patients who require surgery and are at risk from both poor systemic perfusion that may result in stroke or myocardial infarction and also from poor wound healing and infection postoperatively. Some evidence suggests that poor surgical outcomes are associated with anemia.

25. How common is iron deficiency in adolescents?

As many as 11–25% of adolescent girls are iron-deficient, although a much smaller percentage have anemia (whereas only 1% of adolescent boys and men are iron-deficient). A recent double-blind, placebo-controlled trial in an urban population suggests that iron-replete adolescent girls perform better on tests of verbal learning and memory than their placebo-treated counterparts. Given its high prevalence, iron deficiency should be searched for on a regular basis in adolescent girls.

26. When is parenteral iron therapy indicated?

Rarely. The ease of oral iron replacement, despite the issue of compliance, and the risk associated with parenteral therapy should lead to the use of parenteral iron only after careful consideration and clear indications. The most serious risk is anaphylaxis (1–2%); other less serious adverse effects occur in as many as 25% of patients treated with iron dextran. Thus, prudence suggests that parenteral iron therapy should be given only (1) after failure of an oral iron absorption test (administration of an oral bolus of 325 mg ferrous sulfate and measurement of serum iron level of 115 µg/dl higher than the pretest level) or (2) when iron needs cannot be met by oral doses because of continued loss of iron through the gastrointestinal tract or intravascular hemolysis. Intolerance to oral iron therapy should be considered an indication only in rare circumstances (if at all).

BIBLIOGRAPHY

1. Beutler E, Lichtman MA, Coller BS, Kipps TJ (eds): Williams' Hematology, 5th ed. New York, McGraw-Hill, 1993.
2. Bruner AB, Joffe A, Duggan AK, et al: Randomized study of cognitive effects of iron supplementation in non-anemia iron-deficient adolescent girls. Lancet 384:992–996, 1996.
3. Eichner ER: Runner's macrocytosis: Runner's anemia as a benefit versus runner's hemolysis as a detriment. Am J Med 78:321–325, 1985.
4. Goodnough LT, Monk TG, Andriole GL: Erythropoietin therapy. N Engl J Med 336:933–938, 1997.
5. Greenbur AG: Pathophysiology of anemia. Am J Med 101(Suppl 2A):7S–11S, 1996.
6. Guyatt GH, Oxman AD, Willan M, et al: Laboratory diagnosis of iron deficiency anemia: An overview. J Gen Intern Med 7:145–153, 1992.
7. Jandl JH: Blood: Textbook of Hematology, 2nd ed. Boston, Little, Brown, 1996.
8. Krause JR: Blood smear evaluation. Hematol Oncol Clin North Am 8:631, 650, 1994.
9. Looker AC, Dallman PR, Carroll MD, et al: Prevalence of iron deficiency in the United States. JAMA 277:973–976, 1997.
10. Mladenovic J, Roodman D: Normocytic anemia. In Spivak J (ed): Textbook of Hematology. Baltimore, Johns Hopkins Press, 1993, pp 91–100.
11. Swain RA, Kaplan B, Montgomery E: Iron deficiency anemia: When is parenteral therapy warranted? Postgrad Med 100:181–193, 1996.
12. Toh BH, Van Driel IR, Gleeson PA: Pernicious anemia. N Engl J Med 227:1441–1448, 1997.

62. LYMPHADENOPATHY AND SPLENOMEGALY

Jeanette Mladenovic, M.D.

1. Why is it important to know the common drainage patterns of lymph nodes amenable to palpation?

Recognizing common drainage patterns of lymph nodes facilitates assessment of the anatomic location of infectious etiologies and potential serious pathology.

Cervical nodes:	Head, ears, eyes, nose, and throat (HEENT) area
Submental and submandibular area:	Salivary glands and mouth
Pre- and postauricular area:	Eyes, scalp, ears
Supraclavicular nodes:	Intrathoracic and intraabdominal areas, in addition to ears, nose, and throat
Axillary nodes:	Breast and thorax
Epitrochlear nodes:	Hand and forearm
Inguinal nodes:	Lower extremities and genitalia
	Femoral and pelvic area

2. Which palpable lymph nodes suggest a malignancy?

1. Supraclavicular nodes are generally not palpable. When they are enlarged, they suggest thoracic malignancy on the right and thoracic or upper gastrointestinal (GI) malignancy on the left (called a Virchow's node).

2. Enlarged femoral nodes complicating usual inguinal adenopathy should raise suspicion.

3. Enlarged periumbilical nodes (Sister Mary Joseph nodes) signify advanced GI malignancy.

3. Which palpable lymph nodes are probably benign?

1. Palpable nodes (1–2 cm) in the anterior cervical area are common under 12 years and persist with diminishing frequency to age 30 years. In addition, almost all children have palpable axillary and inguinal adenopathy.

2. Mild insignificant bilateral inguinal adenopathy is common throughout life.

3. Isolated posterior cervical lymphadenopathy is usually benign.

4. List the most common causes of generalized diffuse lymphadenopathy in the United States.

Infectious, inflammatory, and malignant diseases account for the majority of lymphadenopathy in clinical practice. Rare storage or lymph node diseases and occasionally hyperthyroidism also may present as generalilzed lymphadenopathy. If a patient has recently traveled to or is from an area with endemic parasitic infections, other causes must be considered.

Infectious diseases	Infectious mononucleosis, cytomegalovirus (CMV), hepatitis A
	Human immunodeficiency virus (HIV), syphilis, toxoplasmosis
	Coccidiomycosis, histoplasmosis
Inflammatory diseases	Sarcoidosis
	Rheumatoid arthritis, systemic lupus erythematosus (SLE), dermatomyositis
	Serum sickness
	Drug reaction (phenytoin)
Malignant diseases	Non-Hodgkin's lymphoma
	Acute or chronic lymphoid or myeloid leukemias
Nonhematologic malignancies	Germ cell tumors, melanoma, breast cancer

5. What is the classic difference between the presentation of Hodgkin's disease and non-Hodgkin's lymphoma?

Non-Hodgkin's lymphoma spreads and often presents with diffuse lymphadenopathy. Classic Hodgkin's disease has a predictable pattern of spread in contiguous groups; thus, isolated lymphadenopathy in contiguously draining areas is more characteristic of Hodgkin's disease.

6. What finding on peripheral blood smear almost always accompanies the diagnosis of infectious mononucleosis?

Mononucleosis is the most common infectious cause of lymphadenopathy in young people. It is often accompanied by pharyngitis and constitutional symptoms. In > 95% of patients the peripheral blood smear shows atypical lymphocytes. Atypical lymphocytes and/or lymphocytosis also may be seen in other conditions, such as CMV, hepatitis, lymphoid malignancy (especially chronic lymphocytic leukemia), toxoplasmosis, serum sickness, and phenytoin lymphadenopathy.

7. For what complications of infectious mononucleosis should corticosteroid therapy be considered?

After a confirmed diagnosis of infectious mononucleosis (monospot or Epstein-Barr virus testing), corticosteroids may be indicated for obstructing tonsillar enlargement, autoimmune thrombocytopenia, severe granulocytopenia, and/or hemolytic anemia. Patients with splenomegaly should limit sports involvement to avoid rupture.

8. When should a lymph node be biopsied?

Biopsy of a lymph node, in most instances, is a minor procedure. The timing of biopsy depends on the clinical presentation, age of the patient, and suspicion of the diagnosis. Certainly, systemic symptoms suggesting malignancy should prompt earlier diagnosis. Careful follow-up is essential, because infectious lymphadenopathy usually improves or recedes in 14 days. Thus, sampling of the lymph node should be performed:

1. When the node is very large or has associated skin changes with matting

2. When the lymph node has increased in size in an area associated with a high incidence of malignancy; or

3. When an isolated lymph node with no clear site of local infection has not receded in 2–3 weeks or when diffuse lymphadenopathy with no clear etiology has not improved in 2–3 weeks.

9. When is lymph node fine-needle aspiration (FNA) not the initial procedure of choice?

FNA is helpful to confirm a suspected diagnosis of infection or metastatic malignancy. It does not provide adequate tissue to distinguish architecture or type of lymphoma or to perform cellular or molecular studies that differentiate tumor origin. Because lymphoma is usually an important diagnostic consideration in many patients undergoing lymph node biopsy, time to diagnosis and treatment should be minimized; thus biopsy is the preferred initial procedure.

10. What is the significance of a nondiagnostic lymph node biopsy?

Lymph node biopsy provides a diagnosis in more than 50% of adults. Up to one-fourth of the patients with nondiagnostic biopsies develop lymphoma in the following year. Thus, careful follow-up of a patient with a nondiagnostic biopsy is mandatory.

11. Does bilateral hilar lymphadenopathy always require a tissue diagnosis?

Isolated bilateral hilar adenopathy in a patient with characteristics and systemic manifestations of sarcoidosis may be followed. The classic patient is an African-American woman with erythema nodosum. However, asymmetry and additional symptoms should prompt aggressive diagnosis, because the differential diagnosis includes lymphoma, lung carcinoma, tuberculosis, and histoplasmosis.

12. How are retroperitoneal lymph nodes evaluated?

Computed tomography (CT) delineates the size of retroperitoneal nodes, including paraaortic nodal areas. The lymphangiogram is now rarely used. Although it may provide more distinct morphology, it does not easily visualize the upper paraaortic areas and is inconvenient and difficult to perform. Once lymph nodes are found on a CT scan, CT-directed lymph node biopsy may be undertaken. Another alternative, depending on the available expertise, is sonographically guided percutaneous biopsy of small lymph nodes in the abdomen, retroperitoneum, and pelvis. In one study, 86% (30/35 specimens) of lymph nodes of 2–2.5 cm were successfully biopsied.

13. What is the significance of massive splenomegaly?

Massive splenomegaly is most consistent with diseases of hematologic origin:

Myeloproliferative diseases
  Myelofibrosis
  Chronic myelogneous leukemia
  End-stage polycythemia vera or essential thrombocythemia
Neoplastic diseases
  Hairy cell leukemia
  Hodgkin's or non-Hodgkin's lymphoma
  Chronic lymphocytic leukemia
  Malignant reticuloendotheliosis

Other less common diseases are usually apparent from other symptoms and signs. Rarely, infiltrative disease (Gaucher's disease), infectious causes (malaria), or inflammatory diseases (sarcoidosis, Felty's syndrome) may present as isolated massive splenomegaly. Massive splenomegaly is seen with thalassemia major, but the majority of other hemoglobinopathies result in lesser splenomegaly.

14. What is the significance of a palpable spleen tip?

A palpable spleen tip usually suggests mild-to-moderate splenic enlargement (except in children) and may be due to any of the diseases that cause diffuse lymphadenopathy, because the spleen is yet another organ of the lymph system. Thus, systemic acute or chronic infection is the most common cause of palpable splenomegaly. Systemic inflammatory diseases that cause lymphadenopathy also may cause splenomegaly, with or without lymph node enlargement (e.g., rheumatoid arthritis, SLE). However, two other categories of diseases should be considered when a spleen tip is palpable:

Congestive diseases: Vascular congestion may be due to portal vein hypertension, hepatic vein thrombosis, or portal or splenic vein thrombosis.

Hematologic diseases: Hemolytic disease due to immune, enzyme, or membrane etiologies. Sickle cell disease of the SS variety is not accompanied by splenomegaly.

15. How can one evaluate the size and function of the spleen?

Besides physical exam, splenic size and consistency (cysts, tumors) may be evaluated by technetium scan, CT, or ultrasound, depending on the level of suspicion. Splenic function may be evaluated by viewing the peripheral blood smear. The finding of Howell-Jolly bodies suggests a nonfunctional spleen. A splenic scan with labeled red cells also may determine size and function.

16. Which patients manifest hypersplenism?

Hypersplenism consists of mild-to-moderate pancytopenia; various cell types are affected to varying detectable degrees. Cells are sequestered in the spleen, as an exaggeration of the spleen's normal function. Thus, anemia with short survival, thrombocytopenia, and leukopenia constitute hypersplenism, which usually complicates diseases that cause splenomegaly by congestion or hypertrophy of the phagocytic elements. Infiltrative diseases (lymphoma, chronic lymphocytic leukemia) usually do not manifest hypersplenism.

17. When is a sentinel node biopsy considered?

In patients with cutaneous melanoma, injection of a radioactive tracer at the site of the primary tumor (before wide excision) delineates the tumor's first draining node. This sentinel node is then removed and examined for metastatic tumor and helps to determine further lymph node dissection and/or therapy.

BIBLIOGRAPHY

1. Brady BS, Coit DG: Sentinel lymph node evaluation in melanoma. Arch Dermatol 133:1014–1020, 1997.
2. Crosby JH: The role of fine-needle aspiration biopsy in the diagnosis and management of palpable masses. J Med Assoc Ga 85:33–36, 1996.
3. Fijlen G: Unexplained adenopathy in family practice: An evaluation of the probability of malignant causes and the effectiveness of the physician's work-up. J Fam Pract 27:373, 1988.
4. Fisher AJ, Paulson EK, Sheafor DH, et al: Small lymph nodes of the abdomen, pelvis, and retroperitoneum: Usefulness of sonographically guided biopsy. Radiology 205:185–190, 1997.
5. Kunitz G: An approach to peripheral lymphadenopathy in adult patients. West J Med 143:393, 1985.
6. Libman H: Generalized adenopathy: Clinical reviews. J Gen Intern Med 2:48, 1987.
7. Pierson FG: Staging of the mediastinum: Role of mediastinoscopy and computed tomography. Chest 103(Suppl 4):3465–3485, 1993.

63. BLEEDING AND THROMBOCYTOPENIA

Jeanette Mladenovic, M.D.

1. What history is important in diagnosing a congenital bleeding disorder?

Careful inquiry into prolonged bleeding with minor common surgeries or insignificant trauma is the most helpful element of the history. Specifically, unusual or prolonged bleeding with circumcision, tonsillectomy, or tooth extraction provides strong clues. A history of hemarthrosis also is suggestive. The common congenital bleeding abnormalities of varying severity that present early or late in life include hemophilia A or B, von Willebrand's disease, and congenital platelet disorders. Of equal importance is the family history in patients who may be suspected of congenital abnormality. Even mild symptoms may be compatible with inherited disorders.

2. What are the major components of the hemostatic system?

The major components of the hemostatic system are platelets, blood coagulation proteins, and structural support of the vasculature. All components should be investigated in a bleeding patient or a patient with evidence of even a mild bleeding abnormality on physical exam. In acute bleeding, a structural lesion (e.g., postoperative bleeders) is likely when platelets and coagulation parameters are corrected. In a patient complaining of recurrent bruisability, failure to consider problems in vascular support may lead to a missed diagnosis (e.g., amyloidosis, vasculitis).

3. What abnormalities on physical examination suggest a bleeding disorder?

Major findings include petechiae and ecchymoses. Isolated thrombocytopenia usually results in petechiae. However, petechiae are seen at lower levels of thrombocytopenia when the platelets are young and highly functional than when the defect is due to poor production and/or dysfunctional platelets, as in myeloproliferative diseases. Ecchymoses, especially in areas not usually subjected to trauma, suggest abnormalities of the coagulation proteins, platelet dysfunction, or vascular fragility. Mucosal bleeding from gingiva or as epistaxis in the absence of other explanations also may suggest a bleeding abnormality. Active oozing from puncture sites is consistent with severe defects in any component of the hemostatic system and also suggests activation of the fibrinolytic system, as in disseminated intravascular coagulation (DIC).

4. What tests measure function of the coagulation system?

The prothrombin time (PT) and the activated partial thromboplastin time (aPTT) measure separate components of the coagulation system in vitro. A normal PT suggests that factor VII and other vitamin K-dependent factors contributing to the common pathway are functionally adequate. A normal aPTT suggests adequate function of factors VIII, IX, and XI. Prolongation of the PT and/or aPTT may be due to inadequate levels of factors or to specific or nonspecific inhibitors.

5. In what circumstances are PT and PTT useful in the initial evaluation of a patient?

PT and PTT are useful in evaluating patients who have the following diseases or history:

Hematologic malignancies   History of bleeding
Hepatobiliary disease   Anticoagulant use
Malnutrition or malabsorption   Systemic lupus erythematosus

6. Are abnormalities of the coagulation system possible in patients with normal PT and PTT?

PT and PTT may be normal in rare patients with mild acquired von Willebrand's disease or abnormalities in factor XIII, alpha-2 plasmin inhibitor, or platelet procoagulant. If a strong history of bleeding (recurrent mucosal bleeding, large muscle hematoma with minimal trauma) is suspected, such disorders are still possible; referral to a hematologist is helpful.

7. List the critical levels of platelets that should direct assessment of bleeding risk.

20,000/mm³: Spontaneous bleeding in the absence of trauma is unusual until platelet counts fall below this level. Spontaneous bleeding is routinely seen with platelets counts of < 5000/mm³.

50,000/mm³: This level is recommended to prevent bleeding after surgery and to maintain hemostasis postoperatively or with trauma.

100,000/mm³: This level, which is compatible with a normal bleeding time, may be required for patients who must undergo major surgery in which hemostasis is paramount (neurosurgery, cardiac surgery) or who have severe defects in the coagulation system or endogenous platelets before surgery.

8. How are platelets evaluated?

Platelets are evaluated by number and function. A low number should be confirmed by viewing the peripheral blood smear and estimating a count of 15,000/mm³ per single platelet viewed on high-power field. The presence of large platelets may help to diagnose immune destruction. Function is evaluated by bleeding time, which also is related to platelet number (100,000 platelets/mm³ are needed for a normal bleeding time). Evaluation of bleeding time, however, is subject to variability in performance and in correlation with bleeding diathesis (especially preoperative or preprocedure evaluation). It may be most helpful in the positive diagnosis of a platelet defect, such as in von Willebrand's disease, or a myeloproliferative disease with thrombocytosis. In addition, the diagnosis of immune thrombocytopenia is corroborated by a short bleeding time with thrombocytopenia.

9. Should patients be screened preoperatively by a bleeding time?
The bleeding time has not proved to be useful in the routine evaluation of patients who are undergoing major surgery as a predictor of intraoperative or postoperative bleeding. A normal bleeding times does not exclude major hemorrhage, nor does it identify patients who have recently ingested aspirin. The best screening tools remain the history and physical examination. In the presence of a bleeding history, evaluation before surgery should include the bleeding time in addition to other tests of coagulation (platelet count, PT, and aPTT initially).

10. What common acquired systemic diseases are associated with bleeding?
Liver and renal failure.

11. List the causes of bleeding in liver disease.
Abnormalities that lead to bleeding in liver disease may be due to structural, hemostatic, or therapeutic causes.
Structural causes
Portal hypertension with varices
Increased incidence of peptic ulceration and gastritis
Hemostatic causes
Decreased hepatic synthesis of procoagulant proteins (fibrinogen, prothrombin, factors V, VII, IX, X, and XI)
Decreased absorption and metabolism of vitamin K
Decreased clearance of activated coagulation proteins
Therapeutic causes
Dilution of proteins and platelets from massive transfusions
Increase in bleeding with therapeutic endoscopy

12. Why are patients with renal failure at risk for increased bleeding?
Chronic uremia is associated with abnormalities in platelet function, which may be improved with dialysis (although the bleeding time does not correct). The bleeding diathesis may be corrected by desmopressin, cryoprecipitate, estrogen, or erythropoietin therapy, depending on which is most appropriate for the patient's clinical needs.

13. What contributes to thrombocytopenia in patients who chronically abuse alcohol?
Direct toxicity of alcohol: Once alcohol is discontinued, the platelet count should rise and return to normal within 1 week in most patients.
Hypersplenism due to portal hypertension: Hypersplenism alone should not lead to a platelet count significantly lower than 50–60,000/mm^3.
Folate deficiency: Folate is required for hematopoiesis; thus folate deficiency may contribute to thrombocytopenia, usually when megaloblastosis and leukopenia are also evident.

14. What diagnosis is likely in a young child with petechiae?
If the complete blood count demonstrates isolated thrombocytopenia, the likely diagnosis is immune thrombocytopenic purpura. This syndrome follows a viral exanthem or upper respiratory illness, and the majority of patients recover spontaneously, usually in 4–6 weeks. Diagnosis is made by the history; by evaluation of the peripheral blood smear, which shows isolated decreased numbers of large platelets; and by bone marrow aspiration, which eliminates an atypical presentation of a more severe hematologic disease as the cause. Transfused platelets are short-lived and sensitize the patient; thus, transfusion should be reserved for severe bleeding. An increased

incidence of central nervous system bleeding is seen with severe thrombocytopenia (< 5–10,000 platelets/mm^3). If needed, prednisone is the drug of choice for initial therapy.

15. What drugs are the most common offenders in drug-induced thrombocytopenia?

Besides alcohol, the best-documented drugs in common practice that cause thrombocytopenia include thiazide diuretics; quinidine and quinine (from tonic water); sulfathiazole; heparin; estrogens; and myelosuppressive chemotherapy. Many other drugs are suspect; the exact cause is documented in only 10% of patients with drug-induced thrombocytopenia. Thus, the best confirmation of drug-induced thrombocytopenia is a prompt rise in platelet count after removal of the drug (in most patients, within 7–10 days). This reaction to a drug should be clearly documented in the patient's chart so that rechallenge does not occur.

16. How is DIC diagnosed?

Clinical setting: DIC should be considered in obstetric catastrophes or in severely ill patients with sepsis, hypoperfusion, nonviable tissue, massive cell breakdown, or malignancy.

Laboratory confirmation: Ongoing activation of the clotting system is evidenced by consumption of coagulation factors, platelets, and secondary fibrinolysis (as demonstrated by circulating dimers, a specific manifestation of plasmin cleavage). Thus, thrombocytopenia or prolongation of the PT and aPTT in the presence of a low fibrinogen level confirms DIC in the appropriate setting. Clinical bleeding correlates best with the fibrinogen level; levels less than 100 µg/ml are likely to require therapy. The presence of nonspecific fibrin degradation products and schistocytes on peripheral blood smear is confirmatory, but their absence does not rule out the diagnosis. However, marked elevation of D-dimers, antigenic fragments released only during plasmin-induced lysis of cross-linked fibrinogen, is a specific marker of DIC. This test provides a reliable laboratory diagnosis of DIC.

17. What is gestational thrombocytopenia?

As a result of automatic platelet counts, asymptomatic thrombocytopenia has been recognized more frequently during normal gestation. The platelet count, normal prior to pregnancy, falls in up to 8% of women during normal gestation. This thrombocytopenia may reach levels as low as 80,000 at delivery but is not accompanied by bleeding or obstetric or fetal complications. The platelet count returns to normal after delivery. Gestational thrombocytopenia is *not* accompanied by hypertension, proteinuria, elevated liver enzymes, or progression to lower platelet counts; thus, it should not be confused with preeclampsia or the HELLP syndrome.

18. What are the complications of platelet transfusions?

Platelet transfusions carry all of the risks of red cell transfusions, with some additions. Febrile, nonhemolytic reactions are more common with platelets (especially with random donor platelets) than with red cells. Although the risk of known viral pathogens has been minimized, platelet transfusions carry a higher risk of bacterial infections—frequently with skin saprophytes.

However, the effectiveness of platelet transfusions is easily decreased by the patient with fever, infection, hypersplenism, DIC, or treatment with amphotericin. Alloimmunization to platelet-specific antigens and HLA may occur with regular transfusions. This problem should be suspected when a platelet increment 1 hour after infusion is less than approximately 7500/U (adjusted for body surface area of the patient).

19. When are patients who have used aspirin no longer at risk for bleeding?

Patients who discontinue aspirin for 3 days are likely to have enough newly produced, unaffected platelets to prevent bleeding. The platelets of such patients also may be used in a donor pool. Total replacement of the platelet pool does not occur until 8–16 days.

BIBLIOGRAPHY

1. American Society of Hematology Practice Guidelines: Diagnosis and treatment of immune thrombocytopenic purpura. Am Fam Physician 54:2437–2447; 2451–2452, 1996.

2. Bell WR, Kickler TS: Thrombocytopenia in pregnancy. Rheum Dis Clin North Am 23:183–194, 1997.
3. Ebert ME, Berkowitz LR: Hemostasis in renal diseases: Pathophysiology and management. Am J Med 96:168–179, 1994.
4. Hassouna HI: Laboratory evaluation of hemostatic abnormalities. Hematol Oncol Clin North Am 7:1161–1249, 1993.
5. Hussein MA, Hoeltge GA: Platelet transfusion therapy for medical and surgical patients. Cleve Clin J Med 63:245–250, 1996.
6. Jandl JH: Blood: Textbook of Hematology, 2nd ed. Boston, Little, Brown, 1996.
7. Kirchner JT: Acute and chronic immune thrombocytopenic purpura. Postgrad Med 92(6):112–118, 125–126, 1992.
8. Kitchens CS: Approach to the bleeding patient. Hematol Oncol Clin North Am 6:983–989, 1992.
9. Mammen EF: Coagulated defects in liver disease. Med Clin North Am 78:545–554, 1994.
10. McMillan R: Therapy for adults with refractory chronic immune thrombocytopenia purpura. Ann Intern Med 126:307–314, 1997.
11. Parker RI: Etiology and treatment of acquired coagulopathies in the critically ill adult and child. Crit Care Clin 13:591–609, 1997.
12. Peterson P, Hayes TE, Arkin CF, et al: The preoperative bleeding time test lacks clinical benefit. College of American Pathologists and American Society of Clinical Pathologists. Arch Surg 133:134–139, 1998.
13. Rutherford CJ, Frenkel EP: Thrombocytopenia: Issues in diagnosis and therapy. Med Clin North Am 78:555–575, 1994.

64. THROMBOSIS AND ANTICOAGULATION

Jeanette Mladenovic, M.D.

1. What are acceptable indications for chronic anticoagulation therapy?

Chronic anticoagulation may be indicated on a short-term (3–6 months) or long-term (lifelong) basis.

Short-term use
Pulmonary emboli
Proximal deep venous thrombosis (DVT)
New bioprosthetic mitral valves with sinus rhythm
Anterior wall transmural infarction with congestive heart failure

Long-term use (1 year or lifelong)
Cardiac disease
Prosthetic mechanical valves
Recurrent (not lone) or persistent atrial fibrillation
Cardiomyopathy with left ventricular (LV) thrombus or emboli
Rheumatic valve disease with embolism, atrial fibrillation, or atrium > 5.5 cm
Recurrent emboli from noninfectious endocarditis or atrial myxoma
Acquired antiphospholipid antibody syndrome with recurrent emboli
Malignancy with recurrent emboli
Inherited disorders of hypercoagulability with recurrent emboli
Systemic emboli from unknown source

2. In what clinical conditions should heparin rather than warfarin be given?

Heparin should be administered in the acute management of thrombosis; for the prevention of thrombosis, especially in operative or hospitalized patients; and in patients in whom sodium warfarin is contraindicated.

Acute management
Venous thrombosis or thromboembolism
Acute thromboembolism
Unstable angina (3–5 days)

Prevention of thromboembolism
>   Preparation for cardioversion
>   General abdominal surgery
>   Orthopedic surgery of the lower extremity
>   Pregnant patients with history of thrombosis
>   Patients with known inherited hypercoagulopathy before surgery, pregnancy, and other situations at high risk for thrombosis

Warfarin contraindicated
>   Maintenance of anticoagulation during invasive surgical procedures
>   Pregnancy, as prevention or treatment for thromboembolism
>   History of warfarin skin necrosis
>   Warfarin failure in malignancy

3. What are the advantages of low-molecular-weight heparin (LMWH) compared with unfractionated heparin?

Because of its lower molecular weight and thus modified pharmacology, LMWH offers several advantages compared with unfractionated heparin:

1. Longer circulating half-life
2. Greater and more predictable bioavailability (less protein and cell binding)
3. Less inhibitory effect on platelets and thrombin
4. Lower incidence of thrombocytopenia
5. Lower incidence of osteoporosis during prolonged administration

These differences translate into less need to monitor therapy and lower costs of care because patients may be managed on an outpatient basis and because they require fewer laboratory tests. Theoretically, heparin-associated bleeding is expected to be lower; however, this advantage has yet to be consistently demonstrated in clinical trials.

4. Can the effect of LMWH be measured?

Yes. A test of anti-Xa activity is required; the effect cannot be measured by the activated partial thromboplastin time (aPTT). However, before initiating therapy with LMWH, the platelet count, PT, and PTT should be measured initially to determine the patient's underlying coagulation status. More importantly, anti-Xa activity should be assessed in patients with unexpected bleeding complications and in patients with renal failure; in addition, anti-Xa activity perhaps should be evaluated in patients weighing < 50 kg or > 80 kg. Although recommendations for the use of LMWH in pregnancy are evolving, if LMWH is used, anti-Xa activity should be monitored during the late stages of pregnancy.

5. Why must heparin be continued during initiation of warfarin therapy?

There is a time lag between the peak level of warfarin, the prothrombin time (PT), and the therapeutic functional anticoagulation. This lag is due to the time required for normal anticoagulation factors to disappear from plasma after their synthesis has ceased. Thus, the PT is maximally prolonged at 72 hours after warfarin administration, when levels of factor VII and protein C fall, but the antithrombotic action does not peak until 7 days, when factors IX and X are significantly depressed. For this reason, heparin administration must continue for 3–5 days while warfarin is instituted. Large loading doses of warfarin are not indicated, because they cannot hasten the initial action.

6. What is the international normalized ratio (INR)?

Warfarin impairs the synthesis of vitamin K-dependent coagulation factors in the liver. Because the PT reflects 3 of the 4 vitamin K-dependent coagulation factors, this test historically has been used to monitor the anticoagulant effect of warfarin. However, standardizing optimal therapeutic regimens has been difficult, because the laboratory reagent used in the test (the thromboplastin) varies widely and thus produces significant variation in results. The INR compares the patient's PT to a population control adjusted for thromboplastin. Thus, the INR allows physicians to follow published recommendations for anticoagulation. Most indications require an

INR of 2–3; the exceptions are patients with mechanical valves, arterial emboli, or recurrent emboli, in whom the INR should be maintained at 3–4.5.

7. When should fibrinolytic agents be considered?

Fibrinolytic agents activate plasminogen and are directed at the site of fibrin thrombi to cause dissolution. Currently streptokinase (in some instances, the more expensive tissue plasminogen activator [TPA]) is indicated in following circumstances: acute coronary occlusion, acute peripheral artery occlusion, and massive pulmonary embolus resulting in hemodynamic compromise. Streptokinase also should be considered in the therapy of axillary vein thromboses and massive iliofemoral vein thromboses. Likewise, thrombolysis with fibrinolytic agents is used locally in thrombosed arteriovenous shunts and arterial or venous cannulas.

8. When is anticoagulation contraindicated?

In general	Active bleeding
	Recent cerebrovascular hemorrhage
	Severe congenital or acquired defects in hemostasis
	Recent major surgery, especially of the central nervous system or eye
	Malignant hypertension
Heparin	Thrombocytopenia with thrombosis
Warfarin	Skin necrosis
	Pregnancy
Fibrinolytic agents	Immediately after external cardiac massage
	Patients with a predisposition to intracranial bleeding: untreated hypertension, head trauma, intracranial neoplasms
Relative contra-indications	Severe hepatic or renal disease
	History of falling or unstable gait
	History of GI, genitourinary, or intracranial hemorrhage
	Requirement of high-dose salicylate or nonsteroidal therapy
	Poor compliance

9. How do other drugs affect the PT?

Numerous drugs affect warfarin therapy by various mechanisms. Recall of all specific drugs effects is impractical; thus, the *Physicians' Desk Reference* (PDR) should be consulted. In addition, the results of drug interactions in individual patients require regular monitoring (every 4–6 weeks when stabilized). However, some general classes of drugs and their effects should be commonly recognized as complicating warfarin therapy.

Increased PT or INR through enhanced potency

Reduced warfarin clearance or binding	Disulfiram
	Metronidazole
	Trimethoprim-sulfamethoxazole
	Phenylbutazone
Increased vitamin K turnover	Clofibrate

Decreased PT or INR through decreased potency

Increased hepatic metabolism	Barbiturates
	Rifampin
Reduced drug absorption	Cholestyramine

10. Which clinical situations are likely to yield increased sensitivity to warfarin or bleeding while on warfarin?

Systemic diseases	Liver disease
	Renal disease
	Hyperthyroidism

Additive to other anticoagulant states   Vitamin K deficiency
                                                Thrombocytopenia
                                                Therapy with heparin
                                                Therapy with aspirin

11. What is the risk of bleeding with use of warfarin?

Up to 10% of patients taking warfarin for 1 year have bleeding complications that require medical intervention. Fatal complications occur as frequently as 1/100 patient years of therapy, despite careful medical management. The highest risk for bleeding is at the initiation of therapy, when patients should be seen frequently. Factors that increase the risk for bleeding are underlying GI, urologic, or neurologic lesions and hypertension. Bleeding usually can be controlled by administration of vitamin K and infusion of fresh frozen plasma.

12. Who is at risk of bleeding from heparin?

Bleeding has not been prevented by frequent monitoring and does not correlate with any clinical assay. Bleeding after surgery or trauma may be severe. Certain patients are at particular risk:
- Patients on drugs that inhibit platelet function
- Patients with renal failure
- Patients with thrombocytopenia
- Postmenopausal women
- Patients with underlying anatomic lesions

Bleeding usually can be managed by discontinuing heparin therapy. However, if necessary, rapid reversal can be accomplished by the slow administration of protamine sulfate, a specific antidote. Although reversal of LMWH by protamine sulfate may not be as complete when measured by persisting anti-Xa activity, clinical cessation of bleeding suggests its efficacy.

13. Should guaiac positivity and hematuria be attributed to vascular mucosal leak from anticoagulant therapy?

No—not until a structural lesion has been ruled out. Several studies have demonstrated the high incidence of demonstrable anatomic lesions in patients who bleed even on therapeutic doses of anticoagulant agents. Thus, the source of bleeding should be carefully evaluated.

14. How should heparin-induced thrombocytopenia (HIT) be managed?

HIT is heralded by a fall in platelet count to 50% of the original count over 5–15 days after initiation of heparin therapy. Because this is an immunologic reaction in patients who have been previously exposed to heparin, a precipitous fall in platelet count may be seen earlier. Management consists of discontinuing heparin immediately. If the patient has an underlying thrombotic disorder, potential treatments include hirudin, vena cava interruption, or danaparoid, a LMWH that has proved effective in one randomized clinical trial. However, this or another LMWH should be tested against the patient's serum for the absence of cross-reactivity. The immediate administration of warfarin is not recommended, because it may exacerbate the HIT procoagulant state. If the patient develops HIT during prophylaxis against DVT, the standard of practice has been to discontinue heparin; however, some data suggest that such patients are also at risk for thrombotic episodes due to the HIT procoagulant state.

15. List ten critical elements of education for all patients on warfarin therapy.

1. Take warfarin at the same time each day; never take extra doses to compensate for missed doses.
2. Report excessive bleeding or ecchymoses immediately.
3. Regularly check for blood in the stool and urine.
4. Notify your provider of all changes in medication.
5. Do not take aspirin or aspirin-containing drugs; use acetaminophen with care.
6. Avoid circumstances that lead to injury in normal daily activities.

7. Limit alcohol to a single beer or 1–2 ounces of liquor daily.

8. Minimize dietary changes and erratic eating.

9. Women of child-bearing age should notify the provider of any delay in menses (3–4 days), when pregnancy may be possible.

10. Prevent epistaxis and learn techniques for its control.

16. List the indications for antiplatelet treatment.

Cardiovascular disease	Unstable angina
	Primary and secondary prevention of myocardial infarction
	Postoperatively for coronary bypass grafting or insertion of certain prosthetic valves
Cerebrovascular disease	Transient ischemic attacks
	Secondary prevention of stroke
Renal disease	Prevention of clotting in arteriovenous fistulas

17. Which systemic diseases are associated with an increased incidence of thrombosis?
• Chronic congestive heart failure
• Carcinoma, especially mucin-producing types
• Hyperviscosity from plasma proteins, red blood cells, or white blood cells
• Nephrotic syndrome
• Hematologic diseases (myeloproliferative diseases, paroxysmal nocturnal hemoglobinuria, hemoglobinopathies such as sickle cell disease)
• Homocystinuria
• Systemic lupus erythematosus (SLE) with lupus anticoagulant

18. What physiologic, environmental, or iatrogenic conditions contribute to a hypercoagulable state?

Physiologic conditions	**Environmental conditions**
Stasis	Smoking
Pregnancy	**Iatrogenic conditions**
Postpartum status	Surgery
Increasing age	Oral contraceptive drugs

19. Who should be screened for an inherited or acquired disorder of hypercoagulability?
The most common inherited disorders that predispose to hypercoagulability are deficiencies of antithrombin III, protein C, and protein S. Proteins C and S are readily assessed either functionally or immunologically. Of patients with recurrent thromboses and a family history of thromboses, about 35% have an identifiable inherited defect in coagulation that appears causative. No known test predicts patients who will thrombose, but the following clinical clues should trigger screening for hypercoagulable states, either inherited or acquired.

Thromboses at age less than 40 years	Thromboses during pregnancy
Thromboses in unusual sites	Warfarin necrosis (protein C)
Recurrent thromboses	Resistance to heparin therapy
Recurrent spontaneous abortions	(antithrombin III)

20. Why is the term lupus anticoagulant a misnomer?
The term is a misnomer because it refers to a group of antiphospholipid antibodies that prolong the aPTT but lead to thromboses in up to 30% of patients. Thus, it is a true hypercoagulable state associated with SLE but also found in other setttings, such as increased age, drug use (phenothiazines), and postinfection states. In women it may present as recurrent spontaneous abortions. However, it also may be found in men, in whom the specificity of the antiphospholipid antibody may differ. Asymptomatic individuals do not routinely require treatment. If thrombosis occurs, heparin therapy and monitoring by heparin assay are indicated.

21. Name the known inherited thrombotic disorders. Which is most common?

It is currently estimated that up to 50% of patients with recurrent thromboses and 1 in 5 patients who present with initial venous thromboembolism may have an inherited hypercoagulable state. These include the following inherited abnormalities:

Abnormalities of activated coagulation factors	Impaired clot lysis
APC resistance (factor V Leiden mutation)	Dysfibrinogenemia
Protein S deficiency	Plasminogen deficiency
Protein C deficiency	**Metabolic defect**
Antithrombin III deficiency	Homocysteinemia, homozygous
Heparin cofactor deficiency	and heterozygous disease

The most common of these to date is factor V Leiden mutation, which has an estimated prevalence of 4–6% in the general population; it is estimated to result in a 5–6-fold increase in thrombotic complications. However, to date no evidence suggests that screening for this defect before surgery, pregnancy, or use of birth control pills is beneficial.

22. When should testing for activated protein C (APC) resistance, protein S or C deficiency, and antithrombin III deficiency be done?

Acute thromboses and therapy with heparin or warfarin may alter levels of proteins C and S. Testing for APC resistance is also sensitive to anticoagulants, liver disease, and antiphospholipid antibodies. Optimally, levels should be measured when the patient is off therapy and asymptomatic. If the patient is on therapy, only a tentative diagnosis may be established if the level is decreased. In addition, because all defects are inherited autosomal dominant traits, confirmation of deficient levels in family members should be pursued. Testing for these deficiencies is best done in the reference laboratory; the results, which may be difficult to interpret, should be reviewed by a hematologist.

23. Should patients with hypercoagulable states be treated with lifelong anticoagulation after the first thrombosis?

No. Common practice is to place patients on chronic warfarin therapy after a second documented episode of thromboses. Patients with low levels of functional proteins and no episodes of thromboses require no treatment.

BIBLIOGRAPHY

1. Antiplatelet Trialists' Collaboration: Collaborative overview of randomized trials of antiplatelet therapy. I: Prevention of death, myocardial infarction, and stroke by prolonged antiplatelet therapy in various categories of patients. BMJ 308:81–106, 1994.
2. Cook DJ, Guyatt GH, Laupacis A, Sackett DL: Rules of evidence and clinical recommendations on the use of antithrombotic agents. Chest 102(Suppl):305–311, 1992.
3. Fihn S, McDonnell M, Martin D, et al for the Warfarin Optimized Outpatient Follow-up Study Group: Risk factors for complications of chronic anticoagulation. Ann Intern Med 118:511–520, 1993.
4. Harris JM, Abramson N: Evaluation of recurrent thrombosis and hypercoagulability. Am Fam Physician 56:1590–1596, 1997.
5. Hirsh J, Poller L: The international normalized ratio: A guide to understanding and correcting its problems. Arch Intern Med 154:282–288, 1994.
6. Jandl JH: Blood: Textbook of Hematology, 2nd ed. Boston, Little, Brown, 1996.
7. Kelton JH, Warkentin TE: Heparin induced thrombocytopenia. Postgrad Med 103:169–178, 1998.
8. Koniaris LS, Goldhaber SZ: Anticoagulation in dilated cardiomyopathy. J Am Coll Cardiol 31:745–748, 1998.
9. Meyer BJ, Chesebro JH: Treatment of arterial thromboembolic disease. Curr Opin Hematol 1:336–340, 1994.
10. Orsinelli DA: Current recommendations for the anticoagulation of patients with atrial fibrillation. Prog Cardiovasc Dis 39:1–20, 1996.
11. Petri M: Pathogenesis and treatment of the antiphospholipid antibody syndrome. Med Clin North Am 81:151–177, 1997.
12. Price DT, Ridker PM: Factor V Leiden mutation and the risks for thromboembolic disease: A clinical perspective. Ann Intern Med 127:895–903, 1997.
13. Raschke RA, Reilly BM, Guidry JR, et al: The weight-based heparin dosing nomogram compared with a "standard care" nomogram: A randomized controlled trial. Ann Intern Med 119:874–881, 1993.
14. Raskob GE, Durcia SS: Treatment of venous thromboembolism. Curr Opin Hematol 1:329–335, 1994.

15. Spandorfer JM, Merli GJ: Outpatient anticoagulation issues for the primary care physician. Med Clin North Am 80:475–491, 1996.
16. Thomas DP, Robert HR; Hypercoagulability in venous and arterial thrombosis. Ann Intern Med 126:638–644, 1997.
17. Weitz JI: Low molecular weight heparins. N Engl J Med 337:682–688, 1997.
18. Welch GN, Lscalzo J: Homocysteine and atherothrombosis. N Engl J Med 338:1042–1050, 1998.

65. SICKLE CELL DISEASE AND OTHER HEMOGLOBINOPATHIES

Jeanette Mladenovic, M.D.

1. How do globin abnormalities result in clinical hemoglobinopathies?

Hemoglobin, the major component of red cells, is a tetramer of four globin chains covalently linked to heme and arranged in two polypeptide chains. Each globin subunit is determined by inherited genes: two alpha genes on chromosome 16 and one nonalpha gene (normally beta) on chromosome 11. Thus, the hemoglobin in each cell may be composed of various globin types, depending on quantitative or qualitative defects in genes inherited from each parent. Remembering the genetic possibilities facilitates an understanding of the common clinical diseases. Alpha globin is inherited on four genes (two from each parent on chromosome 11), and the severity of quantitative defects (alpha thalassemias) increases with each missing gene. Because chromosome 16 contains a single gene not only for beta hemoglobin but also for other normal hemoglobins that are present in varying amounts during fetal and adult life, quantitative and qualitative defects commonly involve the beta gene. In addition, combined abnormalities may arise from quantitative and/or qualitative defects of genes on both chromosomes. The common abnormalities are as follows:

Qualitative defects in the beta gene are structural:

Hemoglobin S, C, E (usually due to specific mutations)

Quantitative defects in both alpha and beta genes are seen with progressive defects in hemoglobin formation as demonstrated by microcytosis and varying clinical severity:

Alpha thalassemias: usually deletions of one or more genes

Beta thalassemias: quantitative defects in the beta gene

Hemoglobin Production

	From the father	From the mother
On chromosome 16:	two alpha genes	two alpha genes
	α and α	α and α
On chromosome 11:	one nonalpha gene	one nonalpha gene
	β, δ^2, γ	β, δ^2, γ
	$\downarrow$	$\downarrow$

Thus the offspring normally inherits globin messages from four alpha genes and two nonalpha genes (β, δ^2, or γ)

$\downarrow$

Heme and four globins form hemoglobin during erythropoiesis. The type formed depends on the age of the individual

$\downarrow$ $\downarrow$

The Majority of Adult Red Cells	Hemoglobin Depends on Age		
	Type	Adult (%)	Newborn (%)
Mostly hemoglobin A: $\alpha_2\beta_2$	A	97	20
A little hemoglobin A_2: $\alpha_2\delta_2$	A_2	2.5	0.5
A little less fetal hemoglobin F: α_2, γ_2	F	< 1	> 80
(Reticulocytes have more F)			

2. Which groups in the United States are at risk for carrying a gene related to one of the common hemoglobinopathies?

S gene	1 in 12 African-Americans
	Combined with beta thalassemia in people from the Mediterranean countries and Africa
C gene	1 in 50 African-Americans
E gene	Southeast Asians, especially from Laos, Thailand, and Cambodia (almost one-fifth of Laotian and Cambodian refugee children in the U.S.)
Beta thalassemia	Americans of African, Italian, and Greek descent
Alpha thalassemia	Americans of African (1/9), Southeast Asian, Chinese, Italian, and Greek descent

3. Why is it important to recognize the populations with high gene frequencies, even though the diseases may be clinically insignificant in patients who are heterozygous carriers?

Affected people may require genetic counseling. Because the genes follow Mendelian inheritance patterns, prevention or early knowledge of the homozygous state (especially sickle cell disease and beta thalassemia major) is possible with prenatal screening.

4. Which defects are lethal in utero or early in life?

Three major defects are severe and require serious genetic counseling or early recognition:

Alpha thalassemia with four deleted genes leads to hydrops fetalis.

Beta thalassemia major (Cooley's anemia), a homozygous variant, leads to severe hemolysis, growth retardation, iron overload, and shortened survival.

Heterozygotes of beta thalassemia and hemoglobin E disease are similar to beta thalassemia major.

5. What abnormality causes sickle hemoglobin?

Because of a structural abnormality in the beta gene, a single amino acid substitution (valine for glutamic acid) creates an unstable hemoglobin instead of the normal beta hemoglobin. When the unstable hemoglobin deoxygenates, the normal biconcave red blood cell (RBC) becomes sickled, stiff, and sticky.

6. How does the primary care provider screen for hemoglobin?

The usual screen is a solubility test (deoxyhemoglobin S is poorly soluble). If the result is positive, a confirmatory test of hemoglobin electrophoresis should be performed. Sickle cell trait or disease is detected by the amounts of hemoglobin S, A, and F. The usual percentage of hemoglobin F and S should be known for patients with homozygous sickle cell disease, because it may be helpful in therapy.

7. Who should be considered for screening and counseling for sickle cell hemoglobin?

All people who are not of Northern European origin should be considered for screening and appropriate counseling before general anesthesia or conception, at diagnosis of pregnancy, and neonatally. Appropriate counseling and screening of partners or family members should be offered if screening is positive.

8. Should persons with heterozygous sickle cell disease be considered at high risk for insurance or employment purposes?

No. Affected people have normal life expectancy and no clinical illness related to hemoglobin. However, they may be unable to concentrate their urine and occasionally (at low oxygen tension) have asymptomatic splenic or renal infarcts; the latter may result in painless hematuria. They are not required to restrict athletic activity.

9. Describe the four major manifestations of sickle cell disease.

1. **Anemia.** Because of markedly shortened RBC survival, each patient has a characteristically low hematocrit (usually between 18 and 30%) with a compensatory reticulocytosis. If the reticulocytosis is depressed by infection or folate deficiency, aplastic crises or critical anemia may develop emergently.

2. **Constitutional symptoms.** Growth and development are delayed because the illness presents in early childhood. In addition, patients soon become functionally asplenic; thus, overwhelming sepsis from encapsulated organisms poses a life-threatening risk.

3. **Acute pain crises.** Vasoocclusive phenomena lead to recurrent and unpredictable pain, which presents most frequently in the abdomen, joints, back, and chest. Patients usually are familiar with their own patterns of precipitating events and periodicity. A prior infection is known to precipitate crises. The chest syndrome is treated as both infection and infarction, because the differentiation is not possible. Abdominal pain is particularly difficult, because it may mimic an acute abdomen. Joint crises may be accompanied by noninflammatory effusions.

4. **End-organ damage.** As patients with sickle cell disease reach adulthood, they experience end-organ damage in essentially all systems because of repeated microvascular occlusions. Most prominently affected are the lungs, heart, kidneys, bones, skin, and eyes. Macrovascular events are particularly apparent in the incidence of cerebral thromboses.

10. How should painful crises be managed?

Acute painful crises should be managed supportively with analgesia and hydration. Oxygen should be administered when low oxygen saturation is present. Infection should be ruled out or treated. Transfusion to decrease the percentage of hemoglobin S or to improve oxygen-carrying capacity should be reserved for severe illness or surgery; it usually is given with consultation of a hematologist.

11. What preventive measures should the primary care provider institute in the care of patients with sickle cell disease?

1. Registration of patients into comprehensive sickle cell programs
2. Immunizations: pneumococcal, *Haemophilus influenzae,* and hepatitis
3. Prophylaxis: penicillin until puberty, malaria for travel to endemic areas
4. Folate supplementation, especially before conception and during pregnancy
5. Counseling of patients to avoid alcohol (dehydration) and tobacco (which may precipitate acute chest syndrome)
6. Awareness of and monitoring for learning disabilities
7. Regular ophthalmologic follow-up
8. Regular foot care and protective shoes
9. Prompt treatment of all minor illnesses, especially those that may lead to dehydration
10. Consideration of supply of analgesics for early prevention of painful crises

12. When should patients with sickle cell disease seek medical help? When should the primary care provider consider hospitalization?

The patient with sickle cell disease should be counseled to seek medical help in the following situations:

1. Persistent fever (over 101° F)
2. Chest pain, shortness of breath, or vomiting
3. Prolonged new headache

The primary care provider should hospitalize the patient with sickle cell disease in the following situations:

1. Tachypnea or signs of lung involvement
2. Neurologic signs
3. Abdominal pain or splenic or hepatic enlargement
4. Swollen, painful joints

   5. Uncontrolled painful crises or loin pain
   6. Congestive heart failure and/or severe pallor

13. What therapies are available to diminish the effect of sickle hemoglobin on the clinical course of the disease?

Therapies are usually aimed at diminishing the percentage of hemoglobin S, often through monitored hypertransfusion programs for unique indications. Although hypertransfusion may appear to be an easy answer to decreasing the percentage of sickle hemoglobin, its routine use leads to iron overload and isoimmunization. Hydroxyurea, in a national multicenter trial, has been shown to reduce the frequency and severity of painful crises and the incidence of acute chest syndrome. In addition, bone marrow transplantation offers the potential for cure. Thus, therapy is available under the direction of specialized clinics or a hematologist.

14. Can sickle cell disease present late in life?

Yes. In some populations, disease severity varies considerably. Thus, hemolytic anemia should raise the possibility of sickle cell disease in a patient who belongs to a susceptible group and has not been screened previously.

15. What are the four major causes of death in patients with sickle cell disease?

Cardiopulmonary failure, renal failure, cerebrovascular events, and infection.

16. Is hemoglobin SS the only genotype associated with the phenotype of sickle cell disease?

No. Two additional disorders may mimic sickle cell disease. Sickle beta thalassemia (one gene for S and one for beta thalassemia) and sickle C (one S and one C gene on each of the two 16 chromosomes) present similarly to sickle cell disease. Sickle beta thalassemia may be seen in Caucasians of Mediterranean descent. If no beta chains are made, this condition may be difficult to distinguish from hemoglobin SS disease on electrophoresis. The life expectancy for patients with SC is approximately two decades longer (seventh decade) than the life expectancy for patients with homozygous SS disease.

17. What inherited hemoglobin abnormalities commonly result in microcytosis?

Prominent microcytosis is seen in three settings: alpha thalassemia trait, beta thalassemia trait, and hemoglobin E (hetero- or homozygous). All may demonstrate a low mean cell volume in routine complete blood counts with no detectable anemia. Alpha thalassemia trait, a common asymptomatic finding in African-Americans, may have a normal electrophoresis. If so, no further evaluation is usually necessary. A silent carrier of alpha thalassemia with one alpha gene missing has no detectable abnormalities. Electrophoresis in patients with beta thalassemia trait usually shows an increase in A_2 hemoglobin. Patients with hemoglobin E, both homo- and heterozygotes, may have microcytosis without anemia or only mild anemia. This condition may be diagnosed by electrophoresis.

18. What happens to patients with alpha thalassemia in whom three genes are missing?

This defect produces a compensated hemolytic disease, with anemia, reticulocytosis, many target cells, and precipitated beta chains in RBCs, called Heinz bodies.

19. What other hemoglobin abnormalities may cause a congenital hemolytic anemia?

The major defects in children or young adults who present with a relatively compensated hemolytic anemia are of three types: RBC enzyme defects (G6PD deficiency); RBC membrane defects; or other mutant hemoglobins. Many other mutants of the beta genes lead to hemolytic anemia and often demonstrate precipitated hemoglobin as Heinz bodies. Whereas these mutants may result in a relatively compensated hemolytic anemia, their structural abnormalities may give rise to hemoglobins that have varying oxygen affinities or that are susceptible to precipitation with oxidant stress by drugs.

20. Which patients are at risk for gallstones?

All patients with congenital hemolytic anemia have an increased incidence of gallstones. In patients with sickle cell disease, the diagnosis is complicated by abdominal pain associated with sickle crisis and liver abnormalities that may result from repeated hepatic infarcts. Generally, cholecystectomy is recommended in symptomatic patients.

21. How may parvovirus affect patients with hemolytic anemia?

Parvovirus has a particular affinity for the developing red cell, resulting in a cessation of mature red cell production. Thus, in patients who require high red cell production, as in all cases of hemolytic anemia, there is a precipitous fall in hemoglobin concentration. Infection with parvovirus is the main cause of aplastic crises in sickle cell anemia but also may cause precipitous anemia in other hemoglobinopathies. It represents a medical emergency in patients with hemolytic anemia. Red cell support and therapy with IgG should be initiated.

BIBLIOGRAPHY

1. Bunn HF: Pathogenesis and treatment of sickle cell disease. N Engl J Med 337:762–769, 1997.
2. Bunn HF: Disorders of hemoglobin. In Isselbacher KJ, Braunwald E, Wilson JD, et al (eds): Harrison's Principles and Practices of Medicine. New York, McGraw-Hill, 1994, pp 1734–1743.
3. Dabrow MB, Wilkins JC: Hematologic emergencies. Management of transfusion reactions and crises in sickle cell disease. Postgrad Med 93:183, 1993.
4. Jandl JH: Blood: Textbook of Hematology, 2nd ed. Boston, Little, Brown, 1996.
5. Davies SC, Oni L: Management of patients with sickle cell disease. BMJ 315:656–660, 1997.
6. Kazazian HH: The thalassemia syndromes: Molecular basis and prenatal diagnosis. Semin Hematol 27:209, 1990.
7. Koshy M, Dorn L: Continuing care for adult patients with sickle cell disease. Hematol Oncol Clin North Am 10:1265–1273, 1996.
8. Steingart R: Management of patients with sickle cell disease. Med Clin North Am 76:669–682, 1992.
9. Weatherall DJ: The hereditary anemias. BMJ 314:492–496, 1997.
10. Weinberger M: Approach to the management of fever and infection in patients with primary bone marrow failure and hemoglobinopathies. Hematol Oncol Clin North Am 7:865–885, 1993.

X. Disorders of the Musculoskeletal System

66. PRINCIPLES OF MUSCULOSKELETAL INJURY AND SPORTS MEDICINE

Richard C. Fisher, M.D.

1. Describe the significant issues in acquiring a history from patients with musculoskeletal injury.

The time course of the injury is most important, particularly to separate acute injuries from chronic, recurrent, and repetitive use mechanisms. Knowing the mechanism of injury in severely traumatized patients often aids in identifying high-risk areas and in determining treatment. High-energy injuries, as in automobile or motorcycle accidents, have profound effects on multiple systems in addition to the musculoskeletal system. Low-energy injuries, such as simple falls, have different implications for patient survival and complications.

2. During the initial evaluation of a severely traumatized patient, what are the important priorities to consider?

As with all patients seen on an emergency basis, the ABCs (airway, breathing, and circulation) should take precedent over other exams. The patient also should be evaluated for chest injuries, abdominal trauma, and head trauma before beginning definitive therapy for musculoskeletal injuries. The most important considerations in the musculoskeletal exam include pelvic fractures, spinal fractures, and long-bone injuries (e.g., femur and tibia). It is also necessary to determine whether any of the fractures are open. Pelvis and open long-bone injuries may entail significant blood loss and be accompanied by significant morbidity and mortality.

3. In evaluating a traumatized extremity, what are the principal tissue priorities to consider?

In order of importance, the six tissues to be considered are the vascular system, neurologic system, skin and underlying soft tissue, muscle-tendon units, joint and ligament complexes, and bone. The ultimate viability of the extremity depends on an intact vascular system, and avascular time is extremely important. Muscle ischemia longer than 6 hours often results in significant damage, which becomes irreversible at 8 hours. Changes in the skin often help to localize problems in an unconscious patient. With open wounds it is extremely important to identify damage to underlying structures such as open fractures, open joints, or lacerations to muscle, tendon, and nerve.

4. How may the vascular integrity of the extremity be evaluated?

Major arteries should be palpated, and the temperature and color of the extremity should be evaluated and compared with noninjured extremities, recognizing that extremities often feel cool in patients with shock. Capillary refill can be evaluated in the nailbeds. If pulses are difficult to palpate, the Doppler may be used. In cases of suspected major vascular injury, arteriography is indicated. High-risk injuries include (1) major injuries about the knee (e.g., knee dislocations, proximal tibia or distal femoral fractures), (2) injuries about the elbow (e.g., distal humeral fractures, which may involve the brachial artery), and (3) penetrating injuries in the vicinity of major vessels.

5. Briefly describe the pathophysiology and common causes of compartment syndromes.

The syndrome is caused by an increase in pressure within the muscle fascial compartments in either the upper or lower extremity. When intracompartmental pressure exceeds perfusion pressure, ischemic changes occur. Healthy muscle undergoes ischemic changes when the intracompartmental pressure is 10–20 mmHg below the diastolic pressure.

In trauma, the usual cause is direct damage to the muscle tissue, which causes swelling within the closed compartment. Other causes include arterial damage, burns, acute and chronic overuse syndromes, and drug overdose. High-risk patients include those with a bleeding diathesis or syndromes that alter state of consciousness, including head injury and drug overdose.

The common clinical symptoms of pulselessness, pallor, paralysis, paresthesia, and pain may be obscured in some patients, and one should keep a keen index of suspicion in high-risk patients. Intracompartmental pressure monitoring should be used.

6. Describe the neurologic evaluation of an injured extremity.

Extremities should be checked for sensation and motor function with an attempt to cover all major peripheral nerves as well as dermatomes. Testing of the deep tendon reflexes also is helpful. Interruption of the tendon or muscle units at times may be mistaken for neurologic injury. Serial exams should be performed because a change in status is a good indicator of developing problems or improvement.

7. What are the stages of injury of a nonfunctioning peripheral nerve? Describe the prognosis for each.

1. **Contusion or neurapraxia** temporarily interrupts nerve conduction, but the nerve cell processes remain in continuity. Function usually returns within 6 weeks.

2. **Crush injury or axonotmesis** causes axon death below the injury. The axon must regrow distally from the point of injury before recovery occurs. Regrowth takes place at about 1 mm/day.

3. **Neurotmesis or complete division** of the nerve is associated with a laceration or injury from the sharp ends of a fractured bone. The nerve will not regain function without surgical repair.

8. Why does an open fracture require emergent management?

Exposure of the bone to outside contaminants has a high incidence of both soft tissue infection and osteomyelitis. The incidence of infection increases dramatically with the extent of the contamination of the wound, type of contamination (especially fecal material as in farm related injuries), and delay in time to definitive debridement. Open fractures should be treated with tetanus prophylaxis and antibiotics as soon as possible. The patient should be transported to the operating room for thorough debridement and irrigation of the fracture to remove all possible contamination. In addition, the fracture should be properly stabilized. The goal is definitive debridement in less than 6 hours from the time of injury.

9. What are the most commonly missed fractures in the polytrauma patient?

The most commonly missed fractures involve the odontoid process, C7 vertebral body, scaphoid, radial head, pelvis, femoral neck, tibial plateau, and talus. The incidence of missed fractures is about 10%.

10. Name some of the systemic conditions that are contraindications to participation in strenuous athletic activity.

Seizure within the past year; history of retinal detachment; active infection; cardiac conditions, such as cardiomegaly, aortic or mitral stenosis, and uncontrolled hypertension; uncontrolled asthma; and uncontrolled diabetes. Other conditions that should be considered carefully include spondylolisthesis with back pain, blood coagulation disorder, and possibly a solitary functioning kidney.

11. Describe the severity rating for muscle strains.

Muscle strains are graded into three stages, depending on the severity of the injury. **First-degree strains** consist of a mildly pulled muscle. The muscle-tendon unit remains intact. The muscle should be protected from use until painless function returns. **Second-degree strains** from a moderate pull to the muscle result in some tearing of muscle fibers, but continuity of the muscle-tendon unit is maintained. Signs and symptoms include impaired muscle function, moderate amounts of pain with muscle use or stretching, swelling, and ecchymosis. **Third-degree strains** are severely pulled muscles that disrupt the continuity of the muscle-tendon unit. Treatment depends on the site of the injury.

12. Any muscle-tendon unit may be injured by direct laceration. List the six most common sites of indirect third-degree muscle tendon injuries.

1. Long head of the biceps tendon at the shoulder
2. Quadriceps tension at its insertion into the patella
3. Patella tendon, which ruptures either from the surface of the patella or in mid-substance
4. Achilles tendon
5. Extensor tendon at the distal interphalangeal (DIP) finger joints
6. Flexor digitorum profundus tendon at the DIP joint

13. Describe the typical signs and symptoms of joint injuries.

A dislocated joint is held in an abnormal position, and because of pain the patient will not allow the joint to be moved. Injured joints usually show a detectable amount of fluid that is either effusion or hemarthrosis; the distinction is made by aspiration. In the presence of ligament injury, careful testing may reveal the associated instability. Testing at times is difficult because of the acute pain and swelling in the joint. The joint should be examined under anesthesia or several days later when the pain subsides.

14. What are the stages of ligament injury?

Stage I injuries involve tearing of some of the ligament fibers without disruption of individual or collective fibers. **Stage II injuries** involve tearing of multiple ligament fibers without disruption of individual or collective fibers. In both stage I and stage II injuries the joint remains stable to testing. In more severe stage II injuries, however, tearing of the ligament fibers may involve partial disruption of the ligament complex. The joint may show mild instability but not complete laxity, and the exam is usually painful. **Stage III injuries** involve complete disruption of the integrity of the ligament, usually with demonstrable instability. Treatment depends on the joint involved but generally is nonsurgical for stages I and II. Stage III injuries may require surgical repair or reconstruction.

15. Describe some of the basic principles for treating ligamentous injuries.

This area remains controversial, but it seems apparent that ligaments heal better and with greater strength with some type of controlled movement across the joint. Gross instability probably requires either surgical stabilization or brace stabilization during the healing process, but, when possible, early controlled motion gives a better long-term result than immobilization. Joint reinjury before completion of healing leads to prolonged disability and a less satisfactory outcome for the involved joint. Thus, early motion with protection against instability, with either surgery or orthoses, seems to give the best ultimate functional recovery.

16. Why does clipping in football invoke a 15-yard penalty?

Clipping is a block from the posterolateral side at the level of the knee. The foot is usually planted on the ground, and a valgus force is produced across the knee. Clipping often results in a tear of the medial collateral ligament, anterior cruciate ligament, and medial meniscus. Treatment is surgical, and rehabilitation is often prolonged. Full functional recovery is not guaranteed.

17. Describe the signs and symptoms of a fractured bone.

Although signs and symptoms vary, the cardinal findings are swelling, point tenderness, visible or palpable deformity, and crepitus at the fracture site. Stress fractures and torus (greenstick) fractures in children may show minimal signs on physical exam. Radiographs are indicated once the area of injury is determined.

18. What principles should be followed in ordering radiographs for musculoskeletal injury?

Generally, plain roentgenograms are indicated after examination of the patient and determination of the site to be examined; 90-90 radiographs are almost always indicated, because deformities may be missed when only one view is taken. In addition, the joint above and the joint below the involved bone should always be included in the exam. Special studies, such as computed tomography (CT) or magnetic resonance imaging (MRI), are indicated to evaluate certain fractures. Injuries most likely to require special imaging studies involve the calcaneus, tibia plateau region, pelvis, and spine. Occult fractures or stress fractures are often diagnosed earliest with bone-scanning techniques.

19. Under what special circumstances does musculoskeletal trauma lead to extreme blood loss that may be missed by the clinician?

Although blood loss needs to be monitored in all trauma patients, musculoskeletal injuries involving the femur, hip, and pelvis and all open fractures are especially prone to large amounts of blood loss. In closed fractures of the femur or pelvis, the loss may not be apparent, and many units of blood may be sequestered before external signs become obvious.

20. Occasionally a patient presenting with a history of trauma in fact may have a preexisting underlying condition responsible for the acute signs and symptoms. Name the more common conditions that may cause problems.

Underlying problems, such as infection and tumor, are often unmasked by simple and seemingly insignificant injury, including pathologic fractures through the lesion and simple contusions that exacerbate symptoms. Gouty arthritis often occurs after trauma and presents as a painful joint at the site or remote from the area of injury. Acute fractures or stress or insufficiency fractures are often the first overt sign of severe osteoporosis. They may occur in older patients and in young patients with abnormalities of bone metabolism, such as estrogen deficiency and osteomalacia.

21. Name the three most common delayed complications after musculoskeletal injury.

Compartment syndrome, fat embolism syndrome, and Sudeck's atrophy. Compartment syndromes usually occur in the region of a long-bone fracture but may occur in remote areas with muscle or crush injuries. Symptoms are usually present within the first 24 hours after injury. Fat embolism syndrome usually presents within 12–72 hours of multiple trauma, long-bone fractures, or burns. Symptoms include confusion, shortness of breath, tachycardia, and petechiae. The partial pressure of oxygen (PO_2) is usually low. Sudeck's atrophy is usually seen late in the course of injury and presents as swelling, redness, and pain out of proportion to the underlying injury.

22. How do the presenting symptoms of a stress fracture differ from those of acute traumatic fractures?

Stress fractures are usually produced by overuse of the extremity and are of gradual onset. The history usually includes an increase in activity levels about 3 weeks before the onset of symptoms, which are exaggerated by repetition of the activity. This pattern of injury occurs commonly in runners when they suddenly increase their distance or time. Some recent data suggest that patients prone to stress fractures have a decrease in bone density. In elite female athletes, decreased production of estrogen may lead to an increased incidence of stress injuries.

23. What are the most common locations for stress fractures?

The location depends to some extent on the activity producing the injury. The stress fracture was first described in the second metatarsal in association with prolonged walking. Fractures of the proximal tibia and mid- and proximal femur are common in runners. Fractures in the area of the femoral neck are especially dangerous and should be stabilized surgically. Fractures of the upper extremities are seen in gymnasts and others involved with prolonged upper extremity activities. Stress fractures associated with osteomalacia also may be seen in the pelvis, scapula, and ribs.

24. Describe the common signs and symptoms of spinal column injury.

The mechanism of injury is important in assessing the potential severity of spinal column and associated injuries. Falls from heights, diving injuries, and motor vehicle accidents are common mechanisms. Pain is usually reported at and below the level of injury, and a careful history should be taken with regard to neurologic symptoms, such as ascending numbness and loss of motor control. The physical exam should include evaluation of cutaneous reflexes, muscle power, muscle tone, deep tendon reflexes, sensation, and anal sphincter tone. The spine should be palpated carefully for areas of tenderness and possible deformity. A multiply injured patient should be treated as if a spinal column injury were present until history, physical exam, and radiographic studies prove otherwise.

25. What are the two most common areas of injury in the spinal column?

The two most common areas are the mobile parts of the column—the cervical spine and thoracolumbar junction.

26. What is the proper management of patients with suspected cervical spine injuries?

Patients should be immobilized initially in a rigid cervical collar, and anteroposterior and cross-table lateral radiographs should be taken. A careful neurologic examination should be performed and the presence or absence of cervical spine pain or tenderness determined. An unconscious patient should be assumed to have a cervical spine injury. In an awake patient with normal radiographs but spine pain and tenderness, the spine should be immobilized until the patient can perform adequate flexion and extension lateral radiographs. These radiographs evaluate soft tissue-ligamentous injury in the absence of acute fracture.

27. Which two injuries most commonly occur in combination with spinal column injuries?

Fractures of the calcaneus associated with lumbar spine fractures and head injuries associated with cervical spine injuries.

28. Describe the common medically important systemic conditions that often interface with musculoskeletal injuries.

The most significant medical illnesses that seem to be found in patients with musculoskeletal illnesses include diabetes, seizure disorders, high-dose steroid use, and various central nervous system disorders, such as stroke or Parkinson's disease.

29. Discuss some of the diagnostic factors and treatment principles that apply to repetitive use disorder or cumulative-trauma disorder.

This problem can be difficult to deal with in the clinical setting. Some of the important features include a chief complaint that is not clear and in which pain is a principal component. At times major psychosocial issues are involved, including depression and dramatization of symptoms. One should search for signs of stress in either the work or home environment and try to define the drug use history, disability, and duration of the symptoms. Treatment decisions should be made after a careful history, physical, and functional evaluation. Evaluation is often best undertaken by a team of people, including primary care physicians, physical therapists, psychologists, and others trained as case managers. Although it is tempting to think that surgical correction is curative, surgery should be approached with great care in patients with this symptom complex. Some of the musculoskeletal conditions that may seem to be part of this complex include carpal tunnel syndrome, cubital tunnel syndrome, thoracic outlet syndrome, and various types of tendinitis in both the upper and lower extremities.

BIBLIOGRAPHY

1. Birrer RB (ed): Sports Medicine for the Primary Care Physician, 2nd ed. Boca Raton, FL, CRC Press, 1994.
2. Browner BD, Jupiter JB, Levine AM, Trafton PG: Skeletal Trauma. Philadelphia, W.B. Saunders, 1992.
3. D'Ambrosia RD: Musculoskeletal Disorder: Regional Examination and Differential Diagnosis. Philadelphia, J.B. Lippincott, 1986.
4. Fabian TC: Unraveling the fat embolism syndrome. N Engl J Med 329:961–963, 1993.
5. Frank CB: Ligament healing: Current knowledge and clinical applications. J Am Acad Orthop Surg 4:74–83, 1996.
6. Iversen LED, Swiantkowski MF: Manual of Acute Orthopaedic Therapeutics, 4th ed. Boston, Little, Brown and Company, 1995.
7. Kasser JR (ed): Orthopaedic Knowledge Update 5: Home Study Syllabus. Rosemont, IL, American Academy of Orthopaedic Surgeons, 1996.
8. Millender LH, Conlon M: An approach to work-related disorders of the upper extremity. J Am Acad Orthop Surg 4:134–142, 1996.
9. Rich BSE: Sudden death screening. Sports Med 78:267–288, 1994.
10. Rockwood CA Jr, Green DP, Bucholz RW, Heckman JD (eds): Fractures in Adults. Philadelphia, Lippincott-Raven, 1996.
11. Whitesides TE Jr, Heckman MM: Acute compartment syndrome: Update on diagnosis and treatment. J Am Acad Orthop Surg 4:209–218, 1996.

67. MONARTICULAR ARTHRITIS

David H. Collier, M.D.

1. List the most common diseases that present with an acutely warm, painful joint (monarticular inflammatory arthritis). Which of these diagnoses is the most critical?

Infections: bacterial, mycobacterial, Lyme disease.

Crystal-related diseases: gout (monosodium urate (MSU), pseudogout (calcium pyrophosphate dihydrate (CPPD), hydroxyapatite deposition disease (basic calcium phosphate (BCP).

Trauma: hemarthrosis, internal derangement.

Other: osteoarthritis, avascular necrosis, foreign-body synovitis, coagulopathy, pigmented villonodular synovitis.

Joint infection is one of the few rheumatologic emergencies. It must be diagnosed and treated quickly. If left untreated, bacterial infections can cause permanent damage to a joint in as early as 1 week. If treated promptly, they will usually resolve without permanent damage. An infectious etiology must be excluded in patients with acute monarthritis of uncertain etiology.

2. What polyarticular diseases occasionally present with a monarticular arthritis?

Rheumatoid arthritis	Ankylosing spondylitis
Juvenile rheumatoid arthritis	Reiter's syndrome
Sarcoid arthritis	Psoriatic arthritis
Viral arthritis	Enteropathic arthritis (associated with ulcerative colitis or Crohn's disease)

3. Which conditions may mimic monarthritic conditions?

Inflammation around a joint, such as in a tendon, ligament or bursa, may mimic a monarthritis. The typical patient with a truly inflamed joint guards the area from movement and will not allow any range-of-motion testing by the examiner. A patient with periarticular inflammation may allow careful movement of the joint and often localizes pain and tenderness to the area around the joint. Common areas of periarticular inflammation include the rotator cuff of the shoulder, olecranon bursa of the elbow, prepatella bursa of the knee, and greater trochanteric bursa of the hip. An effusion may be present in either case.

4. What key information from the history can narrow the differential diagnosis for a monarthritis?

1. **Which joint is involved**. Gout commonly presents in the first metatarsophalangeal joint. Pseudogout and infections commonly present in the knee. Dactylitis is a common presentation of the spondyloarthropathies.

2. **Rapidity of onset**. Septic and crystal-induced arthritis tend to be very rapid onset. Autoimmune or collagen vascular diseases tend to have less rapid onset.

3. **History of trauma, coagulopathy, or operations**, which may point to a traumatic cause or hemarthrosis.

4. **Previous attacks** may point to crystals or other inflammatory joint diseases.

5. **Age and sex**. In young patients think of the spondyloarthropathies and rheumatoid arthritis; in older patients consider gout and pseudogout. In males consider gout, spondyloarthropathies and hemachromatosis; in females think of rheumatoid arthritis and systemic lupus erythematosus.

6. **History of intravenous drug use or recent corticosteroid use** may point to an infection or osteonecrosis of the bone.

5. What is the single most important test to determine the cause of an acute monarticular arthritis?

A sample of the synovial fluid aspirated from the inflamed joint.

6. Explain the helpful information that can be obtained from the evaluation of joint fluid.

Although several tests are available to analyze joint fluid, examination of the fluid for white and red blood cell counts with differentials, assessment of crystals, and microbiologic cultures for infectious organisms are the most useful. White blood cell counts > 2000 white cells/mm³ are consistent with inflammation; the highest counts are seen with septic joints, although crystals and pseudosepsis in rheumatoid arthritis or the spondyloarthropathies may give very high counts. A Gram stain, even in the presence of crystals, should be done; if the results are negative, however, a negative culture is required to exclude suspected diagnosis of septic arthritis. A noninflammatory arthritis is suggested by the finding of < 2000 white cells/mm³.

Examination of the fluid for crystals requires a rose-quartz filter and a polarizing microscope. Gout is confirmed by the presence of negatively birefringent, needle-shaped crystals, which appear yellow with the slow wave of the polarizer parallel to the crystals. Pseudogout is suggested by small, rhomboid positively birefringent crystals, which appear blue with the slow wave of the polarizer parallel to the crystals.

7. Does an overlying cellulitis preclude aspiration through the apparently infected area?

No. A diagnosis of septic arthritis must be pursued, if suspected. However, before the aspiration, systemic antibiotics should be given for the cellulitis. Hemarthrosis, due to a coagulopathy, either congenital or acquired, is a relative contraindication to arthrocentesis. If a septic joint is suspected in this case, try to reverse the coagulopathy before arthrocentesis.

8. What radiographic findings are helpful in the differential diagnosis of arthritis?

Although frequently normal, radiographs may reveal a fracture or osteonecrosis of the bone. Soft-tissue swelling, periarticular osteopenia, and joint space loss followed by erosions at the site of the capsular insertion into the bone are characteristic of inflammatory arthritides. Crystal-induced arthritis may show dramatic erosions or calcified cartilage (pseudogout) with intact cartilage space. In contrast, osteoarthritis demonstrates cartilage loss in stress areas, with sclerosis along the joint line and osteophyte formation. The contralateral joint radiograph may serve as basis for comparison.

9. List other diagnostic studies that are useful in the initial evaluation of monarthritic conditions.

1. **Complete blood count.** Leukocytosis may be seen in bacterial infections of the joint.

2. **Cultures of blood, urine, or a suspected site of infection** is useful when a septic joint is considered because most joints become septic as a result of hematogenous spread.

3. **Serum prothrombin and partial thromboplastin times** when a coagulopathy or hemarthrosis is considered.

4. **Erythrocyte sedimentation rate** is nonspecific but usually elevated in inflammatory processes.

5. **Serum uric acid level** is sometimes helpful in gout. However, a normal serum uric acid level does not exclude gout, nor does a high uric acid level confirm a diagnosis of gout.

10. What are the most likely causes of an acute monarthritis in an elderly person hospitalized for a medical or surgical problem?

The most likely causes are gout, pseudogout, and infection.

11. List additional factors that may precipitate a gouty attack.

1. Drugs that cause a change in uric acid level. Common examples can be remembered by the mnemonic **CAN'T LEAP**:

Cyclosporine	**L**asix (furosemide)
Alcohol	**E**thambutol
Nicotinic acid (niacin)	**A**spirin (low dose)
Thiazides	**P**yrazinamide

2. Exercise, weight reduction, hyperalimentation, and fluid shifts
3. Trauma, hemorrhage, infection
4. Dietary excess of purines
5. Radiation therapy and chemotherapy for malignancies

12. Which joints are most commonly involved in gout?

The first metatarsophalangeal (MTP) joint is involved in > 50% of initial attacks and over time is involved in > 85% of patients (this condition is termed **podagra**). After the MTP, the joints most frequently involved are the joints of the foot, instep, ankles, and heel, followed by the knees, wrists, fingers, and elbows. Gout in the elderly frequently presents as polyarticular inflammation in the fingers and wrists.

13. Does crystal deposition only occur in joints?

No. Deposition of MSU, CPPD, and BCP in periarticular tissue may present as acute attacks of tendinitis or bursitis.

14. Should a fluid-filled bursa be aspirated?

A fluid-filled bursa, especially one that appears inflamed, should be approached in a manner similar to acute monarthritis. Infections, crystalline-induced arthritis, and traumatic causes need to be excluded. Thus, aspiration of fluid for Gram stain, culture, and crystal analysis is indicated in the first episode of bursitis. If infection is clinically suspected, intravenous antibiotics should be administered for 2–4 days, followed by 10–14 days of oral antibiotics covering *Staphylococcus aureus* or streptococci and daily aspiration of the bursa until little fluid is obtained or the white count is low. If sterility of the synovial fluid is assured, bursitis may be treated with aspiration, compression dressing and extensor pads, nonsteroidal antiinflammatory drugs (NSAIDs), or steroid injection, which shortens the course of the disease.

15. How should gout be treated acutely?

Therapy of gout is effective if begun early in the attack. Gout responds well to NSAIDs. Indomethacin is commonly used but should be avoided in patients with congestive heart failure, cirrhosis, renal disease, or a history of gastrointestinal (GI) bleeding. Colchicine, the traditional specific therapeutic intervention, is helpful when the diagnosis is uncertain; however, the frequency of GI side effects usually makes it a less popular alternative. Intravenous colchicine must be used carefully. It has a highly sclerosing effect on veins. Oral colchicine should not be given for 1 week following intravenous colchicine. Oral adrenocorticosteroids are used when NSAIDs and colchicine are contraindicated or in cases resistant to both therapies. If none of these drugs can be used, intraarticular steroids may be considered.

16. Why should the level of uric acid not be treated during an attack of gout?

An acute attack may be prolonged or precipitated when the level of uric acid is treated. Thus, it is wise to wait 4 weeks or more before instituting therapy to lower the level of uric acid. Treatment is begun once it is determined whether the patient is an overproducer or underexcretor of uric acid. Underexcretors are the most common type. Probenecid is a cost-effective drug to treat underexcretors (in the absence of renal disease or tophi); allopurinol treats both underexcretion and overproduction but may cause exfoliative dermatitis.

17. What is pseudogout? How does it present?

Pseudogout is an acute arthritis related to the release of CPPD crystals into the joint. It may mimic a gouty attack, although it tends to be less painful and takes longer to reach peak intensity than gout. It usually affects one joint but may be polyarticular. The most frequently involved joints are large joints, the knee being the most common (this condition is termed **gonagra**). If left untreated, the acute attack usually resolves within 1 month; the patient is asymptomatic between attacks.

18. What is the spectrum of CPPD deposition disease?

Acute synovitis caused by CPPD crystals is not the only presentation of CPPD deposition disease. This disorder may present in a polyarticular fashion, mimicking rheumatoid arthritis; it may complicate osteoarthritis or appear like an atypical osteoarthritis; or it may be noted as calcified hyaline and fibrocartilage on radiographs in asymptomatic patients. Rarely, it may behave as a pseudoneuropathic or pseudo-Charcot joint. These clinical presentations frequently overlap. CPPD deposition increases in incidence with age. Acute attacks are precipitated by the same physical factors that precipitate gouty attacks.

19. How is pseudogout treated?

Therapy for pseudogout is symptomatic and based on NSAIDs. Colchicine also leads to improvement and may be given prophylactically for frequent recurrence. Joint aspiration may provide symptomatic relief, and glucocorticoid injection is an option, although it should be used with care. There is no therapy to prevent crystalline deposition.

20. Which joints are most likely to become bacterially infected?

Usually bacteria are hematogenously spread from a remote focus. Organisms resist serum and reticuloendothelial defenses and colonize synovial tissue. This resistance accounts for the increased likelihood of infection in a damaged joint or impaired host and in joints with the greatest amount of synovium. Therefore, the most commonly affected joints are the knee, hip, shoulder, ankle, wrist, and elbow. The most common joints affected in intravenous drug abusers include the vertebral column, sacroiliac joint, sternoclavicular joint, knee, and ankle, often on the side used for drug injection. Such patients usually have staphylococcal infections, but atypical infections are noted in many case reports.

21. What organisms are commonly responsible for acute pyogenic arthritis in adults?

Organism	Incidence (%)
Neisseria gonorrhoeae	50
Staphylococcus aureus	35
Streptococcus pyogens	10
Gram-negative bacilli	5
Mycobacteria, fungi	<1

Suspicion or diagnosis of septic arthritis requires intravenous antibiotic therapy.

22. What is the definition of chronic monarticular arthritis?

The usual definition is persistence of symptoms in a single joint for longer than 6 weeks. The most likely diagnosis shifts from crystals and bacterial infection to more indolent diseases, such as spondyloarthropathies, mycobacterial or fungal septic arthritis, avascular necrosis, and internal derangement.

23. List the diseases most likely to cause chronic monarticular arthritis.

Inflammatory	**Noninflammatory**
Spondyloarthropathies	Osteoarthritis
Mycobacterial infection	Avascular necrosis of bone
Fungal arthritis	Internal derangement
Lyme arthritis	Synovial chondromatosis
Sarcoid arthritis	Pigmented villonodular synovitis
Unusual presentation of rheumatoid arthritis or systemic lupus erythematosus	Synovioma
Foreign-body synovitis	

24. What other tests should be considered for a chronic monarthritis?

1. Mycobacterial and fungal cultures.

2. Radiograph of the sacroiliac joint to look for spondyloarthropathy.

3. Chest radiograph to look for evidence of sarcoid and possibly evidence of mycobacteria. However, fewer than 50% of chest radiographs are abnormal in patients with mycobacterial arthritis.

4. Tuberculin skin test to document exposure to mycobacteria.

5. Serologic tests for Lyme disease, rheumatoid factor, and antinuclear antibody.

BIBLIOGRAPHY

1. Baker DG, Shumacher HR: Acute monoarthritis. N Engl J Med 329:1013–1020, 1992.
2. Calin A, Taurog JD (eds): The Spondylarthritides. New York, Oxford University Press, 1998.
3. Carias K, Panush RS: Acute arthritis. Bull Rheum Dis 43(7):1–4, 1994.
4. Espinoza L, Goldenberg DL, Arnett FC, Alarcon GS (eds): Infections in Rheumatic Diseases: A Comprehensive Review of Microbial Relations to Rheumatic Disorders. Orlando, FL, Grune & Stratton, 1988.
5. Goldenberg DL, Reed JI: Bacterial arthritis. N Engl J Med 312:764–771, 1985.
6. Ho G, DeNuccio M: Gout and pseudo-gout in hospitalized patients. Arch Intern Med 153:2787–2790, 1993.
7. Klippel JH, Dieppe PA (eds): Practical Rheumatology. London, Mosby-Wolfe, 1995.
8. Mankin HJ: Nontraumatic necrosis of the bone (osteonecrosis). N Engl J Med 326:1473–1479, 1992.
9. McCarty DJ: Crystals and arthritis. Dis Month 40:253–299, 1994.
10. Schumacher HR: Crystal-induced arthritis: An overview. Am J Med 100 (Suppl 2A):46S–52S, 1996.
11. Shmerling RH: Synovial fluid analysis: A critical reappraisal. Rheum Dis Clin North Am 20:503–512, 1994.
12. Shoen RP, Moskowitz RW, Goldberg VM: Soft Tissue Rheumatic Pain: Recognition, Management, and Prevention, 3rd ed. Baltimore, Williams & Wilkins, 1996.

68. POLYARTICULAR ARTHRITIS

David H. Collier, M.D.

1. List the most common diseases that present with acute polyarthritis.

Inflammatory arthritis
Rheumatoid arthritis
Systemic lupus erythematosus (SLE)
Psoriatic arthritis
Reiter's syndrome
Sarcoid arthritis
Polyarticular gout
Juvenile rheumatoid arthritis
Hypertrophic pulmonary osteoarthropathy

Infections
Neisseria gonorrhoeae
Bacterial endocarditis
Lyme disease
Meningococcal
Viral (e.g., hepatitis B and C,
   parvovirus, HIV, rubella)
Acute rheumatic fever

2. List the most common diseases that present as chronic (persisting > 6 weeks) polyarthritis.

Inflammatory
Rheumatoid arthritis
Systemic lupus erythematosus
Psoriatic arthritis
Reiter's syndrome
Polyarticular gout
Pseudogout
Enteropathic arthritis
Sarcoid arthritis
Polymyalgia rheumatica
Polymyositis
Mixed connective tissue disease (MCTD)

Noninflammatory
Osteoarthritis
Hypermobile joint syndrome
Hemachromatosis
Paget's disease
Polyarticular gout
Calcium pyrophosphate deposition disease

3. Describe how age, sex, and family history can be useful in the differential diagnosis of polyarticular disease.

Some types of arthritis are more common in certain age groups and gender.

Young: rheumatoid arthritis, spondyloarthropathies, SLE.

Old: gout, pseudogout, polymyalgia rheumatica.

Male: gout, ankylosing spondylitis, Reiter's syndrome, hemochromatosis.

Female: rheumatoid arthritis, SLE.

Types of arthritis that run in families include rheumatoid arthritis, SLE, spondylo-arthropathies, gout, and osteoarthritis (hereditary generalized osteoarthritis and hereditary Heberden and Bouchard nodes).

4. How may the temporal pattern of joint involvement in polyarthritis be helpful in the differential diagnosis?

Polyarthritic diseases present in three types of temporal patterns. The characteristic arthritides associated with these patterns are as follows:

Migratory pattern. Symptoms and signs appear in joints, then remit and go to other joints. Examples are gonococcal arthritis, rheumatic fever, and early Lyme disease.

Additive pattern. Symptoms and signs appear in some joints and remain as other joints become involved. This pattern is seen in patients with rheumatoid arthritis, SLE, psoriatic arthritis, Reiter's syndrome, and MCTD.

Intermittent pattern. This pattern presents as an acute polyarticular attack with a complete remission, followed by a recurrent bout of a polyarticular attack. Examples of this pattern are gout, pseudogout, sarcoid arthritis and sometimes rheumatoid arthritis, psoriatic arthritis and Reiter's syndrome.

5. Name the two most common causes of chronic polyarthritis.
Osteoarthritis and rheumatoid arthritis.

6. How do the history and physical examination help to determine whether complaints of polyarticular arthritis are more likely due to rheumatoid arthritis or osteoarthritis?

	RHEUMATOID ARTHRITIS	OSTEOARTHRITIS
History		
Morning stiffness	Usually > 1 hr	Usually < ½ hr
Movement	Improves stiffness	Increases pain
Systemic symptoms	Common	Uncommon
Physical examination		
Inflammation	Warm, occasionally red	Rare
Swelling	Invariable	Variable
Symmetry	Characteristic	Variable
Joints	Distal small joints	Variable
Hands and feet	Proximal interphalangeal (PIP) joint, metacarpophalangeal (MCP) joint	Distal interphalangeal (DIP) joint, first carpometacarpal (CMC) joint, first metatarso-phalangeal (MTP) joint

7. Clinical osteoarthritis can be placed into six categories. Name them.
1. **Primary generalized osteoarthritis.** Inheritance is autosomal dominant in women and recessive in men. Commonly affected joints are PIP, DIP, first CMC, knees, and spine.
2. **Inflammatory or erosive small-joint osteoarthritis.** Found primarily in post-menopausal women and in some cases familial; this category of disease involves the DIP and PIP joints. The patient usually has a negative rheumatoid factor, normal sedimentation rate, and no systemic symptoms.
3. **Isolated nodule osteoarthritis** usually begins after age 45 and is inherited. The patient has Heberden nodes over the DIPs and Bouchard nodes over the PIPs.
4. **Unifocal large joint osteoarthritis** usually affects the hip or knee. Congenital hip problems are notable.
5. **Multifocal large joint osteoarthritis** usually affects both hips or knees.
6. **Unifocal small joint osteoarthritis** commonly affects the first CMC or first MTP (bunion).

8. How is rheumatoid arthritis (RA) diagnosed?
RA is diagnosed by a constellation of clinical and laboratory abnormalities, often appearing over a 1-year period. Criteria developed by the American College of Rheumatology have a high sensitivity (90–95%) and specificity (89%) in establishing the diagnosis but cannot be used to exclude early disease. These criteria were developed mainly for studies on patients with RA. Four of the seven following criteria should be observed by a physician for 6 weeks:
1. Morning stiffness of more than 1 hour's duration
2. Polyarticular arthritis (simultaneous involvement of 3 or more joint areas)
3. Arthritis of the hands or wrist
4. Simultaneous symmetric arthritis
5. Rheumatoid nodules
6. Positive rheumatoid factor
7. Typical radiographic changes of rheumatoid arthritis in the hands adjacent to affected joints

9. Is RA a disease only of joints?

No. The spectrum of RA ranges from mild, seronegative disease to high titers of rheumatoid factor accompanied by vasculitis. Patients with RA may have rheumatoid nodules, small and medium vessel vasculitis involving the skin and peripheral nerves, pleuropericardial or pleuropulmonary disease, eye disease (episcleritis, scleritis), and Felty's syndrome. About one-third of patients have associated secondary Sjögren's syndrome or Sicca syndrome with dry eyes and dry mouth. Carpal tunnel syndrome is common.

10. What other diseases in addition to rheumatoid arthritis may have subcutaneous nodules?

SLE	Rheumatic fever
Tophaceous gout	Vasculitis
Erythema nodosum	Panniculitis
Scleroderma with calcinosis	Sarcoid
Juvenile rheumatoid arthritis	Type II hyperlipoproteinemia

11. What is the standard therapeutic approach to patients with RA?

1. Education by trained professionals.

2. Occupational and physical medicine to instruct patient about joint protection, assistive devices, range-of-motion exercises, and use of heat and cold.

3. First-line pharmacologic therapy for control of pain and inflammation is usually nonsteroidal antiinflammatory drugs (NSAIDs), prescribed at optimal doses as tolerated. If the disease is not adequately controlled by NSAIDs, second-line agents should be started. Erosive disease usually becomes evident in the first 2 years of disease. Thus, second-line agents should be started in patients with evidence of progression of the arthritis.

4. The main second-line agents are methotrexate, oral or injectable gold, hydroxychloroquine, sulfasalazine, azathioprine, penicillamine, and cyclosporine. Low doses of prednisone are used as a bridge to control symptoms until the second-line agents take effect.

12. What is the characteristic difference between the arthritis in RA and SLE?

Both are a polyarticular symmetric inflammatory arthritis that most commonly affects the hands (PIPs, MCPs, wrists) and feet. SLE, however, is nonerosive and has reducible deformities. Alignment abnormalities, swelling, pain, and even subcutaneous nodules may be seen in both diseases.

13. What is the "gel" phenomenon?

The gel phenomenon refers to the complaint of stiffening with inactivity and is characteristic of systemic arthritides. Typically, it develops with prolonged sitting or is manifest as morning stiffness that requires loosening with a hot shower or activity. Quantitating the morning stiffness may be helpful in gauging the severity of the disease and its response to therapy.

14. Describe the four major characteristics of the spondyloarthropathies.

1. Seronegative arthritis (absence of rheumatoid factor and nodules).

2. Asymmetric involvement of peripheral joints (often in the lower extremity), accompanied usually by sacroiliitis (whether symptomatic or evident only on radiographs) and often by spondylitis involving the posterior intervertebral apophyseal joints.

3. Involvement of synchondroses (cartilaginous junction between bones), specifically in the vertebral bodies and discs, pubic symphysis, and manubriosternal joints.

4. Enthesopathies or inflammation at insertions of ligaments, tendons, and fibrous structures into the bone.

15. How are the spondyloarthropathies characterized?

Spondyloarthropathies are characterized by the level of involvement of the sacroiliac joint:

Bilateral sacroiliitis	**Unilateral sacroiliitis**
Ankylosing spondylitis	Reiter's disease
Enteropathic arthropathies	Psoriatic arthropathy
due to ulcerative colitis or	
Crohn's disease	

Other diseases, such as Whipple's disease and Behçet's syndrome, may present with sacroiliitis but are not spondyloarthropathies.

16. What five questions about back pain may distinguish an inflammatory cause, as seen with a spondyloarthropathy, from a mechanical one?

1. Did the back pain begin before the age of 40 years? Most mechanical back problems start after 40, whereas most spondyloarthropathies are symptomatic before 40.

2. Was the onset of pain insidious? The pain of ankylosing spondylitis typically has a slow, vague onset, whereas most mechanical back problems start suddenly.

3. Is the duration of the pain over 3 months? More than 80% of acute back injuries improve after 3 months, whereas pain of the spondyloarthropathies is slowly progressive.

4. Is the pain worse in the morning and associated with morning stiffness? A major complaint of most patients with inflammatory problems is severe back stiffness and pain in the morning, which lasts over 1 hour. Mechanical back problems typically improve after a night's rest.

5. Does the pain improve with exercise? Moving the back exacerbates pain due to a mechanical problem, whereas a patient with ankylosing spondylitis may exercise each morning to feel more comfortable and to carry out daily activities.

17. What physical maneuvers may point to a diagnosis of spondyloarthropathies?

1. **Measurement of spinal range of motion**. Mark two points on the back, one at the base of the low back in the L5–S1 area and one 10 cm above this mark. The patient is asked to bend over in an attempt to touch the toes. A normal change between the two marks is 5 cm, or a total range of motion of 15 cm. A smaller change suggests restricted range of motion of the lower spine.

2. **Palpation of the sacroiliac joints**. Pressure on the pelvis while the patient lies on the side or back may elicit pain over the sacroiliac joint. Pain in the sacroiliac joint may be brought out by Gaenslen's maneuver, in which the patient lies on the side, flexes the ipsilateral hip (knee to chest), and then hyperextends the contralateral hip.

18. What five organ systems may be involved in patients with spondyloarthropathies?

1. Eyes: iritis, uveitis, or conjunctivitis
2. Skin: psoriasis, keratoderma blenorrhagicum (similar to psoriasis)
3. Cardiovascular system: aortitis, conduction defects
4. Pulmonary system: apical pulmonary fibrosis
5. Gastrointestinal tract: diarrhea, ulcerations of the small and large intestines

19. What constitutes Reiter's syndrome?

Reiter's syndrome is a type of reactive arthritis. Typically it is an acute, asymmetric arthritis of the lower extremities, sometimes accompanied by dactylitis (sausage digit). It may be isolated to joints or include systemic illness characterized by fatigue, fever, and weight loss. Classic accompanying or intercurrent manifestations involve the following three systems:

1. Urethritis or cervicitis (including prostatitis and salpingitis)
2. Ocular manifestations, ranging from sporadic conjunctivitis to debilitating uveitis
3. Mucocutaneous disease, ranging from painless oral or genital ulceration to keratoderma blenorrhagica, a psoriatic like skin lesion typically on the palms and soles.

20. What organisms have been associated with patients who develop reactive arthritis?

The following organisms have been cultured from stool or genitourinary discharge: *Chlamydia trachomatis, Neisseria gonorrhoeae, Shigella flexneri, Yersinia enterocolitica, Campylobacter jejuni, Borrelia burgdorferi,* and *Salmonella* species. *Salmonella, Borrelia* and *Neisseria* species may cause true septic arthritis as well as reactive arthritis. Other organisms also have been implicated.

21. Psoriatic arthritis can present in five different patterns of joint involvement. Name them.
1. Asymmetrical oligo- or polyarthritis of peripheral joints
2. Chronic symmetrical polyarthritis, with or without skin lesions
3. Rapidly destructive arthritis (arthritis mutilans)
4. Spondylitis, with or without peripheral arthritis
5. Isolated arthritis of distal interphalangeal joints

22. When should the human leukocyte antigen B27 (HLA-B27) be assessed in patients suspected of having a spondyloarthropathy?
Seronegative spondyloarthropathy probably arises from interactions of a susceptible genetic background and an environmental factor that induces the disease. HLA-B27 is strongly associated with the spondyloarthropathies, especially in Caucasians (over 80% of Caucasians with ankylosing spondylitis are HLA-B27–positive). However, in Japanese and Africans HLA-B27 is associated with less than one-half of cases. Of 100 people who are HLA-B27–positive, only 2 have a spondyloarthropathy. Thus, it is a poor screening test. HLA-B27 may be helpful in family counseling or in particularly enigmatic cases in which every piece of evidence may help to determine a probable diagnosis.

23. What skin lesions may lead to the diagnosis of a patient presenting with polyarthritis?
Psoriatic plaque—psoriatic arthritis
Keratoderma blennorrhagicum—Reiter's syndrome
Butterfly rash, discoid lupus, subacute cutaneous lupus, or photosensitive skin rash—systemic lupus erythematosus
Erythema marginatum—acute rheumatic fever
Erythema nodosum—sarcoid arthritis, enteropathic arthropathies
Erythema chronicum migrans—Lyme arthritis
Vesicopustular lesions or hemorrhagic papules—gonococcal arthritis
Heliotrope rash on eyelids or erythema of the upper chest—dermatomyositis
Gottron's papules overlying the extensor aspects of the MCP and PIP joints of the hands—dermatomyositis
Gray/brown skin hyperpigmentation—hemochromatosis
Thickened skin—systemic sclerosis

24. What rheumatic conditions are possible in a patient with Raynaud's phenomena and polyarticular complaints?
Systemic sclerosis (prevalence: over 90%)
Mixed connective tissue disease (prevalence: 80%)
Systemic lupus erythematosus (prevalence: 10–40%)
Sjögren's syndrome (prevalence: 30%)
Polymyositis/dermatomyositis (prevalence: 20%)
Cryoglobulinemia (prevalence: 10%)

25. What tests may be helpful in evaluating a patient with polyarthritis?

Complete blood count	Urinalysis
Erythrocyte sedimentation rate	Synovial fluid analysis
Antinuclear antibodies (ANA)	Radiographs
Rheumatoid factor	Others to consider:
Liver enzymes	Thyroid-stimulating hormone
Serum creatinine	Calcium, phosphorus, albumin
Serum uric acid	Iron studies

CONTROVERSY

26. Are antibiotics of benefit in the therapy of reactive arthritis?

Treatment of reactive arthritis has classically centered on NSAIDs; refractory cases are treated with sulfasalazine, corticosteroids, methotrexate, or other immunosuppressive drugs. In the past antibiotics were thought to play no role. Recently, however, chlamydia-induced disease was shown to respond to a 3-month course of long-acting tetracycline. However, the effectiveness of other antibiotics remains to be determined.

BIBLIOGRAPHY

1. American College of Rheumatology Ad Hoc Committee on Clinical Guidelines: Guidelines for the management of rheumatoid arthritis. Arthritis Rheum 39:713–722, 1996.
2. Bornalaski JS: Acute rheumatologic disorders in the elderly. Emerg Med Clin North Am 8:341–359, 1990.
3. Calin A, Elswood J, Rigg S, Skevington SM: Ankylosing spondylitis—an analytical review of 1500 patients: The changing pattern of disease. J Rheumatol 15:1234–1238, 1988.
4. Calin A, Porta J, Fries JF, Schurman DJ: Clinical history as a screening test for ankylosing spondylitis. JAMA 237:2613–2614, 1977.
5. Epstein JH, Zimmerman B, Ho G: Polyarticular septic arthritis. J Rheumatol 13:1105–1107, 1986.
6. Granfors K: Do bacterial antigens cause reactive arthritis? Rheum Dis Clin North Am 18:37–48, 1992.
7. Harris ED: Rheumatoid arthritis: Pathophysiology and implications for therapy. N Engl J Med 322:1277–1289, 1990.
8. Hochberg MC, Altman RD, Brandt KD, et al: Guidelines for the medical management of osteoarthritis: Part I. Osteoarthritis of the hip. Arthritis Rheum 38:1535–1540, 1995.
9. Hochberg MC, Altman RD, Brandt KD, et al: Guidelines for the medical management of osteoarthritis: Part II. Osteoarthritis of the knee. Arthritis Rheum 38:1541–1546, 1995.
10. Hughes RA, Keat AC: Reiter's syndrome and reactive arthritis: A current view. Semin Arthritis Rheum 24:190–210, 1994.
11. Klippel JH, Dieppe PA (eds): Practical Rheumatology. London, Mosby-Wolfe, 1995.
12. Pinals RS: Polyarthritis and fever. N Engl J Med 330:769–774, 1994.

69. LOW BACK PAIN

Joseph Anderson, M.D.

1. Why should the primary care provider develop expertise in the management of low back pain?

Low back pain is one of the most common presenting symptoms in a doctor's office. Approximately three-quarters of all adults experience back pain during their life. A recent survey found that low back pain accounted for almost 15 million office visits, ranking it as the fifth most common complaint by patients. In addition, disability from chronic back pain is growing at an alarming rate. Practitioners should be prepared to help patients with low back pain maintain functional status and be vigilant about identifying diseases that may present as low back pain, such as aortic aneurysm.

2. Which structures in the body may be a source of low back pain?

Musculoskeletal structures	Visceral structures
Vertebral periosteum	Renal organs
Outer layers of the anulus fibrosus	Gastrointestinal organs
Nerve roots	Pelvic organs (e.g., prostate, ovary, uterus)
Apophyses	Aorta
Posterior longitudinal ligaments	Endocrine organs

3. Which potentially serious diagnoses should be considered in the evaluation of low back pain?

Osteomyelitis, malignancy, aortic aneurysm, and unstable spine fractures.

4. What are the relative frequencies of diseases that cause low back pain?

Unfortunately, a large percentage (up to 85%) of patients cannot be given a definite diagnosis. Less than 5% of all patients with low back pain present with sciatic complaints. Another small fraction (< 5%) have malignancy, infection, fracture, or visceral disease as a cause of pain.

5. In addition to a careful history aimed at determining the organic cause of pain, what additional information should be elicited from the patient with low back pain?

The practitioner should extract a thorough and careful history from the patient, because the differential diagnosis of low back pain encompasses many organ systems. However, it is also important to question the patient about motor vehicle accidents, sports injuries, and previous back surgery. In addition, a full employment history as a date of eligibility for disability should be obtained. The practitioner also should ask about lifestyle behavior such as weight, exercise, and smoking.

6. Most mechanical back pain is relieved by bed rest. What diagnoses may be considered when low back pain persists despite bed rest?

Malignancy and spondyloarthropathy are two diagnoses in which pain may persist even after bed rest. Malignancy also may be suspected in the presence of weight loss and/or previous history of malignant disease. Spondyloarthropathies tend to present with an insidious onset of pain and morning stiffness.

7. What are good predictors of compression fractures?

Steroid use and age greater than 70 years are good predictors for the presence of compression fractures. Although trauma may be a cause, most patients have no history of trauma.

8. What is sciatica? What does it indicate?

Sciatica is a sharp, burning pain radiating posteriorly or laterally down the leg past the knee, often in association with numbness. Such pain is usually increased with coughing and sneezing. The complaint of sciatica is a clue to nerve root irritation and may herald neurologic compromise. The presence of sciatica usually signifies disc herniation, which most commonly occurs at the level of L4–L5 or L5–S1; however, sciatica also may be seen in spinal stenosis.

9. What characteristic history suggests the diagnosis of spinal stenosis?

Spinal stenosis is a degenerative disease of the spine and thus usually begins after the age of 50 years. Patients complain of pseudoclaudication or back pain accompanied by lower extremity pain with parasthesias or dysesthesias that worsen with standing but are not present in the sitting position.

10. What maneuvers should be performed during the physical examination of patients who present with low back pain?

1. Inspection of the back including identifying leg length discrepancies and spinal curvature abnormalities.

2. Palpation of the vertebral column and the sacroiliac joints. Point tenderness may be found in malignancy or infection, whereas sacroiliac (SI) joint tenderness suggests spondyloarthropathies.

3. Range of motion of the spine. Two lines are drawn (at L5–S1 and 10 cm above), and the distance between the two lines is measured during spinal flexion. A distance of less than 15 cm during flexion suggests decreased range of motion and may be one of the earliest manifestations of spondyloarthropathy. This test is called the Schober test.

4. Straight leg-raising. With the patient supine, the examiner raises the affected leg in the extended position. Pain at less than 60° signifies nerve root irritation.

5. Motor exam. See the table below for correlation of nerve with muscle innervation. Foot dorsiflexion testing is particularly useful.

6. Sensory exam. Careful attention must be paid to the dermatomal or lack of dermatomal distribution of numbness. The saddle area must be included.

7. Reflexes, especially ankle reflexes, are diminished when the S1 nerve root is affected. Although ankle reflexes decrease with age, unilateral loss of ankle reflexes at any age should alert the practitioner.

NERVE	MOTOR	SENSORY	REFLEX
L1	Hip flexion	Back/groin	Cremasteric
L2	Hip adduction	Back	Cremasteric
	Hip flexion	Anterior thigh	
L3	Same as L2 and	Back	Patellar
	knee extension	Upper buttock	
		Anterior thigh	
L4	Knee extension	Medial foot/calf	Patellar
L5	Toe extension	Lateral lower leg	Tibialis posterior
	Ankle dorsiflexion	Medial dorsum of foot	
S1	Ankle plantar flexion	Sole/heel	
	Knee flexion	Lateral foot	Achilles
S2	Ankle plantar flexion	Posterior upper and	None
	Toe flexion	lower leg	
S3	No test	Medial buttocks	Bulbocavernosus
S4	No test	Perirectal	Bulbocavernosus
S5	No test	Perirectal	Anal

11. What is the utility of plain radiographs of the spine?

Plain radiographs, although inexpensive, are often not helpful or even misleading. Because by the age of 50 years, two-thirds of adults have narrowing between vertebrae and 20% have osteophytes, radiographs are of greatest use after trauma or when systemic disease is suspected from the history or physical exam.

12. What routine laboratory studies may be helpful clues in the diagnosis of a patient with low back pain?

An elevated sedimentation rate (ESR) suggests malignancy and infection. A complete blood count, urinalysis, and assessment of calcium and alkaline phosphatase levels may be considered in patients who are older than 50 years, have failed conservative management, or have signs or symptoms suggestive of systemic disease.

13. When should an HLA-B27 test be ordered?

The HLA-B27 test should be considered only when the radiographs are normal, but the clinical history, setting and physical exam are perplexing and highly suggestive of a spondyloarthropathy.

14. When are other imaging tests indicated?

A bone scan may detect malignancy or infection before radiograph. However, it is not specific and does not detect lytic lesions. Computed tomography (CT) or magnetic resonance imaging (MRI) should be ordered when surgery is contemplated. Both are sensitive for disc pathology. However, a recent study found evidence of disc herniation in a significant percentage of asymptomatic patients.

15. What is the cauda equina syndrome?

The cauda equina syndrome is the constellation of bowel dysfunction and/or urinary retention, saddle anesthesia, and bilateral leg weakness or numbness. This syndrome constitutes a true surgical emergency.

16. When should back pain result in surgical referral?

Cauda equina syndrome (emergency)

Progressive or severe neurologic deficit at presentation (presence of fever should suggest epidural abscess as an emergency)

Persistent neurologic deficit and sciatica after 4–6 weeks of conservative management

17. How should patients with acute back pain be managed?

1. Education
   - Explanation of symptoms
   - Advise to return for worsening symptoms
   - Strong reassurance about the natural history (resolution expected)
   - Counseling: weight loss, smoking cessation (if applicable)
2. Activity
   - Limit activity only as desired (2–3 days) in patients with neurologic deficits
   - Bed rest should be prescribed for longer periods (up to 1 week) for patients with neurologic deficits
3. Pain control
   - NSAIDs may control inflammation and pain but should be used with caution in elderly patients or patients with renal disease
   - Narcotics and muscle relaxants should be used only for short, well-defined periods (1 week)
   - Heat may be used as desired after the acute injury
4. Follow-up: 1 month–6 weeks if the patient does not improve

18. What is the role of exercise in the treatment of low back pain?

An exercise program, in the absence of neurologic deficit, should be encouraged. Stretching exercises for the lower back and extremities and general aerobic fitness may improve back mobility, increase energy levels, and decrease recurrent acute episodes of back pain. Such a program may begin within 2 weeks of the acute episode, assuming that it has resolved.

19. What are the indications for hospitalization?

The patient should be hospitalized only if surgery is contemplated. Traction has not been shown to be beneficial in the treatment of low back pain.

20. What methods may be used to determine whether the patient is a malingerer?

Waddell reported five ways to elicit nonorganic signs in a patient who amplifies symptoms:

1. Spinal loading or rotation. Lightly press down on the patient's head and rotate the patient's hips and pelvis. These maneuvers should not cause back pain.

2. Nonorganic tenderness. If lightly touching the paraspinal muscles causes pain, the patient may be amplifying the symptoms.

3. Distraction straight leg raising. When the patient is seated, straighten the leg while asking about the knee. This maneuver should produce pain in the back, causing the patient to lean backward, especially if the straight leg-raising test is positive.

4. Inappropriate sensory findings. Check for reproducibility of sensory abnormalities as well as dermatomal distribution.

5. Overreaction during examination.

Kummel recently reported that the finding of limitation of shoulder motion causing low back pain is more specific than Waddell's signs for a poor prognosis for return to work.

21. List five basic principles in treating patients with chronic back pain.

Only 10% of all patients with back pain develop chronic symptoms. Patients must understand that complete resolution of chronic pain is an unrealistic goal. The mnemonic **TREAT** summarizes the approach to preventing chronic back pain:

T = **T**ransfer some responsibility to the patient. The patient must adhere to lifestyle changes such as weight loss and smoking cessation.

R = **R**eassurance. The patient should understand that the back pain is not life-threatening and should not interfere with most activities of daily living.

E = **E**arly mobilization. The patient should understand that activity will not be detrimental and may be beneficial.

A = **A**void drug dependency. It is unrealistic for the patient to expect total relief from medication.

T = **T**itrate medications upward only for short, preset periods during occasional flareups.

22. What therapeutic modalities have a role in chronic back pain?

Steroid injections have been shown to alleviate back pain for short periods (up to 4 months) in patients with sciatic complaints. A recent study of 158 patients confirmed the short-term benefit but failed to show any long-term effect of injection treatment. Patients with disc pain who fail conservative treatment may be candidates for this treatment.

23. What role does chiropractic medicine play in back pain?

Despite methodologic flaws in studies supporting spinal manipulation for low back pain, its use appears to have some efficacy in acute low back pain. A recent study found that the cost per episode of back pain was less for patients who saw a primary care practitioner than those who saw a chiropractor. However, there was a higher rate of satisfaction among patients who went to chiropractors than among patients who saw a primary care practitioner. Thus, chiropractors may have a role in acute back pain.

CONTROVERSY

24. Should strict bed rest be prescribed for all patients with acute low back pain, even if sciatica is present?

Strict bed rest has been the cornerstone of conservative treatment. The rationale is to limit disc pressure so that the disc may resume its previous form. However, most low back pain does not originate with the disc. Furthermore, little evidence supports bed rest as a therapeutic modality. Deconditioning, loss of muscle, and demineralization of bone are among the deleterious effects of just a few days of bed rest. On the other hand, the back must be given sufficient recovery time to prevent chronic injury.

A recent randomized, controlled study found that patients who continued normal activities as tolerated had better recovery than patients who were prescribed bed rest. Statistically significant differences were noted in duration of pain, pain intensity, lumbar flexion, and ability to work.

Thus, it appears unwise to prescribe bed rest for a patient without a neurologic deficit or sicatic complaints. Individualized treatment plans should be the rule with an emphasis on early mobilization. Patients with a neurologic deficit should stand periodically to decrease the negative effect of bed rest. Standing causes only a slight increase in disc pressure over the supine position.

BIBLIOGRAPHY

1. Assendelft W, Koes B, Knipschild P, Bouter L: The relationship between methodological quality and conclusions in reviews of spinal manipulation. JAMA 274:1942–1948, 1995.
2. Borenstein D: Chronic low back pain. Rheum Dis Clin North Am 22:439–454, 1996.
3. Borenstein D: Epidemiology, etiology, diagnostic evaluation and treatment of low back pain. Curr Opin Rheumatol 9:144–150, 1997.
4. Borenstein D, Wiesel S: Low Back Pain: Medical Diagnosis and Comprehensive Management. Philadelphia, W.B. Saunders, 1989.
5. Carette S, Leclaire R, Marcoux S, et al: Epidural corticosteroid injections for sciatica due to herniated nucleus pulposus. N Engl J Med 336:1634–1640, 1997.

6. Carey T, Garrett J, Jackman A, and the North Carolina Back Pain Project: The outcomes and costs of care for acute low back pain among patients seen by primary care practitioners, chiropractors, and orthopedic surgeons. N Engl J Med 333:913–917, 1995.
7. Deyo R, Loeser J, Bigos S: Herniated lumbar intervertebral disk. Ann Intern Med 112:598–603, 1990.
8. Deyo R, Roinville J, Kent D: What can the history and physical exam tell us about low back pain? JAMA 268:760–765, 1992.
9. Hall S, Bartleson J, Onotrio B: Lumbarspinal stenosis. Ann Intern Med 103:271–275, 1985.
10. Hart L, Deyo R, Cherkin D: Physician office visits for low back pain; frequency clinical evaluation, and treatment patterns from a U.S. national survey. Spine 20:11–19, 1995.
11. Jensen M, Brant-Zawadzki M, Obuchowski N, et al: Magnetic resonance imaging of the lumbar spine in people without back pain. N Engl J Med 331:69–73, 1994.
12. Kummel B: Nonorganic signs of significance in low back pain. Spine 21:1077–1081, 1996.
13. Malmivaara A, Hakkinen U, Aro T, et al: The treatment of acute low back pain—bed rest, exercises, or ordinary activity? N Engl J Med 332:351–355, 1995.
14. Spaccarelli K: Lumbar and caudal epidural corticosteroid injections. Mayo Clin Proc 71:169–178, 1996.
15. Waddell G, McCulloch JA, Kummel E, Vernner R: Nonorganic physical signs in low back pain. Spine 5:117–125, 1980.
16. Walvogel F, Vassey H: Osteomyelitis: The past decade. N Engl J Med 303:360–370, 1980.

70. HIP AND KNEE PAIN

Richard C. Fisher, M.D.

1. What are the most important questions to characterize pain in the hip or knee regions?

The purpose of the history is to focus attention on possible causes of the pain. The following areas are the most important:

1. **Localization of pain.** Pain originating in the pelvis is often felt throughout the low back, gluteal muscles, and thigh. Pain from bursae or tendons is sharply localized. Hip joint pain is often felt in the anterior groin area or medial thigh and knee in the distribution of the obturator nerve.

2. **Onset and duration of pain.** Onset is slow in inflammatory conditions but rapid with trauma or infections.

3. **Relation of pain to activities.** It is important to know whether the pain occurs at rest, whether it has changed the lifestyle of the patient, and whether it requires the use of walking support such as a cane or walker.

4. **Associated systemic symptoms.** Of specific importance are back pain, abdominal complaints, other joint involvement, and associated fever, chills, and malaise.

2. What is the first change in the physical examination of a patient with a disorder of the hip joint?

Loss of joint motion, usually internal rotation, is affected first. Motion should be measured with the patient supine and include flexion, extension, abduction, adduction, and internal-external rotation. Loss of motion and pain should be noted. Other findings include a limp and decreased circumference of the thigh due to secondary disuse atrophy. At times, pain with deep palpation is noted over the anterior aspect of the hip joint.

3. List the most common causes of hip joint pain.

Degenerative, inflammatory, and occasionally infectious arthritides	Stress fractures
	Paget's disease
Avascular necrosis of the femoral head	Tumors, especially pigmented
Acute fractures	villonodular synovitis

4. What is the differential diagnosis of traumatic hip pain in elderly patients?

The most obvious consequence of trauma to the hip region in elderly patients is a fracture of the proximal femur. Occasionally the initial films appear normal, but the patient continues to have varying degrees of pain with activity. In such situations establishing the correct diagnosis is important. The most common abnormalities include simple contusion of the soft tissue, fractures of the greater trochanter, occult fractures of the pelvis, and occult fractures of the femoral neck or intertrochanteric region. The latter are the most significant, because an initial occult fracture may become displaced without appropriate treatment. Focused routine radiographs may show a fracture line; if no fracture is seen, the diagnosis may be confirmed with a radionucleotide bone scan. This test, however, may not be diagnostic for as long as 3 days after injury. Magnetic resonance imaging (MRI) scans have been reported to be useful in assessing occult femoral neck fractures immediately after injury.

5. What common problems may masquerade as hip and thigh pain?

Spine problems
Atraumatic pelvis fractures (pelvic insufficiency fractures)
Lower abdominal abnormalities, including tumors and infection
Meralgia paresthetica (compression of the lateral femoral cutaneous nerves)
Claudication of the internal iliac artery

6. Name the common causes of avascular necrosis of the femoral head.

Among the many causes of avascular necrosis, the most common are trauma (e.g., femoral neck fracture or hip dislocation); use of corticosteroid medication; alcohol overuse; rapid decompression (caisson disease); sickle cell disease; and radiation.

7. How is avascular necrosis diagnosed?

MRI evaluation may show the earliest changes. The technetium 99-m bone scan is abnormal before plain radiographs. The scan may show decreased uptake of technetium initially and then increased uptake as revascularization begins. Plain radiographs show changes at a later time when an increase in bone density and subchondral fractures become apparent.

8. Describe the treatment options for avascular necrosis.

Initial treatment should include protective weight-bearing and physical medicine modalities such as range of motion and muscle strengthening. Antiinflammatory medication is of value for symptomatic pain relief. Once structural changes occur in the femoral head, the surgical options should be considered. The value of surgical decompression of the femoral head remains controversial. Decompression in the stage before radiographic changes but after changes on MRI studies may improve the prognosis for revascularization without collapse, but this approach remains unproved. Once the femoral head has begun to deform, decompression may not be helpful. Osteotomy or total joint replacement is indicated at this stage.

9. What are the manifestations of overuse syndromes in the region of the hip and knee?

1. **Stress fractures**. The most commonly seen overuse problem is stress fractures in the proximal or mid femur or proximal aspect of the tibia. Of greatest concern is a stress fracture of the femoral neck and intertrochanteric region, which often results in displaced fractures. Patients with this diagnosis should be removed from weight bearing immediately and considered for referral to an orthopedic surgeon for surgical stabilization.

2. **Soft-tissue injury**. Soft-tissue injuries develop from repetitive motion of the fascia lata over the greater trochanter (greater trochanteric bursitis) and lateral femoral condyle (iliotibial friction syndrome) of the femur.

3. **Tendinitis**. Quadriceps and patella tendinitis are more frequent in young patients at the tendon insertion sites.

10. Briefly discuss the diagnosis approach and treatment options for patients presenting with a painful snapping hip.

The "snapping hip syndrome" is not uncommon, although it is not always painful. The three major causes include (1) the popping of the iliotibial band over the greater trochanter of the femur, often associated with trochanteric bursitis; (2) a popping on the medial side of the hip associated with the iliopsoas tendon; and (3) various intraarticular lesions, including loose bodies, old fractures, labral tears, or hypertrophic synovium. Diagnosis is made largely by the clinical exam, although plain radiographs may show bony fragments within or about the hip joint. Iliopsoas bursography may be confirmatory for popping secondary to the iliopsoas tendon on the medial side of the hip. All conditions are best treated conservatively with rest or avoidance of symptom-producing activities. Antiinflammatory medication and stretching exercises likewise should be part of the rehabilitation program. Steroid injections into the bursal area or iliopsoas tendon may be of value. Surgical treatment is rarely necessary.

11. Which bursae about the hip or knee are more commonly involved in clinical symptoms?

Greater trochanteric bursa, prepatellar bursa, infrapatellar bursa, and pes anserinus bursa seem to be the most commonly involved. Others include the iliopsoas bursa and occasionally the ischiogluteal bursa (with prolonged wheelchair use).

12. Describe the treatment for bursitis and tendinitis.

Initial treatment consists of rest from aggravating activities. Rest may be supplemented with application of ice and use of nonsteroidal antiinflammatory agents (NSAIDs). Various physical therapy modalities are also effective, including ultrasound treatments. When conservative therapy is not effective, injections of corticosteroids into the bursa or tendon sheath may be indicated. The use of steroids about ligaments and tendons should be considered carefully because the alteration of collagen synthesis may lead to tendon or ligament rupture. The same is not necessarily true of bursitis. Surgical excision of the bursa or release of the tendon sheath is occasionally indicated for unremitting and disabling cases.

13. List the more common atraumatic causes of knee pain.

Because knee trauma is extremely common, it is important in evaluation of knee pain to elicit any history of injury. Atraumatic causes of knee pain, which may be associated with an effusion, include inflammatory or infectious arthritis, patella femoral arthritis, gout or other crystal-induced arthropathy, and synovial hypertrophy due to pigmented villi nodular synovitis. Other less common causes, which may not be associated with knee effusions, include avascular necrosis of the femoral or tibial condyles, sympathetic reflex dystrophy, and stress fractures. Intraarticular hip abnormalities often refer pain to the knee area via common obturator nerve innervation.

14. Describe the clinical presentation of a patient with reflex sympathetic dystrophy (RSD) about the knee.

RSD has been recognized for some time in peripheral parts of the extremities but only more recently about the knee area. Typically, the patient has had some minor trauma or an arthroscopic procedure on the involved knee and presents with early loss of motion to the joint. The classic signs include hypersensitivity to touch, pain far out of proportion to physical findings, decreased temperature, swelling, and atrophic skin changes. The most consistent area involved is the patella femoral joint. Radiographic examination shows osteopenia later in the course of the syndrome. Bone scans and tomography are helpful, but perhaps the most reliable diagnostic study is magnetic resonance imaging, particularly in ruling out intraarticular knee pathology as a cause of the pain. Treatment, as with other forms of RSD is usually symptomatic, initially with gentle physical therapy and antiinflammatory medication. If the symptoms progress, diagnostic and/or therapeutic sympathetic block may be indicated.

15. Enlargement about the knee may be associated with bursitis, knee effusion, or generalized swelling. How are the three differentiated?

Prepatellar bursitis causes fluid accumulation between the skin and the patella. A fluctuant area superficial to the bony patella is palpable.

A **knee effusion** elevates the patella, which is readily palpated beneath the skin with no intervening fluid. In addition, the suprapatellar pouch, which extends approximately 3 fingerbreadths above the superior pole of the patella, feels full superiorly, medially, and laterally.

Generalized swelling in the knee, as occurs from acute injuries, is not localizable to either the bony patella or the suprapatellar pouch. Swelling is diffuse, usually extends to the proximal tibia and distal femur, and is often circumferential in nature. It is frequently associated with ecchymosis.

16. What are the most common causes of knee effusions?

1. **Traumatic effusions** usually contain blood or a mixture of blood and synovial fluid. The fluid may contain fat droplets in the presence of an associated fracture.

2. **Posttraumatic effusions** occur after meniscal tears, ligamentous injuries, or other destabilizing injuries of the knee. Posttraumatic effusions show an increased amount of normal-appearing synovial fluid.

3. **Inflammation**, as seen in rheumatoid arthritis or gout, often causes an effusion with an abnormal synovial analysis.

4. **Purulent fluid** is seen in both acute and chronic infections.

17. What are the indications for joint aspiration?

The aspiration should be done for diagnostic purposes. Occasionally, after trauma the knee swells to the extent that it becomes tense and painful. Removing a portion of the bloody joint fluid relieves the patient's pain temporarily. After aspiration, the fluid should be examined visually to determine whether it is purulent, translucent, or bloody and should be sent to the lab for culture, cell count, crystal exam, and other specific tests as needed.

18. Describe the classic signs and symptoms associated with early degenerative arthritis of the knee.

The history usually includes pain with weight-bearing activities. Often patients report removal of a meniscus or a ligamentous injury some years before. A mild effusion may be present, and crepitus is felt with joint motion. The early radiographic changes include flattening of the femoral condyles, osteophyte formation beginning at the joint margins, and narrowing of the cartilage space. Weight-bearing films provide the best roentgenographic evaluation.

19. Describe the history and physical findings associated with patellofemoral disease.

The major finding in the history is pain with walking up or down stairs or inclines, rising from a chair, and kneeling. The pain is felt directly beneath the patella and associated with crepitus or a rough feeling as the patella glides over the femoral condyle. On physical examination the patella may track laterally as the knee reaches full extension. Patellar instability is evaluated by palpation with the quadriceps muscle rested and the knee extended. The patient becomes apprehensive as the patella is pushed to the lateral side.

20. What treatment is available for patella femoral joint pain?

The treatment depends to some extent on the cause of the pain. In general, treatment is symptomatic, as in other inflammatory conditions, and consists of rest, ice or heat, and NSAIDs. Protection of the patella femoral joint is sometimes possible with a patellar orthosis or a special type of taping to correct malalignment. Physical therapy consists primarily of short arc quadriceps-strengthening exercises. In patients with severe malalignment and recurrent subluxations or dislocations, surgical correction protects the underlying articular cartilage. The value of arthroscopic or open patella debridement and shaving remains controversial.

21. When are imaging techniques useful in the evaluation of knee problems?
Imaging techniques are useful for bony lesions such as osteochondritis dessicans, fractures, tumors, and early degenerative changes. Routine radiographs are indicated for the initial evaluation. MRI has become increasingly useful for diagnosing soft-tissue problems such as meniscal and anterior and posterior cruciate injuries and for evaluating possible bony or soft-tissue tumors about the knee. The arthrogram has been largely supplanted by MRI for the evaluation of meniscal injuries, although an arthrogram may still be of value in diagnosing the size and extent of popliteal cysts. Ultrasound is also useful for evaluating popliteal cysts and distinguishing fluid-filled from solid lesions. Computed or plain tomography is of value in evaluation of certain fractures, particularly in the proximal area of the tibia and distal femur.

22. When is total hip or total knee arthroplasty indicated?
Replacement arthroplasty is a serious undertaking and should be used only in patients with no other alternatives for treatment. Failure of arthroplasties may result in either a flail or a fused joint. Arthroplasty should be recommended only as an endstage procedure when the joint is destroyed by an arthritic or traumatic process beyond the point at which conservative measures are effective. The failure rate in young patients is high, and surgery is usually discouraged before the age of 60 years. However, in young patients who have incapacitating joint destruction and are not candidates for either osteotomy or arthrodesis, arthroplasty may be an appropriate procedure.

23. What are the expected outcomes from total hip or total knee arthroplasty?
The expected outcome is return to a pain-free functional status. Rarely does the involved joint regain full motion or become totally pain-free. The goal is return of enough function to allow activities of daily living and low-impact recreational activities. The major short-term complications are infection (reported incidence of 0.5–4%) and mechanical failure (reported incidence of 5% at 2 years). Both complications usually require revision surgery. The major long-term complication is mechanical failure or loosening, which at 10-year follow-up is reported in the range of 10–40%.

24. Discuss the treatment options for pyogenic infections of the hip and knee joint.
The choice of open drainage, arthroscopic drainage, or needle drainage of pyogenic infections remains controversial, although experts agree that some type of drainage is needed. Antibiotics also are mandatory in the treatment of these potentially destructive infections. In general, the two most important considerations are the type of organism involved in the infection and ease of access to the joint. The most destructive organisms include the gram-negative bacilli and staphylococci, whereas streptococci and gonococci are known to be relatively benign. Joint accessibility is important for adequacy of drainage and monitoring of the clinical response.

Pyogenic hip joint infections in children should be treated with open drainage. Treatment of other joints remains controversial. No clear evidence indicates an advantage of one treatment over another for adult hips and knees. If clinical response is not adequate within 3–4 days of aspiration, open or arthroscopic drainage is indicated. Failure of needle drainage is probably related to the virulence of the organism and inability to evacuate loculated areas within the joint. Acute infections following total joint arthroplasty should be treated by open drainage.

BIBLIOGRAPHY

1. Allen WC, Cope R: Coxa Saltans: The snapping hip revisited. J Am Acad Orthop Surg 3:303–308, 1995.
2. Cooper DE, DeLee JC: Reflex sympathetic dystrophy of the knee. J Am Acad Orthop Surg 2:79–86, 1994.
3. D'Ambrosia RD: Musculoskeletal Disorders: Regional Examination and Differential Diagnosis. Philadelphia, J.B. Lippincott, 1986.
4. Ecker ML, Lotke PA: Spontaneous osteonecrosis of the knee. J Am Acad Orthop Surg 2:173–178, 1994.
5. Frymoyer JW (ed): Orthopaedic Knowledge Update 4. Rosemont, IL, American Academy of Orthopaedic Surgeons, 1993.
6. Fulkerson JP, Shea KP: Disorders of patellofemoral alignment. J Bone Joint Surg 72A:1424–1429, 1990.
7. Holder LE, Schwarz C, Wernicke PG, et al: Radionuclide bone imaging in the early detection of fractures of the proximal femur (hip): Multifactorial analysis. Radiology 174:509–515, 1990.
8. Jackson RW: The painful knee: Arthroscopy or MR imaging? J Am Acad Orthop Surg 4:93–99, 1996.

9. McCarty DJ, Koopman WJ (eds): Arthritis and Allied Conditions. Philadelphia, Lea & Febiger, 1993.
10. Teitz CC, Garrett WE, Miniaci A, et al: Tendon problems in athletic individuals. Instructional Course
    Lectures. American Academy of Orthopaedic Surgeons, vol. 46, 1997.
11. Turek SL: Orthopaedics: Principles and Their Application. Philadelphia, J.B. Lippincott, 1984.

71. SHOULDER AND ELBOW PAIN

Richard C. Fisher, M.D.

1. What questions are important in taking a history from a patient presenting with shoulder or elbow pain?

1. Time of onset and patient's perception of the cause of pain, such as a fall or other trauma, overuse, or systemic illnesses
2. Duration of the pain and its change over time
3. Anatomic location of maximal discomfort
4. Activities that increase or decrease the pain
5. Functional limitations caused by the pain, specifically decreased range of motion, inability to use the arm for certain activities of daily living, and difficulty sleeping
6. Treatment modalities that have been tried

2. Describe the measurement of range of motion for the shoulder.

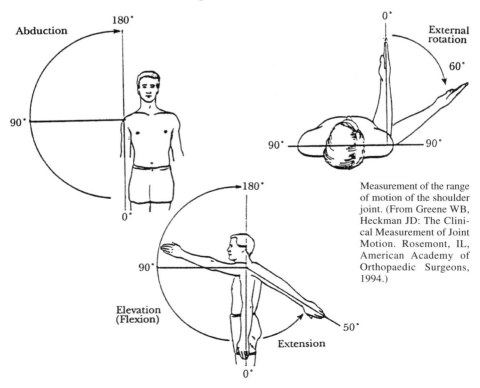

Measurement of the range of motion of the shoulder joint. (From Greene WB, Heckman JD: The Clinical Measurement of Joint Motion. Rosemont, IL, American Academy of Orthopaedic Surgeons, 1994.)

3. Describe the visible deformities that may suggest the cause of the patient's pain.

After trauma, deformity may be seen with acromioclavicular (AC) separations, shoulder or elbow dislocations, and fractures of the clavicle and humerus. AC separations show a prominence and/or swelling at the AC joint and may be accompanied by an abrasion over the tip of the shoulder. Patients with anterior shoulder dislocations have a hollow area inferior to the acromion with a palpable humeral head more distally. The arm is held in abduction and cannot be adducted to the side. Patients with posterior dislocations are unable to rotate externally. Elbow dislocations show a prominence of the distal humerus or olecranon with loss of motion. Fractures of the clavicle are usually in the mid-portion and present with swelling and/or bony angulation. Some fractures of the mid-humerus have visible angular deformity. Pain of neurogenic origin may be associated with muscle atrophy about the shoulder and arm region. The most common abnormality is atrophy of the deltoid muscle after axillary nerve injury or of the supraspinatus and infraspinatus muscles after compression injuries to the suprascapular nerve. Patients with spastic neuropathies often have an internal rotation contracture at the shoulder.

4. Can palpation help to delineate the cause of pain?

Yes. Patients with olecranon and subacromial bursitis have point tenderness over the tip of the elbow or shoulder. Traumatic deformity, even if not visible, often can be delineated by palpation about the clavicle, acromioclavicular joint, shoulder joint, and elbow joint. In patients sustaining acute AC separations, instability of the joint may be palpable with gentle downward stress on the arm. Patients with referred pain often have a diffuse area of discomfort that does not correspond to any specific anatomic abnormality and may have no tenderness at the site at which they perceive the pain.

5. What common sites refer pain to the shoulder and upper arm region?

1. Cervical spine
2. Brachial plexus
3. Thoracoabdominal region, including tumors of the lung, ischemic heart disease, subphrenic abscesses, gastric and gallbladder disease

6. How are the causes of referred pain differentiated?

Referred pain due to cervical spine and brachial plexus abnormalities usually is accompanied by local discomfort that is aggravated by motion of the neck and palpation over the brachial plexus. Neurologic deficits may be present. In thoracic and abdominal problems symptoms are referable to those areas and usually accompanied by physical findings or radiographic abnormalities.

7. Describe the differential diagnosis of a patient presenting with an acute swollen shoulder or elbow that is red, warm, and painful and not associated with recent trauma.

The most important condition to exclude is acute septic arthritis which can be diagnosed by aspiration of the fluid and examination for cell count, crystals, Gram stain, and culture. Other conditions to consider include an inflammatory arthropathy, such as gout or rheumatoid arthritis, and a neuropathic or Charcot joint. The latter is often associated with syringomyelia. Other conditions include diabetes, syphilis, leprosy, Charcot-Marie-Tooth disease, and rarely, congenital-indifference-to-pain syndrome. The diagnosis is usually confirmed by radiographic changes showing osteolysis and osseous fragmentation of the periarticular structures.

8. Name the common locations of compression neuropathies of the shoulder, upper arm, and elbow region.

Suprascapular nerve entrapment occurs as the nerve transverses the suprascapular notch on the superior border of the scapula. The presenting complaint is weakness of shoulder abduction and external rotation as well as diffuse, nonspecific shoulder pain. Atrophy of the scapular fossa muscles is usually present. Suprascapular nerve entrapment is often seen in throwing athletes and patients performing other repetitive motions. **Thoracic outlet syndrome** is commonly associated with pain after using the upper extremity in the elevated or abducted position and with symptoms of ulnar nerve dysfunction. **Ulnar nerve compression** at the olecranon groove of the elbow is one of the most common compression neuropathies of the upper extremity. **Median nerve compression** by the pronator muscle in the proximal forearm is seen less frequently.

9. Describe the diagnostic features of thoracic outlet syndrome.

Usually the patient complains of pain in the shoulder region with radiation into the arm. If the arm is held in the abducted position, the palpable pulse at the wrist decreases, and a bruit may be audible over the subclavian artery. This test also may produce pain and dysesthesias in the upper extremity. The ulnar nerve is most commonly involved, but median and radial nerves also may be affected. Adson's test is performed with the arm at the side and the head turned from one side to the other while the patient inhales. A positive test reproduces the patient's symptoms, and a decreased radial pulse is noted.

10. What are the diagnostic features and treatment options for ulnar nerve entrapment at the elbow?

Diagnostic signs include (1) a positive Tinel's sign (tingling sensation with percussion of the nerve) at the olecranon groove on the medial aspect of the distal humerus and (2) motor and sensory changes in the ulnar nerve distribution distal to the elbow. Electromyography and nerve conduction tests are confirmatory in most cases, if the diagnosis is unclear. Treatment initially consists of rest with a splint or sling and often a trial of antiinflammatory medications. Corticosteroid injections may be used but are somewhat hazardous because of the tight compartment in which the nerve travels at the medial epicondyle. Surgical decompression is indicated for persistent symptoms or progressive neuropathy.

11. Name the most common sites of bursitis in the shoulder and elbow region.

The **subacromial bursa** can be palpated directly distal to the tip of the acromion process on the lateral aspect of the shoulder. If inflamed, it is tender to palpation and painful with shoulder abduction approaching 90°. **Olecranon bursitis** produces swelling directly over the tip of the olecranon process, which is tender to palpation. In acute cases, surrounding skin appears red and indurated. Olecranon bursitis is differentiated from an infected bursa by the lack of systemic signs of infection and by the results of aspiration.

12. How does the cause of bursitis in the subacromial and olecranon bursae differ?

The principles of overuse and compression apply to both bursae. The subacromial bursa is injured indirectly by impingement of the greater tuberosity of the inferior aspect of the acromion when the arm is used in the abducted position. Olecranon bursitis is secondary to direct pressure on the tip of the elbow over the bursa. It may be initiated by an acute traumatic event but most often results from chronic irritation. If an abrasion is present over the bursa, the chances of infection are increased.

13. Discuss the common lesions in the elbow region that are secondary to repetitive trauma.

The most common problem is **lateral epicondylitis** (tennis elbow), which is caused by repetitive use of the upper extremity for a variety of activities, such as tennis or gripping a hammer or saw. **Medial epicondylitis**, although less frequent, results from similar activities, including golf. In both conditions the area directly over the epicondyle at the insertion of the extensor or flexor muscle mass is usually tender. On the lateral side other causes of pain include **entrapment of the radial nerve** just distal to the elbow and **inflammation of the anular ligament** about the radial head.

14. Explain the initial treatment protocol for medial and lateral epicondylitis.

Initial treatment includes avoidance of aggravating activity, ice before and after use, and antiinflammatory medication. Physical therapy modalities and a graded biceps- and triceps-strengthening program are useful. A tennis elbow band, which fits just below the elbow, acts as a damper for the extensor muscle mass and may be beneficial during activity. If noninvasive therapy has not helped, an injection with corticosteroid may be tried. Surgical release and reimplantation of the extensor muscle mass into the lateral epicondyle may be indicated in resistant cases.

15. List the pathologic stages of shoulder impingement syndrome.

The major stages include inflammation, fibrosis and scar formation, and overt tendon rupture. The inflammatory stage results from overuse in the region, which causes swelling about the bursa and/or adjacent tissues so that the greater trochanter impinges on the acromion with abduction and internal rotation of the arm. If treatment fails or repetitive activity continues, the tissues become fibrotic and scarred and lead to a decreased range of motion of the shoulder joint. Once the rotator cuff tendon, which includes the predominantly supraspinatus and infraspinatus muscles, ruptures, shoulder function is greatly altered and abduction is not possible. The late stage impingement syndromes are associated at times with degenerative changes in the acromioclavicular joint, which may lead to osteophyte formation and increased impingement in that region.

16. Describe the treatment for shoulder impingement syndrome.

The inflammatory stage is reversible and is treated with rest, gentle physical therapy, and perhaps steroid injection in selected patients. The stage of fibrosis and scarring is accompanied by a decreased range of motion. This phase is also reversible initially but becomes less so with time and repetitive activities. Treatment should begin with the same modalities as in the inflammatory stage, but some patients may benefit from surgical decompression either open or with the arthroscope. Once the tendons of the supraspinatus and/or infraspinatus and teres major rupture, surgical reconstruction is usually needed to regain function. In some patients, pain can be relieved with nonsurgical modalities.

17. What are the diagnostic features of rotator cuff tear?

A history of decreasing function and increased pain about the shoulder is fairly typical. Often the pain is worse at night or when the patient lies in the supine position. Degenerative tears occur over a long period after repetitive use. Traumatic tears usually are associated with an injury that the patient can identify as the onset of symptoms. The physical examination typically demonstrates the patient's inability to abduct the arm beyond 30–40°. If the arm is passively abducted above 90°, the patient can maintain the arm in this position. On lowering the arm, the patient loses control at about 90°, and the arm becomes painful as it falls. Often patients learn to maneuver the arm into abduction by circumducting the shoulder. Useful imaging techniques include routine shoulder arthrography, computed tomographic arthrography, and magnetic resonance imaging.

18. Describe the common mechanisms of injury in the shoulder region.

Falls onto the outstretched arm and hand commonly result in injuries at many levels, including the radial head, supracondylar area of the humerus, humeral shaft, and midclavicle area. If the arm remains tucked close to the side in a position of adduction, a fracture of the proximal humerus is likely. Such a fall is typical among older people, who may slip while holding a grocery bag. Falls onto the tip of the shoulder, often accompanied by an abrasion, are the classic cause of acromioclavicular separations. This mechanism is common with forward falls from bicycles and horses. Injuries with the arm abducted are associated with shoulder joint dislocations.

19. Explain the functional classification of acromioclavicular (AC) joint injuries.

Grade I injuries are mild and may affect both the coracoclavicular and AC joints. The ligaments are stretched and become painful but remain intact; no separation or deformity is present. Grade II separations involve a partial ligament injury with instability at the AC joint but without gross upward displacement of the clavicle. The coracoclavicular ligaments remain intact. Grade III separations occur secondary to disruption of the coracoclavicular ligaments, and the clavicle is displaced upward. With severe grade III separations, which often are classified as grade V in-juries, the tip of the clavicle penetrates the deltoid and trapezius muscle sling and occupies a sub-cutaneous position. Treatment of grades I, II, and III injuries is usually a sling followed by physical therapy for motion and strengthening. Grade III and V injuries may require surgical stabilization.

20. Why should an axillary radiographic view be obtained of all shoulder injuries?

Dislocations caused by trauma to the abducted arm usually result in an anterior dislocation of the shoulder; the humeral head is anterior and usually inferior to the glenoid cavity. The inci-dence of posterior dislocations due to trauma is about 10%. Seizures, however, result in a much higher incidence of posterior dislocations. Care should be taken in diagnosis, because the joint often appears normal in the anteroposterior radiograph. Thus it is important to obtain an axillary view in all suspected cases of shoulder dislocation. Recurrent dislocations require much less trauma and at times occur with simple reaching activities.

21. Describe the treatment for acute and recurrent dislocations of the shoulder.

The recurrence rate for a first-time shoulder dislocation depends on the age of the patient. Patients in the second and third decades of life at the time of the initial dislocation have a recur-rence rate as high as 70%; the rate decreases with age. Although the efficacy of treatment is con-troversial, the initial step consists of immobilization with the arm in a position of adduction and internal rotation; limited range-of-motion exercises should begin at 2–3 weeks. Abduction and external rotation of the shoulder should be limited for 6–8 weeks, and sporting and other high-risk activities should be avoided. The decision to perform surgical stabilization of the shoulder is based on the number and ease of recurrent dislocations and the inconvenience or risk to the pa-tient caused by repeated dislocation.

22. List some of the common skeletal tumors about the shoulder area that may present with a predominant symptom of pain.

In young people several benign lesions are not uncommon, including chondroblastoma, which usually occurs in the proximal humeral epiphysis; exostosis, which sometimes is associ-ated with multiple familial osteochondromatosis; and unicameral cysts, which are more common in children than adults. Malignant tumors include osteosarcoma and chondrosarcoma. Chondrosarcomas seem to have a predilection for the pelvic and shoulder girdle areas. Metastatic disease is common in the humerus, as is multiple myeloma. Although such lesions are rare, the possibility that they underlie shoulder pain make it especially important to obtain radiographs before proceeding with steroid injections or other treatment for benign conditions.

23. Describe the pattern of involvement of the elbow and shoulder region with the various types of arthritis.

Rheumatoid arthritis and osteoarthritis frequently affect the elbow, shoulder, and AC joints. AC joint disease may follow discreet episodes of previous trauma. The humeral head is a common site of avascular necrosis with collapse and destruction of the humeral articular surface. Poststeroid avascular necrosis seems to be the most common cause. Other less common causes include sepsis, neuropathy (see question 7), Paget's disease, and gout.

24. Briefly describe principles of treatment for arthritis of these joints.

If the arthritis is due to a systemic condition, treatment of the underlying systemic disease is indicated. For degenerative or osteoarthritis, nonsteroidal antiinflammatory agents and gentle physical measures monitored by physical therapy are appropriate. Synovectomy is at times indi-cated for early rheumatoid arthritis in the elbow; resection arthroplasty of the AC joint is a satis-factory procedure that usually follows conservative care and a trial of steroid injections into the joint area. Total joint arthroplasty of the shoulder and elbow are indicated when other treatment has failed.

25. What are the expected results of total shoulder and elbow arthroplasties?

Total shoulder arthroplasty has shown results comparable to those of knee and hip procedures. A 90% relief of pain can be expected initially, but the long-term failure or revision rate is 10–20% at 10 years. The cause of the joint destruction makes some difference in the outcome. Patients with osteonecrosis or degenerative arthritis have better results than patients with rheumatoid arthritis. The worst results are seen in traumatic arthritis following fractures about the shoulder with scarring and interruption of the rotator cuff tendons. Total elbow arthroplasty is less reliable than arthroplasty of the shoulder, but with new techniques it is becoming a more efficacious procedure. Its primary indication is joint destruction due to inflammatory arthritis, but satisfactory results can be expected in patients with posttraumatic arthritis.

BIBLIOGRAPHY

1. Alpert SW, Koval KJ, Zuckerman JD: Neuropathic arthropathy: Review of current knowledge. J Am Acad Orthop Surg 4:100–108, 1996.
2. Crenshaw AH (ed): Campbell's Operative Orthopaedics. St. Louis, Mosby, 1992.
3. D'Ambrosia RD: Musculoskeletal Disorders: Regional Examination and Differential Diagnosis. Philadelphia, J.B. Lippincott, 1986.
4. Dawson DM: Entrapment neuropathies of the upper extremities. N Engl J Med 329:2013–2018, 1993.
5. Frymoyer JW (ed): Orthopaedic Knowledge Update 4. Rosemont, IL, American Academy of Orthopaedic Surgeons, 1993.
6. Greene WB, Heckman JD: The Clinical Measurement of Joint Motion. Rosemont, IL, American Academy of Orthopaedic Surgeons, 1994.
7. Jobe FW, Ciccotti MG: Lateral and medial epicondylitis of the elbow. J Am Acad Orthop Surg 2:1–8, 1994.
8. Kasser JR (ed): Orthopaedic Knowledge Update 5 Home Study Syllabus. Rosemont, IL, American Academy of Orthopaedic Surgeons, 1996.
9. Leffert RD: Thoracic outlet syndrome. J Am Acad Orthop Surg 2:317–325, 1994.
10. Teitz CC, Garrett WE, Miniaci A, et al: Tendon Problems in Athletic Individuals. Instructional Course Lectures. American Academy of Orthopaedic Surgeons, vol. 46, 1997.

72. HAND PAIN

Richard C. Fisher, M.D.

1. What are the most common categories of atraumatic hand pain?

Referred pain from the shoulder or cervical spine	Inflammatory conditions
	Compression neuropathies
Overuse syndromes	Arthritis

2. List the common compression neuropathies involving the forearm and hand.

1. Median nerve compression at the wrist (carpal tunnel syndrome)
2. Anterior interosseous syndrome (pain in the proximal forearm associated with weakness of flexion of the index fingertip)
3. Pronator syndrome (median nerve compression in the region of the pronator teres muscle)
4. Ulnar nerve compression at the wrist joint within Guyon's canal
5. Radial nerve compression at the wrist (Wartenberg's syndrome)

3. How is carpal tunnel syndrome diagnosed?

The classic history includes pain at night, sufficient to wake the patient from sleep. Pain may be referred to the elbow and shoulder. In addition, the patient may have pain with repetitive hand use, a feeling of clumsiness, and numbness and tingling in the median nerve distribution on the radial side of the hand. Physical findings include decreased sensation in the thumb, index and long fingers, and half of the ring finger (with 2-point discrimination > 5 mm); weakness of thumb opposition; dysesthesias with percussion of the median nerve at the wrist (Tinel's sign); reproduction of the carpal tunnel symptoms with acute flexion of the wrist (Phalen's sign); or direct median nerve compression at the wrist. Radiographs may show changes due to an old fracture or other lesion in the bone, but these are rare causes of carpal tunnel syndrome. Electrodiagnostic studies help to confirm the diagnosis by showing prolonged sensory and motor latency and decreased conduction velocity across the wrist.

4. List the general medical conditions that may be associated with carpal tunnel syndrome.

Hypothyroidism	Hemophilia
Rheumatoid arthritis	Pregnancy
Multiple myeloma and amyloidosis	Hemodialysis
Diabetes mellitus	

5. What is the best approach for treating carpal tunnel syndrome?

The primary treatment is to decrease repetitive activities, to use night splints, and to initiate a trial of nonsteroidal antiinflammatory drugs (NSAIDs). Injection of corticosteroids into the carpal canal is controversial but at times may be helpful. About 1 in 5 patients receive long-term benefit from such injection. Results are better if the symptoms are less than 1 year in duration, intermittent, and associated with normal 2-point discrimination. Surgical release, open or endoscopic, of the transverse carpal ligament is usually the definitive procedure.

6. What is reflex sympathetic dystrophy (RSD)?

RSD is characterized by pain, swelling, discoloration, and stiffness in the hand and distal forearm after trauma. The symptoms are usually out of proportion to those expected from the instigating trauma.

1. Pain may be of a cutting or searing nature, usually worsens with range of motion, and usually is felt with light touch.

2. Swelling usually is extensive in and about the hand and often spreads from the point of initiation to encompass the whole distal aspect of the extremity.

3. Discoloration often begins as redness accompanying the swelling, changes to a dusky color in secondary stages, and may become pale in the chronic stages.

4. Stiffness initially is caused by pain with attempted range of motion, but as the fibrosis progresses, the joints become markedly limited in their range of motion. The final stages may actually be painless despite marked limitations of function.

5. Osteoporosis is seen initially as spotty areas of demineralization and later progresses to involve the entire extremity.

7. Explain the relationship of the shoulder-hand syndrome to RSD.

The physical findings in both conditions are similar, but the patient with shoulder-hand syndrome usually reports a history of proximal trauma to the neck or shoulder region, chest injury, cervical spine disc disease, myocardial infarction, gastric ulcer, or Pancoast's tumor. The physical findings in shoulder-hand syndrome include tenderness and stiffness of the shoulder and elbow in addition to the hand symptoms in RSD.

8. What do de Quervain's syndrome and trigger fingers have in common?

Both hand abnormalities result from stenosing tenosynovitis. The two most commonly involved areas are the tendon sheaths of the abductor pollicis longus and extensor pollicis brevis (de Quervain's syndrome) and the flexor tendon sheaths in the palm (trigger finger syndrome).

De Quervain's disease is caused by a repetitive use of the hand, especially the thumb, and characterized by mild swelling over the tendon sheath at the radial styloid as well as tenderness to palpation and pain with adduction of the thumb across the palm. Treatment may consist of splinting, NSAIDs, injection of corticosteroids into the tendon sheath, or surgical release of the tendon sheath on the radial side of the wrist.

Trigger finger deformities involve a tendon nodule at the opening of the flexor sheath at about the level of the distal palmar crease. The nodule becomes entrapped either within or outside the tendon sheath and makes a snapping sensation accompanied by discomfort in the area of the nodule when the fingers or thumb is flexed or extended. Treatment with injection into the sheath has been beneficial and should be tried initially. Surgical release of the sheath opening is indicated for persistent problems.

9. Describe the expected outcome after steroid injections for de Quervain's disease and trigger finger. What are the complications of such treatment?

Injection and immobilization of de Quervain's tenosynovitis show a success rate of about 60%, whereas in trigger finger the success rate is about 90%. The complications of steroid injection in this area include tendon ruptures; subcutaneous atrophy if injection is outside the sheaths and into the subcutaneous fat area; and loss of skin pigmentation if the steroid extravasates beneath the skin. Absolute contraindications are infection in the vicinity of the injection; injection directly into the substance of a tendon or ligament; and noncompliance of the patient in cooperating with a period of postinjection rehabilitation, which includes initial immobilization followed by gradual resumption of activity.

10. Patterns of arthritic involvement of the joints of the hand are somewhat characteristic of the specific diagnosis. Name the regions commonly involved with osteoarthritis and rheumatoid arthritis.

Osteoarthritis involves the distal interphalangeal joints, predominantly with production of Heberden nodes or distal osteophytes. In addition, the first metacarpophalangeal (MCP) joint and the first carpometacarpal joint (Bennett's joint) of the thumb are common sites of degenerative change. Rheumatoid arthritis involves predominantly the proximal interphalangeal and metacarpophalangeal joints of the hand as well as the intracarpal joints at the wrist. Synovial hypertrophy is common at the wrist and digital joints, and late changes typically include swan-neck deformity and ulnar deviation at the MP joints.

11. What are the common causes of posttraumatic midwrist discomfort?

Several entities may follow minimal trauma to the wrist that may be overlooked initially but manifest at a later time. The most common is fracture of the scaphoid bone that has progressed to nonunion, often with avascular necrosis of the proximal fragments. Untreated, it leads to late degenerative changes. Various syndromes of carpal instability that follow intercarpal ligament injury may cause diastasis of the carpal bones. The most common is scapholunate separation. Kienböck's disease (avascular necrosis of the lunate) follows trauma or a congenital discrepancy between the length of the radius and the ulna. Radiographic changes include irregular density of the lunate, often with collapse or change in shape of the bone. In addition, the most common location for ganglion cysts is the dorsal aspect of the wrist, and at times the cysts become painful because of impingement with the extensor tendons. A mass is usually palpable, and its size often changes in relation to activity.

12. List the causes of ulnar wrist pain.

The most significant aspect of the ulnar side of the wrist involves the distal radial ulnar joint in association with the triangular fibrocartilage complex, which completes the articulation of the carpal bones at the wrist. Tears or abnormalities in this cartilaginous complex may lead to pain and a snapping sensation with use. Injuries may be traumatic, resulting in tears of either the ulnar or radial attachment or through the midsubstance of the cartilage plate. Atraumatic injury results from degenerative changes causing tears of the cartilage and subsequent arthritis in the ulnar carpal side of the wrist joint. Initial treatment should consist of rest, nonsteroidal antiinflammatory drugs, and consultation from the occupational therapist. Carefully selected surgical treatment may be necessary. Other causes of pain include dislocation and/or arthritis of the distal radioulnar joint and tendinitis in an unstable extensor carpi ulnaris tendon.

13. A patient presents with swelling and pain about the index and long fingers after being bitten by a playful cat. How should the patient be treated? What are the likely organisms involved?

About 50% of cat bites become infected, and the most prevalent organism is *Pasteurella multocida*, although staphylococcus, streptococcus, and anaerobic organisms are also common. Before obtaining culture results, antibiotic treatment should be directed against these organisms; the first-line therapy is penicillin G and a first-generation cephalosporin. Other acceptable regimens include amoxicillin, or nafcillin plus penicillin. If it is believed that the joint or tendon sheath have been perforated or the bone is contaminated, surgical exploration and irrigation are also indicated. Do not forget tetanus and rabies prophylaxis.

14. Describe the clinical presentation of common hand infections.

Infection usually follows some type of puncture injury and involves several characteristic locations. Perionychia often develops around the nailbed on the dorsal aspect of the digit. Volar infections may involve the closed space of the palmar side of the tip of the digit (felon), which becomes red, swollen, and exquisitely tender. Because of the many spaces in the hands, swelling of the palmar surface with tenderness is the first sign of a deep space infection. If the tendon sheath is involved, the finger is held in a moderately flexed position and becomes painful with attempted passive extension or active flexion. In addition, fullness and tenderness may be palpated in the distribution of the tendon sheath into the palm. Because of the lymph drainage pattern, the swelling secondary to infection eventually involves the dorsal aspect of the hand, although the primary focus of the infection is usually on the palmar surface. Prompt treatment is imperative and usually involves both antibiotics and surgical drainage.

15. Discuss the common tumors that involve the hand.

The common benign lesions include ganglion cysts, giant-cell tumors of tendon sheaths, epidural inclusion cysts, and enchondromas. The first three are soft-tissue lesions that are easily treatable with simple excision. Enchondromas occur most commonly within the bones of the phalanges, usually are not clinically symptomatic until the bone fractures through the cyst, and most often are diagnosed by incidental radiographs. Primary malignant musculoskeletal tumors or metastatic tumors of the hand, although not unknown, are extremely rare.

BIBLIOGRAPHY

1. Abrams RA, Botte MJ: Hand infections: Treatment recommendations for specific types. J Am Acad Orthop Surg 4:219–230, 1996.
2. Chidgey LK: The distal radioulnar joint: Problems and solutions. J Am Acad Orthop Surg 3:95–109, 1995.
3. D'Ambrosia RD: Musculoskeletal Disorders: Regional Examinations and Differential Diagnosis. Philadelphia, J.B. Lippincott, 1986.
4. Fadale PD, Wiggins ME: Corticosteroid injections: Their use and abuse. J Am Acad Orthop Surg 2:133–140, 1994.
5. Green DP (ed): Operative Hand Surgery, vol. 1, 3rd ed. New York, Churchill Livingstone, 1993.
6. Idler RS (ed): The Hand: Examination and Diagnosis. New York, Churchill Livingstone, 1990.
7. Szabo RM: Nerve entrapment syndromes in the wrist. J Am Acad Orthop Surg 2:115–123, 1994.

73. LEG PAIN

Jeffrey M. Sippel, M.D.

1. Aside from obvious trauma, what are the most common causes of acute leg pain?
Bone and joint disorders and deep venous thrombosis (DVT).

2. List the common causes of chronic leg pain.

Intermittent claudication	Muscle cramps
Peripheral neuropathy	Reflex sympathetic dystrophy
Chronic venous insufficiency	Myofascial and rheumatologic illnesses

3. What are risk factors for the development of DVT?
DVT is the formation of a blood clot within the deep venous plexus of the calf or within the popliteal, deep femoral, superficial femoral, or iliac veins. Any component of Virchow's triad—endothelial damage, stasis, or hypercoagulability—increases the risk for developing DVT. Endothelial damage usually results from trauma, stasis due to immobility (as after surgery or prolonged travel), and hypercoagulability due to various protein abnormalities. Age greater than 40 years, congestive heart failure, myocardial infarction, stroke, prior venous thromboembolism, and possibly high-dose estrogen use are other risk factors.

4. What historical and physical findings support the diagnosis of DVT?
Patients who suffer from DVT complain of pain and swelling in the affected limb, usually acute or subacute in duration. Pain often is associated with use of the calf muscles, and frequently warm and erythematous skin is present. However, as many as one-half of patients may be completely asymptomatic. Physical exam focuses on at least four areas:

1. The calf is often tender to compression, and pain sometimes is elicited with forced dorsiflexion of the foot (Homans' sign).
2. Palpation along the superficial femoral vein (medial thigh) and into the popliteal fossa may reveal a palpable venous cord or clot.
3. The affected limb may be swollen with pitting edema; circumferential measurements (traditionally made 10 cm below and 20 cm above the tibial plateau) may objectively verify asymmetry.
4. The skin may be warm and red in the affected leg.

5. How reliable is the physical examination in diagnosing DVT?
Even in the face of abnormal findings, the clinician's ability to diagnose DVT accurately by examination alone is poor, probably not exceeding 50%. Numerous reliable tests are available to facilitate the diagnosis.

6. Discuss the different radiologic tests available for diagnosing DVT and their sensitivity and specificity.
1. **Contrast venography** is considered the gold standard of diagnostic tests for DVT. It is capable of visualizing clots in the deep calf veins as well as in the popliteal and femoral system. Contrast venography is an invasive test and in up to 25% of cases cannot be performed or interpreted for technical reasons. Risks include contrast dye allergy, nephrotoxicity, and induction of thrombosis. For these reasons, contrast venography is generally not the first choice when DVT is considered.
2. **Impedance plethysmography** (IPG) is a noninvasive test that measures changes in blood volume of the legs by using inflationary cuffs on the thighs. It is most sensitive for detecting clots

in the iliac, femoral, and popliteal veins and much less sensitive for clots below the knee. False positives may occur in states of hypotension, congestive heart failure, pregnancy, and severe obstructive pulmonary disease.

3. **Doppler ultrasonography** (US) assesses the patency of veins, looking for alterations in blood flow with direct venous compression. Like IPG, it is most useful for DVTs at or above the knee. It is highly operator-dependent but has excellent sensitivity and specificity when performed by trained personnel. False positives occur with any condition that may cause external compression of the suspected vein, such as hematomas, edema, and popliteal (Baker's) cysts. False negatives may occur with total vein occlusion. Duplex US combines the modalities of Doppler with real-time imaging and has improved sensitivity for clots in the lower leg. In certain cases it also differentiates fresh intraluminal clot from chronic thickening of veins due to old clots.

4. **Radioactive fibrinogen uptake** is not frequently used except in research. It has excellent sensitivity and specificity for DVTs of the calf but is not as accurate for above-the-knee DVTs.

Diagnostic Tests for DVTs (Compared with Contrast Venography)

TEST	SENSITIVITY (%)	SPECIFICITY (%)	LOCATION OF CLOT
IPG	94	94	thigh
Doppler US	76–100	87–100	thigh
Duplex US	92–95	96–100	thigh
Fibrinogen uptake	95	90	calf

7. What complications may arise from an untreated DVT?

Of DVTs in the calf, 10–20% propagate to the popliteal system or higher; once the DVT reaches the level of the knee, the risk of subsequent **pulmonary embolus** (PE) is about 25%. If the DVT remains below the knee, the incidence of PE is less than 2%. Therefore, in patients with contraindications to anticoagulation and DVT limited to the calf, the clot may safely be followed by serial noninvasive testing. If on repeat examinations the DVT does not progress, anticoagulation can be deferred with a low risk for PE, The recurrence rate for inadequately treated DVTs is approximately 50%, regardless of location. The incidence of **postphlebitic syndrome** is greatly increased with inadequately treated DVTs (see question 17). Within the 10 years following DVT, 85% of patients have some clinical evidence of postphlebitic syndrome.

8. Which hospitalized patients should receive prophylaxis for DVT?

The prevalence of hospital-acquired DVT is significant (see table below). Several studies have shown that the incidence of DVT, subsequent pulmonary embolus, and even overall mortality can be successfully reduced. Prophylaxis includes low-dose subcutaneous heparin (LDH), adjusted-dose heparin (ADH), low-molecular-weight heparin (LMWH), intermittent pneumatic compression (IPC), warfarin, and elastic compression stockings (CS).

Prophylaxis for DVT

POPULATION	PREVALENCE OF DVT (%) WITHOUT PROPHYLAXIS	RISK REDUCTION (%) WITH PROPHYLAXIS
Myocardial infarction	24	72 (LDH)
Ischemic stroke	47	45–80 (LMWH, LDH)
General surgery	25	20–80 (LMWH, LDH, IPC, CS)
Knee surgery	50–80	60 (LMWH, IPC)
Elective hip surgery	50–75	20–80 (LMWH, ADH, warfarin)
Hip fracture	50–75	43 (LMWH, warfarin)
Neurosurgery	24	60 IPC, LDH
Acute spinal cord injury	40	83 LMWH, ADH

9. Discuss the use of LMWH in treating DVT.

Hull et al. randomized 432 patients with documented DVT to receive either conventional in-travenous infusion of heparin, followed by oral anticoagulation, or once-daily subcutaneous LMWH, followed by oral anticoagulation. They found a reduced rate of DVT recurrence (2.8% vs. 6.9%), fewer major bleeding complications (0.5% vs. 5%), and an overall lower mortality rate (4.7% vs. 9.6%) with LMWH. The use of LMWH simplifies care and may reduce hospital costs for patients with DVT.

10. Does recurrent DVT with adequate warfarin therapy necessarily mean "failure"?

No. Recurrence of DVT is directly related to the adequacy of heparin therapy immediately after diagnosis. Hull et al. demonstrated that among 115 patients with documented DVT those who did not achieve an activated partial thromboplastin time (aPTT) of 1.5 times control within 24 hours had a 15-fold greater risk of recurrent DVT than those who did (24.5% vs. 1.6%). Heparin dosing nomograms have proven benefit for venous thromboembolic disease and should be used in all patients treated with unfractionated heparin.

11. What are risk factors for intermittent claudication or peripheral arterial disease (PAD)?

Intermittent claudication occurs when oxygen delivery fails to meet the oxygen requirements of a specific muscle group, usually during exertion. Inadequate delivery most commonly results from significant arteriosclerosis in the affected limb. The risks for PAD closely parallel those for coronary artery disease.

1. **Diabetes** carries a relative risk of three; in fact, 13–30% of adult-onset diabetics have lab-oratory evidence of PAD.

2. **Hypertension** is associated with a two- to threefold increase in disease and is seen in one-third of patients with PAD.

3. **Cigarette smoking** increases the risk of disease by two- to sevenfold.

4. **Hypertriglyceridemia** or **low levels of high-density lipoprotein** (HDL) carry a relative risk of two. The prevalence of PAD is approximately 20% in the general population over 70 years of age; PAD reduces life expectancy by 10 years.

12. Describe the typical complaints of patients with intermittent claudication.

Intermittent claudication typically causes a cramping or aching pain in the calf, thigh, or but-tock, reproducibly triggered by mild to moderate walking. Calf pain is the most common. The pain persists throughout walking, often causing the person to reduce or stop activity. Symptoms typically resolve within 10 minutes of rest. Disease of the iliac arteries is generally manifested as thigh, buttock, and calf pain; impotence also may be present. Isolated calf or foot claudication re-flects disease of the femoral, popliteal, or tibial arteries. Symptoms are often severe enough to affect normal daily activities and force a change in lifestyle.

13. Explain the significance of ischemic rest pain.

Ischemic rest pain is caused by tissue hypoxia when the patient is in a resting state; that is, ex-ercise and increased oxygen demand are not necessary to cause hypoxia and subsequent painful is-chemia. With sudden arterial occlusion, as in embolic disease, the pain is acute and severe. In most patients, however, ischemic rest pain results from progressive arteriosclerosis; pain may be subacute in onset, with numbness, paresthesias, and muscle weakness. The presence of ischemic rest pain indicates that a significant number of vessels have become occluded and that collateral flow is inad-equate to meet the basal metabolic demands. Patients with this marker of more severe disease are at greater risk to develop complications of PAD, including infection, focal necrosis, and amputation.

14. What physical findings are present with intermittent claudication?

The initial examination focuses on at least three components:

1. Begin by palpating the arterial pulses of the leg, including femoral, popliteal, dorsalis pedis, and posterior tibial arteries. Check for asymmetry in pulse amplitude and duration. Pulses in legs affected by PAD often are diminished or absent. If pulses are not palpable, a hand-held

Doppler device may be used to auscult the arterial pulse. This technique is also used for calculating ankle-brachial indices (see question 14).

2. Check for asymmetry in leg size that may be due to muscle atrophy in the affected leg. If the patient has bilateral disease, however, this finding may be absent.

3. Cutaneous changes are numerous and include thinning of skin, loss of hair on the digits, and predisposition to developing ulcers. Elevation of the foot produces dependent rubor and blanching. After the leg is lowered, venous filling in the foot may be delayed by 15 or more seconds (delayed capillary refill).

15. What tests help to establish a diagnosis of PAD?

The most commonly used noninvasive screening test is comparison of the ankle systolic pressure with the arm systolic pressure, referred to as the ankle-brachial index (ABI). Doppler ultrasound is used to detect the ankle pressure, over either the posterior tibial or dorsalis pedis arteries. In a normal person, the ratio is near 1.0 and does not decrease after exertion. A resting ratio < 0.94 or a postexertion ratio < 0.73 is suggestive of PAD in the appropriate clinical setting. If available, segmental limb pressures may be used to help in defining a level of blockage; pulse volume recording is helpful in defining sites at which focal calcifications may be present. Lower extremity angiography also may be used in the diagnosis of PAD, but it is not a screening test and generally is not performed unless surgical intervention is considered.

16. Discuss surgical vs. medical management of PAD.

Surgical measures for the treatment of intermittent claudication include percutaneous transluminal angioplasty (PTA) and surgical bypass. The goal of both therapies is to improve symptoms and function and possibly to slow progression of disease, thereby reducing the need for limb amputation. Both modalities have been shown in trials to improve symptoms, walking ability, and hemodynamics. Direct comparisons have shown the two modalities have similar rates of success, complication, and disease progression at 3-year follow-up. However, a population-based study by Tunis et al. showed that the large increase in the number of PTA and bypass procedures over a 10-year period did not decrease the rate of limb amputation, indicating that such invasive procedures may not be effective in limb salvage.

Medical management traditionally includes risk modification, and scheduled walking programs. Smoking cessation has been shown in some studies to improve maximal walking times and to reduce disease progression; although this finding may be inconsistent, smoking cessation is generally recommended. Lipid-modifying regimens have been shown to reduce progression of disease by 66%. Hiatt et al. showed that a supervised progressive treadmill walking program over a 12-week period was associated with improved peak walking time (123%), pain-free walking time (165%), and peak oxygen consumption (30%). In contrast, the control group increased peak walking time by 20%, but other parameters showed no improvement. Other investigators have shown similar benefits from increased walking distance with daily exercise programs. At least one study directly compared PTA and exercise. The 20 patients who underwent PTA showed a significant improvement in ABIs at 9-month follow-up but no increase in walking distances, whereas 16 patients enrolled in an exercise program showed significant increases in walking distances at 18 months without concomitant increases in ABIs.

17. Are any drugs available to treat claudication?

Several drugs have been studied with limited success. In some clinical trials pentoxifylline has been shown to increase pain-free and maximal walking distances by 66%. Other studies show favorable results only in patients with ABIs less than 0.8, and with symptoms for over 1 year. Pentoxifylline is the only agent approved for clinical use in the United States.

18. What causes chronic venous insufficiency? What physical findings are characteristic of this condition?

Chronic venous insufficiency of the legs is characterized by dependent edema and venous engorgement and frequently associated with local pain. Valvular incompetence within the thigh and/or deep venous system of the calf causes venous hypertension, which is responsible for the subsequent skin changes and swelling. Superficial varicosities also may develop, either from valvular incompetence or from inability of the thin wall to support high venous pressure. Skin changes include subcutaneous fibrosis, brawny edema, hyperpigmentation (typically on the medial and lateral aspects of the ankle), and predisposition to developing ulcers. Chronic venous insufficiency caused by DVTs is referred to as the postphlebitic syndrome. In many cases, however, other risk factors are implicated, such as obesity, advanced age, pregnancy, or occupational hazards (e.g., heavy lifting and prolonged standing). Diagnostic tests include ambulatory venous pressure monitors, Doppler venous surveys, and contrast venography.

19. How and why is chronic venous insufficiency treated?

Therapy includes leg elevation to a level above the heart and knee-high compression stockings, both directed at improving venous drainage. In fitting stockings it is important to ensure that a tourniquet effect is not created at the knee by an improperly fitted stocking. In addition, the patient should avoid prolonged periods of standing and elevate the legs several times a day. Because patients are prone to develop skin complications such as ulcers, stasis dermatitis, and bacterial or fungal suprainfections, local skin hygiene is important. Specific therapy for treatment of skin conditions may be found in section 13. When conservative treatment of secondary varicosities fails, surgery should be considered, including ligation and removal of the incompetent valves and varicosities. Sclerotherapy is sometimes used as an adjunct to surgery.

20. Which peripheral neuropathies can cause leg pain?

The most common type of painful neuropathy encountered by the primary care provider is diabetic neuropathy, which typically is a symmetric distal sensory neuropathy but may have mixed sensory and motor findings. Burning pain, numbness, and paresthesias are common in the stocking-glove distribution. Other conditions that may cause painful neuropathy are listed below:

Medical illnesses	Toxins
Chronic liver disease	Cis-platinum
Hypothyroidism	Vincristine
Paraproteinemias	Isoniazid
Multiple myeloma	Lead
Waldenström's macroglobulinemia	Nitrofurantoin
Cryoglobulinemia	Pesticides
Uremia	Phenytoin
Vitamin B_{12} deficiency	

21. What physical findings are present in patients with diabetic neuropathy?

Decreases in vibratory sensation and pinprick vs. light touch as well as impaired two-point discrimination may be demonstrated in patients with diabetic neuropathy. Such sensory findings occur most commonly in a stocking-glove distribution and do not follow dermatomes. Autonomic neuropathy may manifest as orthostatic hypotension or abnormal heart rate/blood pressure responses to maneuvers such as Valsalva, deep inspiration, squatting, or sustained handgrip.

22. Describe muscle cramps.

A true muscle cramp is a palpable and visible muscle contraction caused by a hyperactive motor neuron unit with increased frequency of muscle action potentials. Cramps may occur in a muscle group that is already contracted and commonly involve the gastrocsoleus and plantar foot muscles. They often occur at night and are recurrent. Cramps may be triggered by voluntary isometric contractions of susceptible muscles. Isolated fasciculations are seen in 70% of patients. The prognosis of muscle cramps is good, given an otherwise normal neuromuscular examination. Therapy includes stretching, and trials have shown the efficacy of quinine, methocarbamol, and chloroquine.

23. Can cramps be associated with systemic illnesses?

Yes. Hypoglycemia and hyponatremia may cause true cramps. Thyroid disease may cause cramps, contractures, and myotonia, whereas hypocalcemia, hypomagnesemia, and hyper- or hypokalemia may cause tetany. Drugs such as beta agonists, calcium channel blockers, and ethanol also may be implicated.

24. What are heat cramps?

Heat cramps follow strenuous or repetitive muscle activity, often in supranormal heat with concomitant fluid loss (sweat) and hypotonic fluid replacement. Salt depletion with volume depletion rather than hyponatremia per se is believed to be the cause. Treatment is directed at replacement of salt and fluid.

25. What is reflex sympathetic dystrophy (RSD)?

RSD is an uncommon pain syndrome of an extremity and almost always follows local trauma. In the leg, many types of blunt trauma may cause RSD, especially when nerves are crushed or stretched. Patellofemoral joint injury, including operative intervention, is also a common precipitating event.

26. Describe the historical and physical findings in patients with RSD.

The constellation of symptoms and signs includes burning pain, hyperesthesias, tenderness to palpation of the extremity, autonomic changes, and muscular atrophy. If untreated, the disease progresses through three stages. Stage I is characterized by the gradual onset of pain and burning with allodynia (pain caused by nonnoxious stimuli). The extremity initially is warm and dry, and patients guard against unnecessary movements. In stage II (2–3 months), the skin becomes cold and clammy; accompanying cutaneous changes include loss of hair and thinning of the skin. Osteopenia develops at a higher rate than expected from limb disuse. Stage III includes limb contracture and severely limited range of motion, due to disuse.

27. How is RSD treated?

Therapy centers on early diagnosis with physical therapy directed at improving and maintaining range of motion. Narcotic analgesics are not uniformly helpful, and their use may be complicated by side effects and addiction potential. Although nonsteroidal antiinflammatory drugs are rarely helpful, a trial may be warranted, given the low risk. Regional sympathetic blockade or surgical sympathectomy may be helpful in selected patients.

BIBLIOGRAPHY

1. Clagett GP, Anderson FA Jr, Heit J, et al: Prevention of venous thromboembolism. Chest 108(Suppl):312S–334S, 1995.
2. Coffman JD: Intermittent claudication—be conservative. N Engl J Med 325:577–578, 1991.
3. Creasy TS, et al: Is percutaneous transluminal angioplasty better than exercise for claudication? Preliminary results from a prospective randomised trial. Eur J Vasc Surg 4:135–140, 1990.
4. D'Amico A: Imaging for deep venous thrombosis. Emerg Med Clin North Am 10:121–132, 1992.
5. DeFelice M, Gallo P, Masotti G: Current therapy of peripheral obstructive arterial disease. The non-surgical approach. Angiology 41:1–11, 1990.
6. Ginsberg JS: Management of venous thromboembolism. N Engl J Med 335:1816–1828, 1996.
7. Goldberg RJ, et al: Occult malignant neoplasm in patients with deep venous thrombosis. Arch Intern Med 147:251–253, 1987.
8. Gordon N: Reflex sympathetic dystrophy. Brain Dev 18:257–262, 1996.
9. Heijboer H, et al: A comparison of real-time compression ultrasonography with impedance plethysmography for the diagnosis of deep-vein thrombosis in symptomatic outpatients. N Engl J Med 329:1365–1369, 1993.
10. Hiatt WR, et al: Benefit of exercise conditioning for patients with peripheral arterial disease. Circulation 81:602–609, 1990.
11. Hiatt WR, et al: Diagnostic methods for peripheral arterial disease in the San Luis Valley diabetes study. J Clin Epidemiol 43:597–606, 1990.

12. Hull RD, et al: Continuous intravenous heparin compared with intermittent subcutaneous heparin in the initial treatment of proximal-vein thrombosis. N Engl J Med 315:1109–1114, 1986.
13. Hull RD, et al: Subcutaneous low-molecular-weight heparin compared with continuous intravenous heparin in the treatment of proximal-vein thrombosis. N Engl J Med 326:975–982, 1992.
14. Hyers TM, Hull RD, Weg JG: Antithrombotic therapy for venous thromboembolic disease. Chest 108(Suppl):335S–351S, 1995.
15. Lindgarde F, et al: Conservative drug treatment in patients with moderately severe chronic occlusive peripheral arterial disease. Scandinavian Study Group. Circulation 80:1549–1556, 1989.
16. McGee SR: Muscle cramps. Arch Intern Med 150:511–518, 1990.
17. Miles MP, Clarkson PM: Exercise-induced muscle pain, soreness, and cramps. J Sports Med Phys Fitness 34:203–216, 1994.
18. Radlack K, Wyderski RJ: Conservative management of intermittent claudication. Ann Intern Med 113:135–146, 1990.
19. Regensteiner JG, et al: Functional benefits of peripheral vascular bypass surgery for patients with intermittent claudication. Angiology 44:1–10, 1993.
20. Regensteiner JG, Hiatt WR: Medical management of peripheral arterial disease. J Vasc Interv Radiol 5:669–677, 1994.
21. Sinatra RS, et al (eds): Acute Pain. Mechanisms and Management. St. Louis, Mosby, 1992.
22. Tunis SR, Bass EP, Steinberg EP: The use of angioplasty, bypass surgery, and amputation in the management of peripheral vascular disease. N Engl J Med 325:556–562, 1991.

74. FOOT CARE

Stephen F. Albert, D.P.M.

1. What are the three most common foot problems in the United States?

Based on the 1990 National Health Interview Survey, ingrown nails and other toenail problems, foot infections, and corns and calluses are the three most common foot problems. Each of these problems troubles over 11 million civilian, noninstitutionalized Americans.

Incidence of Foot Problems in the United States, 1990

PROBLEMS	NUMBER IN MILLIONS
Ingrown nails or other toenail problems	11.3
Foot infection, including tinea and warts	11.3
Corns and calluses	11.2
Foot injury	5.6
Flat feet	4.6
Bunions	4.4
Arthritis of toes	3.9
Toes and joint problems	2.5
Bone spurs	0.95
Nerve damage to foot	0.23
Clubfoot	0.16
Others	2.7

2. What are the chances of success when an ingrown nail is treated by avulsion only?

At 1-year follow-up the success rate is poor. Ingrown toenails most commonly affect the great toes, but any digit may be involved. Although the condition may occur in either sex and at any age, it is seen most frequently in boys and young men. A prospective British study randomized 163 patients with ingrown nails into three groups: total nail avulsion, nail edge excision, and nail edge excision with chemical cautery (phenolization) of the germinal nail matrix. The recurrence rates at 1 year were 73%, 73%, and 9%, respectively. Phenolization of the germinal nail matrix can be performed by primary care practitioners, but the technique requires attention to procedural details. Underapplication of phenol may result in a greater than expected rate of recurrence, whereas overapplication may result in a persistent draining periungual wound that is prone to infection.

3. Why is foot care important to patients with diabetes mellitus?

Twenty-five percent of patients with diabetes develop related foot problems. Foot ulcers and amputation rank high among the many disabling complications of diabetes. Multiple foot problems may quickly progress to a critical point; without immediate and definite measures, amputation may soon follow. Of all nontraumatic amputations, 50–70% occur in patients with diabetes. Although the precise location and number of amputations are unknown, it is estimated that 56,000 involve the foot and leg per year.

4. Which factors contribute to amputations in diabetics?

Infection and gangrene are common causes of diabetic amputations. Contributing causes include minor trauma, cutaneous ulceration, and failure of wound healing. All of these factors are exacerbated by the nearly universal occurrence in diabetics of peripheral neuropathy (motor, sensory, and autonomic), peripheral arterial disease, and mechanical dysfunction in the lower extremities.

5. What is the most frequent cause of hospitalization of diabetic patients?

Serious foot or lower extremity problems (1 of 5 admissions of diabetics to hospitals in the United Kingdom).

6. Plantar calluses and plantar warts are often confused. How does the clinician differentiate the two?

Warts (verruca plantaris) result from viral infection, whereas a plantar callus (also called tyloma or plantar keratoma) is a dermal response to the vertical and shear forces of standing and walking on a foot with mechanical dysfunction, osseous plantar prominences, or a thinned plantar fat pad. Both are painful, visible skin lesions that are exacerbated by weightbearing.

Warts may be solitary with a clearly circumscribed border or mosaic with a patchy and irregular border. They have a rough surface with hypertrophic papillae and are tender with side-to-side squeezing. Individual papillae may become darkly colored from capillary hemorrhage secondary to standing and walking. Plantar warts are surrounded and covered by keratotic tissue. They may or may not be associated with an osseous plantar prominence. After paring, a "cauliflower" center is visible, the patient experiences pain, and pinpoint capillary hemorrhages readily appear.

Initial management of discrete plantar warts most commonly involves patient application of 40% salicylic acid plasters every 2–3 days after removal of overlying hyperkeratosis. Removal of macerated hyperkeratosis is best accomplished if the patient soaks the foot for 5 minutes in water and then uses an emory board or pumice stone only on the treated area, avoiding surrounding skin. Salicylic acid pain (10%) with lactic acid (10%) in flexible collodion may be used for mosaic warts or warts that coalesce over larger areas. The paint is commonly applied once daily and again is most effective if the macerated hyperkeratotic tissue is removed. Caution is advised when using salicylic acid at this concentration in patients with neuropathy and peripheral vascular disease. The physician should supervise closely the use of any caustic agents for verruca.

Plantar callus presents as a hyperkeratotic mass at a site of friction or pressure. The lesion consists of raised, often clear, compressed layers of stratum corneum without a definite border. The more severe lesions may be pared below the level of the surrounding skin without pain or pinpoint capillary hemorrhage. Calluses are commonly managed by periodic paring of the hyperkeratosis and use of cushioning innersoles or foot orthoses to alleviate mechanical dysfunction and to accommodate osseous plantar prominences and thinned plantar fat pads.

7. What advice about foot care should be given to vascularly impaired or diabetic patients?
1. Wash and inspect the feet daily.
2. Use foot creams or lubricating oils, except in toe webs.
3. Cut toenails straight; do not bevel the sides.
4. Do not attempt to cut corns or calluses.
5. Avoid self-medication and extreme temperatures.
6. Do not walk barefooted.
7. Wear appropriate shoes and inspect the insides daily.
8. Seek early medical care for all skin lesions.
9. Do not delay medical care for abrupt foot swelling.

8. What guidelines assist a patient in attaining properly fitting shoes?
Properly fitting shoes are necessary to avoid aggravating or precipitating foot problems. A recent study of 356 women aged 20–60 years found that 88% wore improperly fitting shoes. Proper fit implies correct shape and size. The shape of the foot and shoe should match. Both feet should be measured. Size should be assessed while the patient stands in both shoes; there should be approximately 1 cm between the tip of the longest toe and the distal aspect of the shoe, the metatarsal heads should be in the widest part of the shoe (particularly the first metatarsal), and the heel should have a snug fit. In feet with high insteps (pes cavus) laces are preferred. For feet subject to edema, shoes should be purchased later in the day. It is important to be aware that shoe size tends to increase with age.

9. What medical diseases are commonly associated with foot deformity?
Diabetes mellitus, rheumatoid arthritis, and gout.

10. How often does rheumatoid arthritis affect the feet?
Rheumatoid arthritis involves the feet in over 50% of patients. Patients commonly present with hallux valgus, hallux varus, hallux rigidus, hammertoes, fibular deviation at the metatarsophalangeal joints, and/or rheumatoid nodules. The distribution is symmetric, particularly at the distal metatarsals, with warmth, tenderness, and edema. The metatarsal heads often become plantarly prominent as the nonfunctional joints develop mechanical adaptations, including dislocation of the digits and displacement of the plantar fat pad. Radiographs show demineralization at the ends of the metatarsals, with joint space narrowing, articular erosions, soft-tissue edema, joint malalignment, and eventually subluxation. Women are affected more commonly than men.

11. What condition should be suspected in a normal-appearing foot with lateral forefoot pain, a joint of maximal tenderness at the third intermetatarsal space, normal radiographs, and negative laboratory tests?
Intermetatarsal neuroma, also known as Morton's neuroma, is often a diagnostic challenge. Foot radiographs, ultrasound, nerve conduction velocity, magnetic resonance imaging, clinical laboratory tests, and visual appearance of the foot usually reveal nothing out of the ordinary. The diagnosis is made through history and examination of the foot. The patient commonly indicates a sharp lancinating, radiating pain in the lateral forefoot that is relieved by removal of the shoe and massage. Palpation or squeezing of the affected intermetatarsal interspace and numbness or burning in the associated toes are common features.

A neuroma of the foot is an irritative process of the common digital nerve that supplies the plantar aspect of adjacent toes. The term *neuroma* is a misnomer because the entity does not demonstrate neoplastic growth of nerve tissue or fibers; instead, histopathology reveals degenerative changes with perineural fibrosis. Repetitive microtrauma and/or constriction are the presumed underlying causes. Intermetatarsal neuroma occurs in all adult age groups and affects women 9 times more frequently than men. The third intermetatarsal interspace is most often involved. Conservative measures include steroid/local anesthetic injection, accommodative padding to separate the metatarsal heads, physical therapy, and/or orthotics. Neurectomy of the affected area is the treatment of choice; the rate of patient satisfaction is reported to be 93%.

12. Why should cigarette smokers be counseled to stop smoking before undergoing amputation?

In a 1991 study of 88 nonsmokers and 77 smokers undergoing amputation, smokers had a 2–5 times higher risk for infection and reamputation. Thus, amputees should avoid smoking at least 1 week before surgery and during wound healing.

13. What patients should be referred to podiatrists routinely and acutely?

Podiatrists treat the full spectrum of foot problems. They excel in treating the chronic recurring foot problems that tend to increase as people age, particularly when periodic care is required, when prior interventions by the primary care provider have not been successful, or when the diagnosis is unclear. Of the acute presenting foot conditions, by far the most potentially devastating are infections in a diabetic, immunocompromised, or vascularly compromised patient. The primary care provider should be aware that podiatrists' educational credentials, interests, and expertise vary. In general, podiatrists that are hospital-affiliated, residency-trained, and board-certified are better prepared to deal adeptly with acute conditions.

14. What is the likelihood that osteomyelitis underlies a diabetic foot ulcer when the ulcer does not appear inflamed?

In one study, as many as two-thirds of 12 patients had clinically unsuspected osteomyelitis. Many practitioners believe that the radionuclide spatial resolution among the numerous bones and joints of the foot is inadequate and that none of the imaging modalities are entirely specific for osteomyelitis. Many advances in imaging modalities since 1993 allow more accurate diagnosis of osteomyelitis. The use of TC-99 HMPAO-labeled leukocyte scan (Ceretec) and MRI are superior to prior techniques. No matter what imaging modality is used, it is quite difficult to differentiate foot osteomyelitis in diabetics from diabetic osteopathy or osteoarthropathy (Charcot foot).

15. Injections into the foot are often painful for patients. What methods can be used to decrease patient discomfort, excluding systemic medication?

The addition of 6.25% sodium bicarbonate to lidocaine in local anesthesia of the foot decreased pain by 50% in a double-blind study. Adjunctive use of skin refrigerant further decreases the pain involved in the initial needle stick.

16. What is the significance of a normal WBC in a suspected diabetic foot infection?

The diagnosis of diabetic foot infections are made primarily on the basis of clinical signs and symptoms. A study completed by Armstrong found that in patients with active foot infections, 56% had WBC counts within normal limits. Therefore, a WBC should be used as an adjunctive test in diagnosis of diabetic foot infections.

17. What are the clinical manifestations of plantar fasciitis?

Sharp pain, aching, or stiffness at the plantar or plantar medial aspect of one or both heels. The pain is often at its worst upon arising in the morning or after sitting down for an extended period and then resuming activity, creating hobbling or limping for a few minutes before comfortable walking can be resumed. In periods of exacerbation during walking or standing, moderate or severe pain may persist. Palpation of a point of maximal tenderness at the medial plantar calcaneal tubercle is quite common. Dorsiflexion of the foot followed by dorsiflexion of the toes stretches the plantar fascia and usually elicits symptoms.

18. What is the role of night splints and shoe modifications in the treatment of plantar fasciitis?

Several investigators have stated that the use of night splints and shoe modifications are a viable alternative to foot orthotics in the therapy of plantar fasciitis. The use of night splints is often a complicated treatment modality. The night splint device is cumbersome in application and use. The theory that plantar fascial pain is the result of contractures and muscle tightening while sleeping is controversial. The concept behind the night splints is to prevent the plantar fascia from contracting. This theory does not explain the common presentation of increased pain upon activity and relief during rest. Studies show, however, that the use of a functional orthotic for up to 3 months relieved the symptoms of plantar fasciitis in 90–95% of patients.

BIBLIOGRAPHY

1. American College of Foot Surgeons: Ingrown Toenail—Preferred Practice Guidelines. Park Ridge, IL, American College of Foot Surgeons, 1991.
2. Armstrong D, Perales T, Murff R, et al: Value of white blood cell count with differential in the acute diabetic foot infection. J Am Podiatr Med Assoc 86:224–227, 1996.
3. Awbrey BJ, Bernardone JJ, Connoly TJ: Prospective Evaluation of Invasive and Noninvasive Treatment Protocols for Plantar Fascitis. Rehabilitation R & D Progress Report. 1989.
4. Bild DE, Selby JV, Sinnock P, et al: Lower extremity amputation in people with diabetes: Epidemiology and prevention. Diabetes Care 12:24–31, 1989.
5. Blume P, Dey H, Daley L: Diagnosis of pedal osteomyelitis with Tc-99M HMPAO labeled leukocytes. J Foot Ankle Surg 36:120–126, 1997.
6. Boulton AJM: The diabetic foot. Med Clin North Am 72:1513–1530, 1988.
7. Cicchinelli LD, Corey SV: Imaging of the infected foot: Fact or fancy? J Am Podiatr Med Assoc 83:10, 1993.
8. Frey C, Thompson F, Smith J, et al: American Orthopedic Foot and Ankle Society Women's Shoe Survey. Foot Ankle 14:2, 1993.
9. Friedman H, Jules K, Springer K, Jennings M: Buffered lidocaine decreases the pain of digital anesthesia in the foot. J Am Podiatr Med Assoc 87:219–223, 1997.
10. Greenberg L, Davis H: Foot problems in the US: The 1990 National Health Interview Survey. J Am Podiatr Med Assoc 83:8, 1993.
11. Grieg JD, Anderson JH, Ireland AJ, Anderson JR: The surgical treatment of ingrowing toenails. J Bone Joint Surg 73B:1, 1991.
12. Janisse DJ: The art and science of fitting shoes. Foot Ankle 13:5, 1992.
13. Keh RA, et al: Long-term follow-up of Morton's neuroma. J Foot Surg 31:1, 1992.
14. Krupski WC: Growth factors and wound healing. Semin Vasc Surg 5:249, 1992.
15. Lind J, Kramhoft M, Bodtker S: The influence of smoking on complications after primary amputations of the lower extremity. Clin Orthop 267:211, 1991.
16. Luskin R, Battista A: Peripheral neuropathies affecting the foot. In Jahss M (ed): Disorders of the Foot and Ankle, vol. 3, 2nd ed. Philadelphia, W.B. Saunders, 1991, pp 2122–2122.
17. Miller S: Morton's neuroma: A syndrome. In McGlamry D, Banks A, Downey M (eds): Comprehensive Textbook of Foot Surgery, vol. 1. Baltimore, Williams & Wilkins, 1992, pp 309–311.
18. Patton JP, Murdoc DP, Lindsey J, Young G: Rheumatoid arthritic foot. J Am Podiatr Med Assoc 83:5, 1993.
19. Pecoraro RE, Reiber GE, Burgess EM: Pathways to diabetic limb amputation. Basis for prevention. Diabetes Care 13:5, 1990.
20. Rogoff R, Tinkle J, Bartis D: Unusual presentation of calcaneal osteomyelitis. J Am Podiatr Med Assoc 87:125–130, 1997.
21. Schauwecker DS: The scintigraphic diagnosis of osteomyelitis. Am J Roentgenol 158:9, 1992.
22. Sussman KE, Reiber G, Albert SF: The diabetic foot problem—a failed system of health care? Diabetes Res Clin Pract 17:1–8, 1992.
23. Wapner K, Sharkey P: The use of night splints for treatment of recalcitrant plantar fasciitis. Foot Ankle 12:135–137, 1991.

75. FIBROMYALGIA AND RELATED SYNDROMES

Danny C. Williams, M.D., FRCPC, FACP, FACR

1. Define soft-tissue rheumatism.

The term **soft-tissue rheumatism** (i.e., nonarticular rheumatism) defines a heterogenous group of common ailments affecting musculoskeletal structures other than the joints. Symptoms may arise from the muscles, tendons, ligaments and their bony insertion sites (entheses), or bursae. Pain and functional loss are usually attributed to inflammation but may occur in its absence. Soft-tissue disorders are categorized according to their distribution: focal (e.g., bursitis, tendinitis), regional (e.g., myofascial pain syndrome), or diffuse (e.g., fibromyalgia).

2. What is fibromyalgia?

Fibromyalgia is a chronic, generalized musculoskeletal pain syndrome of unknown etiology. Fibromyalgia is not a disease but a distinct, chronic pain syndrome characterized by multiple somatic symptoms and widespread muscle tenderness. The term **fibromyalgia** is preferred over **fibrositis**, the syndrome's previous designation, which erroneously implies an inflammatory disorder. In the clinical setting, fibromyalgia simply identifies a patient population exhibiting similar symptoms and signs.

3. Who develops fibromyalgia?

Fibromyalgia is predominantly a disorder of middle-aged women (80–90%). Although peak age of onset is from 35–50 years, fibromyalgia may occur in anyone, including children (usually adolescents) and elderly people. The prevalence of fibromyalgia is estimated to be 2% in the general population. Familial aggregation has been reported, suggesting the possibility of genetic predisposition.

4. In what settings may fibromyalgia be seen?

Fibromyalgia may develop at any time, either spontaneously or in relation to a stressful life event, such as a flulike illness, whiplash injury, or divorce. Despite temporal association of precipitating events with fibromyalgia inception, no evidence of a causal relationship has been demonstrated. Fibromyalgia also may be seen in patients with established, chronic illnesses such as rheumatoid arthritis, alcoholism, and acquired immunodeficiency syndrome. In patients with chronic diseases (e.g., systemic lupus erythematosus), careful evaluation for fibromyalgia may prevent unwarranted therapeutic alterations (e.g., prescribing corticosteroids) for symptoms actually attributable to the chronic pain syndrome.

5. Describe the clinical features of fibromyalgia.

The essential features of fibromyalgia are diffuse subjective pain and physically demonstrable areas of muscle tenderness (i.e., tender points). Profound fatigue, nonrestorative sleep, and diffuse stiffness are also major manifestations. Other associated symptoms may include headaches (tension or migraine), dizziness, sicca, atypical chest pain, irritable bowel syndrome, irritable bladder, arthralgias with subjective joint swelling, nondermatomal paresthesias, cognitive dysfunction, and depression. Raynaud's phenomenon and mitral valve prolapse are common. Symptoms may be exacerbated by factors such as physical and mental stress, weather changes, inactivity, repetitive exercise, and poor sleep.

6. What are tender points?

Aside from a nonspecific, alpha electroencephalogram (EEG) sleep anomaly, multiple tender points are the only physical finding in patients with fibromyalgia. Tender points are discrete areas

(2–3 cm in diameter) of normal-appearing skin at which application of digital pressure elicits focal pain. Adequate pressure is the pressure required to blanche the thumbnail (4 kg/cm²). Palpation of a tender point should generate pain and frequently causes a sudden withdrawal response—the "jump sign." Control points (e.g., central forehead, anterior mid-thigh, and thumbnail) are used to differentiate fibromyalgia from somatoform disorders and malingering.

7. How does myofascial pain differ from fibromyalgia?

Myofacial pain differs from the diffuse pain of fibromyalgia by being localized to a specific region, usually a single muscle or closely related muscle group (e.g., temporomandibular joint syndrome). Trigger points, which are typical of myofascial pain syndromes, consist of palpable abnormalities (taut band or thickened nodule) usually found in the bellies of traumatized muscles. Palpation of a trigger point produces local tenderness and, unlike palpation of tender points, generates referred pain throughout the involved muscle or muscle group. In general, tender points should not be equated with trigger points, but they may coexist in the same patient.

8. How is fibromyalgia diagnosed?

The clinical diagnosis of fibromyalgia is based on the 1990 American College of Rheumatology classification criteria:
1. Widespread pain ≥ 3 months affecting all four body quadrants and the axial skeleton
2. Palpable, subjective pain in 11 of the following 9 pairs of tender points (see figure)

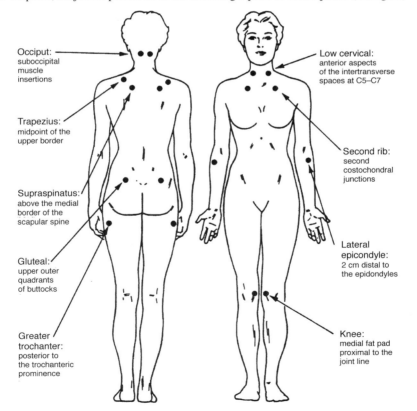

Occiput: suboccipital muscle insertions

Low cervical: anterior aspects of the intertransverse spaces at C5–C7

Trapezius: midpoint of the upper border

Second rib: second costochondral junctions

Supraspinatus: above the medial border of the scapular spine

Gluteal: upper outer quadrants of buttocks

Lateral epicondyle: 2 cm distal to the epidondyles

Greater trochanter: posterior to the trochanteric prominence

Knee: medial fat pad proximal to the joint line

The tender points of fibromyalgia. (From Freundlich B, Leventhal L: The fibromyalgia syndrome. In Schumacher HR Jr, Klippel JH, Koopman WJ (eds): Primer on the Rheumatic Diseases, 10th ed. Atlanta, Arthritis Foundation, 1993, pp 247–249; with permission.)

- Occipital
- Low cervical (posterolateral C5–C7)
- Trapezius (mid, upper fold)
- Supraspinatus (origin)
- Second rib (costochondral junction)
- Lateral epicondyle (2 cm distally)
- Gluteal (upper, lateral quadrant)
- Greater trochanter (2 cm posteriorly)
- Knee (medial fat pad)

A patient is classified as having fibromyalgia if both criteria are present.

Pearls:
- Palpate one tender point at a time.
- Palpate with sufficient pressure to blanche the nailbed.
- Because most of the tender points appear at articulation sites, I frequently locate a tender point at the posterior midcalf to convince the patient that they have a muscle pain syndrome and not arthritis.

9. What is the differential diagnosis of fibromyalgia?

Many systemic illnesses may present with the clinical features of fibromyalgia. Likewise, fibromyalgia may mimic many systemic diseases; however, as a clinical entity, fibromyalgia is not a systemic disorder. There are no consistent physical or laboratory abnormalities in patients with fibromyalgia. Therefore, evidence of inflammation or systemic disease suggests diagnoses other than fibromyalgia. The following select disorders may share features with fibromyalgia:

- Rheumatoid arthritis (early)
- Spondyloarthritis (early)
- Systemic lupus erythematosus
- Sjögren's syndrome
- Polymyositis
- Polymyalgia rheumatica
- Giant cell arteritis
- Generalized osteoarthritis
- Drug-induced myopathy
- Chronic fatigue syndrome
- Myofascial pain syndrome
- Paraneoplastic disorders
- Hyper- or hypothyroidism
- Hyper- or hypoparathyroidism
- Viral infections
- Metastatic cancer
- Somatoform disorders or depression

Caution: Fibromyalgia is not a diagnosis of exclusion because it also may occur in patients with systemic disease.

10. What laboratory screening tests are useful in the diagnosis of fibromyalgia?

In patients with fibromyalgia alone, laboratory investigations and imaging studies are typically normal. Thus, screening tests are performed to determine whether a systemic disease (see above) is generating fibromyalgia-like symptoms. The following investigations are useful in the diagnosis of fibromyalgia:

Essential
- Complete blood count and differential
- Erythrocyte sedimentation rate
- Serum electrolytes, creatinine
- Serum calcium, phosphate, magnesium
- Liver function tests
- Creatine phosphokinase
- Urinalysis
- Thyroid stimulating hormone

Optional (select patients)
- C-reactive protein
- Rheumatoid factor
- Antinuclear antibody
- Hepatitis profile
- Serum protein electrophoresis
- Radiographs
- Bone scan

Note: Formal neuropsychological testing may be appropriate in select patients to exclude subtle organic brain dysfunction.

11. Is polysomnography useful in the diagnosis of fibromyalgia?

Sleep disturbance is common in fibromyalgia (75%), and some patients exhibit electroencephalographic (EEG) alterations during polysomnography testing. A distinct pattern, the alpha EEG sleep anomaly, is observed and appears to be associated with nonrestorative sleep, pain, and fatigue. It represents intrusion of an arousal state pattern (alpha rhythm) onto the nonrapid eye movement (NREM) patterns of restorative sleep. The alpha EEG sleep anomaly is not a consistent or specific finding among patients with fibromyalgia. It has been demonstrated in other disorders and in asymptomatic, normal people. Thus, polysomnography should not be used in the evaluation of fibromyalgia unless symptoms of sleep apnea or narcolepsy are reported.

12. Describe the nonpharmacologic management of patients with fibromyalgia.

Reassurance is a major therapeutic tool for patients with fibromyalgia. Many patients suspect that their symptoms are the result of occult malignancy, crippling arthritis, or an aberrant psyche. The latter suspicion is usually reinforced by the patient's family, friends, and/or physician. Simply providing a diagnosis may be therapeutic. Local measures such as heat packs, gentle massage, gentle stretching exercises, and avoidance of cold may provide temporary relief. The best therapeutic intervention at present is the adoption of a graduated (progressing over 4–6 months) aerobic exercise program. The goal is to perform a low-impact, aerobic activity so that patients exercise 3 times/week, 30 minutes each session, and at 70% of their maximal heart rate. Aquatic aerobics, stationary bicycle riding, and brisk walking seem to be most effective. Older patients or patients with cardiac risk factors may warrant an initial exercise treadmill test to determine exercise tolerance. Other potentially helpful modalities include fibromyalgia self-help groups, biofeedback, stress reduction exercises, vapocoolant spray and stretch techniques, and acupuncture.

Pearl: A useful analogy is the "pain thermostat." I explain to the patient that during the development of fibromyalgia the "pain thermostat" in the brain has been reset so that even mild, external stimuli are abnormally perceived as painful. I state that a routine exercise program serves to reset the pain thermostat threshold to normal limits. The key to the fibromyalgia exercise program is that the patient must progress in minute increments with reasonable goals, akin to losing weight. Too aggressive a program causes postexercise flare and subsequent avoidance of exercise.

13. Is pharmacologic management of patients with fibromyalgia effective?

The pharmacologic management of patients with fibromyalgia assumes a trial-and-error approach because there is no consistent underlying abnormality, symptoms are typically heterogeneous, and individual response is variable. Medical therapy should be tailored to the individual in an effort to relieve specific symptoms that may perpetuate the fibromyalgia condition. Examples include disturbed sleep, anxiety, depression, muscle spasms, and stiffness. The goal of pharmacologic management should be directed toward functional improvement, not eradication of the chronic pain, which may be unrealistic. Functional improvement may foster participation and compliance with an exercise program (see above). The following medications may be effective in some patients with fibromyalgia:

Analgesics	Hypnotics	Antidepressants
• Acetaminophen	• Antihistamines	• Tricyclics
• Aspirin	• Zolpidem	• Serotonin reuptake inhibitors
• NSAIDs	• Melatonin	
• Tramadol	• Antidepressants	**Local therapy**
• Muscle relaxants	• Tranquilizers	• Tender point injection
• Anticonvulsants		• Topical capsaicin

Analgesics and muscle relaxants provide variable relief from the symptoms of fibromyalgia. Narcotics and benzodiazepine derivatives may exacerbate symptoms and are not recommended for patients exhibiting potential for chronic pain. Systemic steroids have no role in the treatment of fibromyalgia. A trial of nonsteroidal antiinflammatory drugs (NSAIDs) is warranted in most patients, but the response is variable and may result only in improved stiffness.

Pharmacologic therapy for fibromyalgia is directed primarily at improving the quality of restorative sleep with low doses of cyclobenzaprine (10–30 mg) or amitriptyline (10–50 mg) administered 2–3 hours before bedtime. If these agents are unsuccessful, other antidepressants may be used in successive trial-and-error fashion. A novel nonbenzodiazepine hypnotic, zolpidem (5–10 mg taken at bedtime), may improve sleep quality in some patients.

Tender point injection with local anesthetics with or without corticosteroids may be effective in select patients, especially if 1 or 2 tender points seem more painful than the rest. Knowing which tender points to inject is the usual dilemma.

Pearl: Fibromyalgia is not amenable to pharmacologic therapy alone. The ideal therapeutic program employs a multidisciplinary approach with education, cardiovascular fitness training, cognitive behavioral therapy, and pharmacologic treatment.

14. What is the prognosis for patients with fibromyalgia?

The few long-term outcome studies suggest that prognosis in fibromyalgia depends on the population studied. For example, patients in community clinics fare better than patients at tertiary care centers. The prognosis for children (73% remission at 30 months) is better than for adults (24% remission at 24 months in community clinics). Overall, most adults continue to have chronic symptoms, regardless of treatment. Remissions are uncommon, but symptoms tend to improve with time. No evidence suggests that fibromyalgia evolves into systemic disease.

CONTROVERSIES

15. Are fibromyalgia and chronic fatigue syndrome the same disorder?

Considerable overlap exists between chronic fatigue syndrome (CFS) and fibromyalgia if patient demographics and clinical features are compared. The greatest difference lies in their diagnostic criteria, not in the patients. The 1994 Centers for Disease Control (CDC) case definition of CFS requires the presence of chronic fatigue ($\geq$ 6 months) and four of the following symptoms ($\geq$ 6 months): impaired memory or concentration, sore throat, tender cervical or axillary lymph nodes, muscle pain, multijoint pain, new headaches, unrefreshing sleep, and postexertion malaise. In contrast to the fibromyalgia classification criteria, there are no physical criteria for CFS in the CDC case definition. Nonetheless, 70% of patients with CFS have tender points. Likewise, 90% of patients with fibromyalgia have fatigue. Because of their clinical similarity, these syndromes are perhaps different manifestations of the same disorder.

Note: No data indicate that a persistent infection (e.g., Epstein-Barr virus) is responsible for CFS or fibromyalgia.

16. Is fibromyalgia a psychological disorder?

It is unlikely that fibromyalgia represents a pure psychological disorder. In tertiary care centers, only 30–35% of patients with fibromyalgia exhibit psychological problems such as increased mental stress, anxiety, or depression. Furthermore, some patients respond to subtherapeutic doses of antidepressants, whereas others have no improvement at all, despite full therapeutic doses. With little evidence for the biomedical model (true tissue pathology) to explain fibromyalgia, attention has been directed to the psychosocial model. This model attempts to relate altered pain perception, sleep disturbance, fatigue, psychological distress, and other symptoms to subtle changes in the neuroendocrine, immune, and psychological systems. The evolving paradigm categorizes fibromyalgia as one of several **affective spectrum disorders**, which share a common but unknown etiology. Examples include fibromyalgia, chronic fatigue syndrome, migraine headache, irritable bowel syndrome, and major depression.

17. Should patients with fibromyalgia receive disability compensation?

Disability for fibromyalgia remains a controversial issue, even though initial consensus guidelines have been established. Most of the controversy stems from an inability to measure objectively the impact of a patient's self-reported symptoms. Another contested issue is whether trauma (i.e., motor vehicle accident) can *cause* fibromyalgia. To date, no studies demonstrate that fibromyalgia can be directly induced by trauma. Symptom severity may be best determined by a combination of health status instruments (e.g., Health Assessment Questionnaire), visual analog scales, psychological testing, and formal functional or work capacity assessments. Tender points, the only objective finding, do not correlate with symptom severity. It is estimated that 10–15% of patients with fibromyalgia have functional impairment severe enough to merit disability; however the majority of patients are able to work productively despite their symptoms. Seeking disability has been shown to affect outcome adversely.

BIBLIOGRAPHY

1. Bennet RM: The fibromyalgia syndrome. In Kelley WN, Harris ED Jr, Ruddy S, Sledge CB (eds): Textbook of Rheumatology, 5th ed. Philadelphia, W.B. Saunders, 1997, pp 511–519.
2. Bennet RM: Fibromyalgia and the facts: Sense or nonsense. Rheum Dis Clin North Am 19:45–59, 1993.
3. Fukuda K, Strauss SE, Hickie I, et al: The chronic fatigue syndrome: A comprehensive approach to its definition and study. Ann Intern Med 121:953–959, 1994.
4. Geel SE: The fibromyalgia syndrome: Musculoskeletal pathophysiology. Semin Arthritis Rheum 23:347–353, 1994.
5. Goldenberg DL (ed): Controversies in fibromyalgia and related conditions. Rheum Dis Clin North Am 22:2, 1996.
6. Goldenberg DL: Fibromyalgia, chronic fatigue syndrome, and myofascial pain syndrome. Curr Opin Rheumatol 8:113–123, 1996.
7. Goldenberg DL: Fibromyalgia and related syndromes. In Klippel JH, Dieppe PA (eds): Rheumatology, 2nd ed. St. Louis, Mosby, 1998, pp 15.1–15.12.
8. Masi AT (ed): Fibromyalgia and myofascial pain syndromes. In Baillière's Clin Rheumatol 8:4, 1994.
9. Moldofsky H: Sleep and the fibrositis syndrome. Rheum Dis Clin North Am 15:91–103, 1989.
10. Sheon RP, Moskowitz RW, Goldberg VM (eds): Soft Tissue Rheumatic Pain, 3rd ed. Baltimore, Williams & Wilkins, 1996.
11. White KP, Manfred H, Teasell RW: Work disability evaluation and the fibromyalgia syndrome. Semin Arthritis Rheum 24:371–381, 1995.
12. Wolfe F: The fibromyalgia syndrome: A consensus report on fibromyalgia and disability. J Rheumatol 23:534–539, 1996.
13. Wolfe F, Smythe HA, Yunus MB, et al: The American College of Rheumatology 1990 criteria for the classification of fibromyalgia: Report of the Multicenter Criteria Committee. Arthritis Rheum 33:160, 1990.

XI. Common Disorders of the Nervous System

76. DEMENTIA

Lawrence A. Meredith, M.D.

1. Define dementia.

Dementia is the persistent loss of previously acquired cognitive skills in 3 of the following 5 categories: memory, language, spatial concepts, personality, and executive function (ability to perform tasks). In general, memory is affected first and foremost by dementing processes. However, as dementia progresses, other brain systems may be affected.

2. How does dementia differ from delirium?

It is important to differentiate dementia from the acute confusional state of delirium. Acute confusional states are characterized primarily by disordered attention. When attention mechanisms are impaired, detailed testing of mental status is difficult and often fruitless. For example, testing of memory is impossible with a patient who cannot attend to the task long enough to encode the information properly.

In acute confusional states arousal mechanisms may be normal, suppressed, or exaggerated and so may give rise to a normally alert, lethargic, or hypervigilant, agitated patient. Patients in various degrees of stupor or coma (i.e., with disorders of arousal) cannot be evaluated accurately for underlying dementia. Demented patients, on the other hand, typically do not exhibit disorders of attention or arousal until late in the course of illness.

3. What is the goal of evaluating dementia?

Finding a potentially reversible cause or component of dementia is the single most important goal.

4. What laboratory evaluation should be included in the initial evaluation of dementia?

All evaluations of dementia should include a brain image (computed tomography [CT] or magnetic resonance imaging [MRI]), assessment of thyroid-stimulating hormone and serum levels of vitamin B_{12}, sedimentation rate, complete blood count, chemistry profile, and syphilis serology. Unfortunately, the yield is low. An electroencephalogram (EEG) is helpful with a history of seizures or blackouts and in patients suspected of cognitive impairment related to depression (so-called pseudodementia).

5. When should a lumbar puncture be performed in the evaluation of dementia?

Lumbar puncture should be strongly considered for patients under age 60 years or patients suspected of infection, meningeal irritation, rapid progression, compromised immunity, or positive syphilis serology. Dementia may occur relatively early in the course of infection with human immunodeficiency virus (HIV) and is an increasingly important consideration, especially in at-risk patients.

6. How do patients with Alzheimer's disease frequently come to the attention of a physician?

Often the family brings the patient because of disorientation in familiar surroundings, problems with the checkbook, or failure at work. Some families clearly observe the loss of memory, whereas others notice only behavioral changes (anger, disinhibition, or social withdrawal). The patient may deny the accusations, but simple testing usually confirms a major impairment in short-term memory despite retention of long-term memory.

7. What is the usual diagnosis for a patient with "idiopathic dementia"?

Alzheimer's disease is the most common nontraumatic cause of dementia, affecting approximately 4% of people aged 70–79 and 11% of those over 80 years. At present, absolute confirmation of the diagnosis depends on pathognomonic brain findings in autopsy specimens. The term "dementia of the Alzheimer type" is sometimes used when the diagnosis is suspected on clinical grounds but not proved pathologically. Experimental work has shown genetic markers for both familial and sporadic cases of Alzheimer's disease. Such research eventually may enable early diagnosis and effective treatments.

8. Why does dementia present acutely?

Although dementia may result from a sudden, severe brain injury, the typical cause is a previously undiagnosed condition unmasked by a stressful event such as moving to a new home, loss of a spouse, hospitalization, illness, or argument. Such dementia initially may be difficult to distinguish from an acute confusional state, to which the elderly are particularly susceptible. Family members or friends often provide the necessary historical clues of prior loss of intellect to reveal an underlying dementia that presents as an acute event.

9. What is MID?

MID is the acronym for multiinfarct dementia, the second leading cause of nontraumatic dementia. In contrast to the gradual, relentless deterioration of cognitive function and general lack of localizing neurologic signs in patients with Alzheimer's disease, patients with MID often exhibit a stepwise progression of mental deficits associated with focal neurologic signs (e.g., clumsiness of one hand, dysarthria, Babinski signs). The physician should be cautious about overuse of this diagnosis without both an appropriate clinical history and supporting radiologic evidence (i.e., focal lesions on CT or MRI scan of the brain). The main goal of therapy is prevention of future strokes through reduction of risk factors, antiplatelet medications (aspirin or ticlopidine), and anticoagulation (if an embolic source is clearly identified). The majority of patients with MID have multiple bilateral, deep lacunar strokes. Multiple large cortical infarcts are a rare cause of MID. At autopsy, many patients with MID have concomitant Alzheimer's disease.

10. How does alcohol lead to dementia?

Alcoholic dementia continues to be a major cause of cognitive dysfunction. Alcoholic cognitive impairment results from two sources: nutritional deficiencies (most notably, thiamine deficiency) and the direct toxic effects of alcohol. Acute alcohol-related thiamine deficiency results in irreversible damage to brain structures and chronic inability to encode new information (Korsakoff's psychosis). Patients with acute alcohol dementia have ophthalmoplegia, gait ataxia, and confusion (Wernicke's syndrome). They require adequate thiamine replacement (100 mg intravenously immediately and 3 times/day) to prevent progression to a severe, permanent deficit in memory.

11. What other structural brain lesions should be considered in the differential diagnosis of a patient with dementia?

Structural brain lesions other than strokes may cause apparent dementia. Only a small percentage of the demented population has a treatable brain lesion. Both CT and MRI can identify such conditions, which are reversible with timely treatment. If stroke coexists with incurable dementia, it is helpful to treat the vascular disorder.

12. How may the primary care provider unknowingly contribute to worsening dementia in an otherwise stable patient?

The brain of elderly patients is highly sensitive to pharmacologic effects. Thus, simple prescription of a new medication may cause an apparent decline in otherwise stable function. Normally innocuous medications, including nonprescription pills, may cause delirium that looks like dementia. The family of the patient must bring in every pill container to which the patient has access so that the physician can evaluate the role of medications in causing apparent dementia. All drugs that act on the central nervous system should be discontinued, if possible.

13. What advice should be given to the family of a demented patient?

Supportive care is necessary, including supervision of activities of daily living, thoughtful management of psychosocial issues, prevention of injury, and judicious use of low-dose medications (haloperidol, thioridazine) to manage aggressive behavior. Support from the family caregiver(s) is also necessary. Memory aids, companionship, and attention to grooming and cleanliness are particularly important.

The family caregiver also needs constant support, including (1) education about anticipated impairments, safety considerations, and the natural history of dementia and (2) encouragement to use respite care as needed (if the demented patient remains in the home) or alternative care settings as appropriate.

14. When is tacrine (Cognex) or donepezil (Aricept) useful in patients with dementia?

Both tacrine and donepezil are centrally active anitcholinesterase inhibitors that modestly improve cognition in mild-to-moderate Alzheimer's disease. Although hepatic intolerance to tacrine is common, requiring slow titration and weekly transaminase testing, donepezil is usually well tolerated with no required laboratory testing. Because donepezil requires no titration and is dosed once daily, it is generally easier to obtain compliance than with tacrine, which requires dosing 4 times/day. Many patients with Alzheimer's disease transiently benefit from tacrine or donepezil, which may delay the necessity of nursing home placement. Unfortunately, neither medication affects the long-term progress.

15. Are newly developed tests for cerebrospinal fluid useful in the diagnosis of dementia?

Several tests that have been recently developed and/or marketed claim to aid in the diagnosis of dementia. In general, experts in dementia remain skeptical about the widespread clinical utility of these tests. The best known test evaluates cerebrospinal fluid for the apoprotein E genotype, which is associated with some forms of inherited Alzheimer's disease. Although testing for such genetic markers may improve the characterization of difficult cases of dementia, they lack the specificity and sensitivity to confirm or eliminate the diagnosis of Alzheimer's disease. In the future the clinical utility of such testing may improve, but for the present the most important use of lumbar puncture in the demented patient is to rule out an infectious process.

BIBLIOGRAPHY

1. Adams RD, Victor M, Ropper A: Degenerative disorder of the nervous system. In Adams RD, Victor M (eds): Principles of Neurology, 6th ed. New York, McGraw-Hill, 1997.
2. Boller F, Duyckaerts C: Alzheimer's disease: Clinical and anatomic aspects. In Feinberg T, Farah M (eds): Behavioral Neurology and Neuropsychology. New York, McGraw-Hill, 1997, pp 521–544.
3. Cummings J, Benson DF: Dementia—A Clinical Approach. Boston, Butterworth, 1992.
4. Katzman R: Delirium and dementia. In Rowland LP (ed): Merritt's Textbook of Neurology, 8th ed. Philadelphia, Lea & Febiger, 1989, pp 3–8.
5. Kaufer D, Cummings J: Dementia and delirium. In Feinberg T, Farah M (eds): Behavioral Neurology and Neuropsychology. New York, McGraw-Hill, 1997, pp 499–520.
6. Kokman E, Whisnaut J, et al: Dementia after ischemic stroke. Neurology 46:154–159, 1996.
7. Mega M, Cummings J, et al: The spectrum of behavioral changes in Alzheimer's disease. Neurology 46:130–135, 1996.
8. Meredith L, Filley C: Acute confusional state. In Jahnigan D, Schrier R (eds): Geriatric Medicine, 2nd ed. Cambridge, MA, Blackwell Science, 1996.
9. Payami H, Montee K, et al: Increased risk of familial late-onset Alzheimer's disease in women. Neurology 46:126–129, 1996.
10. Rogers S, Friedhoff L: The efficacy and safety of donepezil in patients with Alzheimer's disease. Dementia 7:293–303, 1996.
11. Schmand B, Tonker C, et al: Subjective memory complaints may announce dementia. Neurology 46:121–125, 1996.
12. Tierney M, Szalai J, et al: A prospective study of the clinical utility of ApoE genotype in the prediction of outcome in patients with memory impairment. Neurology 46:149–154, 1996.
13. Whitehouse P (ed): Dementia. Philadelphia, F.A. Davis, 1993.

77. TREMOR

C. Alan Anderson, M.D., and Richard Hughes, M.D.

1. Define tremor.

Tremor is an involuntary, unwanted movement characterized by a rhythmic oscillation ranging in frequency between 1 and 12 or more Hz.

2. What four questions help to classify a tremor?

1. Where in the body does it occur? Is it restricted to the hands?
2. Is it unilateral or asymmetric?
3. Does it occur at rest or with movement?
4. Is it affected by sustained posture (postural or static tremor), movement (kinetic, action, or intention tremor), or a specific activity such as writing (task-specific tremor)?

3. What causes rest tremor?

Nearly all resting tremors are related to parkinsonian-like states. Possible diagnoses include Parkinson's disease, drug-induced parkinsonism, focal brain injury from stroke, other degenerative disorders, tumor, trauma, and infections.

The tremor of Parkinson's disease is typically 4–6 Hz, asymmetric, and "pill-rolling" in appearance. The diagnosis of Parkinson's disease is supported by the presence of bradykinesia, rigidity, stooped posture, loss of postural reflexes, and festinating gait. Treatment includes anticholinergic agents (trihexyphenidyl, benztropine), dopamine precursors (levodopa), dopamine agonists (bromocriptine, pergolide), and monoamine oxidase inhibitors (selegiline).

4. Which drugs are most commonly responsible for drug-induced parkinsonism?

Drug-induced parkinsonism most commonly results from neuroleptic or antiemetic agents (e.g., metoclopramide). Occasionally the antidepressant amoxapine is responsible. Treatment of drug-induced parkinsonism is removal of the offending drug.

5. What causes postural tremor?

The most common causes are familial tremor and essential tremor. Essential tremor, which occurs sporadically, and familiar tremor, which follows an autosomal dominant pattern of inheritance, have identical characteristics. The head and distal upper extremities are most often affected. The tremor may begin at any time from childhood to late in life and is slowly progressive. It rarely persists at rest but worsens with use of the limb. Many patients describe temporary improvement of essential or familial tremor with alcohol. This response is so specific that it is helpful diagnostically. Conventional therapy includes beta blockers, primidone, or injections of botulinum toxin.

Parkinson's disease occasionally involves a postural tremor coexisting with a resting tremor. Wilson's disease may present with postural tremor. The tremor of Wilson's disease varies in amplitude and frequency and is more prominent proximally. Patients often have psychiatric problems, liver disease, and other abnormal movement.

6. Why do excitement and caffeine produce tremor?

All people experience a low-amplitude tremor with frequency of 6–12 Hz when they maintain a fixed posture. This normal physiologic tremor may be exaggerated with anxiety, excitement, fatigue, caffeine, thyrotoxicosis, hypoglycemia, alcohol withdrawal, hysteria, and drugs. The most commonly involved drugs are stimulants, lithium, beta-adrenergic agents, theophylline, and valproate. Exaggerated physiologic tremor may be suppressed by removing or minimizing the underlying cause; if necessary and tolerated, beta blockers or anxiolytics may be used.

7. Characterize a kinetic tremor.

Kinetic (or action) tremors are usually irregular, jerky, severe, and ataxic; they are caused by diseases of the cerebellum or its outflow tracts. They may affect the trunk and limbs and interfere with all activities. Specific causes include chronic toxicity from alcohol, phenytoin, or other drugs and structural brain lesions, such as multiple sclerosis, tumors, infection, stroke, and trauma. Hysteria should be considered if no obvious cause is present.

8. What is a task-specific tremor?

A task-specific tremor occurs only with repetitive hand-arm activity, such as writing. It is similar to the focal dystonia known as writer's cramp. Psychological factors are common, but cause and effect remain uncertain. Treatment includes beta blockers, anxiolytics, or anticholinergics, but the best results are achieved with injections of botulinum toxin.

9. What principles should be followed in treating patients with tremor?

Tremor alone is rarely a painful or life-threatening disease. The classification of the tremor should direct treatment, and the clinical response to therapy may help diagnostically. Treatment should be started slowly to minimize side effects, with the response measured over weeks to months.

10. What is the role of botulinum toxin injections?

Botulism is a potentially fatal disease caused by a neuromuscular junction toxin produced by the anaerobic bacterium, *Clostridium botulinum*. The toxin can be purified and injected into muscles to reduce excessive contractions, including those that cause tremor. As experience grows, more tremors are treated with botulinum toxin, but results are mixed at best. Botulinum toxin is best for dystonias, chronic focal tremor, or spasms.

BIBLIOGRAPHY

1. Adams R, Victor M, Ropper A: Tremor, myoclonus, focal dystonias, and tics. In Adams R, Victor M (eds): Principles of Neurology, 6th ed. New York, McGraw-Hill, 1997.
2. Calne D: Treatment of Parkinson's disease. N Engl J Med 329:1021–1027, 1993.
3. Hallett M: Classification and treatment of tremor. JAMA 266:1115–1117, 1991.
4. Jankovic J, Fahn S: Physiologic and pathologic tremor. Ann Intern Med 93:460–465, 1980.
5. Lou J, Jankovic J: Essential tremor. Neurology 41:234–238, 1991.

78. MUSCLE WEAKNESS

Michele A. Ferguson, M.D., and Richard Hughes, M.D.

1. Describe the three patterns of muscle weakness that aid in determining cause.

1. The **upper motor neuron** or **elective pattern** of weakness involves the extensor muscles of the upper extremity and the flexor muscles of the lower extremity. This pattern is seen in cerebral hemisphere lesions, subdural hematomas, stroke, and tumor. The patient assumes a posture of arm flexion and adduction with wrist drop and leg extension that causes a spastic gait and circumduction of the affected leg.

2. **Proximal muscle weakness** involving the muscles of the shoulder and pelvic girdle usually occurs in patients with myopathy, which may be inherited (muscular dystrophy) or acquired (polymyositis, hypothyroidism).

3. A **distal pattern** of weakness involving primarily the hands and feet is seen in peripheral nerve disease associated with diabetes, trauma, and amyotrophic lateral sclerosis (ALS), or an inherited condition.

2. What physical maneuvers permit the best functional assessment of weakness?

Weakness may be evaluated both functionally and formally. Functional testing is carried out by the observation of simple everyday tasks such as walking on heels and toes, arising from a chair without assistance or use of hands, stepping onto a stool or step, raising the arms above the head, buttoning a shirt or closing a zipper, or "burying" eyelashes. Such observation of everyday activities allows an assessment of functional impairment.

3. How is muscle strength graded?

Formal testing of muscle strength involves isolating individual muscles or muscle groups for evaluation. Strength is graded with a 6-point scale developed by the Medical Research Council:

> 5 = Normal power
> 4 = Active movement against gravity and resistance
> 3 = Active movement against gravity only
> 2 = Active movement with gravity removed
> 1 = A trace of flicker of muscle contraction
> 0 = No muscle contraction detectable

This scale has significant shortcomings because of the high degree of interobserver variability and subjectivity; 90% of patients tend to be evaluated at grade four.

4. What is the most common motor neuron disease in adults?

ALS is the most common motor neuron disease in adults. It affects men more commonly than women, typically presents between 40 and 60 years of age, and is primarily a clinical diagnosis. Patients usually complain of weakness, atrophy, fasciculations, and muscle cramps. Some patients also have dysarthria and dysphagia. Diagnosis is based on a combination of diffuse upper and lower motor neuron findings and a rapidly progressive course.

Electromyography (EMG) proves most useful by demonstrating diffuse denervation; studies of the cerebrospinal fluid (CSF) are characteristically normal. Once the diagnosis is confirmed, supportive measures such as physical therapy and symptomatic treatment for aspiration or depression are helpful.

5. In which patients should the physician consider Guillain-Barré syndrome (GBS)?

The most frequent cause of acute muscle weakness from a peripheral neuropathy is GBS. The clinical picture is dominated by acute weakness (duration of hours to days), with only minor asymmetries, that usually begins in the legs and ascends but occasionally begins in the arms or face and descends. Maximal weakness may occur distally or proximally and may involve both bulbar and respiratory muscles, making intubation necessary. Reflexes range from diminished to absent; sensory aberrations and autonomic dysfunction are not uncommon. CSF protein levels may remain normal early in the course of the disease but usually rise after the first week and peak within 4–6 weeks. The protein peak often coincides with the maximal amount of weakness. The CSF may demonstrate a mild leukocytosis. EMG studies support the diagnosis by demonstrating delayed nerve conductions.

Because GBS has an immunopathogenic basis, plasmapheresis or intravenous immunoglobulins are used to limit the severity and duration of disease. Supportive care to maintain respiratory functions and to avoid infections has dramatically reduced the mortality of GBS.

6. Describe the course of botulism.

Botulism occurs 12–48 hours after the consumption of contaminated food. It progresses rapidly over a matter of hours, causing death if respiratory support is not available.

7. What are the first symptoms of botulism?

Symptoms of cranial nerve dysfunction appear first, including diplopia, ptosis, blurred vision, dysphagia, and dysarthria. Dilated fixed pupils are a classic sign of botulism but often are not present. The five cardinal features of botulism, as outlined by the Centers for Disease Control and Prevention, include (1) absence of fever, (2) normal mental status, (3) normal or slow pulse, (4) no sensory dysfunction, and (5) symmetric neurologic dysfunction. Respiratory failure may precede the onset of significant limb weakness. Treatment strategies include the removal of unabsorbed toxin via cathartics and emetics, neutralization of circulating toxins with antitoxins, and compensation for neurologic deficits through vigorous support.

8. How is mysathenia gravis differentiated from botulism?

Mysathenia gravis rarely presents as fulminantly as botulism and typically begins with progressive fatigability accompanied by intermittent diplopia, ptosis, dysarthria, and dysphagia. Most patients report that symptoms worsen throughout the day and improve after periods of rest. Diagnostic tests for myasthenia gravis include the edrophonium chloride test, repetitive nerve stimulation, and measurement of serum antibodies to acetylcholine receptors.

Although both myasthenia gravis and botulism are disorders of neuromuscular transmission, the pathology is quite different. Whereas botulism results from impaired release of acetylcholine at peripheral synapses, myasthenia gravis involves impaired binding of acetylcholine to postsynaptic receptors, which are blocked by antibodies. Treatments for myasthenia gravis include immune modulation and thymectomy.

9. What is the difference between weakness and fatigue?

Patients often complain of "weakness" when in fact they are fatigued. Fatigue is defined as a lessened capacity for work, whereas weakness is a state of reduced power. The diagnosis of weakness is often clarified by a history of decreased strength or decreased muscular contraction with normal force. Some patients have both weakness and fatigue.

Patients with fatigue often state that they are "tired all the time" or "exhausted." They often have decreased interest in otherwise routine exertion and decreased initiative. Fatigue is to be expected with sleeplessness, prolonged exertion, and excessive work. Fatigue associated with a psychiatric disorder is often worse in the morning, increases with mild activity, and generally relates more specifically to some activities than to others. Fatigue is often the first symptom of psychosocial stress and interferes with mental activity.

10. Which medical disorders may present as fatigue?

Medical disorders that may produce fatigue include common viral infections, hepatitis, tuberculosis, Lyme disease, mononucleosis, metabolic or endocrine disorders (e.g., Addison's disease, hypothyroidism, diabetes, hyperparathyroidism, anemia), and occult malignancy. Nutritional deficiencies and other causes of poor health also may present as fatigue. Fatigue is a common problem for patients with multiple sclerosis.

11. What are myopathies?

The myopathies are a heterogeneous group of primary muscle disorders. They are characterized by clinical and laboratory evidence of muscle destruction with or without inflammation.

Inflammatory myopathies include polymyositis, dermatomyositis, inclusion body myositis, and infectious myopathies. They typically present as a chronic proximal muscle weakness accompanied by pain. EMG studies, elevated serum creatine phosphokinase (CPK), and muscle biopsy are helpful in making the diagnosis.

Noninflammatory myopathies include both inherited and endocrine myopathies. Common inherited myopathies include Duchenne's muscular dystrophy and the adult form, Becker's muscular dystrophy, both are which are X-linked and accompanied by calf hypertrophy. Endocrine myopathies include hyperthyroid, hypothyroid, and steroid-induced myopathies.

12. Which myopathies are not accompanied by an elevated level of CPK?

Classically the level of CPK is not elevated in steroid-induced myopathy. It may be elevated in hypothyroidism because of decreased renal clearance and is characteristically elevated in inflammatory myopathies. In common inherited myopathies, although muscles are not painful, the CPK level may be markedly elevated.

13. When may steroid use cause myopathy?

Steroids can induce dramatic proximal weakness. Despite reports of onset within a few weeks or with low doses (e.g., 15 mg of prednisone), myopathy typically occurs in chronic users of high-dose steroids. Many steroids have a discrete dose threshold above which weakness predictably occurs. Similar weakness occurs with excessive endogenous production of glucocorticoids, as in Cushing's disease or ectopic production of adrenocorticotropic hormone (ACTH). Fortunately, such myopathies resolve with correction of the endocrine condition or withdrawal of the steroid.

BIBLIOGRAPHY

1. Adams R, Victor M (eds): Principles of Neurology, 5th ed. New York, McGraw-Hill, 1993.
2. Campbell W, Swift T: Differential diagnosis of acute weakness. South Med J 74:1371–1375, 1981.
3. Dalakas MC: Polymyositis, dermatomyositis, and inclusion-body myositis. N Engl J Med 325:1487–1498, 1991.
4. Riggs JE: Adult-onset muscle weakness. Postgrad Med 78:217–226, 1985.
5. Rowland LP (ed): Merritt's Textbook of Neurology, 8th ed. Philadelphia, Lea & Febiger, 1989.

79. NUMBNESS AND TINGLING

Michele A. Ferguson, M.D., and Richard Hughes, M.D.

1. When should a complaint of numbness and tingling raise the concern of a primary care provider?

Numbness and tingling, also known as paresthesias (or, if painful, dysesthesias), can originate anywhere in the nervous system, either peripheral or central. If severe or clearly localized to a focal brain or spinal cord lesion, the complaint may herald a serious condition, especially if the symptoms are continuous and progressive.

Fortunately, paresthesias are usually of little significance, especially if fleeting. For example, everybody experiences a limb "falling asleep" from compression of the ulnar, sciatic, or peroneal nerves, and simple anxiety with hyperventilation commonly produces paresthesias of the face, hands, and legs.

2. Describe the pathway of sensory fibers.

Sensory information is first registered in various specialized nerve endings in the skin, subcutaneous tissue, and deep tissue. It is then conveyed via the peripheral nerves to the dorsal roots. Here the fibers enter the spinal cord and split into the dorsal columns (proprioception and vibratory sense) and the spinothalamic tracts (pain and temperature). These tracts ascend into the medulla, where the proprioception/vibration fibers synapse and cross over to form the medial lemniscus, whereas the pain/temperature fibers ascend laterally. All sensory information converges in the thalamus. From there the final step is through the deep white-matter tracts of the internal capsule to the sensory cortex, located in the parietal lobe of the brain. A lesion at any point in these pathways may produce sensory symptoms, including paresthesias, hypoesthesia (lack of sensation), or hyperesthesia (increased sensation).

3. What clues suggest that a lesion in the sensory cortex produced the paresthesias?

Lesions in the sensory cortex also produce objective signs. Examples include astereognosis, the inability to identify simple objects (e.g., paper clips, keys) placed in the hand by texture and shape, and graphesthesia, the inability to identify letters or numbers scratched on the palm. Many patients also have mild hemiparesis. Because many processes may affect this area of the brain, neurologic consultation is needed if more than subjective paresthesias are present on examination.

4. When may a cerebrovascular event cause isolated sensory loss?

Lacunar or small strokes result from small-vessel occlusions in the internal capsule, thalamus, or brainstem. The major symptoms of such purely sensory strokes is objective numbness to pain and temperature in the contralateral face, arm, and leg. Thalamic infarction may cause a long-lasting, painful "numbness" that is refractory to treatment.

An unusual but important situation is the lateral medullary infarction, also known as Wallenberg syndrome. Symptoms include numbness of the ipsilateral face but contralateral body. This split sensory loss occurs as the fibers responsible for facial sensation travel to the cervical spinal cord before crossing and synapsing in the thalamus. Other signs and symptoms of lateral medullary syndrome include hoarseness, ipsilateral Horner's syndrome, hiccoughs, vertigo, and ipsilateral ataxia.

5. What signs and symptoms suggest a lesion in the spinal cord?

Spinal cord lesions produce symptoms and signs at or below their cervical, thoracic, or lumbar level. The face is spared. Other clues include back pain, Lhermitte's sign (electric shocks or tingling sensations down the back with forward flexion of the neck), bladder dysfunction, and a discrete level at a sensory dermatome.

6. How common is paresthesia as a presentation of multiple sclerosis (MS)?

Patients with MS commonly complain of unilateral or bilateral paresthesias from demyelinating plaques in the cerebral hemisphere or spinal cord. Paresthesias may be the first symptoms, but typically they are associated with other signs, such as upper motor neuron weakness, incontinence, ataxia, or optic neuritis (blurred vision in one eye).

7. Do herniated discs cause numbness and tingling?

Yes. In addition to pain, herniated discs may produce paresthesias radiating to the shoulder, arm, and hand (cervical) or the buttocks, thigh, and foot (lumbar). Less commonly, other serious lesions may produce sciatica, including epidural abscess, strategically placed tumors, and osteophytes impinging on the neural foramina. Serious causes are usually suspected by the presence of excruciating pain, severe tenderness, fever, or tenderness.

8. Where do the most common causes of numbness and tingling originate?

The most common causes of numbness and tingling originate in the peripheral nerves. Both polyneuropathies and mononeuropathies have paresthesias as prominent symptoms. The causes of polyneuropathy are numerous, but the most common are diabetes, infection with the human immunodeficiency virus (HIV), alcohol abuse, nutritional deficiencies (including vitamin B_{12}), drugs (chemotherapeutic agents), and idiopathic factors. The most common cause of hand paresthesias is carpal tunnel syndrome.

9. Why do polyneuropathies typically follow a stocking-glove pattern?

The patient with polyneuropathy typically has paresthesias in a stocking distribution, because these branches of the nerves are farthest from the cell bodies in the dorsal root ganglion. As neuropathies progress, the patient may experience similar symptoms in a glove distribution in the hands.

10. Which classic polyneuropathy is life-threatening and treatable?

A life-threatening but treatable polyneuropathy is Guillain-Barré syndrome or acute idiopathic demyelinating polyneuropathy (AIDP). Patients experience mild-to-severe symmetric paresthesias in the feet, legs, or thigh in association with progressive paralysis and areflexia. The syndrome may progress to respiratory failure requiring mechanical ventilation. Effective treatments include plasmapheresis or intravenous immunoglobulin. The recurrent form of this process is called chronic idiopathic demyelinating polyneuropathy (CIDP).

11. How does a claw hand deformity develop?

Compressions of the ulnar nerve at the elbow or "funny bone" produce paresthesias in the ulnar aspect of the hand, the fourth and fifth fingers. If the condition is longstanding, atrophy may be seen in the first dorsal interosseous muscle on the dorsum of the hand in the web space between the thumb and the index finger. In a complete palsy, the claw hand deformity develops.

12. What causes a peroneal palsy?

Compression of the peroneal nerve at the fibular head occurs in bedridden patients, habitual leg crossers, and diabetics; it also may be associated with surgery, overly tight compression stockings, and trauma. In the days before soft luggage, peroneal palsy was called palsy of the "suitcase nerve," because hard valises often repetitively traumatized the lateral knee. Patients experience paresthesias and hypoesthesias down the lateral leg to the dorsum of the foot; footdrop may result from weakness of the tibialis anterior muscle.

13. What neural lesions do *not* produce numbness and tingling in the nervous system?

Amyotrophic lateral sclerosis (ALS, motor neuron disease) is a disease of the anterior horn cells and long motor tracts; sensory symptoms directly exclude ALS. **Neuromuscular junction disease** (e.g., myasthenia, botulism) and **myopathies** (polymyositis and muscular dystrophy) produce weakness without sensory symptoms or signs.

14. What clues suggest the hysterical patient?

Be wary of the patient who complains of paresthesias in nonanatomic distributions. On repeated examination, the location of the symptoms often changes. Hysterical patients often note decreased hearing, vision, smell, or taste. Many have typical functional complaints in other organ systems and historically have suffered from depression, anxiety, or stress-related disorders.

15. When should electromyographic (EMG) studies be ordered?

EMG and nerve conduction studies may be helpful in the diagnosis and prognosis of patients with nerve, plexus, and root lesions. EMG is not helpful in patients with diseases of the central nervous system except to exclude concomitant peripheral disease. Its usefulness depends on the clinical setting. Neurologic consultation is advisable before requesting EMG testing.

16. Any closing thoughts?

Remember—try to localize the lesion by the pattern of numbness and sensory loss and by associated findings. Most confusion is due to imprecise descriptions of sensory symptoms. Patients often use "numb" or "dead" for either sensory changes or weakness. With a clear description, good localization, and knowledge of the patient's medical history, the etiology of the numbness or tingling becomes inapparent.

BIBLIOGRAPHY

1. Adams R, Victor M (eds): Principles of Neurology, 6th ed. New York, McGraw-Hill, 1997.
2. Branzis P, et al: Localization. In Clinical Neurology, 2nd ed. Boston, Little, Brown, 1990.
3. Devor M: Neuropathic pain and injured nerve: Peripheral mechanisms. BMJ, 47:619–630, 1991.
4. Kanchardani R, Howe JG: Lhermitte's sign in multiple sclerosis: A clinical survey and review of the literature. J Neurol Neurosurg Psychiatry 45:308–312, 1982.
5. Manusov EG: Late life migraines accompaniments: A case preventative and literature review. J Fam Pract 24:541–544, 1987.
6. Patten JP: Neurological Differential Diagnosis, 2nd ed. London, Springer-Verlag, 1996.
7. Schmahmann JD, Leifen D: Parietal pseudo-thalamic pain syndrome: Clinical features and anatomic correlates. Arch Neurol 49:1032–1037, 1992.

80. CEREBROVASCULAR DISORDERS

C. Alan Anderson, M.D., and Richard Hughes, M.D.

1. What is the difference between a transient ischemic attack (TIA) and a cerebrovascular accident (CVA)?

The nomenclature for stroke is less than ideal. Both CVA and TIA refer to ischemia in the brain that results in neurologic deficits. If the *clinical* deficit resolves by 24 hours, the ischemia is termed TIA. If the deficit is persistent at 24 hours, even if it resolves over a few days, the ischemia is called CVA or stroke. The nomenclature becomes more complicated because 30–50% of patients with *clinically* defined TIA actually have permanent abnormality in the brain on computed tomography (CT) or magnetic resonance imaging (MRI) or at autopsy. Thus TIAs and stroke represent a continuum of ischemic injury to the brain.

2. What is the value of the history and physical examination in patients with obvious stroke?

In most instances the history and physical examination explain the pathophysiology of the event. For example, small-vessel thrombosis or lacunae are associated with a history of hypertension and risk factors for arteriosclerosis (advanced age, high cholesterol, smoking, diabetes). Patients often awaken with the deficit and commonly present with either pure motor or pure sensory findings with proportional involvement (equal impairment of face, arm, and leg). Some patients with cerebral embolism have a history of cardiac arrhythmias, valvular disease, or myocardial infarction. Artery-to-artery embolism is also common, as suggested by the finding of carotid bruits. The onset of an embolic deficit is immediate and usually associated with activity or physical exertion. Because superficial vessels are usually affected, a combination of cortical problems (aphasia, neglect) with motor and sensory findings and nonproportional involvement (greater involvement of face and arm than leg) is common.

3. Can a migraine cause a stroke?

Yes. The rare migraine that causes a stroke, however, must be differentiated from the more common complicated migraine, which presents with a neurologic deficit that resolves within 20–30 minutes. Actual strokes cause persistent symptoms and objective deficit. A careful search for unusual causes of stroke, such as hypercoagulable states and inflammatory conditions, is indicated before stroke is attributed to migraine.

4. How frequently does a CVA or TIA present as a seizure?

A seizure is the first manifestation of ischemia in 5–10% of embolic strokes. A seizure rarely, if ever, complicates a small or lacunar stroke.

5. What other medical conditions can mimic a stroke?

Seizure/Todd's paralysis	Systemic infections	Demyelinating disease
Complicated migraine	Peripheral nerve disease	Toxic/metabolic disorders
Trauma	Transient global amnesia	Meningoencephalitis
Brain abscess	Psychiatric illness	Hypertensive encephalopathy

6. Why should patients with ischemic events be rapidly evaluated?

The risk of recurrent stroke is highest in the first few days and weeks after an initial stroke or TIA. Therefore, it is crucial that patients have an appropriate evaluation to prevent, if possible, a second ischemic event. Furthermore, about 20% of acute cerebral infarcts progressively worsen during the first 24 hours after onset. Rapid, thorough clinical evaluation and management can prevent progressive brain injury.

7. What mistakes during early management of patients with a CVA may worsen injury?

Overtreatment of hypertension	Failure to prevent aspiration
Failure to treat dehydration	Failure to treat concomitant cardiac disease

8. Is contrast CT necessary to evaluate patients with an acute CVA?

Generally not. An acute imaging study, such as a CT scan, is useful mainly to exclude the presence of hemorrhage. If the patient has a history of malignancy that theoretically could metastasize to the brain, a CT scan with contrast or an MRI scan is worthwhile.

9. Is anticoagulation indicated in a patient with acute stroke?

Anticoagulation is indicated to prevent recurrent embolization in either cardiogenic emboli (i.e., atrial fibrillation) or noncardiogenic emboli (i.e., artery-to-artery). It is not clear whether anticoagulation should begin immediately or after a few days. The duration of anticoagulation varies with the risk of recurrence. For example, atrial fibrillation or valvular diseases usually require anticoagulation for life. Transient conditions, such as myocardial infarction or carotid artery injuries (e.g., dissection), may need only short-term anticoagulation.

10. When is thrombolytic therapy indicated in patients with an acute stroke?

Recombinant tissue plasminogen activator (r-TPA) was approved by the Food and Drug Administration for use in acute ischemic stroke in 1996. Recent studies with the thrombolytic agent, streptokinase, demonstrated no benefit and reported a higher mortality rate in patients who received the drug. Streptokinase is contraindicated in stroke.

Approval of r-TPA therapy in acute stroke was based in large part on the results from the National Institute of Neurological Disease and Stroke (NINDS) r-TPA Study Group. The study looked at outcome in patients with acute ischemic stroke treated with intravenous r-TPA given within 3 hours form the onset of symptoms. Outcome at 3 months after stroke was significantly better in the r-TPA-treated group. The patients' age, race, or sex; stroke location; and stroke mechanism did not influence benefit from the drug. There was no significant difference between the r-TPA-treated and placebo groups in mortality, although r-TPA-treated patients fared slightly better, despite a significantly higher incidence of symptomatic hemorrhage during the first 24 hours after treatment. Based on these results, r-TPA is a recommended treatment if it can be given within 3 hours of onset of acute ischemic stroke. If the patient awakens from sleep with deficit, the last time they were known to be well is used to calculate the time from onset. The use of r-TPA requires careful patient selection.

11. What factors contraindicate the use of r-TPA in treatment of stroke?

Onset > 3 hours before therapy	Seizure at onset of stroke
Rapidly improving deficit	Prior intracranial hemorrhage
Isolated, mild neurologic deficits	Use of oral anticoagulants
Possible hemorrhage on CT	International normalized ratio (INR) > 1.7
Early changes of major infarction on CT	Use of heparin within past 48 hours
Stroke in previous 3 months	Prolonged partial thromboplastin time (PTT)
Head trauma in previous 3 months	Blood glucose < 50 mg/dl or > 400 mg/dl
Major surgery within past 14 days	Platelet count < 100,000/ml
Recent myocardial infarction	Pretreatment systolic blood pressure (BP)
Gastrointestinal or urinary tract	> 185 mmHg
bleeding within prior 21 days	Pretreatment diastolic BP > 110 mmHg

A potential alternative in some patients may be the administration of thrombolytics via an angiographic catheter, which permits demonstration of the thrombus and study of the vascular anatomy with contrast injection, followed by delivery of the thrombolytic agent at the site of occlusion. A better understanding of proper patient selection, contraindications, and the benefit of catheter-based thrombolytic therapy relative to intravenous thrombolytic therapy awaits the results of ongoing trials.

12. Does every patient with a CVA or TIA need an echocardiogram?

No. However, the mechanism of the stroke should be defined in every patient. Cardiac ultrasound, either transthoracic or transesophageal, has demonstrated unsuspected cardiac sources for emboli in many patients, including common sources, such as atrial fibrillation, prosthetic valves, endocarditis, and mural thrombi, as well as paradoxical emboli through a patent foramen ovale (PFO). Young victims of stroke (< 45 years old) have a 2–3 times greater prevalence of PFO than age-matched controls, suggesting that PFO plays an important role in causing strokes.

13. How much aspirin is required to prevent stroke?

The initial recommendation was 4 aspirin/day, but recent evidence has demonstrated that 1 aspirin/day is as effective as higher doses. It may be possible to reduce the dose further; for example, 80 mg/day or 1 aspirin 3 days/week may eventually become the standard. Reducing the dose of aspirin reduces the risk of gastrointestinal and perhaps cerebral hemorrhages. Ticlopidine is a newer antiplatelet agent that may be more effective than aspirin in the first year after a stroke or TIA. It is a good alternative when therapy with aspirin or warfarin fails or is contraindicated.

A small number of patients with hyperaggregable platelets need higher doses of aspirin to block platelet aggregation effectively. Currently no standard guidelines specify which patients need platelet aggregation testing. Such testing may be considered in patients in whom aspirin therapy has failed, young patients, migraineurs, or patients without typical risk factors for stroke.

14. Which patients benefit from carotid endarterectomy?

With information from recent clinical trials, carotid endarterectomy has become a less controversial topic. Results from the North American Symptomatic Carotid Endarterectomy Trial (NASCET) and the Asymptomatic Carotid Atherosclerosis Study (ACAS) provide reasonable data for selecting patients for surgery. It has been established that after a successful endarterectomy the risk of a stroke in the affected vascular distribution is reduced, probably for many years. Both studies demonstrated that the risks of surgery increase as the severity of carotid disease increases. Finally, it is clear that the angiographic and surgical morbidity and mortality rates vary greatly among individual patients, institutions, and surgeons.

Symptomatic patients who have had either a TIA or a stroke and have carotid stenosis of 70% or greater benefit from an endarterectomy performed by an experienced surgeon. Because the benefit of the surgery is obvious after a few months, older patients, if robust, are reasonable candidates for the procedure. Asymptomatic patients with carotid stenosis of 60% or greater also benefit from the surgery, but the criteria for patient selection are less clear. Relatively healthy ACAS patients reduced the risk of stroke by one-half over a 5-year period with endarterectomy and aggressive management of modifiable risk factors. The perioperative morbidity and mortality rates were less than 3%. The overall risk of stroke, with or without surgery, is not great, making the option to use medical therapy alone reasonable, even if somewhat less effective. For patients who are fragile, aged, or in poor health, medical therapy is best. For younger, healthier patients, carotid endarterectomy is a reasonable option and should be fully discussed.

BIBLIOGRAPHY

1. Adams H, Brott I, Crowell R, et al: Guidelines for the management of patients with acute ischemic stroke. A statement for healthcare professionals from a special writing group of the Stroke Council. Stroke 25:1901–1913, 1994.
2. Adams RD, Victor M: Approach to the patient with neurologic disease and the major categories of neurologic disease. In Adams RD, Victor M, Ropper A (eds): Principles of Neurology, 5th ed. New York, McGraw-Hill, 1993.
3. European Carotid Surgery Trialists Collaborative Group: MRC European Carotid Surgery Trial: Interim results for symptomatic patients with severe (70–90%) or mild (0–29%) carotid stenosis. Lancet 337:1235–1243, 1993.
4. Executive Committee for the Asymptomatic Carotid Atherosclerosis Study: Endarterectomy for asymptomatic carotid artery stenosis. JAMA 273:1421–1428, 1995.

5. Gent M, et al: The Canadian American Ticlopidine Study (CATS) in thromboembolic stroke. Lancet 1:1215–1220, 1989.
6. North American Symptomatic Carotid Endarterectomy Trial Collaborators: Beneficial effect of carotid endarterectomy in symptomatic patients with high grade carotid stenosis. N Engl J Med 325:445–453, 1991.
7. Sauer J, Starkman S: State of the art medical management of acute ischemic stroke. J Stroke Cerebrovasc Dis 6:189–194, 1997.
8. Special Writing Group of the Stroke Council AHA: Guidelines for thrombolytic therapy for acute stroke: A supplement to the guidelines for management of patients with acute ischemic stroke. Circulation 94:1167–1174, 1996.

81. HEADACHE

Catherine Amlie-Lefond, M.D.

1. How common are migraines?

Migraine affects 1.7% of 7-year-olds, 5.3% of 15-year-olds, 17% of women, and 6% of men.

2. Characterize the four migraine syndromes.

1. **Common migraine** occurs in 5–10% of the population and accounts for about 80% of all migraines. Symptoms include throbbing headache, nausea and vomiting, pallor, and sensitivity to light and noise. The headache usually lasts for hours and often is relieved by sleep.

2. **Classic migraine**, which occurs in about 1% of people, has features of a common migraine as well as preceding or associated neurologic symptoms, which often include visual phenomena, such as scotomata or fortification spectra (zig-zag lines).

3. **Basilar artery migraine** is rare and usually occurs in young women. It is associated with symptoms referable to the territory of the vertebral and basilar arteries, such as vertigo, dysarthria, ataxia, and quadriplegia.

4. **Complicated migraine** is associated with focal neurologic symptoms and signs that outlast the headache and occasionally are permanent. In rare cases migrainous neurologic symptoms may precede the headache or occur without headache.

3. How should migraine headaches be treated?

Therapy for migraine is divided into two stages: (1) treatment of acute migraine and (2) chronic therapy to prevent and reduce severity of headaches. Standard therapy for a moderately severe headache consists of nonsteroidal antiinflammatory drugs (NSAIDs; e.g., ibuprofen, 600 mg every 4 hr), vasoconstrictors (Midrin, Cafergot), or analgesics (Fiorinal, acetaminophen with codeine), often accompanied by a sedating antinausea drug (metoclopramide or hydroxyzine). More severe headaches are treated with dihydroergotamine (DHE-45; 0.5–1.0 mg intramuscularly), usually combined with sedating antinausea supplement. Sumatriptan (6 mg subcutaneously) is highly effective in treatment of acute, severe migraine. It may be self-injected by the patient, thus avoiding emergency department visits. Oral sumatriptan (25 mg) is also available but may not be as efficacious as the subcutaneous form. Chronic therapy to prevent migraines includes tricyclic antidepressants, beta-blocking agents, daily NSAIDs, valproic acid, or methysergide. Most agents have not been irrefutably proved to be effective, however.

4. How does cluster headache differ from migraine?

Cluster and migraine headaches differ in epidemiology, presentation, and treatment. Migraine is more common in young women; cluster headache is more common in middle-aged men. Cluster headache is defined by multiple episodes of unilateral orbital pain that last 0.5–1.5 hours/day over several weeks. The headache may be accompanied by unilateral conjunctival injection, lacrimation, sweating, or even Horner's syndrome.

5. How should cluster headache be treated?

Individual headaches are sometimes relieved by inhaled oxygen (6–8 L/min; 100% oxygen mask for 10–15 minutes), subcutaneous sumatriptan, or dihydroergotamine. Clusters of headaches may be abbreviated with prednisone (60 mg/day for 7 days, followed by a rapid taper) and vera-pamil. Verapamil should be continued until the patient has been headache-free for 2 weeks and then tapered. Chronic cluster headaches can be treated with verapamil, lithium, or valproic acid.

6. Define tension headaches. How are they treated?

The classic dichotomy of vascular (i.e., migraine and cluster) and tension (muscle contrac-tion) headaches is useful but not fully accurate. The typical "bandlike" frontooccipital tension headaches are presumably caused by increased contraction of scalp muscles due to life stress.

Treatment is usually with NSAIDs; rarely are more potent analgesics used. However, many patients have headaches with features of both vascular and tension types. Such headaches are best treated as common migraine.

7. What characteristics of a headache should raise the suspicion of intracranial disease?

No headache is pathognomonic for brain tumor, although the classic triad of headache, vom-iting, and papilledema may be seen. Nonetheless, the physician must recognize the headache that is a sign of intracranial disease. Such headaches may awaken the patient from sound sleep and be more severe in the early morning. The pain usually progressively worsens over days or weeks and is increased by changing posture, cough, or Valsalva effort. Changes in mental status or focal neurologic signs also may be present. New-onset seizures in combination with headache often herald serious brain lesions.

8. When should benign intracranial hypertension (BIH) be considered as a cause of head-ache? Is it in fact benign?

BIH, also pseudotumor cerebri, is elevated intracranial pressure of unknown etiology. It often is associated with obesity, pregnancy, and use of oral contraceptives, vitamin A, tetracy-cline, or steroids. It usually presents in young women as a headache that is worse on waking. The headaches often respond poorly to treatment. Papilledema is present, often along with visual symptoms such as blurring, enlarged blind spot, constricted visual fields, or even blindness.

BIH is not benign. Without proper therapy (weight loss, discontinuance of inciting medica-tions, and treatment with acetazolamide, corticosteroids, lumboperitoneal shunt, or optic nerve sheath fenestration) visual loss may be permanent.

9. What medical emergency is suggested by a unilateral headache in an elderly patient?

Temporal arteritis, or giant-cell arteritis, is a disease of the elderly that presents with headache centered over the temporal artery or around the eye. It also may be associated with fever, anorexia, myalgias, malaise, weight loss, or leukocytosis. On palpation the temporal artery is prominent and tender. The diagnosis is suggested by a sedimentation rate over 50 mm/hr. Definitive diagnosis depends on temporal artery biopsy, which shows granulomatous inflam-mation. The diagnosis represents an emergency because the central artery of the retina, a branch of the ophthalmic artery, may become thrombosed, causing unilateral or bilateral blindness in over 25% of patients. Prednisone, 50–75 mg/day, may diminish headache and help to prevent blindness.

10. What should be done for the patient who complains of intense sharp, stabbing pains through the eye?

Lancinating or "icepick" pains are a common phenomenon. They are sudden, brief (< 10 sec), highly localized, piercing pains, often through or behind one eye, temple, occiput, or ear. They may hit first one spot, then another. They are common in migrainous and anxious patients but occur in many other settings. They are always benign, do not require brain imaging, and are too brief to be treated. The best therapy is to reassure the patient.

11. What condition is suggested by the patient with daily or constant headache who takes daily NSAIDs, acetaminophen, vasoconstrictors, or analgesics?

The patient probably has drug-withdrawal rebound headaches. He or she needs consultation and treatment by a specialist experienced in the management of severe headaches, chronic pain, and drug withdrawal. Hospitalization may be required.

BIBLIOGRAPHY

1. Donaldson JO: Pseudotumor cerebri. In Johnson RT, Griffin JW (eds): Current Therapy in Neurologic Disease, 5th ed. St. Louis, Mosby, 1997, pp 93–95.
2. Raskin NH: Headache. In Appel SH (ed): Current Neurology, vol. 10. Chicago, Year Book, 1990, pp 195–219.
3. Rothner AD: Headaches in children and adolescents. In Johnson RT, Griffin W (eds): Current Therapy in Neurologic Disease, 5th ed. St. Louis, Mosby, 1997, pp 95–99.
4. Saper JR, Silberstein SD, Gordon CD, Hamel RL: Handbook of Headache Management. Baltimore, Williams & Wilkins, 1992.
5. Silberstein SD: Intractable headache: Inpatient and outpatient treatment strategies. Neurology 42(Suppl 2), 1992.
6. Silberstein SD, Young WB, Lipton RB: Headache and facial pain. In Johnson RT, Griffin JW (eds): Current Therapy in Neurologic Disease, 5th ed. St. Louis, Mosby, 1997, pp 85–92.
7. Touchon J, Bertin L, Pilgrim AJ, et al: A comparison of subcutaneous sumatriptan and dihydroergotamine nasal spray in the acute treatment of migraine. Neurology 47:361–365, 1996.

Website

Headache specialist David C. Haas, M.D.: http://www.hscsyr.edu~haasd/index.html

82. DIZZINESS AND SYNCOPE

Richard Hughes, M.D., and B. Jane Disrud, M.D.

1. What is the first thing to do when a patient complains of dizziness?

Because dizziness is a vague term, it is critical to understand the patient's definition. The first task is to distinguish dizziness from complaints referable to weakness, visual disturbances, or seizures. The second task is to distinguish between vestibular and nonvestibular types of dizziness. Vestibular dizziness or vertigo is accompanied by a sensation of movement, whereas nonvestibular dizziness is often described as a sensation of lightheadedness or imbalance.

2. What are the most common causes of dizziness?

The key role of the primary care physician is to identify the common causes of dizziness: postural hypotension, positional vertigo, hyperventilation, and multiple sensory deficits. Thus unnecessary referrals and expensive testing are often avoided.

3. What historical data are important in suggesting the cause of dizziness?

Vestibular causes are suggested by episodic attacks that may be precipitated by positional changes and often are accompanied by nausea and vomiting, with or without hearing loss or tinnitus. Nonvestibular causes usually result in a prolonged sensation of lightheadedness brought on by stress, hyperventilation, or standing and perhaps accompanied by palpitations, perspiration, paresthesias, and pallor. Syncope may result. The patient should be questioned about a history of head injury, recent viral infections, diabetes, or psychiatric disturbance.

4. Which medications most notably cause dizziness?

Antibiotics (e.g., gentamicin, streptomycin), anticonvulsants, high-dose salicylates, antiparkinsonian agents, and antihypertensives may be responsible. Any sedative medication may cause fatigue and unsteadiness that some patients call "dizziness."

5. Describe the specific elements of the evaluation of the dizzy patient.

The cardiovascular examination pays special attention to pulse and blood pressure (standing and supine), murmurs, arrhythmia, and carotid bruits. The examination also should focus on evidence of impacted wax and ear infection as well as a brief assessment of hearing loss. Hyperventilation for 2–3 minutes may reproduce the symptoms and confirm the diagnosis of primary hyperventilation. A careful neurologic exam with special attention to cranial nerve and cerebellar function is critical to exclude signs of a focal process.

6. When are laboratory tests helpful in evaluating the patient with dizziness?

Laboratory tests are dictated by the history and examination. A complete blood count and electrolyte panel are needed when the patient equates dizziness with "feeling generally unwell." A routine electrocardiogram (EKG) should be performed to search for evidence of cardiac disease. An imaging study (computed tomography [CT] or magnetic resonance imaging [MRI]) is useful when focal brainstem abnormalities, such as acoustic neuromas or multiple sclerosis, are suspected. Audiometry is useful in patients with hearing loss and tinnitus. Other tests, such as electromyogram, electroencephalography (EEG), brainstem-evoked potentials, and cervical spine films, are usually not needed.

7. Once a diagnosis of dizziness of vestibular origin is made, is the patient treatable?

Yes. Most dizziness or tinnitus of vestibular origin is self-limited. Symptomatic treatment with transdermal scopolamine, meclizine (Antivert), or dimenhydrinate (Dramamine) is helpful for vertigo. Promethazine hydrochloride (Phenergan) or trimethobenzamide (Tigan) is usually effective for controlling associated nausea. Vestibular exercise therapy may be useful in benign positional or posttraumatic vertigo.

8. Which serious central nervous system diseases may cause new-onset vertigo?

1. **Posterior circulation cerebrovascular disease** typically is associated with brainstem or occipital lobe complaints.

2. **Acoustic neuroma**, when unilateral, typically is associated with hearing loss in the telephone range.

3. **Other posterior fossa tumors** are associated with slow onset and coordination difficulties.

4. **Multiple sclerosis** typically is associated with more than one neurologic abnormality as well as episodic symptoms.

9. Can seizures cause dizziness?

Yes. **Complex partial seizures** may present with an aura of dizziness, vertigo, or unsteadiness. Without clear evidence of epilepsy, the diagnosis may require EEG monitoring. Complex partial seizures are easily treated with appropriate anticonvulsants. **Basilar migraine**, an odd variant of complicated migraine, may be accompanied by lightheadedness, vertigo, or ataxia.

10. What systemic disorders may cause dizziness or even brief alterations of consciousness?

Hypoglycemia, allergic reactions, drug or alcohol blackouts, and orthostasis due to loss blood, volume, or electrolytes (adrenal insufficiency).

11. Describe syncope.

Syncope is a brief loss of consciousness that occurs while standing and causes the patient to collapse to the floor. Syncope is usually preceded by a warm or "floating" feeling and perhaps by changes in vision. Such premonitory symptoms typically last a fraction of a second but on occasion may be prolonged. When patients experience premonitory symptoms and sit or lie down to prevent syncope, the condition is termed "presyncope."

Once the patient hits the floor, unconsciousness lasts from a few seconds to a minute. During the period of unconsciousness muscle twitches, called myoclonic jerks, may be observed. When prominent, they are mistaken for seizures. Only rarely, however, does syncope induce a truly generalized tonic-clonic seizure. When patients try to stand too quickly, syncope commonly recurs; the autonomic system may require a few minutes to recover sufficiently to allow maintenance of an erect posture. Typically patients are not confused or disoriented.

12. Is it important to discover the cause of syncope?

Most causes of syncope in the United States are not serious. Episodes of simple fainting or vasovagal syncope account for approximately 50% of all events. For the neurologist or cardiologist who sees a small subset of high-risk patients with syncope, a serious diagnosis is more common, accounting for another 20% of cases. This bias explains the variation in opinion on the seriousness of syncope, which depends on which group of patients is seen. Approximately 20% of patients have no known diagnosis after evaluation.

13. How do I know who is safe?

Perhaps the most important role of the primary care physician is to recognize and treat appropriately (or leave alone) simple vasovagal syncope or fainting. A good history includes the instigating event (if any), premonitory symptoms, and typical resolution of the syncopal episode. If the neurologic and cardiovascular examinations are normal, little more needs to be done.

Common triggering mechanisms include heat and dehydration combined with physical stress or startle. Examples include fainting at the sight of blood or instrumentation, micturition syncope, tussive syncope, Valsalva syncope (e..g, diving, weightlifting, trumpet playing), and the notorious tendency of people to faint at church services or weddings. Military recruits often faint during routine immunizations. If the patient cannot recall a triggering event, a witness may help.

14. Which cardiovascular abnormalities are associated with syncope?

Cardiac syncope requires a 50% drop in cardiac output and thus is a harbinger of serious cardiac disease. Mechanical, ischemic, and arrhythmic etiologies may lead to syncope. Mechanical lesions include aortic and pulmonary obstruction, including hypertension. Arrhythmias, including complete heart block, sick sinus syndrome, and brady- or tachycardias, may cause syncope. Ischemia due to myocardial infarction or aortic dissection also may present with syncope. Thus, any syncopal patient over the age of 50 years or with known cardiac abnormalities on EKG or physical examination requires further evaluation.

15. When should prolonged EKG monitoring be performed in the evaluation of syncope?

Certainly patients with a history, physical examination, or routine EKG suggestive of cardiac disease should have prolonged EKG monitoring. However, prolonged EKG monitoring provides diagnostic information in only 20% of syncopal patients older than 50 years with no clues pointing to cardiovascular disease. Further study is needed to determine the cost-benefit ratio.

16. What is the value of invasive testing in the diagnosis of syncope?

A thorough history and examination, an EKG, and 24-hour cardiac monitor should be performed in older patients. If no abnormalities or clues are found, additional invasive testing, such as electrophysiology or coronary angiography, head CT, or EEG, seldom adds significant information.

17. How useful is the tilt table?

Unfortunately, a tilt table can make anyone faint, regardless of what symptoms they may have had in church last week. Perhaps the most useful information results from inducing a faint in the patient with an unexplained loss of consciousness, which confirms that the episode was indeed a faint rather than another type of spell (such as hysteria). Many investigators have remarked on the negative electrophysiologic studies of patients who have simple faints on the tilt table. However, the tilt table is not a good screening device to determine who may need a more involved evaluation.

18. Define "drop" spells.

Drop spells are vaguely defined attacks that usually affect older patients, especially women. Patients experience a sudden "giving way" of the legs, fall, and may injure themselves but do not lose consciousness. The cause is not known. Once a thorough history, physical, and EKG are performed, no additional evaluation is needed.

19. Can strokes or neurologic problems cause syncope?

Yes. Patients with basilar artery ischemia may lose consciousness but usually have vertigo, unsteadiness, dysesthesia, weakness, or blindness. Furthermore, basilar artery ischemia usually involves a longer period of unconsciousness than simple syncope. Epilepsy is always a concern in patients whose syncope was unwitnessed or who do not recall the event. Typical postictal clues, such as headache, confusion, fatigue, tongue biting, or incontinence, are found. Many neurologic disorders cause fainting by loss of normal blood pressure and pulse responses to standing. Both central degenerative disorders (e.g., Alzheimer's disease, Parkinson's disease, Shy-Drager syndrome) and peripheral nerve disorders induce autonomic impairment sufficient to cause syncope.

20. What is the natural history of syncope?

Because most syncope occurs in the older population, mortality may be high. For simple vasovagal syncope the 1-year mortality rate is less than 5%, whereas the 1-year mortality rate for cardiac syncope is 20–30%. Electrophysiologic testing has probably increased understanding of the disorder more than it has changed mortality rates.

BIBLIOGRAPHY

1. Adams RD, Victor M: Principles of Neurology, 5th ed. New York, McGraw-Hill, 1993.
2. Brandt TH, Daroff RB: Physical therapy for benign paroxysmal vertigo. Arch Otolaryngol 42:290–293, 1980.
3. Hart GT: Evaluation of syncope. Am Fam Physician 51:1941–1952, 1995.
4. Kapoor WN: Workup and management of patients with syncope. Med Clin North Am 79:1153–1170, 1995.
5. Kapoor WN, Hammil SC, Gersch BJ: Diagnosis and natural history of syncope and role of invasive electrophysiologic testing. Medicine 69:160–175, 1990.
6. Kaufmann H: Neurally mediated syncope: Pathogenesis, diagnosis and treatment. Neurology 45(5):S12–S18, 1995.
7. Manolis AJ, Linzer M, Salem D, Estes NAM: Syncope: Current diagnostic evaluation and management. Ann Intern Med 112:850–863, 1990.
8. McGee SR: Dizzy patients: Diagnosis and treatment. West J Med 162:37–42, 1995.
9. Samuels MA: Manual of Neurology, 4th ed. Boston, Little, Brown, 1991.
10. Troost BT, Patton JM: Exercise therapy for positional vertigo. Neurology 42:1441–1444, 1992.

83. SEIZURE DISORDERS

Archana Shrestha, M.D., and Richard Hughes, M.D.

1. Define epilepsy.

The International League of Epilepsy defines epilepsy as an ongoing propensity to have seizures in the absence of provoking circumstances. Thus withdrawal seizures, childhood febrile seizures, and seizures during cardiorespiratory arrest do not constitute epilepsy.

2. When does the onset of epilepsy most frequently occur?

Although the onset of seizure disorders may occur at any age, the incidence of first seizure has been found to be highest in patients below the age of 20 years.

3. Describe the different forms of epilepsy.

Primary generalized epilepsies begin in a widespread fashion, involving the entire cortex (i.e., generalized rather than focal pathology). They often follow an autosomal dominant pattern of inheritance with incomplete penetrance. The onset is usually in childhood (for example, 5–7 years of age for absence seizures or puberty for juvenile myoclonic epilepsy). Patients typically have a normal neurologic examination and normal IQ. The possible types of seizure include absence (petit mal), generalized tonic-clonic (grand mal), atonic (often called "drop attacks"), and myoclonic (often described simply as "jerks").

Acquired epilepsies begin focally but often invade the entire brain (generalized), thus making the focal onset difficult to confirm. Genetic factors may create a predisposition, but the onset is highest under age 20 and over age 60 years. Although some patients with acquired epilepsy have clear evidence of a focal brain lesion by history, examination, or neuroimaging, most are normal. Common seizure types include complex partial seizures (which affect mentation without loss of consciousness), simple partial seizures (which do not alter mentation), and secondarily generalized seizures (grand mal seizures immediately preceded by a brief complex partial or simple partial seizure).

4. When do traumatic seizures usually occur?

When the cause of trauma to the cortex is known, the onset of seizure disorder is most likely to occur within 1 year of injury, although it may occur several years later.

5. Should prophylactic anticonvulsants be given to patients with significant head trauma?

No. The prophylactic administration of currently available anticonvulsant medications after trauma or disease of the central nervous system (CNS) probably does not alter the risk of developing a seizure disorder.

6. When is CNS imaging warranted in the evaluation of new-onset seizure?

When the clinical manifestations of seizure disorder fit one of the syndromes of primary generalized epilepsy, with an appropriate family history, response to medications, and electro-encelphalographic (EEG) findings, imaging of the brain may be unnecessary, unless specific findings or elements of the history suggest coexisting focal neuropathology. In contrast, evaluation of acquired seizure disorders always includes an imaging study of the brain in an attempt to elucidate the cause of the presumed focal cortical injury. The differential diagnosis is voluminous and includes almost all illnesses and mechanisms known to cause injury to the cortex.

7. How is epilepsy treated?

Treatment depends on whether the patient has a primary generalized or acquired seizure disorder. All of the seizures associated with primary generalized epilepsies, including absence, generalized tonic-clonic, atonic, and myoclonic seizures, may be effectively treated with Depakote (divalproex sodium). Absence seizures are also successfully treated with Zarontin (ethosuximide), which has little value in treatment of other seizure types. Lamotrigine is currently being studied for its use in primary generalized epilepsies; preliminary results look promising.

Treatment of acquired seizure disorders is equally successful with either Tegretol (carbamazepine) or Dilantin (phenytoin). Newer medications include lamotrigine, gabapentin, and felbamate. Topirimate and tiagabine were approved by the Food and Drug Administration in 1997, and vigabatrin was approved in 1998 as add-on treatment of partial onset seizures.

Although inexpensive and effective against most types of seizures, barbiturates such as phenobarbital, primidone, and mephobarbital are less favored because of sedation, cognitive impairment, and emotional depression.

8. Are two drugs better than one in the treatment of seizures?

No. In general, polypharmaceutical treatment of seizures is not necessary and may be disadvantageous. Although it is true that the beneficial effects of most of the antiepileptic medicines may be additive, the side effects are synergistic and typically accumulate faster than the benefits.

Most patients have the best profile of benefit/side effects with the use of a single, appropriately chosen, optimally titrated medication.

9. Can generic drugs be used to treat seizures?

No. Most classes of medications do not require the precise degree of titration that is necessary in antiepileptic drugs. Because most antiepileptic drugs have narrow therapeutic windows, the differences in bioavailability among various generic preparations often cause clinically important fluctuations in serum levels. For these reasons, generic antiepileptic medications should not be used.

10. What are possible causes for an increase in seizure frequency?

Possibilities include medication, noncompliance, changes in antiepileptic medication (including generic substitution), addition of another medication that may interact with the antiepileptic medication, or any physical, psychological, or emotional stress. Examples include infections and sleep deprivation.

11. What are common causes of nonepileptic seizures?

This broad list includes almost all illnesses and mechanisms known to cause acute injury to the cortex. Common causes include electrolyte and other metabolic disturbances, CNS infections, trauma, tumors, stroke, drug effects, and alcohol.

12. Can some patients eventually discontinue their seizure medications?

Yes. However, patients with a primary generalized seizure disorder generally have to be on life-long medication. Patients with an acquired seizure disorder who have a normal neurologic exam, a normal imaging study, and a repeat EEG (prior to stopping medication) that has no epileptiform activity and who have remained seizure-free for approximately 2 years may attempt slow titration off anticonvulsant medication.

13. How frequently should laboratory tests be used to monitor patients on therapy?

In general, a complete blood count, assessment of electrolytes, and liver function tests should be obtained before initiating therapy with antiepileptic medications and repeated 1–2 months later. The value of routine repetition of these tests in patients who are doing well with antiepileptic therapy is debatable. A single assessment of serum levels may be useful when titration appears to be successful to document the appropriate level for the patient. This level then may be maintained. If seizure control decreases or side effects increase, serum levels of medication should be assessed. Remember the tried and true aphorism: "Treat the patient, not the laboratory." Patients occasionally do best (no seizures or side effects) at levels below or above the usual laboratory range.

14. What is status epilepticus?

Convulsive status epilepticus is a life-threatening emergency defined as generalized tonic-clonic seizure or a series of generalized tonic-clonic seizures without return of consciousness over a period of 30 minutes. Nonconvulsive status epilepticus involving partial or absence seizures is not associated with the poor outcomes common to generalized status epilepticus.

15. Do women with epilepsy have increased obstetric risks?

Because of the many misunderstandings about pregnancy in patients with epilepsy, it is important to educate all women of childbearing age who have seizure disorders. Whereas approximately 2% of all births in the United States involve fetal malformation, the incidence in infants born to epileptic mothers is 4–6%. This increased risk may be attributed to three causes: the underlying illness, if any, that created the mother's seizure disorder; the seizures themselves; and the medications taken by the mother to control the seizures.

As long as the mother does not experience trauma secondary to a seizure, nonconvulsive seizures have little, if any, significance to the fetus. Generalized tonic-clonic seizures in the mother have been shown to be associated with decelerations in fetal heart rate and thus place the fetus at significant risk. Therefore, patients with generalized tonic-clonic seizures should continue with antiepileptic medications from conception through delivery. The risks and benefits must be assessed on a case-by-case basis.

Folic acid supplementation is recommended for all pregnant women, but for women taking valproic acid or carbamazepine, a higher dose of 1 mg/day is generally recommended. Carbamazepine, phenytoin, and barbiturates may cause a transient and reversible deficiency of vitamin K clotting factors in neonates. Therefore, a 20-mg oral dose of vitamin K is recommended in the last few weeks of pregnancy along with 1 mg intramuscular vitamin K for the neonate immediately after birth.

16. Should antiseizure medications be changed during pregnancy?

Although the teratogenicity of the various anticonvulsant medications differs, the current recommendation is to continue the regimen that has been most effective (best control with least toxicity) in the past. Because of changes in hepatic function, it is usually necessary to make gradual incremental changes in dosages of medications metabolized in the liver. Serum levels during the mother's monthly prenatal visit should guide drug dosage. At the time of delivery, the dosage should be restored to prepregnancy levels.

Epileptic mothers taking ethosuximide or barbiturates should be advised that these medications appear in breast milk in significant concentrations; thus breast feeding is inadvisable.

17. May patients with epilepsy drive a car?

The laws regarding driving (not including commercial or interstate driving) vary from state to state. Epileptics should not drive until it is clear that medication completely controls their seizures. The usual standard is a seizure-free period of 6–12 months.

18. What advice should be given to patients with epilepsy?

Routine "seizure precautions" include the advice to abstain from all activities, situations, or circumstances in which the patient may be injured (or injure others) in the event of a seizure. Although certain risky activities, such as using power tools, climbing ladders, or swimming, are likely to be self-evident, other less obvious activities, such as exposure to hot tap water, may pose significant risk to the patient with an active seizure disorder.

19. Do epileptics need to quit their jobs?

No. Most patients with epilepsy are able to continue working. Like patients with other chronic health problems, they are well advised to understand the Americans with Disabilities Act. Because of old fears and ignorance, employers, teachers, and/or family also may benefit from education.

20. Where can patients with epilepsy get more information?

The Epilepsy Foundation of America, which can be reached at 1 (800) EFA-1000, may be of importance to patients, families, caregivers, and clinicians who provide medical care for patients with seizure disorders.

Disclaimer: All treatment guidelines are made with the understanding that the ultimate responsibility for all evaluation and treatment decisions rests exclusively with the treating physician. The authors take no responsibility for outcome or appropriateness of treatment guidelines.

BIBLIOGRAPHY

1. Delgado-Escueta AV, Janz D: Consensus guidelines: Preconception counseling, management, and care of the pregnant woman with epilepsy. Neurology 42(Suppl 5):149–160, 1992.
2. Dodson WE: Level off [editorial]. Neurology 39:1009–1010, 1989.
3. Hauser WA, Hesdorffer DC: Epilepsy: Frequency, Causes and Consequences. New York, Demos Publications, 1990.

4. Hauser WA, Kurland LT: The epidemiology of epilepsy in Rochester, Minnesota, 1935 through 1967. Epilepsia 16:1–66, 1975.
5. Mattson RH, Cramer JA, Collins JF, et al: Comparison of carbamazepine, phenobarbital, phenytoin, and primidone in partial and secondarily generalized tonic-clonic seizures. N Engl J Med 313:145–151, 1985.
6. Salazar AM: Jabbari B, Vance SC, et al: Epilepsy after penetrating head injury. I: Clinical correlates: A report of the Vietnam Head Injury Study. Neurology 35:1406–1414, 1985.
7. Sato S, White BG, Penry JK, et al: Valproic acid versus ethosuximide in the treatment of absence seizures. Neurology 32:157–163, 1982.
8. Spitz MC, Towbin JA, Shantz D: Risk factors for burns as a consequence of seizures in patients with epilepsy. Epilepsia 35:764–767, 1994.
9. Temkin NR, Dikmen SS, Wilensky AJ, et al: A randomized, double-blind study of phenytoin for the prevention of post-traumatic seizures. N Engl J Med 323:497–502, 1990.
10. Treiman D: VA Cooperative Study (in press).
11. Turnball DM, Rawlins MD, Weightman D, Chadwick DW: A comparison of phenytoin and valproate in previously untreated adult epileptic patients. J Neurol Neurosurg Psychiatry 45:55–59, 1982.
12. Weiss GH, Salazar AM, Vance SC, et al: Predicting posttraumatic epilepsy in penetrating head injury. Arch Neurol 43:771–773, 1986.
13. Young B, Rapp RP, Norton JLA, et al: Failure of prophylactically administered phenytoin to prevent late posttraumatic seizure. J Neurosurg 58:236–241, 1983
14. Yerby MS: Pregnancy, teratogenesis, and epilepsy. Neurol Clin 12:749–764, 1994.

XII. Common Disorders of the Chest

84. DYSPNEA

Benjamin T. Suratt, M.D., and Elizabeth L. Aronsen, M.D.

1. Define dyspnea.

Simply defined, dyspnea is the uncomfortable sensation of breathing. Normally breathing is an automatic function that involves no conscious effort. Patients may describe the symptom variously as "difficulty getting air in," "chest tightness," a feeling of "breathlessness," or perhaps a lack of "good air" or "air hunger."

2. What are the pathophysiologic mechanisms of normal breathing?

1. **Cortical brain**. The sensory cortex receives and processes afferent signals.

2. **Brainstem**. Chemoreceptors in the medulla respond to changes in hydrogen ion, carbon dioxide, and oxygen concentrations.

3. **Carotid body**. This peripheral chemoreceptor signals changes in hydrogen ion, carbon dioxide, and oxygen concentrations.

4. **Respiratory muscles**. Muscle spindles in intercostal muscles release afferent signals to spinal reflexes. Central respiratory drive is influenced by tendon organs in the diaphragm.

5. **Mechanoreceptors**. The airways and lung parenchyma have at least three types of mechanoreceptors that influence respiration:
   - Stretch receptors respond to changes in lung volume.
   - Irritant receptors along the bronchial walls respond to inhaled substances.
   - C-fibers in the interstitium respond to changes in interstitial fluid.

3. What are the mechanisms of dyspnea?

The mechanisms of dyspnea are incompletely understood. It is thought that signals from receptors described above contribute to varying degrees to patients' descriptions of dyspnea:

1. **Chemoreceptors**, sensitive to excessive serum hydrogen ions (metabolic acidosis), increased carbon dioxide (respiratory acidosis or increased production), or decreased oxygen (hypoxemia) may signal a need for increased minute ventilation, perceived as breathlessness.

2. **Mechanoreceptors**, activated by hyperinflation, inhaled toxins, or perhaps increases in lung water, may trigger a cascade of events eventually described by the patient as chest tightness or pressure.

3. **Respiratory muscle** dysfunction, whether due to weakness or mechanical disadvantage, may be described by the patient as increased work of breathing or respiratory effort.

4. The **sensory cortex** must integrate a wide variety of signals. Dyspnea may be due to "afferent mismatch" between discordant outgoing motor signals to the respiratory muscles and subsequent incoming afferent information.

4. What is the differential diagnosis of acute dyspnea?

The entire list of causes of dyspnea is extensive. However, one may think of the differential diagnosis in terms of contributing mechanisms or in broad categories such as the following:

1. **Cardiac disorders**
   - Dysrhythmias (paroxysmal supraventricular tachycardia, atrial fibrillation or flutter, bradycardia, nonsustained ventricular tachycardia)

- Valvular disease (aortic or mitral stenosis or regurgitation)
- Pericardial disease (restrictive pericarditis or tamponade)
- Obstruction to outflow (idiopathic hypertrophic subaortic stenosis or atrial myxoma)
- Dysfunction (ischemia or hypertension with congestive heart failure or pulmonary edema)
- Shunt

2. **Pulmonary disorders**
   - Upper airway obstruction (foreign body aspiration, angioedema, epiglottitis)
   - Bronchoconstriction (chronic obstructive pulmonary disease [COPD] or asthma exacerbation)
   - Alveolar filling disease (pneumonia, edema, hemorrhage)
   - Interstitial disease (fibrosis, inflammation)
   - Vascular disease (embolism, vasculitis, venoocclusive disease)
   - Inhalation injury
   - Pneumothorax (spontaneous or secondary to trauma or an underlying disease such as COPD, asthma, cystic fibrosis, *Pneumocystis carinii*, or neoplasm)

3. **Other disorders**
   - Deconditioning
   - Anemia
   - Thyroid disease
   - Metabolic acidosis (of any cause)
   - Hyperventilation syndrome

5. How is dyspnea affected by position?

Postural effects on dyspnea are frequent and likely due to changes in respiratory mechanics and/or gas exchange (ventilation-perfusion mismatching) related to body position. Positional dyspnea is described as (1) **orthopnea** (dyspnea in a supine position), (2) **trepopnea** (dyspnea in the right or left lateral decubitus position), (3) **platypnea** (dyspnea that worsens in the upright position and improves in the supine position).

6. Describe a reasonable and cost-effective work-up of the patient with dyspnea.

Work-up of any chief complaint begins with a complete history and physical examination. Diagnostic tests may then be used to narrow the differential or to confirm the diagnosis.

History. The characteristics and circumstances of the dyspnea may provide clues to the principal diagnosis and the mechanism of the dyspnea. Associated symptoms, current and recent medications (including over-the-counter, illegal, or herbal compounds), potential toxic exposures, and past medical history are also important.

Physical exam. Although it should always be complete, the physician may want to focus especially on the head and neck, neurologic, cardiopulmonary, and skin exams.

Chest radiograph (CXR). Many patients may have an entirely normal physical exam but an abnormal CXR that accounts for the dyspnea. If one has not been performed previously while the patient has been dyspneic, a CXR should be done at the initial evaluation.

Electrocardiogram (EKG). Because cardiac abnormalities account for a great number of causes of dyspnea, a resting EKG should be performed early in the assessment.

Resting and exercise saturation by pulse oximetry (R/E SpO_2). Although some offices are not equipped to perform R/E SpO_2, it is helpful to perform this test early in the evaluation of dyspnea. Most cardiopulmonary causes of dyspnea result in exercise desaturation, whereas many noncardiopulmonary causes do not.

Laboratory tests. Laboratory tests may include a hemogram to exclude anemia or leukemia, chemistries to evaluate renal, liver, or metabolic causes of dyspnea, and assessment of thyroid-stimulating hormone.

7. What is hyperventilation syndrome (HVS)?

Hyperventilation syndrome (HVS) is a poorly understood entity that predominantly affects young women without underlying cardiopulmonary disease or other causes of dyspnea. It is characterized by fluctuating, recurrent episodes of dyspnea (often described as "breathlessness") without relation to exertion, often associated with atypical chest pain and other vague complaints. Stress at home or at work can precipitate an episode. Secondary complaints, often related to respiratory alkalosis caused by hyperventilation, include dizziness, faintness, or tingling and numbness of the fingers and toes. The only laboratory abnormality typically is respiratory alkalosis with a normal alveolar-arterial (A-a) gradient on arterial blood gas. HVS is a diagnosis of exclusion.

8. What is the differential diagnosis of dyspnea in patients with cancer?

Fifteen percent of patients with cancer present with dyspnea as the initial complaint. Dyspnea occurs in as many as 65% during the course of the illness. For these reasons it is important to have in mind an understanding of cancer-specific dyspnea. Causes include the tumor itself, treatment of the malignancy, and anxiety relating to the diagnosis.

1. **Cancer-related causes**
   - Upper airway obstruction
   - Superior vena cava syndrome
   - Lung effacement by tumor
   - Pleural effusion
   - Pericardial effusion
   - Lymphangitic spread of tumor
   - Ascites or hepatomegaly obstructing normal diaphragmatic excursion
2. **Treatment-related causes**
   - Radiation pneumonitis
   - Lung injury from chemotherapies
   - Pulmonary insufficiency following lobectomy or pneumonectomy

9. What more specialized testing is used to evaluate dyspnea?

Causes of dyspnea not diagnosed by routine testing generally require consultation with a subspecialist. However, further tests often include:

1. **Pulmonary function tests (PFTs).** Full PFTs include spirometry or lung mechanics, lung volumes, diffusing capacity, flow-volume loop, and, if requested, arterial blood gases (ABGs).

2. **High-resolution computed tomography of the chest (HRCT).** HRCT provides a detailed examination of lung interstitium without the morbidity of tissue biopsy and is often performed in patients with suspected interstitial lung disease even with a normal CXR.

3. **Cardiopulmonary exercise testing (CPET).** CPET may be used to distinguish occult cardiac and pulmonary diseases from simple deconditioning.

10. When should the patient with chronic dyspnea be referred for cardiopulmonary exercise testing?

1. When the exact cause of dyspnea remains unclear despite complete pulmonary function testing.

2. When the patient has both pulmonary and cardiac disease and the contribution of either needs to be determined.

3. When the patient's symptoms are out of proportion to the severity of physiologic impairment.

4. When obesity, deconditioning, or anxiety is suspected as a cause of chronic dyspnea.

11. What therapeutic modalities may be used to help alleviate dyspnea associated with COPD?

Based primarily on our current understanding of the pathophysiology of dyspnea in COPD, three general approaches may be pursued:

1. **Improve ventilatory capacity** by standard therapeutic methods, which include bronchodilation, antiinflammatories, and respiratory muscle training. Bronchodilation is achieved with beta agonists, anticholinergics, and theophylline. Antiinflammatory agents include cromolyn,

nedocromil, and inhaled or systemic steroid. Respiratory muscle training is usually most effective in patients with demonstrable muscle weakness.

2. **Reduce ventilatory demand** by supplemental oxygen therapy, with exercise training to enhance mechanical efficiency and, in certain circumstances, with anxiolytic and dyspneolytic agents such as benzodiazepines or opiates.

3. **Mechanically unload inspiratory muscles** with negative pressure ventilation or low-level continuous positive-pressure ventilation.

12. Are narcotics or anxiolytics useful in the treatment of profoundly dyspneic patients?

Treatment of the underlying disease is obviously the first choice in the therapy of dyspnea. Relief of breathlessness is often incomplete, however, leading to consideration of pharmacologic agents to improve symptoms of profound dyspnea. Narcotics and anxiolytics may alter the perception of breathlessness, although they do not treat the underlying cause. Concern about their use centers on their potential to depress respiratory function and to worsen gas exchange. Most of the knowledge about such agents results from treatment of patients with COPD (dyspnea refractory to standard medical therapy) or patients with terminal cancer and intractable dyspnea.

Narcotics. Opiates have been used with variable efficacy to relieve dyspnea. Their major mechanism of action is respiratory depression through direct effects on the respiratory center of the brainstem. They not only alter the perception of breathlessness but also may reduce ventilatory drive. Exercise tolerance may increase without increased sensation of breathlessness. However, because of their frequent side effects (e.g., nausea, vomiting, constipation, drowsiness) and potential for addiction, they should be used only for the most severe cases of dyspnea in preterminal patients.

Anxiolytics. Anxiety and panic are often confounding factors in severely dyspneic patients. Because benzodiazepines act as anxiolytics and reduce respiratory drive, they are potentially beneficial in the treatment of refractory dyspnea. Early reports showed a subjective improvement in both dyspnea and exercise tolerance. However, the majority of the literature has not demonstrated consistent benefit in improving symptoms of breathlessness, exercise tolerance, or arterial blood gas values. In general, benzodiazepines are not indicated in treatment of dyspnea and should be used with extreme caution in patients with profound breathlessness and anxiety.

CONTROVERSY

13. Is the disproportionate dyspnea seen in some patients with breathlessness psychological in origin?

It has been suggested that depression, anxiety, and hysterical reactions may cause disproportionate symptoms. In patients with COPD and comparable degrees of respiratory impairment, the severity of breathlessness may vary considerably. Such variations in the level of dyspnea probably occur because dyspnea is a subjective sensation dependent on numerous factors, including past behavioral influences, the situation in which breathlessness occurs, and the patient's ability to describe breathlessness.

For: Comparisons between patients with and without disproportionate dyspnea found that significant numbers of patients with disproportionate breathlessness have depression (52%), anxiety (22%), and hysterical reactions (26%), whereas the other group suffers from no formal psychiatric disorder. Furthermore, successful treatment of the psychiatric disorder 2–3 years later revealed complete or partial resolution of dyspnea in patients with disproportionate symptoms. Finally, some data suggest that the threshold for detection of resistive ventilatory loads is greater in anxious patients.

Against: Differences among patients in perception of changes in respiratory effort, thoracic displacement, or respiratory muscle force offer a physiologic explanation for differences in the sensation of dyspnea. In addition, successful treatment of psychiatric symptoms with no improvement in disproportionate dyspnea has been reported. This suggests that the psychiatric disorders are a consequence and not a cause of dyspnea.

BIBLIOGRAPHY

1. Manning HL, Schwartzstein RM: Pathophysiology of dyspnea. N Engl J Med 333:1547–1553, 1995.
2. Harver A, Mahler DA: The symptom of dyspnea. In Mahler DA (ed): Dyspnea. Mount Kisco, NY, Futura, 1990, pp 1–53.
3. Elliot MW, et al: The language of breathlessness: Use of verbal descriptors by patients with cardiopulmonary disease. Am Rev Respir Dis 144:826–832, 1991.
4. Smith K, et al: Respiratory muscle training in chronic airflow limitation: A meta-analysis. Am Rev Respir Dis 145:533–539, 1992.
5. O'Donnell DE: Breathlessness in patients with chronic airflow limitation: Mechanisms and management. Chest 106:904–912, 1994.
6. Cherniak NS, Altose MD: Mechanisms of dyspnea. Clin Chest Med 8:207–214, 1987.
7. Mahler DA: Dyspnea: Diagnosis and management. Clin Chest Med 8:215–230, 1987.
8. Mahler DA: Diagnosis of dyspnea. In Mahler DA (ed): Dyspnea. New York, Marcel Dekker, 1988, pp 221–253.
9. Smoller JW, Pollack MH, Otto MW, et al: Panic anxiety, dyspnea, and respiratory disease. Theoretical and clinical considerations. Am J Respir Crit Care Med 154:6–17, 1996.
10. Dudgeon DJ, Rosenthal S: Management of dyspnea and cough in patients with cancer. Hematol Oncol Clin North Am 10:157–171, 1996.

85. HEMOPTYSIS

Jeffrey M. Sippel, M.D.

1. Define scant hemoptysis (blood streaking), frank hemoptysis, massive hemoptysis, and pseudohemoptysis.

Scant hemoptysis is sputum that contains trace amounts of blood but is composed primarily of mucus. Frank or gross hemoptysis is expectoration of blood that originates in the lower respiratory tract (lung parenchyma, bronchi, and trachea). Scant and frank hemoptysis are the most common types in the outpatient setting. Massive hemoptysis is expectoration of more than 600 cc of blood in 24 hours or any amount that causes respiratory distress, hemodynamic compromise, or anemia. Pseudohemoptysis is expectoration of blood that does not originate from the lower respiratory tract. Sources include hematemesis or blood aspirated from the gastrointestinal (GI) tract and blood that collects in the hypopharynx or trachea from the oral cavity, sinuses, or nasopharyngeal source.

2. What is the differential diagnosis of hemoptysis based on the quantity of blood present?

Hemoptysis commonly arises from diseases affecting the lung parenchyma or tracheo-bronchial tree, which may be either focal, such as bronchogenic carcinoma, pneumonia, and tuberculosis, or diffuse, such as pulmonary vasculitis and collagen vascular diseases. Cardiovascular or hematologic disorders, such as mitral stenosis or thrombocytopenia, also may be implicated, although less commonly. Although the differential diagnosis may be rather large, certain patient populations are associated with a higher frequency of specific illnesses. For example, an elderly male cigarette smoker has a much higher prevalence of lung cancer than a young woman who is more likely to have pulmonary vasculitis or collagen vascular disease. In addition, the various causes of hemoptysis may produce different amounts of bleeding. The list below is not exhaustive but focuses on the more common etiologies of hemoptysis:

Scant hemoptysis (blood streaking)
- Bronchitis
- Bronchiectasis
- Lung cancer
- Tuberculosis

Frank and massive hemoptysis
- All of the above
- Arteriovenous malformations
- Pulmonary embolus or infarct
- Pulmonary vasculitis

- Bleeding diathesis or coagulopathy
- Cystic fibrosis
- Goodpasture's syndrome
- Mitral stenosis
- Necrotizing or cavitary pneumonia

- Systemic lupus erythematosus
- Wegener's granulomatosis
- Iatrogenic (pulmonary artery catheter,
  tracheoinnominate fistula)

Pseudohemoptysis
- Upper GI bleed with aspiration or expectoration of blood
- Sinus, oral, pharyngeal, or laryngeal bleeding site

3. What are the most common causes of hemoptysis in the outpatient setting?

The etiology of hemoptysis has changed over the last 50 years. Tuberculosis and bronchiectasis were the most common causes of hemoptysis before effective antimicrobial chemotherapy. According to recent studies, however, bronchitis (22–44%), bronchogenic carcinoma (6–29%), and idiopathic hemoptysis (22–33%), are now the three most common etiologies. Tuberculosis is seen in only 1.5–7% of patients and bronchiectasis in 1%. The populations in these epidemiologic studies were predominantly male, cigarette smokers, and over the age of 50 years; the etiologies may vary with the population studied.

4. What are the most common causes of hemoptysis among patients with human immunodeficiency virus (HIV) infection?

Hemoptysis is caused by bacterial pneumonia in 66% of cases, and no specific cause can be identified in 22% of cases. Tuberculosis causes 6–16% of hemoptysis in HIV-infected patients, which may be higher than in the general population. Other causes include Kaposi's sarcoma, other malignancies, fungal infections, and, rarely, *Pneumocystis carinii* pneumonia. Hemoptysis occurs in about 2% of hospitalized HIV-infected patients, and the frequency rises to 10% among those with lung abscess.

5. What factors, in combination with hemoptysis, are risks for pulmonary malignancy?

RISK FACTOR	PREVALENCE OF RISK FACTOR WHEN MALIGNANCY PRESENT
Cigarette smoking	45–100% have more than 40 pack-year history
Age over 40 years	Nearly 100%
Abnormal chest roentgenogram	25–80%
Symptoms for over 1 week	50–80%
Male gender	58–99%

6. What should be included in the initial evaluation of hemoptysis in the outpatient setting?

A thorough history focuses on quantity and duration of hemoptysis, cigarette smoking, presence of cough and sputum production, fever or other constitutional symptoms, and cardiovascular symptoms. The physical examination focuses on the nares, sinuses, oropharynx, heart, lungs, and extremities. If available, mirror laryngoscopy should be performed; if laryngoscopy is negative, a chest roentgenogram is obtained. If history and physical examination suggest an etiology other than acute bronchitis or if symptoms are recurrent, appropriate tests include sputum cytology, arterial blood gases, blood and platelet counts, prothrombin time, partial thromboplastin time, tuberculin skin test, urinalysis, and creatinine level. Pending results of these studies, further evaluation may include fiberoptic bronchoscopy and other radiographic techniques.

7. What is the role of fiberoptic bronchoscopy in the evaluation of hemoptysis?

Bronchoscopy provides diagnostic information in 10–69% of cases, depending on the subset of patients. The diagnostic yield of bronchoscopy generally increases in patients who are smokers, male, or over the age of 40 years or who have prolonged symptoms. Fiberoptic bronchoscopy is an integral part of the evaluation when malignancy is suspected because tissue biopsies can be performed. Bronchoscopy provides a histologic diagnosis in over 75% of malignancies when the chest roentgenogram is abnormal. Bronchoscopy also permits collection of lavage or brush specimens for mycobacterial and fungal cultures and may be useful for localizing the anatomic site of bleeding if hemoptysis is ongoing.

8. What is the role of computed tomography (CT) in the evaluation of hemoptysis?

If the chest roentgenogram is normal or nonlocalizing, chest CT scans yield additional information that suggests an etiology in 39–68% of cases. Chest CT is a reasonable alternative if malignancy is suspected and bronchoscopy is not available. Chest CT findings are abnormal in nearly 100% of patients with bronchogenic carcinoma; however, chest CT scans do not obviate the need for tissue diagnosis if malignancy is suspected. Likewise, chest roentgenogram and fiberoptic bronchoscopy fail to suggest malignancy in only 3% or less of cases. CT scans are more sensitive than either roentgenogram or fiberoptic bronchoscopy for the diagnosis of bronchiectasis.

9. Do diffuse infiltrates on chest roentgenogram always imply a diffuse process as the cause of hemoptysis?

No. Although bilateral infiltrates suggest that hemoptysis may be due to a more widespread process or systemic illness, a focal hemorrhage may cause the same radiographic appearance if the patient aspirates blood.

10. What is idiopathic hemoptysis? How should it be managed?

Idiopathic hemoptysis is a diagnosis of exclusion and should be made only after a thorough investigation has yielded no specific diagnosis. The incidence of idiopathic hemoptysis is estimated at 22–33%, and the disorder carries an overall favorable prognosis. Adelmann et al. followed 67 patients with hemoptysis, a normal or nonlocalizing chest roentgenogram, and nondiagnostic fiberoptic bronchoscopy for 3 years. The hemoptysis resolved within 6 months in 90% of patients and recurred in only 5%. Bronchogenic carcinoma was diagnosed at 20-month follow-up in only 1 patient (1.5%). The average patient age was 54 years; 72% smoked or had smoked cigarettes; 39% had a diagnosis of COPD; and 46% were tuberculin skin test-positive. A study by Santiago et al. confirmed the low rate of pulmonary malignancies: only 3 of 119 patients (2.5%) developed cancer within follow-up of 2–5 years.

11. What systemic illnesses may cause hemoptysis?

Amyloidosis	Mitral stenosis
Coagulation disorders	Pulmonary-renal syndromes
(iatrogenic and acquired)	Sarcoidosis
Congestive heart failure	Systemic lupus erythematosus
Metastatic cancer	Vasculitis

12. How do the initial evaluation and management differ in massive and frank hemoptysis?

Major complications of massive hemoptysis include hemodynamic instability and death from asphyxiation. Immediate management, therefore, must focus on hemodynamic stabilization and prevention of asphyxiation by aggressive airway control The patient may require emergent endotracheal intubation. If hemorrhage is localized to one lung, either placement of a double-lumen endotracheal tube or bronchoscopic-directed selective mainstem intubation may help to isolate and preserve gas exchange in the nonhemorrhaging lung. The nonhemorrhaging lung also may be protected by placing the patient in the decubitus position, bleeding side down; if the hemorrhage is of unknown or diffuse origin, the patient should be placed in the Trendelenberg position. Subsequent assessment should include a complete serologic evaluation, fiberoptic or rigid bronchoscopy, and surgical consultation.

13. What treatments are available for ongoing hemoptysis?

Bronchoscopy frequently identifies the bleeding site and provides therapeutic options, including selective bronchus intubation and, in appropriate cases, either topical fibrin application or balloon tamponade. Arteriography and embolization should be used in patients who continue to bleed despite bronchoscopic therapy. Emergent surgical intervention should be considered in operative candidates with unilateral bleeding when embolization is not available, when bleeding continues despite embolization, or when bleeding is associated with persistent hemodynamic and respiratory compromise.

CONTROVERSY

14. Should bronchoscopy be performed early (within 48 hours) in patients with hemoptysis?

For early bronchoscopy:

1. The procedure has minimal risk and is tolerated well by most patients.
2. The diagnostic yield for visualizing the site of bleeding is greater while the patient is actively hemorrhaging.
3. Therapeutic options after visualization include endobronchial tamponade, selective mainstem intubation, and surgical resection, all of which are facilitated by localizing the site of bleeding.

Against early bronchoscopy:

1. Early bronchoscopy induces coughing, which may worsen hemoptysis.
2. Although early bronchoscopy more frequently reveals a source of bleeding (40% early vs. 10% delayed), clinical management and outcome are not affected.

BIBLIOGRAPHY

1. Adelman M, et al: Cryptogenic hemoptysis. Clinical features, bronchoscopic findings, and natural history in 67 patients. Ann Intern Med 102:829–834, 1985.
2. Berger R, Rehm SR: Bronchoscopy for hemoptysis. Chest 99:1553, 1991.
3. Cahill BC, Ingbar DH: Massive hemoptysis: Assessment and management. Clin Chest Med 15:147–167, 1994.
4. Freitag L, Tekolf E, Stamatis G, et al: Three years experience with a new balloon catheter for the management of haemoptysis. Eur Respir J 7:2033–2037, 1994.
5. Gong H, Salvatierra C: Clinical efficacy of early and delayed fiberoptic bronchoscopy in patients with hemoptysis. Am Rev Respir Dis 124:221–225, 1981.
6. Jackson CV, Savage PJ, Quinn DL: Role of fiberoptic bronchoscopy in patients with hemoptysis and a normal chest roentgenogram. Chest 87:142–144, 1985.
7. Johnston H, Reisz G: Changing spectrum of hemoptysis. Underlying causes in 148 patients undergoing diagnostic flexible fiberoptic bronchoscopy. Arch Intern Med 149:1666–1668, 1989.
8. Naidich DP, et al: Hemoptysis: CT-bronchoscopic correlations in 58 cases. Radiology 177:357–362, 1990.
9. Najarian KE, Morris CS: Arterial embolization in the chest. J Thorac Imaging 13:93–104, 1998.
10. Nelson JE, Forman M: Hemoptysis in HIV-infected patients. Chest 110:737–743, 1996.
11. O'Neil KM, Lazarus AA: Hemoptysis. Indications for bronchoscopy. Arch Intern Med 151:171–174, 1991.
12. Poe RH, et al: Utility of fiberoptic bronchoscopy in patients with hemoptysis and a nonlocalizing chest roentgenogram. Chest 92:70–75, 1988.
13. Santiago S, Lehrman S, Williams AJ: Bronchoscopy in patients with haemoptysis and normal chest roentgenograms. Br J Dis Chest 81:186–188, 1987.
14. Santiago S, Tobias J, Williams AJ: A reappraisal of the causes of hemoptysis. Arch Intern Med 151:2449–2451, 1991.
15. Set PA, Flower CD, Smith IE, et al: Hemoptysis: Comparative study of the role of CT and fiberoptic bronchoscopy. Radiology 189:677–680, 1993.
16. Weaver LJ, Solliday N, Cugell DW: Selection of patients with hemoptysis for fiberoptic bronchoscopy. Chest 76:7–10, 1979 [see also editorial, 1–2].

86. COUGH AND SPUTUM PRODUCTION

Carlos E. Girod, M.D., and Michael E. Hanley, M.D.

1. What are the components of the cough reflex?

The cough reflex protects the lung from injury and infection by clearing large bronchial airways of foreign material or accumulated secretions. The cough reflex requires interaction of three components: sensory nerves, the cough center in the central nervous system, and motor nerves. The sensory component of the cough reflex includes cough receptors located not only in the respiratory system but also in extrapulmonary sites, including the pleura, ear canal, nose, paranasal sinuses, stomach, pericardium, and diaphragm.

2. What pathophysiologic stimuli contribute to cough?

Activation of the cough reflex occurs through inflammatory, mechanical, chemical, and thermal stimuli. Inflammation of the pharynx, upper airway, trachea, and bronchi activates the cough reflex by exposing superficial sensory nerves that are abundant throughout the epithelium of the respiratory system. Mechanical stimuli, such as foreign objects, impacted mucopurulent material, postnasal drip, and airway manipulation, activate the cough reflex through stimulation of myelinated or nonmyelinated sensory nerves in the larynx or the rapidly adapting stretch receptors in the lung. Examples of chemical stimuli that may activate the cough reflex include gastric acid from gastroesophageal reflux, chlorine gas, and other irritant reducing or oxidizing agents. Thermal stimuli (cold or hot air exposure) promote cough in patients with underlying reactive airway disease.

3. What are the four most common causes of chronic cough?

Cough is the fifth most common chief complaint encountered by office-based physicians. The prevalence of chronic cough in nonsmoking adults ranges from 14–23%. Chronic cough is defined as troublesome cough that lasts more than 3 weeks. More than 90% of patients with chronic cough have one or more of the following etiologies: postnasal drip, 41%; occult asthma, 24%; gastroesophageal reflux, 21%; and chronic bronchitis, 5%. A large percentage of patients have a nonpulmonary disorder as the main cause of cough. In most cases, therefore, the diagnosis of chronic cough can be made without referral to a pulmonologist.

4. What are the less common causes of chronic cough?

Less common causes of chronic cough include postviral cough, bronchiectasis, bronchogenic carcinoma, left ventricular failure, sarcoidosis, esophageal diverticuli, tuberculosis, and use of angiotensin-converting enzyme (ACE) inhibitors. Most of these conditions can be diagnosed by careful history, physical exam, and chest roentgenogram. Nevertheless, some authors report that even after extensive work-up for chronic cough 12% of patients remain undiagnosed.

Rare causes of chronic cough, such as vocal cord dysfunction, laryngeal polyps, foreign body aspiration, bronchostenosis, or broncholithiasis, may require invasive, specialized procedures for diagnosis (direct laryngoscopy or fiberoptic bronchoscopy). On the other hand, chronic cough may be due to a trivial diagnosis such as loose hair in the external ear canal that impinges on the tympanic membrane and stimulates cough receptors located in the auditory canal mucosa.

5. What drugs may be associated with chronic cough?

The awareness that certain drugs may promote cough has increased. Beta blockers were once the most common medications associated with chronic cough, especially in patients with underlying or previously asymptomatic bronchial hyperreactivity. The mechanism is bronchoconstriction through direct blockade of beta-2 receptors in the airways.

More recently, a new class of widely used drugs with vasodilator and antihypertensive effects—the ACE inhibitors—have been associated with a high incidence (5–25%) of chronic cough. ACE inhibitor-induced cough may occur as early as 3 weeks or as late as 1 year after start of therapy. The pathophysiologic mechanism is believed to be the accumulation of prostaglandins, kinins, and/or substance P, which directly or indirectly excites cough receptors that initiate the cough reflex. The diagnosis can be eliminated or confirmed with a short 4-day trial of withdrawal of the medication and careful observation for resolution or improvement of cough. Therapy consists of removal of the offending medication. Attempts to treat ACE inhibitor cough with the addition of nonsteroidal inflammatory agents or change to another ACE inhibitor are not recommended.

6. What is psychogenic cough?

Psychogenic cough is a rare condition in which chronic cough is believed to be consciously or unconsciously mediated by the patient. It is usually seen in children or adolescents during periods of high emotional stress. Psychogenic cough is a diagnosis of exclusion. Clues to the diagnosis include complete absence of cough during sleep and ability to reproduce the cough pattern at the examiner's request. In most cases, psychogenic cough is self-limited and resolves in a few months. A unique therapeutic technique involves placement of a chest harness or folded bedsheet around the chest with a large knot over the sternum and negative reinforcement through sharp commands to stop coughing. This technique was successful in 31 of 33 pediatric patients.

7. What are the roles of sinus radiographs, pulmonary function tests, and other laboratory evaluations in the diagnosis of chronic cough?

The most helpful part of the evaluation of patients with chronic cough are the history and physical examination. In a recent study of 102 patients, Irwin et al. delineated the clinical usefulness of the following tools in the diagnosis of chronic cough:

1. History	70%	5. Upper GI series	21%
2. Physical exam	49%	6. Esophageal pH monitoring	16%
3. Pulmonary function tests	26%	7. Sinus radiographs	15%
4. Methacholine inhalation challenge	23%	8. Chest radiograph	7%
		9. Bronchoscopy	4%

Sinus radiographs, pulmonary function tests, methacholine inhalational challenge, upper GI series, and ambulatory pH monitoring are helpful only if the initial history and physical examination suggest sinus disease, occult asthma, or gastroesophageal reflux, respectively. A useful diagnostic protocol, called the anatomic diagnostic protocol, for the evaluation of chronic cough is based on this strategy:

1. All patients must receive a careful history and physical examination focused on the anatomic location of cough receptors. Chest radiograph is recommended for all patients.

2. In smokers and patients with occupational or environmental exposures, initial steps include elimination of the irritant and observation, with no further diagnostic studies for at least 4 weeks.

3. Other imaging studies and pulmonary physiologic evaluation depend on the suspected cause after initial evaluation by history, physical examination, and chest radiograph. For example, if postnasal drip and chronic sinus disease are suspected, sinus roentgenogram and allergy evaluation should be ordered first. If occult asthma is suspected, pulmonary function tests and methacholine inhalation challenge are recommended. If no cause is suggested by the history and physical examination, the next appropriate step is pulmonary function testing before and after administration of a bronchodilator or methacholine.

4. If the above strategy suggests no cause, tests for the evaluation of gastroesophageal reflux are recommended, including esophagogram and, if available, ambulatory pH monitoring, even in the absence of symptoms. If these studies are negative, bronchoscopy and/or cardiac function imaging studies are recommended.

5. If one or more possibilities are discovered, specific therapy should be initiated to pinpoint the exact cause of the cough.

8. How does a history of excessive sputum production help in the evaluation of chronic cough?

Previously, it was believed that chronic cough accompanied by excessive sputum production indicated a primary pulmonary condition such as chronic bronchitis, emphysema, bronchiectasis, and cystic fibrosis. A recent prospective study reported by Smyrnios, et al. (1995), however, clearly demonstrated that this is not the case. The most common cause of chronic cough with excessive sputum production continued to be postnasal drip syndrome (PNDS) in 40% of patients. Other common causes paralleled those seen in patients with no sputum production and chronic cough: asthma, 24%; gastroesophageal reflux disease, 15%; bronchitis, 11%; bronchiectasis, 4%; left ventricular failure, 3%; and miscellaneous causes, 3%. Therefore, the diagnosis should proceed as for all patients with cough. However, the evaluation may be more extensive and require longer to reach a specific diagnosis in patients with excessive sputum production.

9. When does a cough that follows an upper respiratory tract illness warrant evaluation?

Viral infections of the upper respiratory tract may promote or activate the cough reflex by injuring the airway epithelium and exposing sensory nerves that represent the afferent loop of the cough reflex. Approximately 77% of patients affected by a viral upper or lower respiratory tract infection have a cough that lasts up to 3 weeks. In such patients, bronchial hyperactivity, as demonstrated with inhalational challenge, persists for up to 7 weeks after viral infection. In a significant number of patients, chronic cough may last longer than 8 weeks from the onset of viral infection. Therefore, full evaluation for chronic cough after viral upper and lower respiratory infection is not recommended unless the cough lasts longer than 8 weeks or is significantly troublesome to the patient. Persistent cough after upper respiratory tract illness is best treated by a short course of corticosteroid and/or inhaled ipratropium bromide.

10. When does a cough in a cigarette smoker require evaluation?

The evaluation of chronic cough in smokers may lead to multiple unnecessary and expensive diagnostic procedures. Useful guidelines for full evaluation of chronic cough in a smoker include (1) change in or development of sputum production, (2) increase in frequency of cough, (3) hemoptysis, or (4) constitutional symptoms, such as weight loss and fatigue. Evaluation should focus on exclusion of lung cancer, emphysema, and chronic bronchitis. The physician also must use this opportunity to reinforce the need for smoking cessation.

Evaluation should follow the diagnostic protocol described in question 7, focusing on history, physical exam, and chest radiograph. If the results are negative, no other diagnostic tests are recommended before complete cessation of smoking. If cough persists after 4 weeks of smoking cessation, fiberoptic bronchoscopy should be considered.

11. What complications are associated with cough?
1. Musculoskeletal: torn chest muscle, rib fractures
2. Pulmonary: pneumothorax, pneumomediastinum
3. Psychological: self-consciousness, fear of public appearances
4. Cardiovascular: syncope or near syncope
5. Neurologic: cough headache
6. Genitourinary: urinary incontinence
7. Constitutional: fatigue, poor appetite, weight loss
8. Miscellaneous: wound dehiscence, hoarseness

12. When and how should chronic cough be treated empirically?

The anatomic diagnostic protocol delineated by Irwin et al. (question 7) leads to a specific diagnosis and treatment for chronic cough in more than 90% of patients. Failure of specific therapy is likely due to incorrect diagnosis or undertreatment. Therefore, empirical therapy for chronic cough is seldom necessary.

When complications are serious or diagnostic tests are not available, chronic cough should be treated in the absence of a diagnosis. However, the cough reflex should not be suppressed if it benefits the patient by clearing the airway of purulent secretions. When empirical therapy is indicated, the most studied and efficacious nonspecific antitussives should be used: narcotics (codeine or codeine-derived cough suspensions), nonnarcotics (most commonly dextromethorphan), and inhaled ipratropium bromide.

Certain clinical scenarios of chronic cough also merit empirical therapy. In some patients diagnosis of gastroesophageal reflux may require 24-hour ambulatory pH monitoring, which is not readily available in most medical centers. Ing et al. performed 24-hour ambulatory pH monitoring on 13 patients with chronic cough of unclear etiology. The majority had reflux episodes associated with onset of cough, and 11 of 13 patients responded to at least 2 weeks of therapy with histamine blockers. Therefore, in patients suspected of having gastroesophageal reflux, empirical therapy with histamine blockers and antireflux techniques should be instituted with careful observation of changes in the cough pattern.

Because of the high incidence of chronic cough due to occult asthma, many authors recommend a short course of oral corticosteroids for chronic cough with no obvious cause. Empirical steroids also may be helpful in treating postviral cough by relieving the associated airway inflammation and reactivity.

13. What is the role of mucolytic therapy in the management of chronic cough and sputum production?

Conditions associated with chronic cough and accompanied by sputum production include emphysema, chronic bronchitis, bronchiectasis, cystic fibrosis, and diseases of the large airways. Although its benefits have not been well documented, mucolytic therapy frequently is used in such clinical settings. Most common mucolytic agents work by thinning hyperviscous mucus. Examples include nebulized water and hypertonic electrolyte solutions, iodides and organic iodine compounds, guaifenesin, ipecacuanha, bromhexine, N-acetyl cysteine (Mucomyst), and proteolytic enzymes. Clinical studies have shown that many of these agents have no benefit in the treatment of chronic sputum-producing conditions, and most must be given at high, nauseating doses to achieve mucolytic action. Nevertheless, mucolytic agents may be helpful in short-course treatment of acute viral respiratory infections and in acute exacerbations of chronic sputum disorders.

CONTROVERSY

14. Is fiberoptic bronchoscopy of value in the evaluation of chronic cough?

In the early 1970s, chronic, severe, unexplained cough was an indication for fiberoptic bronchoscopy. Most of the controversy surrounding bronchoscopy for chronic cough is due to this uncorroborated indication, which was based on anecdotal reports of high yields of endobronchial abnormalities or carcinoma. In the 1980s and 1990s, many careful studies of patients with chronic cough demonstrated that bronchoscopy in a patient with a normal chest radiograph results in a low yield (approximately 4%) of diagnoses. Irwin et al. performed fiberoptic bronchoscopy in 51 of 109 patients with chronic cough and made a diagnosis of occult bronchogenic carcinoma in only one. Fiberoptic bronchoscopy is recommended if the chest roentgenogram is abnormal, but it should not be included routinely in the evaluation of chronic cough.

On the other hand, Sen and Walsh performed bronchoscopy in 25 patients with undiagnosed chronic cough despite careful examination, chest radiograph, and trial of empirical therapy. Fifty percent of the patients were older (> 50 years) smokers with extensive prior work-up for cough. In approximately one-fourth, bronchoscopy yielded a diagnosis of broncholithiasis, tracheobronchopathia, tuberculous bronchostenosis, laryngeal dyskinesis, or laryngeal polyps. The authors recommend bronchoscopy in selected older patients with undiagnosed cough that lasts more than 2 months and is refractory to empirical therapy.

15. Can the history obtained from patients delineating the character, timing, quality, and complications of chronic cough determine its cause?

For: The medical literature has many examples of features of the history that suggest the etiology of chronic cough: paroxysms of cough suggest asthma; cough in supine position or sleep, gastroesophageal reflux; sputum production, chronic bronchitis or bronchiectasis; and a loud "brassy" cough, large airway diseases.

Against: A recent prospective study conducted by Mello et al. (1996) demonstrated only two statistically significant correlates: (1) "wet" or productive cough was associated with bronchiectasis, and (2) "barking" or paroxysmal cough negatively correlated with asthma. Other historical features did not correlate with a specific etiology for chronic cough.

BIBLIOGRAPHY

1. Cohlan S, Stone SM: The cough and the bed sheet. Pediatrics 74:11–15, 1984.
2. Fuller RW, Jackson DM: Physiology and treatment of cough. Thorax 45:425–430, 1990.
3. Ing AJ, Mgu MC, Breslin ABX: Chronic persistent cough and clearance of esophageal acid. Chest 102:1668–1671, 1992.
4. Irwin RS, Curley FJ, Pratter MR: The effects of drugs on cough. Eur J Respir Dis 71(Suppl 153):173–181, 1987.
5. Irwin RS, Zawacki JK, Curley FJ, et al: Chronic cough as the sole presenting manifestation of gastroesophageal reflux. Am Rev Respir Dis 140:1294–1300, 1989.
6. Irwin RS, Curley FJ, French CL: Chronic cough: The spectrum and frequency of causes, key components of the diagnostic evaluation, and outcome of specific therapy. Am Rev Respir Dis 141:640–647, 1990.
7. Irwin RS, Curley FJ: The treatment of chronic cough: A comprehensive review. Chest 99:1477–1484, 1991.
8. Israili ZH, Hall WD: Cough and angioneurotic edema associated with angiotensin-converting enzyme inhibitor therapy: A review of the literature and pathophysiology. Ann Intern Med 178:234–242, 1992.
9. Mello CJ, Irwin RS, Curley FJ: Predictive values of the character, timing, and complications of chronic cough in diagnosing its cause. Arch Intern Med 156:997–1003, 1996.
10. O'Connell EJ, Rojas AR, Sachs MI: Cough-type asthma: A review. Ann Allergy 66:278–282, 1991.
11. Poe RH, Israel RH, Utell MJ, Hall WJ: Chronic cough: Bronchoscopy or pulmonary function testing? Am Rev Respir Dis 126:160–162, 1982.
12. Poe RH, Harder RV, Israel RH, Kallay MC: Chronic persistent cough: Experience in diagnosis and outcome using an anatomic diagnostic protocol. Chest 95:728–732, 1989.
13. Sen RP, Walsh TE: Fiberoptic bronchoscopy for refractory cough. Chest 99:33–35, 1991.
14. Smyrnios NA, Irwin RS, Curley FJ: Chronic cough with a history of excessive sputum production. Chest 108:991–997, 1995.
15. Widdicombe JG: Mechanisms of cough and its regulation. Eur J Respir Dis 153(Suppl):173–181, 1987.
16. Zanjanian MH: Expectorants and antitussive agents: Are they helpful? Ann Allergy 44:290–295, 1980.

87. UPPER RESPIRATORY TRACT INFECTIONS AND SINUSITIS

Gayle S. Cekada, M.D., and Thomas R. Vendegna, M.D.

1. What is an upper respiratory tract infection?

Upper respiratory tract infections (URI) consist of the common cold, pharyngitis, otitis, and sinusitis. These illnesses are the most common human diseases; an average adult acquires 1–4 infections per year. In addition to their morbidity, they account for more than 5 billion dollars spent per year in the United States, a tremendous economic cost.

2. Why are colds so common?

The common cold consists of six different viral families, each with a different serotype: rhinovirus, coronavirus, respiratory syncytial virus, adenovirus, parainfluenza virus, and influenza virus. Rhinovirus, the most common (30–40%), has 100 different serotypes, and adenovirus (10–15% of cases) has 47 serotypes. Therefore, one person can have one cold per year without exhausting the different strains. Furthermore, because most people have an incomplete or short period of immunity against an individual strain, reinfection is possible.

3. Who is at risk for a common cold? What is the pathogenesis of the infection?

Despite everything mothers and fathers say, cold temperatures and dampness do not contribute to cold acquisition or severity. A study performed 40 years ago divided volunteers in three groups: chilled and wearing wet socks, chilled alone, and normal. Within each group of volunteers one-half received direct nasal inoculation. All groups with direct inoculation had an equal rate of cold acquisition and severity; the rest were not susceptible. Several studies have looked at psychological stress and cold acquisition and severity; more recent data indicate a positive correlation. Cigarette smokers experience the same incidence of infections but have a more severe course.

Analysis of nasal biopsies reveal minimal epithelial damage and inflammation. It has been suggested that viral particles promote the release of inflammatory cytokines that create vascular leak and systemic symptoms. Recent studies have confirmed the elevation of interleukin-1 (IL-1), kinins, IL-6, and IL-8 in nasal lavage of volunteers after nasal inoculation. Studies are underway to see whether cold symptoms and severity decrease with cytokine blockade.

4. How do we catch a cold?

Viral shedding occurs predominantly in the first 3 days of symptoms. The viral families that produce the common cold are hardy and may remain infectious for up to 3 hours after drying on hard surfaces. In one study, subjects became infected after a 10-second handshake with someone with a known URI. Consequently, infection from hand-to-hand contact is effective and probably the most common form of transmission. Infection from aerosolized large particles produced during coughing and sneezing is less effective at transmission and requires prolonged exposure (up to hours). Kissing is also an ineffective means of transmission; a recent study demonstrated an 8% infection rate. The viral particles most commonly cause infection from hand-to-nose or hand-to-eye contact.

5. What are the clinical features of a cold?

The diagnosis of a cold is not difficult. In order of occurrence, symptoms include nasal discharge, sneezing, sore throat, headaches, cough, myalgias, and low-grade temperatures. Symptoms tend to peak in 3 days and often last for 1 week. Colds are known precipitants of asthma (especially in children) and chronic obstructive pulmonary disease (COPD) and may lead to a secondary otitis, sinusitis, bronchitis, and pneumonia.

6. What is the effect of vitamin C on the common cold?

Multiple studies have demonstrated no prophylactic effect of vitamin C against the common cold. Vitamin C may decrease the duration of symptoms, but these studies may be flawed by the lack of objective measures. Beneficial effects are believed to be secondary to its antioxidant properties. Vitamin C is safe, but most people experience diarrhea at doses of 4–10 gm per day.

7. Is zinc the cure for the common cold?

Enthusiasm for zinc centered on a recent trial by Mossad et al., which demonstrated a decrease in cold symptoms from 7.6 days in controls compared with 4.4 days in subjects treated with 13.3-mg lozenges every 2 hours. Subjects were enrolled within 24 hours of symptom onset. Zinc-treated patients reported a higher frequency of bad taste, mouth irritation, and nausea. In addition, the doses taken are far in excess of the daily recommended allowance of 15 mg. Although zinc may decrease the duration of symptoms, further studies are needed to establish its safety.

8. What is the treatment for the common cold?

Multiple modes of therapy exist to treat the common cold, including many home remedies. Other than the above study with zinc lozenges, no study demonstrates a decrease in duration of symptoms. First-generation antihistamines, decongestants (pseudoephedrine hydrochloride), aspirin, nonsteroidal antiinflammatory agents, acetaminophen, nasal ipratropium bromide, and nasal sodium cromoglycate have been shown to decrease symptom severity. Unfortunately, physicians often prescribe antibiotics (no proven efficacy) for colds at a cost of $37.5 million dollars per year. There is no recommended therapy for the common cold, but the above agents may improve symptoms. Patients should be educated about modes of transmission, including recommendations for good handwashing and avoidance of shared glassware or dishware.

9. How often do common cold viruses involve the sinuses?

Recent studies have confirmed that the common cold can involve the sinuses in 87% of cases. Therefore, the common cold should be thought of as viral rhinosinusitis and not simply as rhinitis. Traditionally, sinusitis was thought of as a bacterial infection, but a more accurate spectrum should include both viral and bacterial etiologies.

10. What is sinusitis?

This simple question lacks a focused definition; thus, a diagnosis of sinusitis is made primarily on clinical terms. As stated above, most common colds involve the sinuses, and cold symptoms predominate. Symptoms specific to the sinuses include cough, purulent discharge, facial pain, fever, headaches, and teeth pain. Imaging studies are sensitive in detecting abnormalities, especially CT scans of the sinuses, but they lack specificity (sinus thickening is seen in 90% of patients with a cold) and are not routinely recommended. Because the sinuses are normally sterile, sinus aspiration culture is the gold standard for detecting bacterial sinusitis but is rarely needed in the proper clinical setting.

11. What are the proper clinical settings for sinusitis?

Sinusitis presents in three clinical scenarios. The most common is after a common cold when symptoms of colored nasal discharge, facial pressure, and cough precede 8–10 days of rhinitis. The common cold leads to acute bacterial sinusitis in 2% of patients, presumably as a result of sinus obstruction and secondary bacterial contamination (possibly created by obstruction). In fact, proponents of antihistamines and decongestants speculate that these agents decrease sneezing, which may seed the sinuses; however, studies have yet to demonstrate prospectively that these agents decrease the incidence of secondary bacterial sinusitis.

A less common cause of sinusitis is acute bacterial sinusitis without a prior viral syndrome. This form may follow dental infection or occur in patients predisposed to sinus obstruction. Finally, contiguous spread from meningitis, brain abscess, or orbital cellulitis may lead to sinusitis, but these etiologies are less common.

12. What conditions predispose to sinusitis?

Anatomic conditions such as septal deviation, osteomeatal occlusion, and polyposis (often allergic) are the most frequent conditions associated with sinusitis. Smoking interferes with ciliary function and sinus clearance, and seasonal allergies may cause polyposis or ciliary disruption, which may predispose to sinusitis. Finally, certain diseases often lead to sinusitis, including HIV infection, cystic fibrosis, primary ciliary dyskinesia, and IgG deficiencies.

13. What are the most common organisms in bacterial sinusitis?

Approximately 60% of patients yield bacteria on sinus aspirate in the proper clinical setting. The organisms most commonly cultured include *Staphylococcus pneumoniae*, *Haemophilus influenzae*, *Morexella catarrhalis*, and anaerobes.

14. How should sinusitis be treated?

An agent active against the above spectrum of bacteria is the most effective. Recommendations include an oral second-generation cephalosporin (such as cefuroxime) and amoxicillin/clavulanate. The course should be 10–14 days or 7 days beyond improvement in symptoms.

Nasal swabs should not be used to guide therapy because they lack sensitivity and specificity. Additional agents such as antihistamines, decongestants, anticholinergics, and analgesics may relieve symptoms but are not proved to shorten the course of disease. If chronic symptoms develop, a prolonged course of antibiotics may be necessary with a focus on anaerobes. In addition, predisposing factors should be investigated, such as mechanical obstruction; if any is found, referral to an ear, nose, and throat specialist is recommended.

15. What are the complications of sinusitis? When should they be investigated?

Serious complications include subperiosteal abscess, orbital cellulitis, meningitis, and cavernous vein thrombosis. These complications occur more commonly when the frontal, ethmoid, and sphenoid sinuses are infected. Warning symptoms include fever, eye pain, orbital erythema, and conjunctival injection. CT scans are recommended if complications are suspected.

16. When should fungal causes of sinusitis be considered?

Immunocompromised patients and patients with diabetes mellitus are at risk for fungal infections of the sinus, which may cause rapid invasion.

BIBLIOGRAPHY

1. Aberg N, Aberg B, Alestig K: The effect of inhaled and intranasal sodium cromoglycate on symptoms of upper respiratory tract infections. Clin Exper Allergy 26:1045–1050, 1996.
2. Brook I: Microbiology and management of sinusitis. J Otolaryngol 25:249–256, 1996.
3. Carrol K, Reimer L: Microbiology and laboratory diagnosis of upper respiratory tract infections. Clin Infect Dis 23:442–448, 1996.
4. Chester AC: Chronic sinusitis. Am Fam Physician 53:877–887, 1996.
5. Gwaltney JM: Acute community-acquired sinusitis. Clin Infect Dis 23:1209–1225, 1996.
6. Hayden FG, Diamond L, Wood PB, et al: Effectiveness and safety of intranasal ipratropium bromide in common colds. Ann Intern Med 125:89–97, 1996.
7. Herr RD: Acute sinusitis: Diagnosis and treatment update. Am Fam Physician 44:2055–2062, 1991.
8. Lukes D, Anderson MR: Antihistamines and the common cold. J Gen Intern Med 11:240–244, 1996.
9. Lorber B: The common cold. J Gen Intern Med 11:229–236, 1996.
10. Mainous AG, Hueston WJ, Clark JR: Antibiotics and upper respiratory infection. J Fam Pract 42(4):357–361, 1996.
11. Mossad SB, Macknin ML, Medendorp SV, Mason P: Zinc gluconate lozenges for treating the common cold. Ann Intern Med 125:81–88, 1996.
12. Smith MBH, Feldman W: Over-the-counter cold medications: A critical review of clinical trials between 1950–1991. JAMA 269:2258–2263, 1993.

88. ASTHMA AND CHRONIC OBSTRUCTIVE PULMONARY DISEASE

Michael E. Hanley, M.D., and Jerry A. Nick, M.D.

1. What are the important historical considerations in asthma?

Asthma is usually easy to diagnose by its periodicity and characteristic symptoms. Chest tightness, breathlessness, and wheezing are reported most commonly. In some patients, especially children and adolescents, cough may be the only symptom. Once the diagnosis is made, emphasis should turn to identification of triggers that may be avoidable or treatable. A personal or family history of atopy, with symptoms triggered by inhalation of readily identifiable allergens, is common. Exercise, cold air, and inhaled irritants or fumes are other common triggers. Esophageal reflux and chronic sinusitis may worsen asthma; a history of such disorders should be pursued aggressively.

Some patients may have poor control because of concomitant use of beta blockers or nonsteroidal drugs. Others may experience symptoms after exposure to metabisulfite in wines and salad bars. If the patient works in a high-risk occupation or reports improvement in symptoms during holidays and weekends, occupational asthma should be suspected.

2. Is there a difference in the pathophysiology of intrinsic and extrinsic asthma?

No. Asthma is an inflammatory disease of the airways characterized by reversible airflow limitation. The pattern of inflammation is similar in allergic (extrinsic) and nonallergic (intrinsic) asthma. The airways are infiltrated with eosinophils and lymphocytes. Release of inflammatory mediators results in airway edema, smooth muscle hypertrophy, and mucus secretion. Mast cell activation and histamine release are probably important in the early bronchoconstrictor response to allergens and other stimuli but not critical in the more chronic late-phase inflammatory reaction, which causes bronchial hyperresponsiveness.

3. When is bronchoprovocation testing useful in the diagnosis of asthma?

The pathophysiology of asthma includes both reversible airflow obstruction and airway hyperreactivity. Demonstration of reversible airflow obstruction by spirometry is highly supportive of the diagnosis of asthma. However, many patients have normal spirometry between exacerbations, even though they remain mildly symptomatic. In this setting demonstration of hyperreactive airways by bronchoprovocation testing is highly suggestive of the diagnosis. Testing involves measuring spirometry before and after inhalation of escalating doses of nonspecific irritants (methacholine or histamine). Patients with airway hyperreactivity experience significant declines in spirometry at much lower doses than normal subjects.

4. Is airway hyperreactivity unique to patients with asthma?

No. COPD, respiratory dysfunction following inhalation of smoke or chemical irritants, chronic bronchiectasis, sarcoidosis, and chronic lung disease after an episode of acute respiratory distress syndrome are characterized by airway hyperreactivity. In general, however, asthma is associated with the most severe degrees of airway hyperreactivity.

5. Should patients with asthma undergo inhalation challenge to identify offending allergens?

No. Identification of potential allergens by inhalation challenge may provoke acute, life-threatening bronchospasm. It should be performed only in extreme circumstances in laboratories specially staffed and equipped to handle respiratory emergencies.

6. When may patients benefit from immunotherapy for asthma?

Immunotherapy may have a role in treating extrinsic asthma when the patient's history correlates well with skin-test results, when avoidance of allergens is not possible, or when symptoms are difficult to control with inhaled corticosteroids and bronchodilators. If desensitization therapy is selected, higher doses of antigen and longer duration of treatment probably produce the best results. However, evidence that some asthmatics improve with desensitization therapy is limited.

7. When should occupational asthma be considered?

Occupational asthma is a condition characterized by reversible airflow limitation that results from exposure to certain chemicals and antigens in the workplace. Over 200 substances are known to produce the syndrome. Symptoms usually develop within a few years of steady exposure. The typical patient experiences relief outside the workplace (e.g., over the weekend or during vacations) but relapses on return to work. Frequent peak-flow monitoring throughout the workday and on weekends for 3–4 weeks may be necessary to make the diagnosis, because patients with predominantly late-phase asthmatic reactions do not become symptomatic until hours after exposure, typically when they are at home. Patients with preexisting asthma who experience exacerbations due to nonspecific irritants in the workplace do not qualify for the diagnosis of occupational asthma. Treatment hinges on avoidance of the antigen; continued exposure may translate into progressive disease. If changing jobs is not an option, the use of a respirator and standard asthma therapy must be strongly considered.

8. What are the goals of pharmacotherapy in asthma?

Treatment of asthma depends on its severity. Patients with mild intermittent asthma have infrequent symptoms and rare exacerbations. They can be managed adequately with short-acting inhaled bronchodilators as needed. Mild, moderate, and severe persistent asthma are characterized by escalating severity and frequency of symptoms and exacerbations. The principal goals of pharmacotherapy in such patients is to prevent acute exacerbations by improving airway hyperreactivity and to maintain near-normal daily lung function while avoiding the unwanted effects of polypharmacy. Patients with mild persistent asthma generally can be managed with a single, low-dose antiinflammatory agent (either inhaled corticosteroid or, in children, cromolyn) administered daily; a short-acting inhaled bronchodilator is used on an as-needed basis for breakthrough symptoms. For moderate persistent asthma the dose of daily inhaled corticosteroid is increased. In addition, a long-acting bronchodilator (preferably inhaled) is also prescribed on a daily, regularly scheduled basis. Patients with severe persistent asthma require daily high-dose inhaled corticosteroids and a long-acting bronchodilator administered on a regularly scheduled basis. Patients with severe persistent asthma whose symptoms are not well controlled on this regimen may also need daily oral corticosteroids. However, before beginning therapy with chronic oral corticosteroids, inhaled corticosteroid and long-acting bronchodilator therapy should be maximized, metered dose inhaler (MDI) technique should be evaluated, and a careful search for reversible triggers should be made.

9. What long-acting bronchodilators are available for treatment of asthma?

Sustained-release theophylline, oral sustained-release albuterol, and inhaled salmeterol are long-term bronchodilators. Of these medications, inhaled salmeterol is the agent of choice based on the strength of its bronchodilating effect and low toxicity. Its sustained effect makes it especially valuable in patients with moderate and severe persistent asthma and patients with significant nocturnal symptoms. However, because its onset of action is slow, patients must still be prescribed and educated to use a short-acting inhaled bronchodilator for breakthrough symptoms.

10. What are leukotriene modifiers?

Leukotriene modifiers are new antiinflammatory agents that interrupt the inflammatory cascade by blocking leukotriene receptors or inhibiting the production of leukotrienes. They also have modest bronchodilating effects. Most of the clinical trials evaluating their efficacy in asthma have been conducted in patients with mild-to-moderate persistent asthma. These studies indicate that leukotriene modifiers may be an alternative to low-dose inhaled corticosteroid therapy in mild asthma. Although it is becoming increasing popular to add these drugs as an additional antiinflammatory agent in patients with severe persistent asthma, their efficacy in this setting has not been studied.

11. Is magnesium indicated in the management of status asthmaticus?

Intravenous magnesium sulfate, 1–2 gm administered over 20 minutes, has been advocated as rescue therapy in patients with status asthmaticus. However, multiple large, randomized, placebo-controlled trials have failed to demonstrate any difference in hospitalization rates, duration of emergency department treatment, or changes in peak expiratory flow rates or FEV_1 in magnesium-treated and untreated patients. Thus, routine use of magnesium sulfate is not indicated in the treatment of status asthmaticus.

12. How should patients with asthma be educated?

Patient education is a critical component of management of asthma, especially for patients with moderate-to-severe persistent disease. Education involves helping patients to understand the disease and to practice the skills necessary to manage it. Information should include the pathophysiology of asthma, especially signs and symptoms, and the need to identify and avoid triggers. In addition, the importance of close monitoring of airway function with peak-flow meters and early intervention when attacks begin must be stressed. Finally, patients must be educated about therapeutic approaches, including the mechanism of action of medications, potential side effects with acute and chronic use (including misconceptions), proper use of inhalers, indications for emergency care, and written plans for managing acute exacerbations.

13. Is peak flow monitoring useful in asthma?

Studies have suggested a reduction in the severity of asthma and reduced airflow variability when peak flows are monitored for several months and therapy is adjusted accordingly. Peak flow meters simply measure the maximal rate of expiratory airflow after inspiration to total lung capacity. Because peak flows are highly dependent on personal effort, patients must be well motivated. If effort is good, serial peak flows provide an objective measurement of airway function and are useful in monitoring respiratory trends in moderate and severe asthma. Such monitoring is important because many patients cannot subjectively detect changes in airflow. Optimal benefit from peak flow monitoring requires keeping a diary that records simultaneous symptoms. The patient should record peak flows each morning and evening (before and after use of a bronchodilator) and whenever chest symptoms occur. Normally, some diurnal variation is seen, with morning values lower than evening values. The degree of hyperresponsiveness in asthmatics has been shown to correlate with early morning peak flows, the gap between morning and evening values (normally < 15%), and the amount of improvement in flow rates after bronchodilator use. If a trend toward increased hyperresponsiveness is seen, the dose of inhaled steroid may be augmented. The converse also may be true.

14. When should a patient with asthma be hospitalized?

The decision to hospitalize an asthmatic patient depends on several factors, including the nature and persistence of the inciting stimulus, the severity of prior attacks (history of hospitalizations, intubation, steroid dependence), severity of symptoms, severity of airflow obstruction, medication use at the time of the exacerbation, access to medical care, adequacy of support at home, and psychiatric stability. Indicators of severe obstruction include tachycardia (> 110 bpm), extensive use of accessory muscles of respiration, pulsus paradoxus ≥ 15, and inability to complete a sentence. An initial force expiratory volume in 1 second (FEV_1) < 40% of the predicted value is an ominous sign. Impending arrest is suggested by cyanosis, altered mental status, normal-to-high $PaCO_2$, low pH, exhaustion, bradycardia, or a silent chest. If signs and symptoms do not improve within 20–30 minutes of aggressive beta-adrenergic therapy, the patient should be admitted. If discharge from the emergency department (ED) is considered, improvement in symptoms and spirometry must be significant and sustained with a rise in FEV_1 to at least 40% of the predicted value after 60–90 minutes. With a history of brittle asthma, relapsing course over the previous weeks or months, or prior ED visits during the current exacerbation, the patient should be considered for admission, regardless of the acute response to bronchodilators and steroids.

15. What is the proper way to use an MDI?

After shaking the inhaler, the patient should exhale normally to functional residual capacity (FRC), place the device about 4 cm in front of the mouth, simultaneously depress the canister, and begin a slow inhalation. Inspiration continues to total lung capacity (TLC), at which point the breath is held for at least a few seconds. Inspiration faster than 4–5 seconds causes excessive deposition of particles in the oropharynx and large airways. Breath-holding is also crucial to allow aerosolized particles to settle on the mucosal surface of the targeted small airways. When used properly, MDIs are at least as effective as nebulizers. Spacers decrease the amount of medication lost to the air or deposited in the oropharynx and should be used routinely during severe exacerbations when slow inspiration and prolonged breath-holding are difficult to perform. They also are useful if proper MDI technique cannot be mastered.

16. What is chronic obstructive pulmonary disease (COPD)?

COPD has no precise definition. It is a nonspecific term that refers to conditions generally characterized by cough expectoration, dyspnea, and progressive reduction in expiratory air flow. The term refers to a spectrum of disease that includes asthmatic bronchitis, chronic bronchitis, and emphysema and recognizes that these diseases share a common pathophysiology with varying clinical presentations. Chronic bronchitis is a clinical diagnosis defined as the presence of a productive cough for three or more months in at least 2 consecutive years without a known underlying cause other than cigarette smoking. Histologically, inflammation of the airway mucosa and hypertrophy of submucosal glands occurs as a result of chronic exposure to inhaled irritants. Emphysema is a pathologic diagnosis defined as the irreversible enlargement of airspaces distal to terminal bronchioles with destruction of gas-exchanging surfaces. As alveolar septae are destroyed, radial traction on small airways is lost. This loss of elastic recoil results in hyperinflation, excessive collapse of airways during expiration, and chronic airflow limitation. Cigarette smoking is by far the most important risk factor in the development of COPD, but only 10–15% of smokers develop clinically significant disease.

17. Is it important to differentiate clinically or physiologically between blue bloaters and pink puffers?

Patients with chronic bronchitis, often referred to as "blue bloaters," present with cough and copious sputum production. They are typically overweight and tend to have more upper respiratory infections as well as worse matching of ventilation and perfusion than patients with emphysema. Hypoxemia and hypercapnia are worse, and complications such as cor pulmonale and polycythemia are more prevalent. Because patients with predominant bronchitis are not markedly hyperinflated and have a tendency toward superimposed hypoventilation, dyspnea (which is related to work of breathing) may not be a major complaint.

Patients with predominant emphysema, often referred to as "pink puffers," are typically thin. Lung volumes are considerably elevated due to air trapping, and dyspnea is a major complaint. Pursed lip breathing and use of accessory muscles of respiration are common, and breath sounds are markedly diminished. In contrast to patients with chronic bronchitis, diffusing capacity may be severely reduced, indicating a major disturbance at the alveolar-capillary interface. Ventilation and perfusion deficits are relatively balanced, however, resulting in only mild or moderate hypoxemia. Hypercapnia usually occurs only during acute exacerbations or in end-stage disease. Consequently, the emphysematous patient experiences fewer complications of chronic hypoxia and hypercapnia and generally lives longer but has more disability related to breathlessness.

Although pure examples exist, chronic bronchitis and emphysema typically coexist in varying proportions within the same patients. In the endstage patient, it is particularly difficult to distinguish between the two.

18. What is the National Lung Health Education Program (NLHEP)?

NLHEP is an ambitious new national education program aimed at primary care providers. A major focus of NLHEP is to improve early identification and intervention in COPD and related disorders through reduction of risk factors. This program was motivated in large part by the Lung Health Study, which confirmed that smokers most at risk for developing COPD can be identified before the onset of clinical disease by office spirometry and that smoking cessation in this group successfully altered the natural course of the disease. A critical concept of this project is that pulmonary function in smokers most at risk for developing COPD is characterized by acceleration of the age-related decline in FEV_1/FVC ratio. The Lung Health Study proved that the excessive rate of decline in FEV_1 in this population can be stopped by smoking cessation. The NLHEP encourages primary care providers to perform office spirometry on smoking patients and to redouble efforts at risk reduction (primarily but not exclusively smoking cessation) in patients with evidence of early airflow obstruction. Patients should "test your lungs, know your numbers."

19. What concerns arise in administering oxygen therapy in patients with COPD?

A common worry associated with administering oxygen in patients with COPD is that life-threatening hypercapnia will result from increased dead space ventilation. When oxygen is administered, hypoxic bronchoconstriction is reduced throughout the lung, including areas that are poorly perfused because of destruction of septal capillaries. The result is increased dead-space ventilation, usually accompanied by a modest rise in carbon dioxide tension. In general, however, the increase in dead-space ventilation and $PaCO_2$ is minimal. Indeed, some patients show an increase in minute ventilation as a result of the rising $PaCO_2$. When oxygen therapy is instituted, the flow rate should be titrated gradually upward to maintain a PaO_2 of 60 and oxygen saturation of 90% without overcorrection. Any adjustment should be accompanied by measurement of arterial blood gases. Oxygen must not be withheld from a hypoxic patient because of fear of a rising $PaCO_2$.

20. Are bronchodilators indicated in patients with COPD if spirometry does not improve acutely after their administration?

Unfortunately, many patients with COPD are labeled as nonresponders in the pulmonary testing laboratory when, on one occasion, they fail to show improvement after beta-adrenergic treatment. Although patients with COPD rarely respond to bronchodilators as dramatically as patients with asthma, most have a component of airway hyperreactivity that improves with treatment. Benefit may be indicated over a few weeks of treatment by improvement in FEV_1, decreased hyperinflation (with or without improved flow rates), reduction in dyspnea, or improved exercise tolerance. Additionally, in patients with stable COPD, anticholinergic agents such as ipratropium bromide produce more bronchodilation than conventional doses of beta agonists and do not lose efficacy over time. Anticholinergics are especially useful in patients with chronic bronchitis, because they reduce the volume of sputum without changing its viscosity. However, because maximal benefit is not achieved for 30 minutes or more after use, these agents are less convenient for testing and often are not used in the pulmonary function laboratory.

21. Are corticosteroids effective in patients with chronic, stable COPD?

Although corticosteroid therapy in some form is essential in managing all patients with moderate or severe asthma, it is often ineffective in patients with COPD. A meta-analysis of 43 studies indicated that only 10% of patients with chronic, stable COPD experienced an increase of 20% or more in FEV_1 after being placed on oral corticosteroids. It is difficult to predict who will respond to corticosteroids. A clinical trial is therefore warranted in patients with moderate-to-severe disease after cessation of smoking and institution of maximal bronchodilator therapy. Pulmonary function testing should be performed before and after the trial to assess objectively the effect on airflow limitation. Prednisone, 40 mg/day (or the equivalent) for 4 weeks, is a reasonable trial. If the patient shows significant objective improvement, the dose should be tapered to the lowest effective maintenance level. If no improvement occurs with corticosteroid therapy, it should be discontinued. No definitive evidence supports the use of inhaled corticosteroids in patients with COPD.

22. What can be done to improve quality of life in patients with severe COPD?

Despite cessation of smoking and optimal medical therapy (including oxygen), patients with severe COPD often continue to complain of breathlessness. Patients begin to avoid physical activity because of anticipated dyspnea and their level of conditioning worsens. Some patients reap great benefits from a program of education and rehabilitation that addresses these issues. After screening for heart disease and exercise-induced hypoxia, daily exercise training may be initiated (e.g., stationary bicycle, walking) to build endurance and to increase the patient's ability to perform activities of daily living. Instruction in diaphragmatic and pursed-lip breathing may be of further assistance. Occupational therapists often suggest energy-saving devices and help to plan daily schedules that include rest periods. Furthermore, mental health professionals may play a key role in managing the reactive depression that is common in patients with severe COPD.

23. What is lung volume reduction surgery (LVRS)?

LVRS is an experimental surgical therapy for COPD. It is based on the concept that lungs in patients with COPD anatomically consist of areas of well-preserved lung tissue interspersed with regions with enlarged airspaces (bullae). Bullae contribute to dyspnea through hyperinflation, represent wasted ventilation that does not contribute to gas exchange, and worsen gas exchange further by compressing adjacent areas of normal lung. Goals of LVRS include improvement of symptoms and gas exchange through surgical resection of bullae with decompression of neighboring lung units. Studies evaluating the efficacy of this surgical approach have been hampered by lack of appropriate randomized controls and a potentially significant placebo effect. Although preliminary studies suggest that surgery results in at least a transient improvement in clinical symptoms and spirometry, it is not known whether this effect persists over the long term or translates into improved survival.

CONTROVERSIES

24. Should anticholinergic agents be used with beta agonists in patients with asthma?
   For:
   1. By inhibiting cholinergic tone and dilating the large airways, anticholinergic agents theoretically may improve penetration of beta agonists into the lungs.
   2. Occasionally patients who respond poorly to beta agonists respond well to ipratropium or combination therapy (especially older patients).
   3. Anticholinergics are preferred in the treatment of psychogenic asthma, because they block the parasympathetically mediated bronchospasm triggered by emotional factors.
   Against:
   1. No synergistic effect has been proved.
   2. Combination therapy results in substantially greater cost and inconvenience to the patient.
   3. In most patients, anticholinergic agents are clearly less effective than beta agonists in producing bronchodilation.

25. Are inhaled corticosteroids completely safe?
   For:
   1. Because systemic absorption is slight, hypercortisolism does not occur.
   2. Suppression of the pituitary-adrenal axis has not been reported in adults, even with high doses.
   3. Worsening of diabetes mellitus has not been reported.
   4. Oral candidiasis is a local complication that can be prevented with use of spacers and rinsing/gargling after use.
   Against:
   1. Some studies in children have documented measurable suppression of the pituitary-adrenal axis, possibly related to the higher dose/kg of body weight.
   2. Increased bone turnover (as measured by bone metabolites) occurs with doses that do not suppress cortisol production. It is not known whether this effect will translate into significant osteoporosis after sustained use.
   3. It is not known whether long-term use of inhaled corticosteroids may increase the risk of developing cataracts.
   4. Use may be associated with the development of thrush and dysphonia.

26. Is theophylline beneficial in the management of patients with asthma and COPD?
   For:
   1. Patients with prominent nocturnal symptoms may be greatly helped by 24-hour theophylline preparations given once daily in the early evening.
   2. Theophylline may be used as a steroid-sparing measure in patients with chronic severe asthma.

3. Theoretical benefits include reduced diaphragmatic fatigability, positive inotropy, and improved mucociliary clearance.

4. Theophylline is a central respiratory stimulant and may benefit a subset of patients with COPD who hypoventilate even though their resistive loads are not extreme (i.e., blue bloaters).

5. Some studies suggest improved performance and quality of life not necessarily related to improved spirometry.

Against:

1. During acute exacerbations, no improvement in spirometry or symptoms results when theophylline is added to maximal beta-agonist therapy, but side effects usually increase.

2. Theophylline has a narrow therapeutic window and levels may be affected by many commonly prescribed drugs as well as by smoking.

3. The theoretical benefits are modest at best and of uncertain clinical importance.

27. Are oral beta agonists indicated in patients with asthma?

For:

1. Long-acting preparations are particularly useful for relief of nocturnal asthma.

2. Many small children and some adults cannot be trained to use MDIs effectively.

Against:

1. At doses resulting in equivalent bronchodilation, oral beta agonists have 4 times the incidence of side effects as inhaled agents.

2. For patients who cannot use MDIs properly, spacer devices, nebulizers, and rotacaps are available as an alternative to oral beta agonists.

3. Long-acting inhaled beta agonists, such as salmeterol, are available for the treatment of nocturnal symptoms.

BIBLIOGRAPHY

1. Ahmed T: Preventing bronchoconstriction in exercise-induced asthma with inhaled heparin. N Engl J Med 329:90, 1993.
2. Anthonisen NR, Connett JE, Kiley JP, et al: Effects of smoking intervention and the use of an inhaled anticholinergic bronchodilator on the rate of decline of FEV_1: The Lung Health Study. JAMA 272:1497–1505, 1994.
3. Bousamra M, Haasler GB, Lipchik RJ, et al: Functional and oximetric assessment of patients after lung reduction surgery. J Thorac Cardiovasc Surg 113:675–681, 1997.
4. Braman SS, Corrao WM: Bronchoprovocation testing. Clin Chest Med 10:165, 1989.
5. Chan Yeung M, Lam S: State of the art: Occupational asthma. Am Rev Respir Dis 133:686, 1985.
6. Chapman KR: Therapeutic algorithm for COPD. Am J Med 91:4A–17S, 1991.
7. Clark NM, Evans D, Mellins RB: Patient use of peak flow monitoring. Am Rev Respir Dis 145:722, 1992.
8. Corbridge TC, et al: The assessment and management of adults with status asthmaticus. Am J Respir Crit Care Med 151:1296, 1995.
9. Ferguson GT, Cherniack RM: Management of chronic obstructive pulmonary disease. N Engl J Med 328:1017–1022, 1993.
10. Gross NJ: COPD: Current concepts and therapeutic approaches. Chest 97:19S, 1990.
11. Gross NJ: Leukotriene modifiers: What place in asthma? J Respir Dis 19:245–261, 1998.
12. Groth ML, Hurewitz AN:Diagnosing and managing bronchial asthma. Emerg Med Sept 19, 1992.
13. Guidelines for the Diagnosis and Management of Asthma. Expert Panel Report II. National Institutes of Health Pub no. 97-4051. Bethesda, MD, 1997.
14. Idris AH, et al: Emergency department treatment of severe asthma. Chest 103:665, 1993.
15. Li JT, Reed CE: Proper use of aerosol corticosteroids to control asthma. Mayo Clin Proc 64:205, 1989.
16. Listello D, Glauser F: COPD: Primary care management with drug and oxygen therapies. Geriatrics 47:28, 1992.
17. Make B: COPD: Management and rehabilitation. Am Fam Physician 43:1315, 1991.
18. Middleton E, Reed CE, et al: Allergy: Principles and Practice. St. Louis, Mosby, 1993.
19. Murray JF, Nadel JA: Textbook of Respiratory Medicine. Philadelphia, W.B. Saunders, 1992.
20. National Asthma Education Program: Guidelines for the Diagnosis and Management of Asthma. Bethesda, MD, National Heart, Lung, and Blood Institute, 1991.
21. Petty TL: The National Lung Health Education Program. Chest 113:123S–161S, 1998.

22. Petty TL, Weinmann GG: Building a national strategy for the prevention, management, and research in chronic obstructive pulmonary disease. JAMA 277:246–253, 1997.
23. Ries AL, Kaplan RM, Limberg TM, Prewitt LM: Effects of pulmonary rehabilitation on physiologic and psychosocial outcomes in patients with chronic obstructive pulmonary disease. Ann Intern Med 122:823–832, 1995.
24. Weiss EB, Stein M: Bronchial Asthma, 3rd ed. Boston, Little, Brown, 1993.

89. PULMONARY FUNCTION TESTS

Michael E. Hanley, M.D.

1. When are pulmonary function tests (PFTs) indicated?

The primary purposes of PFTs are diagnostic (to uncover clinically undetected disease and to determine the nature of physiologic dysfunction), quantitative (to determine severity of dysfunction), and monitory (to follow response to therapy or progression of disease). Common indications for pulmonary function testing in the primary care setting include evaluation of patients with unexplained dyspnea, cough, hypoxemia, right-sided congestive heart failure, or abnormal chest roentgenogram suggestive of diffuse lung disease. Pulmonary function tests are particularly useful for chronic monitoring of patients with conditions characterized by infiltrative processes or airflow limitation.

2. Describe the myriad of PFTs.

Simple spirometry, lung volumes, diffusion capacity of the lungs for carbon monoxide (DLCO), flow-volume loops, and arterial blood gases are available in most laboratories. More extensive tests, including pressure-volume curves, airway resistance and conductance, inhalational challenge, exercise testing, ventilatory drive studies, maximum inspiratory and expiratory pressures (PI_{max} and PE_{max}), and polysomnography, are available in specialty laboratories.

3. What constitutes simple spirometry?

Simple spirometry consists primarily of forced vital capacity (FVC), forced expiratory volume in one second (FEV_1), FEV_1/FVC ratio, forced expiratory flow between 25 and 75% of vital capacity ($FEF_{25-75\%}$), and peak expiratory flow rate (PEFR). Simple spirometry also includes measurement of these parameters after bronchodilator treatment. Additional flow rates, such as forced expiratory flow at 25%, 50%, and 75% of vital capacity ($FEF_{25\%}$, $FEF_{50\%}$, and $FEF_{75\%}$) are occasionally reported but do not add significantly to the sensitivity of the other tests.

4. How is simple spirometry interpreted?

The patient's ability to perform the tests must be evaluated first. Abnormal results are occasionally obtained because patients are either unable (because of poor comprehension of instructions, altered mental status, or abnormal oral anatomy that precludes a good spirometer interface) or unwilling to cooperate with testing. Clues to poor patient cooperation include inability to produce consistent results (spirometry is generally measured at least 3–5 times during a test session), the presence of artifacts on flow-volume loops or spirograms, and written comments of the technician performing the tests. Although all parameters measured in simple spirometry depend on patient effort, the FEV_1 and FVC are the most reproducible and therefore offer the most reliable information.

If patient cooperation is good, the next step is to determine if the results are normal. Absolute PFT values obtained in normal subjects are influenced by several factors, including age, height, and sex. Regression equations are used to calculate published predicted normal values for a given patient on the basis of these factors. Other factors, in particular race, also influence predicted normal values but are not routinely considered in published standards. In general, predicted values for patients of African or Asian heritage tend to be 8–13% lower than those for Caucasians, but the optimal correction factors are controversial and not well defined.

Finally, if the results of FEV_1 or FVC are not within the normal range, the pattern of dysfunction should be determined by consideration of the FEV_1/FVC ratio and other flow rates (see questions 5 and 6).

5. Define "obstructive" lung diseases. How are they diagnosed?

Obstructive lung diseases are characterized anatomically and physiologically by obstruction of airflow (airflow limitation). Airflow depends on the lung volume at which it is measured (lower rates occur at smaller lung volumes), resistance of the airways, and pressure that generates flow (driving force determined by elastic recoil of the lung-thoracic cage unit). Common obstructive lung diseases caused primarily by increased airway resistance include asthma, chronic bronchitis, and chronic bronchiectasis; airflow limitation in emphysema is largely secondary to decreased elastic recoil. Because the FEV_1 depends on the rate of airflow more than the FVC, the FEV_1 is generally decreased out of proportion to the FVC in obstructive lung processes. Thus, the FEV_1/FVC ratio is decreased, usually below 0.7.

6. What are restrictive lung diseases?

Restrictive lung diseases are characterized by a reduced total lung capacity (TLC). The differential diagnosis is complex but can be simplified by organizing restrictive disorders into four categories: (1) parenchymal infiltrative disease (interstitial and/or alveolar); (2) chest wall abnormalities; (3) pleural disease; and (4) neuromuscular weakness involving ventilatory muscles.

Restrictive diseases are characterized by decreased lung volumes and, with the exception of neuromuscular weakness, increased elastic recoil of the lung-thoracic cage unit. Thus, although absolute measures of airflow are decreased (because of lower lung volumes), airflow corrected for lung volume is normal or increased. The FEV_1/FVC ratio is therefore normal or increased in patients with restrictive lung disease.

7. Define lung volumes.

Lung volumes measure the absolute volumes of the lungs at various points in the respiratory cycle. Commonly reported volumes include total lung capacity (TLC; volume of gas in the lungs after total inspiration), residual volume (RV; volume of gas in the lungs after total expiration), and function residual capacity (FRC; volume of gas remaining in the lungs at end expiration during tidal volume breathing). When FRC is measured by body plethysmography (body box), it is referred to as thoracic gas volume (TGV).

As with simple spirometry, normal values are influenced by age, height, sex, and race. Thus, results are reported as both absolute values and as a percentage of the predicted normal value.

8. What approach is used in interpreting lung volumes?

Measurement of lung volumes is especially sensitive to patient effort. Of the three commonly measured volumes, FRC (or TGV) is the least effort-dependent and the most reliable; thus it should be considered first. In severe obstructive lung diseases, all three volumes are usually increased, whereas in severe restrictive diseases, they are usually decreased. Demonstration of a decreased TLC and an increased RV (regardless of FRC) suggests poor patient effort (inability or unwillingness to perform maneuver).

9. When are lung volumes indicated?

Simple spirometry differentiates obstruction from restriction in most patients. Similarly, spirometry alone is adequate to monitor most patients' clinical condition and response to therapy over time. Therefore, lung volumes, which add significant expense to PFTs, are seldom required. Lung volumes are indicated (1) to evaluate patients with pulmonary symptoms and normal spirometry; (2) to quantitate more accurately the severity of restriction or obstruction; (3) to evaluate patients with both obstruction and restriction; and (4) to evaluate patients with severe obstruction and a markedly reduced FVC. In patients in the fourth category, lung volumes can clarify whether the decrement in FVC is due to obstruction alone or a coexistent restrictive process.

10. What does DLCO measure?

DLCO measures the diffusion of carbon monoxide (CO) across the alveolar-capillary membrane and is thought to reflect the efficiency of gas exchange. Although the permeability (and therefore thickness) of the membrane affects the value of DLCO, other factors are also important, including the surface area of the membrane (and therefore the lung volume at which it is measured), the hemoglobin (Hb) concentration in blood (Hb binds CO), and matching of ventilation and perfusion. Absolute values for DLCO are usually corrected for some of these factors. Specifically, DLCO-Hb corrects DLCO for hemoglobin concentration, and DLCO/VA corrects for the lung volume at which it is measured.

11. What diseases are associated with an abnormal DLCO?

DLCO is decreased in lung diseases characterized by thickening of the alveolar-capillary membrane (pulmonary infiltrative disorders), destruction of the membrane (emphysema or pulmonary vasculopathies), and mismatching of ventilation and perfusion. Thus, an abnormal DLCO is nonspecific.

Conditions characterized by increased DLCO include congestive heart failure (prolonged capillary blood transit time increases the time for absorption of CO) and significant alveolar or airway hemorrhage.

12. What is the value of screening spirometry in asymptomatic cigarette smokers?

Smokers most at risk to develop COPD experience a long, asymptomatic period characterized by an accelerated loss of pulmonary function. Such patients can be identified by measuring the FEV_1/FVC ratio with office spirometry. Several studies have demonstrated that pulmonary function tests in patients with the most rapid decline in pulmonary function are characterized by an FEV_1/FVC ratio < 70%. Successful intervention during this time interval can return patients to the normal age-related rate of pulmonary function decline before the onset of symptomatic COPD.

13. What is the effect of smoking cessation on pulmonary function in smokers most at risk to develop COPD?

FEV_1 declines at a rate of 70–90 cc/yr in asymptomatic smokers who have an FEV_1/FVC ratio < 70%. The 5-year Lung Health Study demonstrated that the rate of change in FEV_1 returned to the normal age-related rate of 20–30 cc/yr after smoking cessation. In addition, FEV_1 increased significantly during the first 2–3 years after smoking cessation.

14. Should PFTs be obtained in the acutely ill patient?

The timing of PFTs depends on the clinical scenario. Physiologic evaluation during an acute exacerbation of a chronic illness may be valuable to diagnose the cause of previously unexplained dyspnea, hypoxemia, or cough or to monitor response to therapy in exacerbations of chronic obstructive disease. However, if the diagnosis is already known or readily apparent from other clinical data, PFTs in the acutely ill patient add little useful information but considerable unnecessary expense. For comparative purposes it is generally more valuable to determine severity of illness when patients are at baseline function. Return to baseline may require up to 6 weeks of convalescence after an acute exacerbation of obstructive disease. In addition, response to therapy in acutely ill patients is more efficiently and economically accomplished by monitoring PEFR alone.

15. Is the diagnosis of asthma confirmed by demonstration of improved airflow after administration of bronchodilators?

One of the clinical hallmarks of asthma is reversibility of airflow obstruction. Reversibility is indicated by significant improvement in FEV_1 and/or FVC after administration of an inhaled bronchodilator, usually a beta-2 agonist. Significant is defined as an increase > 15–20% with an absolute increase of at least 200 cc in either parameter. However, other obstructive lung diseases, such as chronic bronchitis and emphysema, occasionally demonstrate similar improvement. Furthermore, PFTs in patients with severe asthma may not demonstrate acute reversibility until parenteral corticosteroids have been administered for several months. Thus, the diagnosis of asthma requires thorough consideration of all available clinical, physiologic, radiographic, and pathologic data and not solely the response to bronchodilator therapy.

BIBLIOGRAPHY

1. American College of Physicians: Preoperative pulmonary function testing. Ann Intern Med 112:793–794, 1990.
2. Anthonisen NR, Connett JE, Kiley JP, et al: Effects of smoking intervention and the use of an inhaled anticholinergic bronchodilator on the rate of decline of FEV_1. The Lung Health Study. JAMA 272:1497–1505, 1994.
3. Burrows B, Knudson RJ, Camilli AE, et al: The "horse-racing effect" and predicting decline in forced expiratory volume in one second from screening spirometry. Am Rev Respir Dis 135:788–793, 1987.
4. Clausen JL: Pulmonary Function Testing Guidelines and Controversies. Equipment, Methods, and Normal Values. New York, Academic Press, 1983.
5. Cotton DJ, Soparker GR, Grahan BL: Diffusing capacity in the clinical assessment of chronic airflow limitation. Med Clin North Am 80:549–564, 1996.
6. Crapo RO: Pulmonary-function testing. N Engl J Med 331:25–30, 1994.
7. Enright PL, Lebowitz MD, Cockroft DW: Physiologic measures: Pulmonary function tests. Asthma outcome. Am J Respir Crit Care Med 149:S9–20, 1994.
8. Gardner RM, Hankinson JL, Clausen JL, et al: Standardization of spirometry—1987 update. Am Rev Respir Dis 136:1285–1298, 1987.
9. Petty TL: The predictive value of spirometry. Identifying patients at risk for lung cancer in the primary care setting. Postgrad Med 101:128–140, 1997.
10. Rossiter CE, Weill H: Ethnic differences in lung function: Evidence for proportional differences. Int J Epidemiol 3:55–61, 1974.
11. Screening for adult respiratory disease: Official American Thoracic Society Statement. Am Rev Respir Dis 128:768–774, 1983.
12. Subramanian D, Guntupalli KK: Diagnosing obstructive lung disease. Why is differentiating COPD from asthma important? Postgrad Med 95:69–85, 1994.
13. Wanger J, Irvin CG: Office spirometry: Equipment selection and training of staff in the private practice setting. J Asthma 34:93–104, 1997.

90. HYPOXEMIA AND OXYGEN THERAPY

Michael E. Hanley, M.D., and Jerry A. Nick, M.D.

1. List the five pathophysiologic causes of hypoxemia.

(1) Reduction in inspired partial pressure of oxygen (P_iO_2), (2) hypoventilation, (3) diffusion impairment, (4) ventilation-perfusion (V-Q) mismatch, and (5) shunting.

2. When does decreased inspired PO_2 contribute to hypoxemia?

1. In patients receiving an inadequate fraction of oxygen in inspired gas (FiO_2) on mechanical ventilation.

2. In persons who travel to or live at an altitude at which inspired PO_2 is decreased because of lower barometric pressure.

3. How does hypoventilation cause hypoxemia?

Arterial PO_2 is determined in part by the partial pressure of oxygen in the alveolus (P_AO_2). P_AO_2, in turn, is determined by the total pressure in the alveolus (essentially barometric pressure) and the fraction of alveolar gas that is oxygen. Hypoventilation results in increased alveolar carbon dioxide (CO_2). As alveolar CO_2 increases, the proportion of alveolar gas that is oxygen falls. Therefore P_AO_2 is lower, and hypoxemia develops.

4. Why is isolated diffusion impairment unlikely to cause hypoxemia?

In diseases such as pulmonary fibrosis, an abnormally thickened alveolar-capillary membrane may impair oxygen diffusion. However, blood in the pulmonary capillaries of normal people is in contact with the alveolus approximately 3 times longer than is necessary to reach oxygen equilibrium. Thus, abnormalities in the alveolar-capillary membrane must be quite severe before hypoxemia results from diffusion impairment alone. In addition, diffusion impairment does not occur alone. Parenchymal lung processes that cause diffusion impairment generally are also associated with either V-Q mismatch or shunt.

5. What is the most common cause of hypoxemia?

V-Q mismatch is the most common cause of clinically noted hypoxemia. Optimal gas exchange requires balanced ventilation and perfusion throughout the lung. Blood passing through poorly ventilated areas of the lung is inadequately oxygenated and contributes to hypoxemia. Because of the characteristics of the oxygen dissociation curve, hyperventilation of normal areas of the lung cannot correct the hypoxemia.

6. When does shunt occur?

Shunt occurs when blood crosses the venous to the arterial circulation without receiving ventilation. Anatomic defects such as atrial or ventricular septal defects, patent ductus arteriosus, or arteriovenous malformations result in shunting. More common causes of shunting include atelectasis and airspace-filling disorders, such as pneumonia or pulmonary edema.

7. When should acute hypoxemia be suspected?

Clinically, acute hypoxemia is manifest by abnormal function in some organs and compensatory changes in others. Disturbance of the central nervous system (CNS) is usually the first clinical sign of hypoxemia. Initially, malaise and impairments of short-term memory and judgment are detectable. As hypoxemia worsens, cognitive and motor function become more compromised until eventually the patient loses consciousness. Cardiovascular compensation for mild-to-moderate hypoxemia includes tachycardia and increased stroke volume, but as hypoxemia worsens, rhythm disturbances develop. Hypoxic stimulation of the carotid body results in increased minute ventilation. Severe hypoxemia results in declining renal function and urine output and development of metabolic acidosis due to anaerobic metabolism. Many patients who are hypoxemic appear cyanotic. Cyanosis, a bluish discoloration of the skin and mucous membranes, is present when the concentration of reduced hemoglobin in capillary blood reaches 5 g/100 ml.

8. What are the pitfalls in the observation of cyanosis?

Because the detection of cyanosis is determined by the amount of reduced hemoglobin in capillaries, a severely anemic patient may not appear cyanotic despite significant hypoxemia, because of insufficient hemoglobin. Conversely, a patient with polycythemia may have hemoglobin in excess of oxygen-carrying needs and appear cyanotic despite a normal blood oxygen content. Furthermore, cyanosis may be caused by disorders other than systemic hypoxemia, such as peripheral vasoconstriction (e.g., Raynaud's disease) and methemoglobinemia.

9. What physical signs and laboratory results suggest chronic hypoxemia?

Hypoxemia results in pulmonary vasoconstriction, which, when chronic, causes pulmonary hypertension. Pulmonary hypertension increases right ventricular workload and eventually leads to right heart failure. In addition, chronic hypoxemic states result in elaboration of erythropoietin, which causes polycythemia. A patient with chronic hypoxemia may manifest signs of pulmonary hypertension and right heart failure, depending on the extent and duration of hypoxemia.

Such signs include a right ventricular heave, loud pulmonic component to the second heart sound, right ventricular S3, murmur of tricuspid regurgitation, jugular venous distension, hepato-jugular reflux, and lower extremity edema. Laboratory tests reveal polycythemia. The electrocardiogram shows signs of right ventricular hypertrophy.

10. What is critical hypoxemia?

The first issue that must be addressed in hypoxemic patients is whether the hypoxemia is acute or chronic. Acute and subacute hypoxemia frequently require immediate hospitalization to diagnose and treat the cause. A $PaO_2 < 50$ places the patient at risk for arrhythmias and further decompensation. Hospitalization also should be considered for patients with clinical signs or organ dysfunction, such as tachypnea, tachycardia, or CNS disturbance. Chronic hypoxemia, if severe enough, has long-term detrimental effects but usually does not require urgent intervention.

11. What factors may lead to false analysis of arterial blood gas (ABG) samples?

Air bubbles in the syringe, if greater than 5% of the sample size, may artifactually raise PaO_2 and lower $PaCO_2$ readings toward ambient air values. In addition, if ABGs are not processed promptly, gas may diffuse through plastic syringe walls, altering readings. Lastly, extreme leukocytosis may result in pseudohypoxemia because of oxygen consumption by the white blood cells in the syringe.

12. How is the alveoloarterial oxygen (A-a O_2) gradient calculated? When is it useful?

The A-a O_2 gradient is the difference between the alveolar PO_2 (P_AO_2) and the arterial PO_2 (PaO_2). The arterial PO_2 is measured on routine blood gas analysis, but the alveolar PO_2 must be calculated with the alveolar air equation:

$$P_AO_2 = FiO_2 (P_B - P_{H_2O}) - \frac{PaCO_2}{0.8}$$

where FiO_2 is the proportion of oxygen in inspired air, P_B is barometric pressure, P_{H_2O} is water vapor pressure (47 mmHg), and $PaCO_2$ is the CO_2 tension in arterial blood. A normal A-a O_2 gradient is 5–15 torr. The gradient helps to distinguish hypoxemia due to cardiopulmonary disorders from other causes and to identify patients with significant lung pathology but a "normal" arterial oxygen tension because of hyperventilation.

13. How does the A-a gradient differentiate the various pathophysiologic causes of hypoxemia?

An elevated A-a O_2 gradient reflects an abnormality in gas transfer between alveoli and pulmonary capillaries. The A-a O_2 gradient is normal if hypoventilation or decreased FiO_2 is present. Hypoventilation is distinguished from decreased inspired O_2 by the presence of elevated $PaCO_2$. Most patients with V-Q mismatch, diffusion impairment, or shunt are able to increase minute ventilation sufficiently to normalize $PaCO_2$ in acute or subacute settings. Therefore, as long as an increased minute ventilation is maintained, blood gases reveal hypoxemia with normal or low $PaCO_2$. V-Q mismatch and shunt can be distinguished by assessing the effect of supplemental O_2 on hypoxemia. Increasing the FiO_2 improves hypoxemia if V-Q mismatch is the cause but does not significantly alter hypoxemia caused by shunting.

14. What are the limitations of pulse oximetry?

Oxygen saturation is estimated in pulse oximetry by measuring optical differences between oxidized and reduced hemoglobin. Because it is rapid, noninvasive, and simple to perform, it is commonly used in emergency departments, intensive care units, and office practices as a method of assessing patients for hypoxemia. It is accurate within 3–5% in patients with saturations above 70%. The main limitation of pulse oximetry is that it provides no measure of $PaCO_2$, a value that is critical both diagnostically and therapeutically. For example, an oxygen saturation of 96% is considered normal unless it is associated with a reduced $PaCO_2$, indicating that the patient must hyperventilate to maintain normal saturation. In addition, carboxyhemoglobin, methemoglobin, abnormal acid-base status, poor perfusion, and bright external light may complicate the interpretation of pulse oximetry.

15. How severe must COPD be before hypoxemia results?

In general, there is a poor correlation between the severity of COPD, as determined by spirometry, and alterations in blood oxygen tension. Patients with severely reduced FEV_1 may maintain normal oxygen tension, whereas others with less severe airflow limitation may be hypoxic. This poor correlation is due to two factors:

1. Although the primary mechanism of hypoxemia in patients with COPD is V-Q mismatch, alterations in airflow as measured by spirometry do not necessarily parallel alterations in V-Q balance. Emphysema and chronic bronchitis, which contribute to airflow limitation to varying degrees, do not result in equivalent degrees of V-Q mismatching. Thus, a patient whose obstruction is primarily emphysematous may not have as severe a V-Q disturbance as a patient with equal obstruction due primarily to chronic bronchitis.

2. Individual patients have varying abilities to compensate for hypoxemia related to pulmonary parenchymal abnormalities by recruiting minute ventilation or cardiac output.

16. When is oxygen therapy indicated?

Supplemental oxygen is used for treatment of tissue hypoxia. Clinical scenarios characterized by presumed tissue hypoxia include acute myocardial infarction, acute anemia, carboxyhemoglobinemia, methemoglobinemia, conditions in which oxygen transport is compromised, and hypoxemia with a $PaO_2 < 60$ mmHg or arterial O_2 saturation $< 90\%$. In chronic settings, long-term oxygen therapy should be initiated if a clinically stable patient on an optimal medical regimen demonstrates a $PaO_2 \leq 55$ mmHg or a $PaO_2 \leq 59$ mmHg in the presence of cor pulmonale or polycythemia. Many authorities also recommend supplemental oxygen therapy for patients who are not hypoxemic at rest but desaturate with exertion or during sleep.

17. What three questions must be answered in patients considered for long-term oxygen therapy?

1. Will the patient benefit from home oxygen therapy?
2. What delivery system is best for the patient?
3. What oxygen flow rate is required at rest, with sleep, and during exertion?

18. What are the advantages and disadvantages of different home oxygen supply and delivery systems?

Home oxygen supply systems include bulk supplies stored as either liquid oxygen or compressed gas and oxygen concentrators. Oxygen concentrators extract oxygen from ambient air. They require less frequent servicing (there is no tank that needs to be refilled) but are more expensive, not readily portable within the home, and require a dependable electrical source. Oxygen concentrators are most appropriate for patients requiring only nocturnal oxygen or sedentary patients on lower oxygen flow rates. Most home oxygen is supplied as liquid oxygen. Liquid oxygen reservoirs have three times the capacity as compressed gas tanks and require less frequent refilling. Liquid oxygen reservoirs are also more portable (the reservoirs have wheels that allow them to be moved easily around the home environment), easier to use to fill portable tanks, and less bulky. However, liquid oxygen is more expensive than compressed gas oxygen.

Oxygen is delivered by either face mask or nasal cannula. Face masks are used primarily in patients requiring a very specific fraction of inspired oxygen or extremely high fractions of inspired oxygen. Masks are uncomfortable and poorly tolerated, limiting their long-term application. Most patients receive home supplemental oxygen via a nasal cannula.

19. What are oxygen-conserving devices?

Most long-term home oxygen therapy is delivered as continuous-flow oxygen. This type of delivery is inefficient because oxygen continues to flow throughout the respiratory cycle. Oxygen that flows during expiration is wasted. Oxygen-conserving devices limit the flow of oxygen to inspiration. They consist of pulsed inspiratory flow monitoring devices and reservoir systems. Pulsed inspiratory metering systems sense each breath and limit flow only to inspiration.

Reservoir systems pool oxygen in a reservoir near the nose that fills during expiration and empties during inspiration. The advantage of these systems is that adequate oxygen saturation can be achieved at lower flow rates, resulting in less frequent servicing of stationary equipment and increased longevity of portable systems.

20. Should all patients with chronic obstructive pulmonary disease (COPD) who are newly diagnosed with hypoxemia be placed on chronic supplemental oxygen?

As many as 50% of patients with COPD who are hypoxic but not on medical therapy are no longer hypoxic once proper therapy is established. Therefore, only patients who are clinically stable and receiving appropriate medical therapy should be considered for supplemental oxygen. Such patients should be placed on long-term supplemental oxygen if the criteria listed in question 16 are met. Chronic supplemental oxygen is associated with improved survival, hemodynamics, and neuropsychological function in chronically hypoxemic patients. Maximal benefit is achieved with continuous oxygen delivery (i.e., 19–24 hr/day).

21. What is transtracheal oxygen therapy? List its benefits and risks.

Transtracheal oxygen therapy is an oxygen delivery system in which a catheter is placed transcutaneously into the trachea at the level of the second or third tracheal ring. The transtracheal delivery system has been shown to have several benefits: improved cosmesis and comfort, decreased oxygen flow rate requirement, improved exercise tolerance, improved patient compliance, and fewer hospitalizations. The most common complications include accidental catheter displacement, obstruction of the end of the catheter with a mucus plug, and mild local cellulitis.

22. What issues are involved with air travel in patients with pulmonary disorders?

Although commercial aircraft cruise between 22,000 and 44,000 feet, passenger cabins are maintained at pressures equivalent to altitudes of 5,000–8,000 feet. It is difficult to estimate the PaO_2 of a particular patient at these altitudes because of patients' varying abilities to compensate. However, in a stable normocapneic patient with COPD, a sea level $PaO_2 > 72$ mmHg usually results in a $PaO_2 > 50$ at 8,000 feet. The patient's expected PaO_2 at a particular altitude can be determined more accurately with the hypoxia altitude simulation test (HAST), which uses normobaric hypoxic breathing to simulate altitude and may be performed in PFT laboratories.

23. What advice should be given to a pulmonary patient who wishes to travel to the mountains?

Atmospheric oxygen is fairly constant at 21% of total barometric pressure at any altitude. However, barometric pressure decreases as altitude increases, resulting in a lower partial pressure of inspired oxygen P_iO_2. The P_iO_2 is 149 at sea level but decreases by approximately 4 mmHg/1,000 feet of elevation. Normal persons respond to the acute hypoxia of altitude by increasing minute ventilation to maximize alveolar PO_2. A healthy person can maintain a PaO_2 of 50–60 mmHg at 8,000–10,000 feet. Mild tachycardia also develops, increasing cardiac output and maintaining oxygen delivery to tissues. Blood flow to the brain is maintained as hypoxic vasodilatation overcomes the vasoconstrictor effect due to respiratory alkalosis. Such issues should be kept in mind in counseling a pulmonary patient about travel to high altitudes. Patients with borderline oxygenation at sea level may become hypoxic, depending on the altitude to which they travel. Such patients may require supplemental oxygen, especially if they have a history of co-morbid conditions such as angina pectoris, congestive heart failure, or cerebrovascular disease. In addition, patients already receiving supplemental oxygen may need to increase their oxygen flow rate.

24. Is chronic supplemental oxygen therapy indicated for patients who desaturate only with exercise or during sleep?

Many patients with COPD have normal or near-normal oxygen tension at rest but desaturate with exercise and during sleep. No clinical trials have evaluated the benefits of oxygen therapy on survival in this subset of patients. Therefore the role of supplemental oxygen in this setting is not well defined. Because patients with COPD generally spend only a small percentage of their day participating in exercise, it may be unlikely that exercise desaturation contributes significantly to morbidity or mortality. However, some patients report an increase in exercise tolerance with supplemental oxygen. To the extent that supplemental oxygen improves quality of life, it may be reasonable to prescribe oxygen for such patients. Small studies have demonstrated that nocturnal oxygen prevents sleep associated transient increases in pulmonary artery pressure and reduces the frequency of dysrhythmias. Although it is not known whether this benefit translates into long-term clinical benefit, many authorities use this rationale to justify the use of nocturnal oxygen in patients who desaturate only during sleep.

BIBLIOGRAPHY

1. Cooper CB: Long-term oxygen therapy. In Casaburi R, Petty TL (eds): Principles and Practice of Pulmonary Rehabilitation. Philadelphia, W.B. Saunders, 1993.
2. Danztker DR: Pulmonary gas exchange. In Bone RC, et al (eds): Pulmonary and Critical Care Medicine. St. Louis, Mosby, 1993.
3. Gong H: Air travel and oxygen therapy in cardiopulmonary patients. Chest 101:1104–1113, 1992.
4. Hagarty KM, Skorodin MS, Langbein E, et al: Comparison of three oxygen delivery systems during exercise in hypoxemic patients with chronic obstructive pulmonary disease. Am J Respir Crit Care Med 155:893–898, 1997.
5. Phillips Y, Kristo D, Kallish M: Writing the take-home oxygen prescription in COPD. J Crit Illness 13:112–120, 1998.
6. Rochester CL, Ferranti R: Long-term oxygen therapy: What benefits for your patient? J Respir Dis 19:133–151, 1998.
7. Rochester CL, Ferranti R: Lont-term oxygen therapy: What role in chronic disease? J Respir Dis 19:133–151, 1997.
8. Tarpy SP, Celli BR: Long-term oxygen therapy. N Engl J Med 333:710–714, 1995.

91. SOLITARY PULMONARY NODULE

Michael E. Hanley, M.D.

1. Why is it important to distinguish between a pulmonary nodule and a pulmonary mass?

A solitary pulmonary nodule (SPN) is a well-circumscribed, approximately round lesion on chest roentgenogram that is less than 4–6 cm in diameter. By definition it is completely surrounded by aerated lung, thus excluding pleural- or mediastinal-based lesions. It is distinguished from a pulmonary mass by size (mass > 4–6 cm in diameter). Although this distinction is arbitrary, it has clinical significance in that the probability of malignancy increases with the size of the lesion.

2. Does a coin lesion differ from an SPN?

No. SPN and "coin lesion" are synonymous terms. Coin lesion, however, is a misnomer, because it implies a two-dimensional lesion, whereas SPNs are three-dimensional.

3. What is the differential diagnosis of an SPN?

The differential diagnosis of SPNs is quite extensive. The major diagnostic consideration is to distinguish benign from malignant processes.

Neoplastic lesions

Malignant
1. Primary lung
   - Bronchogenic carcinoma
   - Alveolar cell carcinoma
   - Adenoma
   - Sarcoma

Benign
1. Hamartoma
2. Teratoma

- Lymphoma
- Hodgkin's disease

2. Solitary metastases

Nonneoplastic lesions

Infection
1. Tuberculosis
2. Coccidioidomycosis
3. Histoplasmosis
4. Blastomycosis
5. Nocardiosis
6. Actinomycosis

Inflammatory process
1. Wegener's granulomatosis
2. Organizing pneumonia
3. Rheumatoid necrobiotic nodule
4. Pulmonary infarct

Vascular lesions
1. Arteriovenous malformations
2. Pulmonary vein varix

Miscellaneous
1. Bronchial cyst
2. Bronchopulmonary sequestration
3. Pulmonary hematoma
4. Lipoid pneumonia
5. Other

4. What is the differential diagnosis of an SPN in HIV-seropositive patients?

Although HIV-seropositive patients may have an increased incidence of primary bronchogenic carcinoma, SPNs in this population most commonly have an infectious etiology. In a review limited by a small number of patients, 60% of the SPNs in HIV-seropositive patients were due to infections (*Pneumocystis carinii* pneumonia, cryptococcosis, nocardiosis, cytomegalovirus, mucormycosis, hydatidosis). The incidence of non-Hodgkin's lymphoma presenting as an SPN was only 10%.

5. Which three constellations of factors favor a benign nodule?

Calcifications of the lesion, absence of a history of tobacco use, and age less than 35 years are important factors that strongly correlate with benign nodules. Noncalcified lesions may be benign or malignant. Absence of smoking history does not entirely exclude a malignant process because of potential exposure to other carcinogens (e.g., radon gas, asbestos, chromium) and second-hand smoke (passive smoking). Indeed, 15% of primary lung cancers occur in nonsmokers. Patients under age 35 years are more likely to have a benign lesion; however, this association is not absolute. A diagnostic work-up may be necessary in the presence of other malignant risk factors, such as enlarging lesions or heavy tobacco use beginning at an early age.

6. Why is regular follow-up of a calcified pulmonary nodule important?

Six common patterns of calcification of SPNs are recognized: diffuse, central, popcorn, laminar, stippled, and eccentric. The first four are almost always benign, whereas the latter two may be either benign or malignant. However, even benign calcification does not exclude the presence of coincidental malignancy in adjacent tissue or the subsequent degeneration of a previously benign process into a malignant lesion ("scar" carcinoma). For this reason, close observation with serial chest roentgenograms every 6 months for at least 2 years is prudent for nodules with benign patterns of calcification.

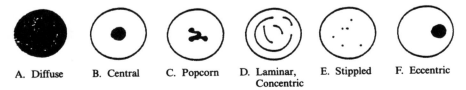

A. Diffuse   B. Central   C. Popcorn   D. Laminar, Concentric   E. Stippled   F. Eccentric

Six common patterns of calcification occur in SPNs. Patterns A–D are associated with benign conditions; patterns E and F occur in both benign and malignant conditions. (Adapted from Webb WR: Radiologic evaluation of the solitary pulmonary nodule. AJR 154:701–708, 1990; with permission.)

7. What other radiographic clues help to differentiate between benign and malignant lesions?

Cavitating lesions, lesions with multilobulated or spiculated contours, and lesions with shaggy or extremely irregular borders tend to be malignant. However, none of these associations is strong enough to determine accurately the nature of a lesion.

8. What is the most valuable test in evaluating an SPN?

The most valuable diagnostic test is comparison with an old chest roentgenogram. Benign nodules tend to grow at either very slow or very rapid rates. In contrast, malignant processes grow at steady, predictable, exponential rates. The growth rate of a nodule is conventionally defined as the doubling time (i.e., the time required for its *volume* to double) and corresponds to an increase in diameter by a factor of 1.26. In general, doubling times > 16 months or < 1 month (20–25 days) are associated with benign processes. Intermediate doubling times require additional evaluation to determine the nature of the lesion. If a nodule has not increased in size over a 2-year period, the probability that it is benign is greater than 99%.

9. What other radiographic tools may help to differentiate malignant and benign SPNs?

Both high-resolution computed tomography (HRCT) and positron emission tomography (PET) have been proposed as additional tools to aid in differentiating malignant and benign pulmonary nodules. Enhancement of the lesion by infusion of iodinated contrast during HRCT correlates with a higher probability of a malignant etiology. In preliminary studies, contrast enhancement had a sensitivity approaching 100%, a specificity of 70%, and a positive predictive value of 90%. The negative predictive value was 92%. Uptake of 18F-fluorodeoxyglucose (FDG) during PET imaging also correlated with a malignant etiology. The sensitivity of FDG-PET imaging for SPN greater than 2 cm in diameter was 81% with a specificity of 80–100%. FDG-PET imaging was significantly less reliable if the lesion was smaller than 2 cm.

10. Does sputum cytology aid in the diagnosis of an SPN?

Sputum cytology has a low yield (5–20%) and is of limited value.

11. What are the pros and cons of the invasive tests available for diagnosing an SPN?

Absolute determination of the true nature of an SPN necessitates obtaining tissue for histologic evaluation. Three options are available:

1. Resection of the nodule by either **open thoracotomy or video-assisted thoracoscopy** (VAT) unequivocally determines the nature of the lesion but is associated with significant perioperative morbidity and occasional mortality.

2. **Fiberoptic bronchoscopy with transbronchial biopsy** is relatively safe (incidence of pneumothorax and significant hemorrhage < 3%), but its sensitivity in diagnosing malignancy depends on the size of the lesion. Overall, the yield is approximately 10–40% for lesions 1–2 cm in diameter, 60% for lesions 2–3 cm, and 80% for lesions > 3 cm. These figures, however, depend heavily on the operator's skill. Addition of transbronchial brushing, washing, and needle aspiration improves the yield.

3. **Percutaneous transthoracic needle aspiration** has a higher sensitivity in diagnosing malignancy than transbronchial biopsy but is associated with more morbidity. The diagnostic yield exceeds 90% for malignancy. However, subsequent pneumothorax occurs in 25% of patients, one-half of whom require tube thoracostomy. In addition, the sensitivity for diagnosing benign lesions is even lower than that for transbronchial biopsy. Because the specific yield of both transbronchial biopsy and transthoracic needle aspiration for benign lesions is low, nonmalignant but nonspecific results do not exclude malignancy with certainty.

12. When should a patient with an SPN be referred for invasive tests?

Initial evaluation of an SPN by the primary care provider consists of a thorough history and physical examination, laboratory tests to screen for potential metastases, and comparison with previous chest roentgenograms. If the presence or pattern of calcification is not readily apparent on a plain chest roentgenogram, computed tomography (CT) of the chest should be obtained.

Patients with a high probability of malignancy should be referred for invasive tests. Patients with a low probability of malignancy (based on characteristics of the nodule and risk factors) should have a repeat chest radiograph in 1 month. If no change is seen, the patient should be followed closely with a serial chest roentgenogram (every 3–6 months) until radiographic stability of the nodule has been demonstrated for at least 2 years.

13. What factors determine whether a malignant SPN should be resected?

Issues that determine whether resection should be performed include the potential for cure and whether the patient can tolerate surgery. The potential for cure is influenced by the histologic nature of the lesion as well as the clinical stage. Ascertaining the ability of a patient to tolerate surgery requires an assessment of cardiovascular and pulmonary risk factors. This assessment includes at minimum performance of a detailed history and physical examination and analysis of the patient's electrocardiogram, chest radiograph, arterial blood gases, and pulmonary function tests. Any abnormalities in these parameters should prompt referral to a cardiologist or pulmonologist for additional evaluation.

CONTROVERSIES

14. Do all patients undergoing thoracotomy for an SPN require CT of the chest before surgery?

For:

Potential benefits of CT scans include identification of a benign pattern of calcification not evident on the plain chest roentgenogram, identification of additional nodules, and identification of mediastinal pathology (lymphadenopathy or direct metastases).

Against:

Demonstration of additional peripheral nodules or mediastinal lymphadenopathy by CT does not confirm that such lesions are malignant (especially when mediastinal lymph nodes are less than 1 cm in diameter). Furthermore, the probability that chest CT will reveal previously unrecognized mediastinal pathology is low if the mediastinum appears normal on the plain chest roentgenogram.

15. Should patients who have an SPN with a high risk of cancer and who also are good surgical candidates be managed by immediate resection of the nodule by either open thoracotomy or VAT rather than subjected to invasive, exclusively diagnostic procedures?

For:

Diagnosis of malignancy by transbronchial biopsy results in subsequent referral for therapeutic thoracotomy, whereas nonmalignant results are usually nonspecific, do not exclude malignancy, and result in referral for a diagnostic thoracotomy. Results of several studies indicate that staging fiberoptic bronchoscopy rarely identifies airway lesions that preclude surgery and potentially curative resection.

Against:

Prethoracotomy fiberoptic bronchoscopy allows staging of the major airways by screening for metachronous endobronchial malignancies that may preclude or alter the extent of subsequent surgery. In addition, 5% of malignant SPNs are small-cell carcinomas that are not treated with surgery. Finally, morbidity and mortality are much lower for transbronchial biopsy and percutaneous transthoracic needle aspiration than for thoracotomy; although the yield for benign lesions is low, the higher risk of thoracotomy justifies an attempt at diagnosis by less invasive approaches, especially for patients who are psychologically reluctant to undergo surgery or at high risk from thoracotomy or VAT.

BIBLIOGRAPHY

1. Dewan NA, Shehan CJ, Reeb SD, et al: Likelihood of malignancy in solitary pulmonary nodules: Comparison of Bayesian analysis and results of FDG-PET scan. Chest 112:416–422, 1997.

2. Dholakia S, Rappaport DC: The solitary pulmonary nodule: Is it malignant or benign? Postgrad Med 99:246–250, 1996.
3. Gasparini S, Ferretti M, Secchi EB, et al: Integration of transbronchial and percutaneous approach in the diagnosis of peripheral pulmonary nodules or masses. Experience with 1,027 consecutive cases. Chest 108:131–137, 1995.
4. Khouri NF, Meziane MA, Zerhouni EA, et al: The solitary pulmonary nodule. Assessment, diagnosis, and management. Chest 91:128–133, 1987.
5. Lillington GA: Management of solitary pulmonary nodules: How to decide when resection is required. Postgrad Med 101:145–150, 1997.
6. Pugatch RD: Radiologic evaluation in chest malignancies: A review of imaging modalities. Chest 107:294S–297S, 1995.
7. Swensen SJ: What is the significance of finding calcifications in pulmonary masses on CT scans? AJR 164:505–506, 1995.
8. Swensen SJ, Brown LR, Colby TV, et al: Lung nodule enhancement at CT: Prospective findings. Radiology 201:447–455, 1996.
9. Torrington KG, Kern JD: The utility of fiberoptic bronchoscopy in the evaluation of the solitary pulmonary nodule. Chest 104:1021–1024, 1993.
10. Webb WR: Radiologic evaluation of the solitary pulmonary nodule. AJR 154:701–708, 1990.
11. Worsley DF, Celler A, Adam MJ, et al: Pulmonary nodules: Differential diagnosis using 18F-fluorodeoxyglucose single-photon emission computed tomography. AJR 168:771–774, 1997.

XIII. Common Disorders of the Skin

92. ECZEMATOUS DERMATITIS

Loren E. Golitz, M.D., and Meg A. Lemon, M.D.

1. Define eczema.

Eczema is the final common manifestation of dermatitis of several etiologies, including atopic dermatitis, allergic and irritant contact dermatitis, and various other clinical forms of dermatitis. Papules, macules, and vesicles often coalesce with weeping and crusting. Eventually, thickening and scaling, called lichenification, result.

2. What rules should be considered in using topical steroid therapy?

1. Topical steroid preparations of low-, mid-, and high-potency must be carefully distinguished. Examples: desonide 0.05% (low), triamcinolone acetonide 0.1% (mid), fluocinonide 0.05% (high).

2. Ointments are more effective in dry, thickened skin than creams.

3. Potent topical steroids (especially fluorinated) should not be applied to intertriginous areas or to the face and neck.

4. Potent topical steroids should be avoided in young children because of the possibility of systemic absorption.

5. Potential side effects from the prolonged use of potent topical steroids include cutaneous atrophy, development of striae, and suppression of the hypothalamus-pituitary-adrenal (HPA) axis. The risk of systemic absorption and suppression of the HPA is increased by high-potency preparations, prolonged use, application to large areas, and occlusive dressings.

3. When are systemic corticosteroids indicated?

In general, systemic steroids are indicated in self-limited, steroid-responsive disorders that present acutely with severe symptoms in an otherwise healthy patient. For example, prednisone may be started at a dose of 40 mg/day and tapered over 3 weeks in acute, severe cases of contact dermatitis (e.g., poison ivy). A rapid taper over 5 days will result in recurrence of rash. Systemic steroids should be avoided, if possible, in chronic illnesses such as psoriasis and atopic dermatitis.

4. What substances are the most common causes of allergic contact dermatitis?

Poison ivy, poison sumac, and poison oak are the three most common plants that cause contact dermatitis in the United States. Topical medications, including neomycin, ethylenediamine, topical anesthetics, and thimerosal, are commonly indicated. Nickel is a common culprit because of its ubiquitous use in jewelry. Chromium may be implicated in patients with industrial exposures to substances such as cement. Rubber, epoxy glue, cosmetics, perfumes, and formaldehyde also may cause allergic contact dermatitis. Paraphenylenediamine in permanent black hair dye may cause severe scalp dermatitis.

5. How is contact dermatitis diagnosed?

The clinical history, including exposures at work and at home, is the most important element in making the diagnosis. The acute episode often follows contact with the allergen by approximately 48 hours. Hobbies are an important source of contact allergens. Any chemical that gets on the hands is readily transferred to the eyelids and genitalia.

6. Describe the classic presentation of poison ivy.

Poison ivy presents with a mixture of vesicles, bullae, and crusting. The blisters often appear in a linear arrangement at points where the broken stem or leaf of the plant has touched the skin. The rash is associated with intense pruritus.

7. Which parts of the hands and feet are commonly affected by contact dermatitis?

Contact dermatitis of the hands and feet usually involves the dorsal aspects, because the palms and soles are relatively protected by the thick layer of keratin.

8. What treatments are effective for contact dermatitis?

Treatment of allergic contact dermatitis includes cool compresses with a Burow's solution (a 1:20 solution is made by diluting 1 package of powder in 1 pint of cold water). The area should be soaked for 10–15 minutes and then patted with a towel. A topical steroid in the form of a cream or ointment may be applied to the skin 2–4 times/day. Once a patient is allergic to a specific chemical, the allergy is maintained throughout life; thus avoidance of contact with the agent is important.

9. In what instances are patch tests useful?

Patch testing may establish the specific cause of an allergic contact dermatitis. Screening trays allow testing of multiple potential allergens. Tests normally are read 48 or 72 hours after application. Patch tests may be used to support the diagnosis of contact dermatitis, to identify the specific allergen, or to exclude the diagnosis. Difficulties include false-positive and false-negative results as well as positive results with unclear clinical significance. Test results must be correlated with the patient's exposures. A common cause of false-negative testing is a delayed reaction after the usual 48-hour reading. A second reading 4–7 days after the application is recommended. Patch tests should not used during an episode of severe extensive dermatitis.

10. Does atopic dermatitis affect adults?

Usually atopic dermatitis is a disease of infancy and childhood, beginning before age 6 months and diminishing in adulthood. However, up to 60% of patients with childhood atopic dermatitis have some form, albeit more limited, in adulthood. Pruritus, the major symptom, is accompanied by dry, lichenified patches on the flexor surfaces of elbows, knees, wrists, ankles, and the periorbital region. The condition is usually idiopathic; exacerbating factors include extreme temperature, dry climates, cutaneous infections, and chemical irritants (e.g., soap).

11. What is the relationship of atopic dermatitis to other atopic states?

Up to 70% of patients have a personal or family history of asthma, hay fever, or dermatitis. Severe atopic dermatitis is seen in the hyperimmunoglobulin E (IgE) syndrome. Thus, diagnosis is usually made by the clinical and family history, examination of the lesions, and, in severe cases, assessment of the IgE level.

12. What is the mainstay of treatment of atopic dermatitis?

The mainstays of treatment are skin hydration and topical steroids. Patients should apply emollients to damp skin after bathing and repeatedly during the day. Topical steroids should be applied 2–4 times each day; ointments of mid-to-high potency, such as triamcinolone acetonide 0.1%, may be required. Occlusive dressings may be used to treat stubborn lesions.

13. What possibilities should be considered when atopic dermatitis fails to respond to therapy?

1. The patient is not meticulous about the frequency of therapy.

2. The patient is allergic (sensitized) to the topical agent. This possibility is especially likely when the treated area coincides with worsening disease.

3. Superinfection with *Staphylococcus aureus* is present. True infection is difficult to determine in the absence of cellulitis. However, vesicles, pustules, and large exudative lesions may warrant therapy with systemic antistaphylococcal agents.

4. The diagnosis is allergic contact dermatitis rather than atopic dermatitis, and the patient continues to be exposed to the allergen. Patch testing may be diagnostic.

14. What causes a pruritic, dry, and scaly dermatitis in elderly patients?

Pruritic, dry, and scaly dermatitis in elderly patients, usually called asteatotic eczema or "winter itch," is related to decreased skin lipids. Drying climate, frequent bathing, and diuresis exacerbate the areas of dryness. Skin fissuring and erythema, most commonly on the anterior legs, dorsum of the hands, and interscapular region, are accompanied by pruritus. Emollients to hydrate the skin, low-potency topical steroids, and decreased soap use usually provide relief.

15. Who is at risk for irritant hand dermatitis?

Irritant hand dermatitis, as opposed to allergic contact dermatitis, appears on the palmar aspect of the hand. Persons at risk include (1) patients with a history of atopic dermatitis or other skin disease and (2) housekeepers, health care professionals, and others who chronically expose hands to water and detergents.

16. Describe the therapy for irritant hand dermatitis.

Hand dermatitis may prove particularly difficult to clear, but the following steps usually are helpful:

1. Use of vinyl gloves, avoidance of chemicals, and addition of lubricant
2. Use of cool compresses and mid-potency steroids
3. Aggressive treatment of secondary bacterial infection

In addition, dermatophyte infection should be ruled out with a potassium hydroxide (KOH) preparation and culture.

17. How are antibiotics useful in flares of dermatitis?

When the epidermal barrier is disrupted in disease states (e.g., atopic, irritant, and contact dermatitis, psoriasis), fissures in the skin allow bacteria to enter and cause local infection. Antigenic portions of these bacteria stimulate the immune response (specifically T-cells) and worsen the dermatitis. A 10–14-day course of oral antibiotics with good staphylococcal and streptococcal coverage (e.g., dicloxacillin, cephalexin, erythromycin) shortens the recovery period.

BIBLIOGRAPHY

1. Fitzpatrick TB, et al (eds): Dermatology in General Medicine, 4th ed. New York, McGraw-Hill, 1993.
2. Halbert AR, et al: Atopic dermatitis: Is it an allergic disease? J Am Acad Dermatol 33:1008–1018, 1995.
3. Leung DY: Atopic dermatitis: Immunobiology and treatment with immune modulators. Clin Exp Immunol 107(Suppl 1):25–30, 1997.
4. Moschella SL, Hurley HJ (eds): Dermatology, 3rd ed. Philadelphia, W.B. Saunders, 1992.
5. Phillips TJ, Dover JS: Recent advances in dermatology. N Engl J Med 326:167–178, 1992.
6. Rothe MJ, Grant-Kels JM: Atopic dermatitis: An update. J Am Acad Dermatol 353:1–13, 1996.
7. Sulzberger MB: The patch test: Who should and should not use it and why. Contact Dermatitis 1:117, 1975.

93. MACULOPAPULAR ERUPTIONS

Mark E. Fogarty, M.D., and Loren E. Golitz, M.D.

1. What is meant by the terms morbilliform and scarlatiniform?

Erythematous macules and papules are referred to as morbilliform, whereas diffuse erythematous macular lesions are scarlatiniform. A morbilliform rash is due to either a viral exanthem or a drug eruption. A scarlatiniform rash, classically seen in scarlet fever, is also seen in patients with toxic shock syndrome and Kawasaki's disease.

2. Describe the typical appearance of a drug eruption.

The most common drug eruption is a morbilliform rash on the trunk, extremities, palms, and soles. The rash may become confluent and is usually quite pruritic. Mild fever may accompany the eruption. The reaction usually begins within a week of starting the drug and may last up to 2 weeks. Drug eruptions also may manifest as urticarial or photosensitive eruptions. Most drugs are suspect, but common etiologic agents include penicillin, barbiturates, allopurinol, and trimethoprim-sulfamethoxazole (a common cause of drug rashes in patients infected with the human immunodeficiency virus [HIV]).

3. How are drug rashes treated?

Treatment involves discontinuation of the drug and avoidance of further exposure. Desensitization is effective in some cases and may be considered when alternative regimens are ineffective (e.g., trimethoprim-sulfamethoxazole desensitization in patients with AIDS who need *Pneumocystis carinii* prophylaxis). Pruritus is treated with antihistamines such as hydroxyzine hydrochloride, 25–50 mg 4 times/day. Severe, generalized drug eruptions may be treated with a short course of oral prednisone.

4. Which three classic childhood exanthems result in a predominant morbilliform rash?

1. **Measles.** A rash beginning on the forehead and hairline follows a prodrome of coryza, cough, and development of small white lesions with blue centers on the oral mucous membranes (Koplik's spots).

2. **Rubella.** Pale maculopapular lesions start on the face and spread downward; lymphadenopathy (occipital and postauricular) is a consistent finding.

3. **Fifth disease** (erythema infectiosum). This parvovirus infection presents with a slapped-cheek appearance and often is accompanied by a mild fever, followed by a diffuse, reticular rash that spreads to the extremities.

5. What diagnosis is suggested when a morbilliform rash develops in a patient treated with ampicillin for pharyngitis?

The probable diagnosis is infectious mononucleosis, which is caused by Epstein-Barr virus. In this instance, a drug-virus interaction results in the eruption. This interaction occurs with much greater frequency (up to 95% of patients treated) than a reaction to ampicillin alone.

6. What diagnosis should be considered when a maculopapular eruption of palms, soles, ankles, and wrists follows a febrile syndrome?

The initial eruption of **Rocky Mountain spotted fever** follows this distribution. Although lesions eventually become classically purpuric, early recognition of this tick-borne infection is important to appropriate management. **Atypical measles** also may present in this manner, especially in immunized adults.

7. What other viral entities cause morbilliform exanthem?

Epstein-Barr virus, coxsackievirus, echovirus, and adenovirus.

8. Why is it important to think of Kawasaki's disease in a child with a morbilliform or scarlatiniform rash?

Kawasaki's disease is a multisytem disorder of young children that results in coronary artery aneurysms in as many as 25% of patients. Early recognition of the disease may permit appropriate therapy (high-dose intravenous gammaglobulin and aspirin) to reduce the incidence of coronary arteritis. Hallmarks of the disease include rash (often leading to desquamation), conjunctival injection, nonsuppurative cervical lymphadenopathy, oral erythema with strawberry tongue, and fever.

9. How is scabies diagnosed?

The rash is not always diagnostic. Look for mite burrows, which appear as scaling lines (especially easy to find in the web spaces of hands and feet as well as the volar wrists, nipples, glans penis, and ankles). The burrows should be scraped onto a slide with a scalpel and immersed in either KOH or mineral oil. The diagnosis is made by finding mites, mite eggs, or mite feces on light microscopy of lesional keratin scrapings.

10. When should the provider consider scabies as a diagnosis?

Scabies is caused by the human mite and characteristically presents with linear burrows 1–2 cm wide and < 1 cm long. Papules are typically located in skinfolds, between the fingers, on the male genitalia, and on the buttocks. Burrows are often replaced by excoriations. Family members and close contacts are often affected. Severe pruritus is usually the presenting feature and often worsens at night.

11. What is appropriate therapy for scabies?

Treatment must include all household and sexual contacts in addition to the patient. Gamma benzene hexachloride (lindane: Kwell) is applied to the dry skin of the entire body below the neck for 4 hours and then washed off. This application may be repeated once in 5 days to eliminate hatching ova. All family members should be treated simultaneously. Patients should be instructed that the pruritus may persist for 3–4 weeks after treatment is completed. Pruritus can be managed with medium-potency topical steroids (triamcinolone cream, 0.025%) and oral hydroxyzine hydrochloride, 25 mg 4 times/day. Gamma benzene hexachloride should not be used in children younger than 1 year. Alternatives include permeathrin (Elimite) or sulfur ointment, 5%. Lindane resistance has been reported.

12. Do other mites affect humans?

Occasionally cat and dog mites (*Chylietella* sp.) may bite humans but do not cause invasive disease like scabies. The diagnosis is made when the patient's veterinarian finds mites on the family pet.

BIBLIOGRAPHY

1. Fitzpatrick TB, et al (eds): Dermatology in General Medicine, 4th ed. New York, McGraw-Hill, 1993.
2. Moschella SL, Hurley HJ (eds): Dermatology, 3rd ed. Philadelphia, W.B. Saunders, 1992.
3. Paules SJ, Levisohn D, Heffron W: Persistent scabies in nursing home patients. J Fam Pract 37:82–86, 1993.
4. Phillips TJ, Dover JS: Recent advances in dermatology. N Engl J Med 326:167–178, 1992.

94. PAPULOSQUAMOUS SKIN LESIONS

Mark E. Fogarty, M.D., and Loren E. Golitz, M.D.

1. What characterizes papulosquamous skin lesions?

This major category of skin disorders is characterized by raised (papular) lesions with scales (squamous). They may or may not be pruritic.

2. Name the three most common diseases seen in primary care practice that present with a generalized papulosquamous rash.

Psoriasis, pityriasis rosea, and lichen planus. These diseases are often mistaken for tinea. A potassium hydroxide (KOH) preparation of dead skin cells helps to clarify the diagnosis.

3. Describe the presentation of psoriasis.

Psoriasis is usually a slowly progressive inflammatory disease that manifests as demarcated erythematous plaques covered with silvery scales and symmetrically distributed over extensor surfaces of elbows and knees, the gluteal cleft, and scalp.

4. When is the Koebner phenomenon seen?

The Koebner phenomenon, which refers to the development of plaques in the area of previous trauma, is commonly seen in patients with psoriasis and lichen planus.

5. What other findings are associated with psoriasis?

Nail-pitting is found in over 50% of patients, along with onycholysis and thickened nails. Joint manifestations are typically rheumatoid factor-negative, asymmetric, and often limited to distal interphalangeal joints.

6. What should be the initial therapy for psoriasis?

Skin hydration and mid-potency steroids are standard therapy for limited skin plaques. A kerolytic agent (salicylic acid) or a tar gel may enhance steroid effectiveness. When the disease becomes less responsive or widespread (especially if erythroderma is present), more aggressive treatment with ultraviolet light or systemic methotrexate may be required. Such patients should be seen by a dermatologist to consider the most appropriate mode of therapy.

7. What is a herald patch?

A herald patch is an anular lesion 2–6 cm in size that "heralds" the onset of pityriasis rosea by a few days.

8. What causes pityriasis rosea?

The cause of this self-limited, seasonal disease (seen in spring and fall) is unknown. A truncal papulosquamous eruption of oval brown lesions parallel to skinfolds follows the herald patch. Treatment for pruritus is symptomatic; topical steroids may be used, if needed. Resolution is expected by 6–8 weeks.

9. What disease may pityriasis rosea mimic?

The lesions of pityriasis are similar to those of secondary syphilis. However, pityriasis rosea does not involve the palms and soles, both of which are commonly involved in secondary syphilis. A serologic test for syphilis should be performed in all patients to exclude syphilis.

10. Where do lesions of lichen planus occur?

The pruritic, violaceous, papulosquamous lesions of lichen planus favor the wrists, shins, lower back, and genital area. Such lesions also commonly involve the oral mucosa, presenting as a white reticulated patch in the buccal area. Scalp involvement may lead to hair loss.

11. What causes lichen planus?

The cause of lichen planus is unknown. Similar lichenoid eruptions may result from a reaction to several drugs, including diuretics, antimalarials, and phenothiazines. Most cases, however, are idiopathic and spontaneously remit within 2 years. Topical steroids are often helpful.

12. What disease is characterized by severe dandruff and greasy, scaly, erythematous plaques over the central area of the face?

Seborrheic dermatitis, which also affects the eyelids, eyebrows, external ear, and glabella and occasionally is even more widespread.

13. What types of people are particularly susceptible to seborrheic dermatitis?

1. Infants— "cradle cap"
2. Patients with Parkinson's disease
3. Patients who previously suffered a cerebrovascular accident
4. Patients infected with the human immunodeficiency virus (HIV)

14. How should seborrheic dermatitis be treated?

1. Nonfluorinated topical steroid solutions of low potency
2. Shampoos with salicylic acid, coal tar, or pyrethione zinc

15. What is the role of infection in seborrheic dermatitis?

Many investigators believe that *Pityrosporum orbiculare* is a causative organism in patients with seborrheic dermatitis. *P. orbiculare* (or *Malassezia furfur*) is a yeastlike fungus that lives in the stratum corneum. The addition of topical antifungal creams to the treatment regimen frequently helps to clear the eruption.

16. Why should a chronic scaly patch or plaque in the swimming-trunk distribution be considered for biopsy?

Such nonspecific lesions, which often appear psoriatic, may be a prodromal or heralding lesion of mycosis fungoides (a T-cell lymphoma). Although the trunk distribution is common, lesions also may appear on extremities.

17. How is mycosis fungoides diagnosed?

The history and physical examination point to the diagnosis. Patients have usually been treated for "eczema" for a prolonged period (up to 10–20 years). The diagnosis is made histologically. Biopsy initially may be nonspecific, but eventually a mononuclear cell infiltrate with Pautrier's abscesses may be found. Multiple biopsies may be necessary before a definitive diagnosis is made.

BIBLIOGRAPHY

1. Bunn PA, Hoffman SJ, et al: Systemic therapy of cutaneous T-cell lymphomas. Ann Intern Med 121:592–602, 1994.
2. Fitzpatrick TB, et al (eds): Dermatology in General Medicine, 4th ed. New York, McGraw-Hill, 1993.
3. Hay RJ, Graham-Brown RA: Dandruff and seborrheic dermatitis: Causes and management. Clin Exp Derm 22:3–6, 1997.
4. Lim KK, et al: Cyclosporine in the treatment of dermatologic disease: An update. Mayo Clin Proc 71:1182–1191, 1996.
5. Millikan LE, Shrum JP: An update on common skin diseases. Postgrad Med 1(6):96–98, 101–104, 107–110, 1992.
6. Moschella SL, Hurley HJ (eds): Dermatology, 3rd ed. Philadelphia, W.B. Saunders, 1992.
7. Phillips TJ, Dover JS: Recent advances in dermatology. N Engl J Med 326:167–178, 1992.
8. Skinner RB Jr, et al: Double-blind treatment of seborrheic dermatitis with 2% ketoconazole cream. J Am Acad Dermatol 12:852–856, 1985.
9. van de Kerkhof PC: Biological activity of vitamin D analogues in the skin, with special reference to anti-psoriatic mechanisms. Br J Dermatol 132:675–682, 1995.

95. VESICULAR AND BULLOUS SKIN ERUPTIONS

Mark E. Fogarty, M.D., and Loren E. Golitz, M.D.

1. What is the difference between a vesicle and a bulla?

Both are blisters of the skin filled with serous fluid, but vesicles are < 0.5 cm and bullae > 0.5 cm in diameter. Some diseases are predominantly vesicular or bullous, whereas others involve a spectrum of lesions.

2. What is the differential diagnosis of a disseminated vesicular rash in children?

A vesicular rash is varicella (chickenpox) until proved otherwise. The diagnosis is suggested by history of exposure (90% attack rate in seronegative people) and crops of maculopapular lesions that progress to vesicles within hours, beginning on the trunk and face, and are accompanied by pruritus. Patients are contagious 48 hours before eruption and until all vesicles are crusted.

Other less likely possibilities, often distinguished by the appropriate history and setting, include (1) infections with coxsackievirus or echovirus, (2) rickettsialpox (which may be distinguished by a herald spot at the site of the mite bite), (3) disseminated herpes simplex infection (which may be seen in patients with atopic dermatitis), and (4) allergic contact dermatitis.

3. What advice should the provider give to patients with chickenpox infections?

1. Lukewarm soaks and compresses relieve pruritus and prevent secondary infection.
2. Close clipping of fingernails prevents excoriations.
3. Aspirin should be prevented because of the risk of Reye's syndrome.
4. Oral acyclovir should be given to adolescents and adults with chickenpox of < 24 hours' duration.
5. New-onset respiratory symptoms require medical assessment.

4. What is shingles?

Shingles or herpes zoster disease results from varicella virus that has been latent in the dorsal root or cranial nerve ganglia. It presents as isolated pain followed by a unilateral vesicular eruption in a dermatomal distribution. Shingles occurs sporadically in the elderly population but rarely recurs. Cranial nerves may be involved, leading to mucosal, ear, and eye lesions.

5. What can be done to decrease the incidence of postherpetic neuralgia?

Up to 50% of older patients have dermatomal pain months after resolution of the vesicular lesions of zoster infection. This pain may be prevented by treatment with 7–10 days of acyclovir; the efficacy of steroids is less clearly established. Symptomatic relief with analgesics and amitriptyline may be attempted.

6. Which patients are at high risk of dissemination from varicella infections?

Immunocompromised patients, including those with HIV/AIDS or Hodgkin's lymphoma; patients who receive bone marrow transplant; and newborns are at risk of dissemination from varicella virus. Immune prophylaxis should be given to exposed patients; intravenous acyclovir is indicated for evidence of disease.

7. What four classic diseases should be considered in the differential diagnosis of a bullous eruption?

The four bullous diseases are pemphigus vulgaris, bullous pemphigoid, erythema multiforme, and dermatitis herpetiformis, which often can be diagnosed by clinical appearance.

Diagnosis is confirmed by routine biopsy or by immunofluorescence microscopy of frozen tissue. Because treatment is somewhat different in each, correct diagnosis is crucial.

8. What is the typical appearance of erythema multiforme?

Erythema multiforme, the most common of the four classic bullous diseases, affects predominantly children and young adults. Cutaneous lesions vary from fixed erythematous papules to anular and bullous lesions. The classic lesion is the target (also termed an iris lesion), which most often occurs on the distal extremities and is characterized by a dusky gray center and an erythematous rim. Involvement of mucous membranes, especially the oral mucosa, is common. Less often the ocular and genital mucosa are affected.

9. What are the most common causes of erythema multiforme?

The most common cause of erythema multiforme minor is recurrent herpes simplex infection (about 90% of patients). The rash of erythema multiforme occurs 7–10 days after a lesion of herpes simplex. Because herpes simplex is frequently recurrent, erythema multiforme also may recur. The second most common cause of erythema multiforme minor is drugs, especially sulfa drugs, barbiturates, and antibiotics such as tetracycline.

10. What is Stevens-Johnson syndrome?

Erythema multiforme major, a more severe form of erythema multiforme, also is known as Stevens-Johnson syndrome. The majority of cases are caused by drugs, particularly sulfa drugs. Patients with Stevens-Johnson syndrome are often very ill and may require hospitalization. The diagnosis is made when erythema multiforme-like lesions are accompanied by the involvement of 2 or more mucous membrane sites in the clinical setting of severe systemic symptoms. Mucous membranes often show severe involvement. If the ocular mucous membranes are involved, an ophthalmologist should be consulted to prevent permanent eye damage.

11. How are erythema multiforme and Stevens-Johnson syndrome treated?

The treatment of erythema multiforme minor is generally symptomatic, because the condition is self-limited. Triamcinolone creams (0.025%, applied 2–4 times/day) and hydroxyzine hydrochloride (for pruritus) are usually effective in relieving the symptoms. In patients with frequent recurrences of herpes simplex and erythema multiforme, long-term suppressive therapy with oral acyclovir may be indicated. If the etiologic agent is a drug, it should be discontinued. The management of Stevens-Johnson syndrome includes hospitalization, aggressive fluid and electrolyte replacement, and surveillance for and treatment of bacterial, yeast, or fungal infections.

12. What diagnosis does a recurrent, severely pruritic vesicular eruption suggest?

Dermatitis herpetiformis is characterized by extremely pruritic vesicles grouped on the elbows, interscapular areas, lower back, and knees. Excoriations are often evident. Approximately 80% of patients have a gluten-sensitive enteropathy, but most are asymptomatic. A routine biopsy of a fresh blister confirms the diagnosis. Mucous membranes are not involved.

13. Describe the treatment of dermatitis herpetiformis.

Therapy with dapsone, 50–100 mg/day, produces a dramatic improvement in the pruritus. The vesicles rapidly heal, and patients usually become asymptomatic. If the patient can maintain a gluten-free diet, the dose of dapsone often may be reduced or eliminated. However, because patients usually do not have bowel symptoms, it is difficult to keep them on a gluten-free diet. Dapsone often needs to be maintained for a long duration at the lowest possible dose. Before initiating dapsone therapy, patients should be evaluated for deficiency of glucose-6-phosphate-dehydrogenase because of the risk of methemoglobinemia. Dapsone causes a mild hemolysis of red blood cells in most patients. Rarely, bone marrow suppression or hepatitis may result. Therefore, patients should be monitored with appropriate laboratory tests.

14. What does pemphigus vulgaris look like?

Pemphigus vulgaris is an autoimmune skin disease in which the patient forms antibodies to the cellular bridges between keratinocytes. The antibodies cause the epidermis to fall apart in response to shear forces. Almost all patients have oral erosions at some point in the disease. Cutaneous lesions show denuded skin, much like a burn. The epidermis pulls away from the dermis with minimal friction. Occasionally flaccid bullae are seen, but they readily rupture, leaving the characteristic erosions.

15. How is pemphigus vulgaris treated?

Before the development of systemic corticosteroids, pemphigus vulgaris was considered to be a uniformly fatal disease. Therefore, treatment needs to be relatively aggressive to control the disease as quickly as possible. Once the correct diagnosis is established, patients should be treated with prednisone, 60–80 mg in a single daily dose. Antacids and H_2 blockers should be used in patients with a history of peptic ulcer disease. In most cases, a steroid-sparing drug, such as azathioprine, should be started at the initiation of prednisone therapy. The full steroid-sparing effect of azathioprine requires approximately 6 weeks. Once the cutaneous lesions of pemphigus vulgaris show complete healing, the dosage of prednisone is slowly reduced. The goal should be to keep the patient on the lowest dose of alternate-day prednisone that controls the disease. It may require several months before the prednisone and azathioprine can be completely discontinued.

16. Describe the presentation and treatment of bullous pemphigoid.

Bullous pemphigoid is typically a disease of middle-aged and elderly patients. At one time, it was referred to as bullous disease of the aged. It is characterized by large tense blisters with a predilection for the intertriginous areas such as the inner thigh and axillae. The blisters show much less tendency to rupture than those of pemphigus vulgaris. Blisters may occur in the mouth but, unlike pemphigus vulgaris, mucosal lesions usually follow the onset of skin disease. Often the tense blisters of bullous pemphigoid are situated on red urticarial plaques. Bullous pemphigoid is less likely to be a life-threatening disease than pemphigus vulgaris. Therefore, the dose of oral prednisone and steroid-sparing agents, such as azathioprine, may be more conservative. An initial prednisone dose of 40–60 mg/day is usually adequate. The disease responds to treatment more rapidly than pemphigus vulgaris.

BIBLIOGRAPHY

1. Fitzpatrick TB, et al (eds): Dermatology in General Medicine, 4th ed. New York, McGraw-HIll, 1993.
2. Huff TC: Erythema multiforme and latent herpes simplex infection. Semin Dermatol 11:207–210, 1992.
3. Huff JC, Weston WL: Recurrent erythema multiforme. Medicine 68(3):133–140, 1989.
4. Moschella SL, Hurley HJ (eds): Dermatology, 3rd ed. Philadelphia, W.B. Saunders, 1992.
5. Phillips TJ, Dover JS: Recent advances in dermatology. N Engl J Med 326:167–178, 1992.
6. Tatnall FM, et al: A double-bind, placebo-controlled trial of continuous acyclovir therapy in recurrent erythema multiforme. Br J Dermatol 132:267–270, 1995.

96. URTICARIA

Mark E. Fogarty, M.D., and Loren E. Golitz, M.D.

1. What is acute urticaria?

Acute urticaria is a localized, transient, white or erythematous swelling of the skin of less than 6 weeks' duration. Individual lesions, also called hives or wheals, are frequently anular or polycyclic. The swelling is due to a localized increase in capillary and venule permeability mediated by histamines and other cytokines. Individual wheals usually resolve within 24 hours but may be present in multiple stages of evolution. Lesions are commonly associated with pruritus or a stinging sensation. Papular urticaria, which is caused by hypersensitivity to anthropod bites, begins as umbilicated red papules and may progress to anular lesions or plaques.

2. What is the difference between angioedema and urticaria?

Urticaria involves the superficial aspect of the skin, whereas angioedema involves the deeper layers, including the subcutaneous tissue. Both may occur separately or together. Demarcation of lesions is less evident in angioedema, which also may involve the upper respiratory tract, presenting as bronchospasm, and the gastrointestinal tract, manifesting as gastrointesintal colic. Thus the caregiver should ask about such symptoms in patients with the complaint of urticaria.

3. When should the provider suspect acute urticaria as a manifestation of anaphylaxis?

Anaphylaxis is a life-threatening response of the sensitized individual to a specific antigen. Respiratory distress followed by vascular collapse may be heralded by or accompanied by pruritus and urticaria, with or without angioedema. The most important aspect in ascertaining the diagnosis of anaphylaxis is an acute history documenting the onset of signs and symptoms within minutes of exposure to an antigen. Early recognition is paramount, because death from anaphylaxis may occur within minutes to hours.

4. Name the most common causes of acute urticaria.

Urticaria with or without angioedema may be immunoglobulin E (IgE)-dependent, complement-mediated, or due to direct release of histamine from mast cells. The most common identifiable causes are medications, arthropod bites, and infections. However, in the majority of patients a definite cause is not identified.

5. What is the mainstay of treatment for acute urticaria?

Treatment involves elimination of the cause, if known. The mainstays of medical therapy are histamine-1 (H_1) receptor blockers, including classic H_1 antihistamines (e.g., diphenhydramine and hydroxyzine) and nonsedating H_1 antihistamines (terfenadine, astemizole, and loratadine). Such agents should be initiated at standard doses and titrated as tolerated. Doxepin hydrochloride, a tricyclic antidepressant with powerful H_1 antagonist activity, also may be useful. H_2 antihistamines administered in combination with H_1 blockers may be more effective than H_1 antihistamines alone in some patients. Disodium cromoglycate, terbutaline, and calcium channel blockers also may have a role in the treatment of some patients. In rare patients, a 1- to 2-week course of systemic corticosteroids may be needed.

6. Is epinephrine ever indicated in the treatment of acute urticaria?

Yes. In severe cases of urticaria or when anaphylaxis is suspected, subcutaneous epinephrine (0.3 cc of a 1:1000 solution) should be administered and may be repeated at 30-minute intervals for severe reactions. Intravenous or intramuscular administration of epinephrine is required in patients with airway involvement, anaphylaxis, or cardiovascular collapse.

7. What should be done for patients who manifest urticaria to bee stings?

It is important to determine the patient's potential risk of anaphylaxis. If no history is easily obtainable to assess risk, a skin test should be considered. Potential for anaphylaxis correlates with a positive skin test. After assessing the risk for anaphylaxis, the following steps should be provided:

1. **Instruction in prevention.** Lifestyle should be modified to avoid exposure to bees (wearing of shoes, avoidance of eating or wearing perfume in high-risk areas, limitation of unnecessary yard work, especially hauling trash).

2. **Instruction in emergency measures.** Unexpired epinephrine kits should be readily available at home and in the car, and informational bracelets and tags should be used.

3. **Desensitization.** In patients with a history or serious risk of anaphylaxis, venom immunotherapy may be undertaken until the skin test is negative. Desensitization is not required for children who experience a systemic reaction limited to the skin, because progression to anaphylaxis is unlikely.

8. Define chronic urticaria.

Chronic urticaria is defined as urticaria lasting longer than 6 weeks. It may be continuous or episodic.

9. Which conditions may be mistaken for chronic urticaria?

- Systemic or subacute lupus erythematosus
- Erythema multiforme
- Erythema anulare centrifugum
- Bullous pemphigoid
- Drug eruptions
- Urticarial vasculitis, a form of leukocytoclastic vasculitis associated with hypocomplementemia

10. What are the most common causes of chronic urticaria?

Causes of chronic urticaria include chronic infection (e.g., sinusitis, vaginitis, otitis, hepatitis), drugs, neoplasia, mastocytosis, collagen-vascular diseases, hyperthyroidism, contact urticaria, pressure urticaria, and psychogenic urticaria. Urticaria may be prominent in skin disorders such as bullous pemphigoid. In most cases of chronic urticaria, the specific cause cannot be determined.

11. Describe the initial evaluation of patients with chronic urticaria.

A thorough history and physical examination are the most important parts of the work-up, Key historical features include the pattern of occurrence and relationship to medications, diet, and activity. Medication usage, including nonprescription drugs and home or "natural" remedies, should be reviewed. Physical examination should rule out signs of systemic disease and physical urticaria. Screening laboratory tests should include complete blood count, liver and renal function tests, erythrocyte sedimentation rate, and urinalysis. Further testing is usually not necessary, unless suggested by positive findings from the history or physical examination (e.g., antinuclear antibodies, stool for ova and parasites, hepatitis-B serology, thyroid function studies, thyroid antibodies).

12. When is a skin biopsy indicated?

If individual lesions of urticaria are purpuric or persist for days, a skin biopsy should be considered to rule out urticarial vasculitis or any other disease mistaken for urticaria.

13. What common disease is associated with urticaria?

Urticaria may be associated with sinusitis. If symptoms of sinusitis are present with urticaria, sinus radiographs are a cost-effective diagnostic procedure. Chronic sinusitis may require an extended course of antibiotics (see chapter 87).

14. How is dermatographism diagnosed and treated?

Dermatographism is the most common cause of physical urticaria. Linear wheals develop rapidly after blunt, firm stroking of the skin and resolve within 1 hour. About 5% of the population has asymptomatic simple dermatographism; symptomatic dermatographism is much less common. Patients with atopic dermatitis have an increased incidence of dermatographism. For symptomatic patients, the pruritic wheals may last for several hours. Treatment consists of oral antihistamines and avoidance of trauma to the skin. Delayed dermatographism presents with linear, red nodules that develop 3–6 hours after stimulation and persist for 24–48 hours.

BIBLIOGRAPHY

1. Bush RK (ed): Clinical allergy. Med Clin North Am 76:805–840, 1992.
2. Charlesworth EN: Urticaria and angioedema: A clinical spectrum. Ann Allerg Asthma Immunol 76:484–495, 1996.
3. Copper KD: Acute and chronic urticaria and angioedema. J Am Acad Dermatol 25:146–154, 1991.
4. Fitzpatrick TB, et al (eds): Dermatology in General Medicine, 4th ed. New York, McGraw-Hill, 1993.
5. Huston DP, Bressler RB: Urticaria and angioedema. Med Clin North Am 76:805–840, 1992.
6. Kennard CD, Ellis CN: Pharmacologic therapy for urticaria. J Am Acad Dermatol 25:177–189, 1991.
7. Moschella SL, Hurley HJ (eds): Dermatology, 3rd ed. Philadelphia, W.B. Saunders, 1992.
8. Phillips TJ, Dover JS: Recent advances in dermatology. N Engl J Med 326:167–178, 1992.
9. Rothe MJ, et al: The mast cell in health and disease. JAMAC Dermatol 23:615–624, 1990.
10. Yecies LD, Kaplan AD: Urticaria. In Parker CW (ed): Clinical Immunology. Philadelphia, W.B. Saunders, 1980, pp 1283–1315.

97. SKIN INFECTIONS

Mark E. Fogarty, M.D., and Loren E. Golitz, M.D.

1. Describe the presentation and treatment of impetigo contagiosa.

Impetigo contagiosa is an infectious disorder of the skin that begins as small vesicles and progresses rapidly to erosions covered by a thick, honey-colored crust. Exposed parts of the body, such as the face and arms, are commonly involved. Most patients are children. Over the past decade, *Staphylococcus aureus* has replaced beta-hemolytic streptococci as the most common organism and accounts for approximately 85% of positive cultures. Treatment includes regular cleansing with antibacterial soap and treatment with oral erythromycin, cephalosporin, and dicloxacillin. Topical antibiotics such as mupirocin may be used instead of systemic antibiotics if skin involvement is not extensive.

2. What is ecthyma?

Ecthyma is similar to impetigo but is deeper and produces a shallow ulcer covered by crust. The causative organisms are the same as for impetigo contagiosa. The lower legs are most commonly affected, and the condition is more prevalent in warm, humid climates. Low-grade fever and lymphadenopathy commonly occur. Treatment includes warm compresses to remove the crust and oral erythromycin, cephalosporin, or dicloxacillin. With appropriate therapy the lesions of impetigo and ecthyma usually heal within 1 week.

3. What is secondary pyoderma?

Secondary pyoderma is a bacterial infection of skin associated with preceding dermatologic disorders such as atopic dermatitis, neurodermatitis, scabies, or traumatic lesions. *Staphylococcus aureus* is the causative organism in approximately 80–85% of cases; in the bulk of the remaining cases, the infectious agents are streptococci. Gram-negative organisms, including *Proteus* sp., *Pseudomonas* sp., and *Escherichia coli*, may colonize the skin in patients with other debilitating conditions, such as diabetes mellitus.

4. How is secondary pyoderma treated?

Treatment includes systemic antibiotics based on culture results and removal of crust and purulent drainage. Abscesses may need to be surgically drained. Antipruritic agents, such as hydroxyzine hydrochloride (25 mg 4 times/day), are useful in the presence of extensive excoriations. Once the infection is under control, the underlying dermatosis should be treated with topical corticosteroids, such as triamcinolone acetonide cream.

5. Describe the typical appearance and treatment of dermatophyte infection of the scalp.

Tinea capitis is a fungal infection of the scalp most commonly seen in children between the ages of 4 and 14 years. *Trichophyton tonsurans* is the most common causative organism in the United States. Infection begins as a small erythematous papule around a hair shaft and then spreads to involve surrounding hairs. Involved hairs often break off at the scalp surface, producing the appearance of black dots. Kerion, an inflammatory plaque associated with hair loss and purulent drainage, also may be caused by *T. tonsurans.*

6. Which simple clinical tests help to make the diagnosis of tinea capitis?

Wood's lamp examination of lesions caused by *Microsporum* sp. shows bright green fluorescence of hair shafts just above the skin surface of the scalp. Hair shafts and scale should be obtained for microscopic examination and culture on Sabouraud's agar. Infected areas may be scraped with a scalpel, or hairs in the infected area may be plucked. The specimen should be examined microscopically after the addition of 20–25% potassium hydroxide (KOH) solution. Hyphae and spores are seen on or within the hair shaft. The differential diagnosis include seborrheic dermatitis, atopic dermatitis, psoriasis, alopecia areata, trichotillomania, and secondary syphilis.

7. How should tinea capitis be treated?

Systemic antifungal agents are required for the treatment of tinea capitis. Adults should receive 1 gm/day of microsize griseofulvin in divided doses with meals; 6 weeks to 3 months of therapy is usually required to produce clinical resolution and negative cultures. In children, the dose of microsize griseofulvin is 10–20 mg/kg/day. Adjunctive therapy with selenium sulfide shampoo may reduce the transmission of tinea capitis to others. Inflammatory tinea capitis (kerion) should be treated with the same dose of griseofulvin plus systemic corticosteroids to reduce the inflammation that often results in areas of permanent hair loss and scarring. Although kerion resembles a purulent bacterial infection, systemic antibodies are not effective.

8. How do dermatophyte infections of the hands and feet present?

Tinea pedis and tinea manuum are fungal infections of the feet and hands, respectively. Tinea pedis occurs most commonly in the summer months. Infections are transmitted from one person to another by the use of communal pools and baths. The most common etiologic fungi include *Trichophyton rubrum* (which causes a dry, mocassin-type eruption), *Trichophyton mentagrophytes* (which may cause vesicles), and *Epidermophyton floccosum* (which is rare and usually limited to the toe webs). Cases of tinea pedis with prominent interdigital maceration and hyperkeratosis may have a secondary bacterial infection. Occasionally, a dermatophyte may involve both feet and one hand (the two-feet, one-hand syndrome). Diagnosis is based on the clinical appearance, positive culture, and a KOH preparation showing branching, septate hyphae.

9. How is a KOH preparation performed?

Unlike vaginal and mucosal KOH preparations, the keratinized epidermis requires special methods to see the hyphae within the cells. The simplest procedure is to use two glass slides, one to scrape dead skin cells and the other to "catch" the cells. The cells are then covered with a cover slip, a few drops of 20% KOH are added, and capillary action is allowed to pull the KOH under the cover slip. The specimen must then be gently heated (with a match lighter or alcohol lamp). Do not allow the KOH to boil because it will crystallize and destroy the specimen. The heat breaks down the keratinized cell wall and allows hyphae to be seen microscopically. Hyphae should cross cell walls. Focusing up and down quickly helps to differentiate between cell walls and hyphal elements.

10. How are tinea pedis and tinea manuum treated?

Treatment includes reduction of excessive moisture with talcum or antifungal powders. Eradication can be achieved with a systemic antifungal agent, such as griseofulvin (1 gm/day in divided doses with meals), but recurrence is common. Topical agents for tinea pedis or tinea manuum include tolnaftate, clotrimazole, miconazole, ketoconazole, and terbinafine. An economic topical treatment for chronic tinea pedis of the dry, mocassin type is 10% salicylic acid ointment, applied twice daily.

11. Describe the appearance of tinea corporis.

Tinea corporis includes fungal infections of glabrous skin, except the hands, feet, and groin. The most common etiologic organisms are *T. rubrum, Microsporum canis*, and *T. mentagrophytes*. Infection may be acquired from contact with infected humans or animals. Tinea corporis most commonly presents as anular lesions with an erythematous scaly border and central clearing. Animal ringworm (i.e., *M. canis*) is often inflammatory or pustular. The differential diagnosis includes other ringlike eruptions, such as erythema anulare centrifugum, nummular eczema, and granuloma anulare.

12. Can dermatophyte infection involve the face?

Yes. Dermatophyte infection of the face, called tinea faciei, may mimic lupus erythematosus, seborrheic dermatitis, and contact dermatitis. Microscopic examination of a KOH preparation of scrapings obtained from the border of the lesions shows branching, septate hyphae. A positive KOH examination may be difficult to demonstrate in the inflammatory variants of tinea. Combining fungal culture and KOH examination increases the likelihood of making the definitive diagnosis.

13. How are tinea corporis and tinea faciei treated?

Localized cases are treated with topical antifungal agents (see question 10), whereas inflammatory and widespread lesions often require treatment with griseofulvin. Because treatment of tinea corporis with griseofulvin usually requires a course of at least 6–8 weeks, the drug should be prescribed only for patients with a positive KOH examination or culture.

14. What is tinea cruris?

Tinea cruris, commonly referred to as "jock itch," begins in the groin fold and progresses with a raised, scaly border. In contrast to inguinal candidiasis, the scrotum and labia are rarely involved, the color is rarely beefy red, and satellite vesicopustules are usually absent. Scrapings of scales are usually positive for hyphae with the KOH examination. Reduction of moisture with talcum powders and application of topical antifungal agents (see question 10) are generally effective. Extensive cases may require 6–8 weeks of therapy with oral griseofulvin.

15. Describe the differentiation of cutaneous candidiasis and tinea cruris.

Infections caused by *Candida albicans* most commonly involve skinfolds, including the axilla, genitocrural, gluteal, submammary, and perianal areas. Candidiasis of the skinfold has a beefy red color and often shows satellite pustules. Obesity, diabetes mellitus, and chronic occupational exposure to excessive moisture are the most common accompanying factors. Presentation may be atypical in immunocompromised patients and may not be limited to intertriginous areas. Other manifestations of candidal infection include thrush, vulvovaginitis, and balanitis. The diagnosis is based on a KOH preparation, which shows round- or oval-budding yeast and pseudohyphae. The organism is easily cultured on Sabouraud's medium.

16. How is cutaneous candidiasis treated?

Treatment of cutaneous candidiasis includes correction of predisposing conditions such as heat and moisture and use of topical antifungal creams or ointments. Powder or cream containing nystatin may be helpful in the treatment of moist intertriginous areas. Occasionally, treatment of the gastrointestinal tract with oral nystatin, in combination with topical agents, is helpful for treating candidiasis of the anogenital area. Oral nystatin is not absorbed and is not useful alone in treating cutaneous candidiasis. Systemic antifungals (itraconazole, fluconazole, terbinafine) may be indicated for patients with chronic infections or patients with underlying immunosuppression (e.g., AIDS).

BIBLIOGRAPHY

1. Abdel-Rahman SM, Nahata MC: Oral terbinafine. A new antifungal agent. Ann Pharm 31:445–456, 1997.
2. Aly R, Berger T: Common superficial fungal infections in patients with AIDS. Clin Infect Dis 22(Suppl 2):S128–S132, 1996.
3. Fitzpatrick TB, et al (eds): Dermatology in General Medicine, 4th ed. New York, McGraw-Hill, 1993.
4. Lesher JL Jr: Recent developments in antifungal therapy. Dermatol Clin 14:163–169, 1996.
5. Moschella SL, Hurley HJ (eds): Dermatology, 3rd ed. Philadelphia, W.B. Saunders, 1992.
6. Phillips TJ, Dover JS: Recent advances in dermatology. N Engl J Med 326:167–178, 1992.

98. ISOLATED SKIN LESIONS

Mark E. Fogarty, M.D., and Loren E. Golitz, M.D.

1. How do common warts present?

Common warts (verrucae vulgares) appear as sharply marginated keratotic papules with a rough surface. They may appear anywhere on the skin but are most common on the dorsal surfaces of the hand and fingers. Common warts are a neoplasm caused by the human papillomavirus.

2. Describe the two common treatments for warts.

1. Twice daily application of 17% salicylic acid solution (Compound W, Wart-Off) results in sloughing of keratin. Prolonged therapy is usually required. Salicylic acid plaster (Mediplast) can be trimmed to cover the wart and left in place for up to 1 week at a time. Gentle debridement of the dead tissue followed by retreatment with the plaster usually results in resolution of the wart within 6–8 weeks.

2. Cryotherapy with liquid nitrogen may be applied with a probe, pressurized spray, or cotton swab. The wart and a narrow rim of normal skin should be frozen for 20–30 seconds, allowed to thaw, and frozen a second time. The treatment is associated with mild burning pain. The double freeze-thaw method should be repeated at 7–10-day intervals until the warts are eliminated. Patients should be told that formation of a blister is an expected effect. The fluid should be drained and the area kept clean.

3. What topical agents are useful in the treatment of genital warts?

For most genital warts (condylomata acuminatum), 25% podophyllin in tincture of benzoin may be applied in the office. Petroleum jelly then should be applied to the normal skin to protect it from irritation. The podophyllin must be washed off in 4 hours. The treatment is repeated weekly until the condylomata are gone. Podophyllin should not be given to patients for home treatment because of the potential for severe reactions. Podofilox may be used topically on genital condylomata and has the advantage that the patient may apply it at home. Less commonly used therapies include 5-fluorouracil and intralesional interferon or bleomycin.

4. How does basal cell carcinoma present?

Basal cell carcinoma, the most common cutaneous malignancy, is found predominantly in patients with a history of chronic sun exposure; 80-90% of lesions are found on the head and neck. Lesions typically are nonkeratinized papules with a smooth translucent surface and telangiectatic vessels. Large lesions commonly have central ulceration and crusting. Basal cell carcinomas may be heavily pigmented and difficult to differentiate from malignant melanoma.

5. Describe the appearance of actinic keratosis.

Actinic keratosis is an isolated macule or papule in a sun-exposed area that is red-brown in color and has a dry, rough adherent scale.

6. Why should actinic keratosis be distinguished from seborrheic keratosis?

Actinic keratosis is a premalignant lesion that leads to squamous cell carcinoma of the skin and thus should be removed. Seborrheic keratosis, which appears on both the face and trunk, is a brownish papule with "stuck-on" appearance and has no particular implication (other than cosmetic).

7. Describe the typical appearance of squamous cell carcinoma.

Squamous cell carcinomas also arise in sun-damaged skin such as the head, neck, or arms. Lesions appear as firm skin-colored or slightly erythematous nodules with a distinct margin. The surface is rough or verrucous, and ulceration is common. Squamous cell carcinomas of the skin often develop from preexisting actinic keratoses.

8. How does the clinical course of squamous cell carcinoma of the lip differ from that of typical squamous cell carcinoma?

Squamous cell carcinomas that develop on the lower lip, in burn scar, or in areas of prior radiation therapy tend to behave in a more aggressive manner and may metastasize.

9. How are basal and squamous cell carcinomas diagnosed and treated?

The definitive diagnosis is based on histologic examination of a biopsy specimen. Metastases are rare in basal cell carcinomas and squamous cell carcinomas in chronically sun-damaged skin. However, both tumors may be locally aggressive. Treatments include surgical excision, curettage and electrosurgery, micrographic surgery, and radiotherapy. Referral to a dermatologist is appropriate.

10. What is the most life-threatening cutaneous malignancy?

Malignant melanoma, although less common than basal and squamous cell carcinoma, has a much higher mortality rate.

11. Who is at risk for the development of melanoma?

- People who are fair-skinned, blue-eyed, red-haired, and freckled
- People with dysplastic nevi (atypical moles)
- Patients with a family history of melanoma
- People with a large congenital melanocyte nevus
- Immunocompromised patients

12. What features of a pigmented skin lesion suggest the diagnosis of malignant melanoma?

The **ABCD rule** can be used to evaluate a pigmented lesion for the possibility of melanoma or melanoma precursor (dysplastic nevus):

Asymmetry	Color variegation or dark color
Border irregularity	**D**iameter > 0.6 cm

The ABCD features are more common in melanomas than in benign pigmented lesions. Ulceration, pruritus, pain, new lesions, or changes in existing pigmented lesions also should arouse suspicion.

13. How should pigmented skin lesions be evaluated?

Clinically atypical lesions should be excised to the level of fat and submitted in their entirety for histologic evaluation. Sampling a portion of a pigmented lesion is not recommended, because a sampling error may occur. Shave biopsies of potentially malignant lesions destroy the pathologist's ability to measure tumor depth and thus interfere with prognostication. Patients with many pigmented lesions or a personal or family history should be evaluated by a dermatologist with special interest in pigmented lesions.

14. How can a hemangioma be distinguished from a nodular melanoma?

Both lesions may appear as a reddish-bluish, dome-shaped nodule. However, compression of a hemangioma (with a glass microscopic slide) results in blanching. Biopsy is indicated to make a definitive diagnosis.

15. How is the prognosis of melanoma established?

Definitive diagnosis of a suspicious lesion is made by excisional biopsy. Prognosis of localized melanoma (localized to the skin) is based largely on tumor thickness, which is measured histopathologically. Lesions less than 0.76 mm in thickness are associated with a favorable 5-year survival rate.

16. What treatment and follow-up are indicated?

Stage I melanoma is treated with surgical excision. Recent studies have shown that wide surgical margins usually are not necessary. Lesions up to 1 mm thick can be treated with 1-cm margins, whereas 2-cm margins may be indicated for thicker lesions. Prospective, randomized studies of prophylactic regional lymph node dissection have shown no survival benefit. Patients should have regular follow-up for local recurrence, metastases, and second primary melanomas. Patients with melanoma are best followed by oncologists, dermatologists, or other specially trained physicians.

BIBLIOGRAPHY

1. DeDavid M, et al: A study of large congenital melanocytic nevi and associated malignant melanomas. J Am Acad Dermatol 36:409–416, 1997.
2. Fitzpatrick TB, et al (eds): Dermatology in General Medicine, 4th ed. New York, McGraw-Hill, 1993.
3. Gallagher RP, McLean DI: The epidemiology of acquired melanocytic nevi. A brief review. Dermatol Clin 13:595–603, 1995.
4. Greenstein DS, Rogers GS: Management of stage I malignant melanoma. Dermatol Surg 21:927–937, 1995.
5. Koh HK: Cutaneous melanoma. N Engl J Med 325:171–182, 1991.
6. Millikan LE, Shrum JP: An update on common skin diseases. Acne, psoriasis, contact dermatitis and warts. Postgrad Med 91(6):96–98, 101–104, 107–110, 1992.
7. Moschella SL, Hurley HJ (eds): Dermatology, 3rd ed. Philadelphia, W.B. Saunders, 1992.
8. Preston DS, Stern RS: Nonmelanoma cancers of the skin. N Engl J Med 327:1649–1662, 1992.
9. Wang CY, et al: Skin cancers associated with acquired immunodeficiency syndrome. Mayo Clin Proc 70:766–772, 1995.
10. Whiteman D, Green A: Melanoma and sunburn. Cancer Causes Control 5:564–572, 1994.

99. ACNE

Mark E. Fogarty, M.D., and Loren E. Golitz, M.D.

1. Describe the pathogenesis of acne vulgaris.

Follicular orifices become filled with debris and may or may not become inflamed, pustular, or even cystic. Inflammation is due to colonization with lipophilic bacteria. Hormonal influences contribute to the initiation of these lesions.

2. Do adults experience acne?

Yes. Although acne vulgaris is usually a disease of young adults, up to 20% of adults may experience some form of acne. In addition, acne rosacea, characterized by central facial erythema and pustules (without comedones), is an adult-onset disease more common in women. Acne rosacea may lead to connective tissue overgrowth (rhinophyma) and inflammatory lesions of the eye.

3. What external factors aggravate acne?

1. Trauma from overvigorous skin scrubbing or irritant contact (athletic gear, picking acne lesions)

2. Topical agents (cosmetics and industrial compounds that are comedone-forming, such as lanolin, paraffin oil, and oleic acid)

4. What drugs may cause an acneiform eruption or exacerbate underlying acne?

Glucocorticoids (topical or systemic), phenytoin, phenobarbital, isoniazid, and lithium.

5. What topical agents are effective therapies for acne vulgaris?

The treatment of acne vulgaris includes various topical agents, which may be more effective when used in combination. Benzoyl peroxide formulations function as topical antibacterial agents. Classic topical antibiotic agents include clindamycin and erythromycin. Topical vitamin A (tretinoin) interferes with the hyperkeratinization that plugs pilosebaceous units to produce comedones. The combination of 5% benzoyl peroxide in the morning and tretinoin (0.05% cream) at bedtime seems to work better than a single topical agent in many patients.

6. What are the indications for oral antibiotics?

Oral antibiotics are indicated in patients with moderate-to-severe acne or mild-to-moderate acne that does not respond to topical therapy. Oral antibiotics decrease the number of *Propionibacterium acnes* in the pilosebaceous units. The organisms break down triglycerides to free fatty acids, thus increasing inflammation. The oral antibiotics most commonly used are tetracycline and erythromycin at doses of 500–1000 mg/day in divided dosages. The dose may be decreased to 250 mg/day after 1–2 months if skin shows improvement.

7. Are there contraindications to the use of tetracycline?

Yes. Tetracycline is contraindicated in pregnant women and in children under 10 years of age because of its effects on developing teeth and bones. Tetracycline may interfere with the effectiveness of oral contraceptive agents. Dairy products reduce the absorption of tetracycline, which is best taken on an empty stomach.

8. What are the indications for second-line antibiotics in the treatment of acne?

In patients who fail to improve after 2–3 months of oral tetracycline or erythromcycin, other antibiotics, such as minocycline, should be considered.

9. When should isotretinoin (Accutane) be used?

Isotretinoin is indicated for severe nodulocystic acne refractory to standard therapy. Because of potential severe side effects, patient reliability is important. Doses usually range from 0.5–1.0 mg/kg/day with doses up to 2.0 mg/kg/day for severe truncal involvement. Therapy should be continued for 15–20 weeks and discontinued after 70–80% improvement is achieved. Monthly visits with close monitoring of side effects, response, and blood work are usually necessary.

10. What are the most common side effects of isotretinoin therapy?

Cheilitis occurs in almost every case. Other side effects include dry mouth, xerosis, conjunctivitis, vertebral hyperostoses, elevated serum lipids, mental depression, and hepatic toxicity. The most important side effect is severe fetal malformation.

11. What precautions should be taken before prescribing isotretinoin to women of childbearing age?

Women of childbearing age should receive isotretinoin only after reading the educational material provided by the manufacturer and giving informed consent, because it has been associated with a 25-fold increase in the risk of severe fetal abnormalities. Women of childbearing age should use two reliable methods of birth control simultaneously and continuously, starting at least 1 month before initiation of therapy. A negative serum pregnancy test should be obtained before initiating therapy, and patients should receive counseling about contraception. Pregnancy should be avoided for approximately 1 year after completing therapy with isotretinoin. Monthly pregnancy tests are imperative.

BIBLIOGRAPHY

1. Fitzpatrick TB, et al (eds): Dermatology in General Medicine, 4th ed. New York, McGraw-Hill, 1993.
2. Leyden JJ: Therapy for acne vulgaris. N Engl J Med 336:1156–1162, 1997.
3. Moschella SL, Hurley HJ (eds): Dermatology, 3rd ed. Philadelphia, W.B. Saunders, 1992.
4. Phillips TJ, Dover JS: Recent advances in dermatology. N Engl J Med 326:167–178, 1992.

100. DISORDERS OF THE NAILS AND HAIR

Mark E. Fogarty, M.D., and Loren E. Golitz, M.D.

1. How does fungal infection of the nail present?

Onychomycosis, which is most commonly caused by *Trichophyton rubrum* and *Trichophyton mentagrophytes*, usually begins at the distal edge of the nail and causes hyperkeratosis beneath the nailplate and distal separation of the nailplate from the nailbed. The fungus grows proximally, leading to thickening and crumbling of the nailplate. Usually some nails are spared. Concomitant tinea pedis or tinea manuum is common. As a general rule, the feet should be examined when a patient presents with a rash of the hands or fingernails.

2. When is treatment of onychomycosis indicated?

Onychomycosis most commonly has cosmetic sequelae. But thickened nails can be painful and usually disabling. Treatment with griseofulvin and ketoconazole is common and results in high failure and recurrence rates. New systemic antifungals (itraconazole, tertinadine) are more effective and safer to use. A positive fungal culture of nail keratin is necessary before committing the patient to prolonged therapy because many other conditions may mimic onychomycoses. Topical therapy for fungal infection of nails or hair is ineffective.

3. What diseases are associated with pitting of the nailbed?

Psoriasis causes pitting of the surface of the nailplate due to involvement of nail matrix. Discoloration, thickening, and distal onycholysis also may be seen. Dermatitis of the posterior nailfold skin may cause pitting or irregularity of the nailplate. Alopecia areata, a form of patchy nonscarring hair loss, also may be associated with nail pitting.

4. What do Beau's lines signify?

Acute illness, such as systemic infection or thyrotoxicosis, may cause temporary malfunction of the nail matrix, leading to development of transverse grooves called Beau's lines. The distance of Beau's lines may date the patient's illness; nails grow at the rate of approximately 1 mm/month.

5. How specific are splinter hemorrhages for subacute bacterial endocarditis (SBE)?

Splinter hemorrhages are seen in patients with SBE but also may be caused by local trauma in otherwise healthy people. Splinter hemorrhages also have been reported with mitral stenosis, glomerulonephritis, vasculitis, cirrhosis, and various other diseases. Rheumatoid arthritis may cause excessive ridging and beading of the nails; systemic sclerosis (scleroderma) causes abnormalities in the capillary arcade of the nailbed, resulting in telangiectatic dilatations that can be seen with a hand-held magnifying glass.

6. What are the common causes of scarring and nonscarring alopecia?

The first distinction to make in a patient with alopecia is whether the hair is scarring or nonscarring. In nonscarring alopecia, the skin appears and feels normal. Examination of the skin in patients with scarring alopecia reveals atrophy, lack of visible follicular openings, and often erythema and hyperpigmentation or hypopigmentation. Causes of nonscarring alopecia include alopecia areata, androgenic alopecia (common baldness), and telogen effluvium (hair loss often seen in women 2–3 months after childbirth). Examples of scarring alopecia include discoid lupus erythematosus, lichen planopilaris (a form of lichen planus), and folliculitis decalvans.

7. Name three common causes of patchy alopecia.

The second major question to be answered in the clinic is whether the alopecia is patchy or diffuse. Three examples of patchy alopecia are alopecia areata, trichotillomania, and discoid lupus erythematosus. Alopecia areata shows round areas of hair loss without scarring. At the periphery of the patches, one may identify small hair shafts (approximately 3–4 mm long) that taper toward the skin surface (exclamation point hairs). Trichotillomania, which may be difficult to distinguish from alopecia areata, often occurs in children and adolescents. Hair loss is patchy, usually without scarring. However, careful examination of the patch of hair loss reveals broken hairs of variable length and often superficial excoriations and areas of scale. In addition to the scalp, eyebrows and eyelashes also are commonly involved. Invariably the patient denies pulling out the hair. Discoid lupus erythematosus is a form of patchy alopecia with scarring. A round or disklike area typically shows central hypopigmentation and atrophy with a hyperpigmented active margin. The surface is scaly, and often hair follicles are plugged with keratin, resembling the open comedones seen in acne. Other forms of patchy alopecia include trauma, radiation therapy, and metastatic carcinoma, particularly breast cancer in women.

Syphilis may cause patchy alopecia in its secondary phase. The classic presentation is a nonscarring, "moth-eaten" appearance to the scalp. Other signs of secondary syphilis may or may not be present. A positive serologic test for syphilis confirms the diagnosis.

8. What causes alopecia at the periphery of the scalp, usually in women?

Occasionally alopecia involves primarily the periphery of the scalp in the areas of the temples and above the ears. This form of alopecia is almost always secondary to traction, such as ponytails, corn-rowing, or tight hair curlers.

9. Which systemic illnesses may result in diffuse alopecia?

Telogen effluvium is the term given to the diffuse alopecia that results when many scalp follicles suddenly enter a resting phase, leading to fall-out of hair shafts. Typically this change occurs 2–3 months after an acute illness, major surgery, childbirth, or severe emotional breakdown. Systemic diseases such as hyper- and hypothyroidism and systemic lupus erythematosus also may cause telogen effluvium. The skin appears normal. Patients can be assured that the hair will grow back, although regrowth may take several months.

10. What nutritional deficiencies may cause hair loss?

Biotin, iron, protein, and zinc.

11. Characterize androgenic alopecia.

Androgenic alopecia (male- and female-pattern baldness) is usually classified as diffuse alopecia, although hair loss is accentuated in the areas of the temples and crown. The thickness of hair behind the ears usually appears normal. Most patients have a family history of first-degree relatives with significant androgenic alopecia. Androgen-producing tumors are a relatively rare cause of androgenic alopecia. On rare occasions, alopecia areata may present as diffuse alopecia.

BIBLIOGRAPHY

1. Abdel-Rahman SM, Nahata MC: Oral terbinafine: A new antifungal agent. Ann Pharm 31:445–456, 1997.
2. Fitzpatrick TR, et al (eds): Dermatology in General Medicine, 4th ed. New York, McGraw-Hill, 1993.
3. Hull PR: Onychomycosis—treatment, relapse, and re-infection. Dermatology 194(Suppl I):7–9, 1997.
4. Lesher JL Jr: Recent developments in antifungal therapy. Dermatol Clin 14:163–169, 1996.
5. Moschella SL, Hurley HJ (eds): Dermatology, 3rd ed. Philadelphia, W.B. Saunders, 1992.

101. DERMATOLOGIC MANIFESTATIONS OF SYSTEMIC DISEASES

Jeanette Mladenovic, M.D., and Meg A. Lemon, M.D,

1. What conditions should be considered when a patient complains of pruritus but no rash is present?

Chronic renal disease. Up to 80% of patients undergoing hemodialysis have pruritus. The cause is unclear, and pruritus has no clear relationship to renal function tests. Patients undergoing dialysis have an increased number of intradermal mast cells and increased pruritus in response to histamine injection. Treatment with antihistamines is usually ineffective. A recent study demonstrated a marked improvement of pruritus in patients treated with erythropoietin. In some patients with secondary hyperparathyroidism, the pruritus may resolve after parathyroidectomy. Therapy with oral psoralen and long-wave ultraviolet light (PUVA) has been effective in some cases of pruritus related to renal failure, possibly through an effect on cutaneous mast cells.

Cholestatic liver disease. Although itching is correlated with increased levels of unconjugated bilirubin, the amount of pruritus is not. Biliary drainage or treatment with bile salt binders (colestipol or cholestyramine) often improves the pruritus.

Endocrine diseases. Thyrotoxicosis may present with generalized itching. Pruritus in hypothyroidism is probably related to dryness of the skin. Diabetes mellitus is usually not a cause of itching, although it may be associated with candidiasis or folliculitis.

Malignancy. With the exception of Hodgkin's lymphoma and polycythemia vera (PV), malignancies rarely cause significant pruritus. One study of 360 patients with Hodgkin's lymphoma found that 5.8% presented with generalized pruritus. "Bath itch" is a diffuse prickling sensation that occurs in 50% of patients with PV 30–60 minutes after a bath or shower. The occurrence of pruritus may precede the development of PV by several years.

Senescence. Itching occurs in many older patients. Most cases are not associated with systemic disease and are believed to be related to dry skin. The mainstay of treatment is hydration of the skin with water and moisturizing creams and avoidance of drying soaps.

Psychogenic disorders. Generalized or localized pruritus (commonly anogenital) may be a manifestation of anxiety. The diagnosis is made after primary skin diseases and systemic disorders are excluded. Extensive excoriation may produce areas of neurodermatitis. Patients with severe psychiatric illnesses may present with parasitophobia manifested by the sensation of worms crawling on or under the skin.

2. Describe the evaluation of patients who have pruritus without rash.

The history should focus on medications, underlying diseases, and dry skin. The physical examination should evaluate for adenopathy and organomegaly. Screening laboratory tests may include complete blood count, chest radiograph, and liver, renal, and thyroid function tests. Patients who have pruritus without a rash should be followed for evaluation of symptoms. Therapy is based on treatment of the underlying disorder. In idiopathic cases, a trial of emollients and oral antihistamines, such as hydroxyzine hydrochloride, is indicated.

3. Why is it important to distinguish palpable purpura from purpura?

Palpable purpura is always a manifestation of systemic disease, whereas purpuric lesions may result from abnormalities in the clotting system or, less commonly, may be isolated cutaneous lesions, with the exception of fat or cholesterol emboli.

4. What types of diseases should be considered in patients with palpable purpura?

Palpable purpura results from vasculitis or embolic disease. Lesions due to vasculitis are seen in patients with polyarteritis nodosa and leukocytoclastic vasculitis. Embolic diseases include meningococcemia, disseminated gonococcemia, ecthyma gangrenosum (due to *Pseudomonas* sp. or other gram-negative organisms), and Rocky Mountain spotted fever. Leukocytoclastic vasculitis is strongly associated with hepatitis C virus infection.

5. Describe erythema nodosum.

Erythema nodosum presents as red subcutaneous nodules, most commonly on the shins. The nodules become bluish as they resolve. Erythema nodosum is often idiopathic; however, the most common systemic associations are streptococcal infection, sarcoidosis, inflammatory bowel disease, and, less commonly, fungal infections (e.g., coccidioidomycosis, tuberculosis, histoplasmosis) and drug toxicity.

6. What is the significance of acanthosis nigricans?

Acanthosis nigricans is an acquired velvety hyperpigmentation in the axilla and groin. It is most often associated with obesity, although it may be associated with other endocrinopathies as well as malignancy, usually of the gastrointestinal tract. Thus, in patients with idiopathic onset and no clearly ascribable cause, a search for malignancy (with attention to appropriate screening for age) should be considered.

7. What does vitiligo imply?

Patients with vitiligo have an increased incidence of autoimmune disorders, especially hypothyroidism, Graves' disease, and pernicious anemia. Less frequently, a variant of melanoma may present with truncal vitiligo.

8. What systemic diseases should be considered in patients with nonhealing ulcers?

In addition to evident vascular diseases (arterial insufficiency of any etiology, microvascular disease of diabetes, venous insufficiency), nonhealing ulcers may be associated with (1) local malignancy, (2) hemoglobinopathies and blood dyscrasias (spherocytosis, cryoglobulin), (3) pyoderma gangrenosum (although the appearance of this entity is characteristic), and (4) vasculitis (rheumatoid vasculitis, Raynaud's phenomenon, Behçet's disease).

9. What diseases are characterized by photosensitivity reactions?

A number of skin diseases, lupus erythematosus, and dermatomyositis are aggravated by the sun. However, true acquired photosensitivity reactions evidenced by erythema, fragility, telangiectasias, recurrent blistering, bullae, and desquamation in sun-exposed areas is limited to a short differential diagnosis: drug sensitization (both topical and systemically administered), porphyria cutanea tarda, and, on rare occasions, acquired metabolic defects. Photoallergy differs in that an eczematous picture develops, again most commonly in response to drug sensitization.

10. What disorder is associated with yellow plaques surrounded by erythematous halos on extensor surfaces of the extremities?

Such lesions may represent xanthomata, which may be associated with lipid disorders such as hypertriglyceridemia. Common xanthelasma of the eyelids are usually *not* associated with defects in lipid metabolism or cardiovascular disease.

BIBLIOGRAPHY

1. Daoud MS, et al: Chronic hepatitis C and skin diseases: A review. Mayo Clin Proc 70:559–564, 1995.
2. Fitzpatrick TR, et al (eds): Dermatology in General Medicine, 4th ed. New York, McGraw-Hill, 1993.
3. Isselbacher KJ, Brownwald E, Martin JB, et al: Harrison's Principles of Medicine, 13th ed. New York, McGraw-Hill, 1994.
4. Moschella SL, Hurley HJ (eds): Dermatology, 3rd ed. Philadelphia, W.B. Saunders, 1992.
5. Sontheimer RD, Provost TT: Cutaneous manifestations of rheumatologic disease. Baltimore, Williams & Wilkins, 1996.

XIV. Care of Special Patients

102. THE ADOLESCENT PATIENT

Roberta K. Beach, M.D., M.P.H.

1. What is special about adolescence?

Adolescence is a time of dramatic physical and developmental changes that challenge the coping skills of adolescents, families, health professionals, and communities to a greater degree than any other age. For convenience, the age range of 13–19 years is often specified as adolescence, but this transitional phase between childhood and adulthood lasts for over a decade, beginning around age 10 years and extending through age 21 years or later. Dynamic changes in three areas are of special interest:

1. **Physical changes.** The growth spurt, development of adult body physique, hormonal changes, sexual development, and the ability to reproduce come with puberty, although there is marked variation in timing and progression of physical growth.

2. **Psychosocial (developmental) changes.** Essential tasks of adolescence include emancipation from family, development of peer relationships and sexual intimacy, determination of educational and vocational goals, and establishment of identity and self-responsibility. Major social milestones ares achieved. The legal rights to drive, vote, and drink and cultural rites of passage such as leaving school, leaving home, first sexual relationship, and first job have immense social significance to the adolescent.

3. **Cognitive changes.** The adolescent progresses from concrete operational thinking ("here and now") to abstract operational thinking with a maturing ability to engage in deductive reasoning, to understand risk and benefit, and to appreciate future consequences of current choices.

2. Characterize the adolescent personality.

Although adolescents are frequently portrayed as hostile, rebellious, and alienated, in fact they have many positive attributes. Adolescents are intensely idealistic and often have a passion for fairness and social justice. They are energetic and enjoy peak physical health. They tend to be optimistic about the future and excited about dreams, plans, and goals. They have a tremendous resilience and capacity for growth, and even serious problems can be converted into learning experiences and opportunities for change. The majority (about 80%) of adolescents progress through this stage of life with only modest difficulty and without serious social problems.

3. How do I get an adolescent patient to talk to me?

Although caregivers often consider them difficult to interview, adolescents are actually eager to find someone "safe" to talk to about their concerns. Because they often believe that "no one understands me," they are highly sensitive to disapproval or being judged negatively. Several techniques help to establish a sense of trust that promotes the therapeutic alliance:

- **Privacy.** Interview the adolescent alone and with full attention in a setting free of interruptions.
- **Confidentiality.** Clarify the policy on confidentiality, and assure patients that nothing will be shared without permission, unless it is life-threatening (such as a suicide attempt) or legally mandated (such as child abuse).

- **Listening skills.** Listen much more than you talk, interrupt rarely, do not lecture, and pay attention to body language, both yours and the patient's.
- **Nonjudgmental approach.** Avoid assumptions, respect differences, and show genuine interest.
- **Open-ended questions.** Use open-ended, nonthreatening questions early in the interview ("Tell me what a typical day in your life is like").
- **Third-person examples.** Lead into sensitive questions by using third-person examples ("Have any of your friends experimented with drugs?").
- **Direct questions.** Once rapport is established, ask direct questions for specific information ("Have you had sex in the past 3 months? Do you think you could be pregnant?").
- **Hidden agenda.** Although the chief complaint is the "entrée to care," frequently an underlying concern motivates the visit. Hidden agendas often relate to sexual concerns.
- **Reflective listening.** If the adolescent is unwilling to talk, reflective listening techniques are the most helpful approach ("You seem very sad," "You said you hate being here … hate?"). Wait patiently for answers.
- **Positive reinforcement.** Adolescents are hungry for honest praise and support ("It took a lot of courage for you to talk about this. Thank you").

4. What are the three developmental stages of adolescence?

Psychosocial development is a dynamic process that continues throughout the lifespan. Adolescence is commonly divided into three developmental stages: **early** (11–14 years), **middle** (15–17 years), and **late** (18–21 years). Age ranges are approximate, and girls tend to progress through the stages earlier than boys. At each stage, characteristic changes take place in cognitive thinking, behaviors, typical health concerns, and the most effective caregiver approach to the patient. Behavioral issues are usually subdivided into the four task areas: family, peers, school/vocation, and self-perception/identity. The following table briefly summarizes the characteristics of each stage.

Adolescent Developmental Stages

	EARLY ADOLESCENCE (11–14 YR)	MIDDLE ADOLESCENCE (15–17 YR)	LATE ADOLESCENCE (18–24 YR)
Cognitive thinking	Concrete thinking: here and now. Appreciate immediate reactions to behavior but no sense of later consequences.	Early abstract thinking: inductive/deductive reasoning; ability to connect separate events; understand later consequences	Abstract thinking: adult ability to think abstractly; philosophical; intense idealism about love, religion, social problems
Psychosocial task areas			
1. Family—independence	Transition from obedient to rebellious Ambivalence about wishes (dependence/independence) Hero worship of other adults	Insistence on independence, privacy May have overt rebellion or sulky withdrawal Much testing of limits	Emancipation (leave home) Reestablishment of family ties Become legally responsible for care
2. Peers—social/sexual	Same-sex "best friend" "Am I normal?" concerns Sexual intercourse not normal at this age; indicates family dysfunction	Dating Sexual experimentation Risk-taking actions Need to please significant peers (of either sex)	Partner selection (serial monogamy) Mature friendships True intimacy possible only after own identity is established

(Table continued on following page.)

Adolescent Developmental Stages (Continued)

	EARLY ADOLESCENCE (11–14 YR)	MIDDLE ADOLESCENCE (15–17 YR)	LATE ADOLESCENCE (18–24 YR)
Psychosocial task areas *(Cont.)*			
3. School—vocation	Middle school Need structured setting Goals unrealistic, changing Want to copy favorite role model	High school Need choices, electives, more flexibility Beginning to identify skills, interests Start part-time jobs	Full-time work or college Identify realistic career goals Watch for apathy (no future plans) or alienation; correlated with negative outcomes, such as unplanned pregnancy or juvenile crime
4. Self-perception—identity	Poor self-image Losing child's role but do not have adult role; hence low self-esteem Tend to use denial (it can't happen to me)	Confusion about self-image Seek group identity Very narcissistic Impulsive, impatient	Realistic, positive self-image Able to consider others' needs, less narcissistic Able to reject group pressure if not in self-interest
5. Values	Stage II values (back-scratching): good behavior in exchange for rewards	Stage II values (conformity): behavior that peer group values	Stage IV values (social responsibility): behavior consistent with laws and duty
Chief health issues (other than acute illness)	Psychosomatic symptoms Fatigue and "growing pains" Concerns about normalcy Screening for growth and development problems	Outcomes of sexual-experimentation (prevention of pregnancy, STDs, AIDS) Health-risk behaviors (smoking, drugs, alcohol, driving) Crisis counseling (e.g., runaways, acting-out, family problems)	Health promotion/healthy lifestyles Contraception and STD/AIDS prevention Self-responsibility for health and health care Transition to adult care settings
Professional approach	Firm, direct support Convey limits—simple, concrete choices Do *not* align with parents, but be an objective, caring *adult* Encourage parental presence in clinic, but interview adolescent alone	Be an objective sounding board (but let them solve own problems) Negotiate choices Ensure confidentiality Adapt system to walk-ins, impulsiveness, testing of limits	Allow mature participation in decisions Act as a resource Idealistic stage; convey "professional" image Can expect patient to examine underlying wishes, motives regarding behavior

5. What are the physical stages of physical growth?

Compared with the complexities of psychosocial development, physical development during adolescence tends to be orderly and straightforward. Growth is divided into five stages from pre-pubertal to adult. Originally called Tanner stages after John Tanner's classic descriptions, they are now referred to as sexual maturing ratings (SMR) 1 through 5. The onset of puberty is highly variable but in girls normally begins between 8 and 14 years and in boys between 9 and 16 years. Physical growth continues for 5–6 years until adult stature is achieved. In girls, the progression usually begins with breast budding at **thelarche** (SMR 2), followed by pubic hair at **pubarche** (SMR 3), first menses at **menarche** (SMR 4), and, finally, completion of pubic hair and breast growth (SMR 5). The average age of menarche in American girls is 12.3 years. The peak female growth spurt occurs immediately before menarche (SMR 2–3). Bone epiphyses close approximately 2 years after menarche, and growth is completed. In boys, the progressions begins with early enlargement of the testes (SMR 2), followed by growth of pubic hair (SMR 3), penile growth (SMR 3–4), peak growth spurt (SMR 3–4), and, finally, facial hair and completion of genital and pubic hair growth (SMR 5). The average age of first nocturnal emission (wet dream) in boys is 13–14 years. In both boys and girls, pubic hair extends onto the thighs during SMR 5 and heralds the completion of physical growth.

6. When is puberty considered precocious?

Sexual precocity is the appearance of sexual maturation before age 8 years in girls and age 9 years in boys. Pubertal development that is out of phase with peers is a cause of great concern to early adolescents. Early pubertal development (too soon) is usually a concern of girls. Delayed pubertal development (too late) is typically a concern of boys.

Breast budding in girls is normal from age 8 years. It may be unilateral, causing concern about a "breast tumor" when noted in an 8- or 9-year-old girl. However, a breast bud should *never* be biopsied (removal destroys future breast growth). Menarche may occur as early as 9 or 10 years, especially in overnourished girls. Complete puberty in girls before the age of 8 years is termed precocious puberty and is caused by the presence of gonadotropins and sex hormones (estrogens and androgens). The differential diagnosis includes hormone-secreting tumors (brain, liver, adrenal gland, ovary); exogenous administration of estrogen, anabolic steroids, or androgens; and hypothyroidism, neurofibromatosis, congenital adrenal hyperplasia, and other rare disorders. Virilization of a young girl indicates an endocrine disorder.

7. When should delayed puberty be evaluated?

If there are no signs of puberty by age 16 years, delayed puberty should be evaluated. The most common causes of delayed puberty include familial short stature, constitutional growth delay, and chronic illness. A rare cause is gonadal failure (Kallman syndrome) in which hypogonadotrophic hypogonadism results in permanent absence of pubertal development. Boys with genetic short stature tend to grow at a rate below but parallel to the third percentile throughout childhood and adolescence. They often begin puberty at the same time as their peers. They will always be short. In constitutional growth delay, the onset of puberty is delayed, but the patient eventually catches up in growth. Growth hormone deficiency should be considered if height is 3–4 standard deviations below the mean. In delayed puberty, the most important aspects of evaluation are the family history, past growth pattern, SMR stage, medical history, bone age radiographs, and measurement of 8-AM serum testosterone in boys or serum follicle-stimulating hormone in girls.

8. Which chronic illnesses are responsible for delayed puberty?

Chronic illnesses that may delay puberty include severe asthma, other pulmonary disorders, renal disease, cardiac disorders, and inflammatory bowel disease.

9. What are the primary health issues of adolescents?

Major morbidity and mortality during adolescence relate to risk-taking behaviors and experimentation. Health concerns result from complex behavioral decisions and include pregnancy, substance abuse, sexually transmitted diseases, infection with human immunodeficiency virus (HIV), depression, suicide, violence, and motor vehicle injuries.

10. What are some ways to screen for adolescent substance abuse?

Primary caregivers should routinely screen adolescents for alcohol and other drug use. Studies show that 90% of high-school students have tried alcohol and one-half of students have used illicit drugs. Adolescent substance use occurs along a continuum, ranging from **experimental use** (a normal developmental variation) to **regular use** (often in a social context), **problematic use** (resulting in negative consequences), **substance abuse** (loss of control and continued use despite harm), and, finally, **addiction** (physiologic and psychologic dependency). Interventions are most effective if adolescents who are risk of developing a substance abuse disorder can be identified during the first three stages. Four questions have good ability to predict which adolescents may be at risk:

1. Do you smoke cigarettes?
2. Have you ever been suspended from school?
3. Has anyone (parent, teacher, friend) ever thought you had a problem with alcohol or drugs?
4. Have you ridden in a car driven by someone (including yourself) who had been using alcohol or drugs?

Adolescents at high risk also include those whose closest friends drink or use drugs or who have a close family member who has a problem with alcohol or drugs.

One of the most useful tools to screen for serious drug and alcohol problems is the **CAGE** series of questions validated in adults and modified for adolescents:

C = Have you ever felt the need to **cut down** on your use of alcohol or drugs?

A = Have you ever gotten **annoyed** by someone's criticism of your alcohol or drug use?

G = Do you ever feel **guilty** or bad about your alcohol or drug use?

E = Do you ever need an **eye-opener**, a drink or drinks in the morning before you go to school?

Two or more "yes" answers have a high degree of sensitivity and specificity in diagnosing substance abuse or dependency.

11. Which adolescents are at risk of suicide?

Suicide is the third leading cause of death among adolescents, exceeded only by motor vehicle accidents and homicide. Adolescent suicide rates have doubled in the past 20 years, and national studies indicate that 5% of boys and 13% of girls have attempted suicide. Suicide attempts have been found to be associated with depression, substance use, overall number of life stressors, gender, and impulsive behaviors. Clinicians should recognize that adolescents at risk of suicide often have a cluster of other health risk behaviors, including lack of seat belt use, physical fighting and gun carrying, tobacco use, and illicit substance use. A history of suicide in a close family is also a high risk factor. The single biggest risk factor in the medical history is a previous suicide attempt.

Over one-half of adolescents who attempt suicide make contact with a physician in the month preceding their attempt. Although no brief screening questionnaires have been validated to be highly predictive for suicide risk, two questions are widely recommended for office use:

1. Have you felt sad or depressed for more than 3 days in a row (or much of the time)?
2. Have you thought of killing yourself in the past 3 months?

More subtle warning signs include a history of declining school performance, increasing family conflict, and persistent psychosomatic complaints. Recognizing a suicidal adolescent is difficult, but if risk factors and warning signs are present, prompt intervention is essential.

12. How do health supervision visits for adolescents differ from traditional health maintenance visits for adults?

Primary care providers should respond to the health consequences of risk-taking behavior by making preventive services a major component of the clinical approach to adolescents. The American Medical Association, in cooperation with the Centers for Disease Control and Prevention, published *Guidelines for Adolescent Preventive Services* (GAPS), a comprehensive set of recommendations that provide a framework for the organization and content of preventive health services. Health supervision visits for adolescents differ from traditional health maintenance visits in six ways:

1. The provider actively complements health guidance that adolescents receive from school, family, and community.
2. Preventive interventions target "new morbidities," such as alcohol, drugs, and sexual risk-taking, rather than emphasize biomedical problems.
3. The provider screens for "comorbidities," which are clusters of risk-taking behaviors, rather than treats categorical health conditions.
4. Annual health supervision visits are recommended to provide anticipatory guidance and early intervention rather than episodic visits such as those for immunizations or sports exams.

5. Comprehensive physical examinations are recommended at each of the three stages of development: early, middle, and late adolescence. Sexually active adolescents need annual screening for sexually transmitted diseases, including an annual Papanicolaou test in sexually active young women.

6. Parents of adolescents should receive specific counseling about parental concerns and adolescent needs at least twice during their child's adolescence.

13. What are the most important positive health behaviors to stress?

Primary caregivers have a critical role in ensuring that all adolescents are competent and motivated to make wise choices as they form life-long habits. The Centers for Disease Control/Division of Adolescent and School Health selected six priority health behaviors for youth based on risk factors that are a major source of morbidity and mortality, highly prevalent, modifiable, and measurable. Other areas of great concern for mortality, such as suicide and homicide, are difficult to reduce to a single, achievable behavioral goal and therefore are not addressed in the six priority behaviors.

Priority Health Behaviors for Adolescents*

1. Use seat belts.	4. Do not smoke.
2. Do not drink (or use drugs) and drive.	5. Eat a low-fat diet.
3. If you have sex, use condoms.	6. Get regular aerobic exercise.

* These six golden rules are the most effective and achievable lifetime behaviors that will reduce years of potential life lost to the major killers: motor vehicle accidents, AIDS, cardiovascular disease, and cancer.

14. How can anticipatory guidance (office counseling) be given without lecturing?

Office counseling is most effective if it actively engages the adolescent in problem-solving. Four steps are involved:

1. **Define the problem.** Ask the adolescent to describe the situation and any feelings or fears about it ("What if your pregnancy test were positive today?").

2. **Explore the options.** Ask the adolescent to describe some ways to solve the problem. The provider simply listens ("Tell me at least three choices you would have if you were pregnant"). Suggest other options if appropriate.

3. **Analyze the consequences.** Ask the adolescent to review the most likely positive and negative consequences of the best solutions considered ("What will be the best thing and the worst thing for you if you placed your baby for adoption?"). Then mention any major consequences or responsibilities overlooked by the adolescent.

4. **Develop an action plan.** Ask the adolescent to identify the specific steps to take after leaving your office. Include a plan for follow-up.

Remember that adolescents are not motivated by the long-term consequences; they are more concerned about immediate rewards and consequences and are particularly motivated by what gives them status and prestige in the eyes of their peers.

15. List the most common medical diagnoses for adolescent office visits.

Common causes of adolescent medical visits include acne, asthma, headache, abdominal pain, fatigue, and musculoskeletal pain.

16. List four common principles applicable to the care of adolescents with symptomatic complaints.

1. Adolescents may have excessive concerns about "Am I normal?" Therefore, they need large amounts of reassurance.

2. Adolescents often have underlying anxiety that they are to blame for the condition because of some behavior about which they feel guilty, such as experimenting with sex or drugs.

3. Adolescents may be very concerned about confidentiality and often want to obtain care independently without parental involvement.

4. Adolescents may need extra support to achieve compliance with treatment plans. They frequently test limits, act impulsively, and discontinue treatment in an effort to "be like everyone else."

In general, adolescents require extra time, more education, and closer follow-up than other age groups.

17. Where do adolescents go for health care?

Of adolescents who have seen a physician in the past two years, approximately one-third see pediatricians, one-third see family practice or internal medicine providers, and one-third utilize local emergency departments. Adolescents have long been recognized as an underserved population who are particularly difficult to reach with health services. Issues of emancipation, independence, and a desire for confidential care create significant barriers for adolescents in the traditional health care system. In general, adolescents visit a health care provider less than once every 2 years, and those visits tend to be primarily for episodic illness or emergency care. With five million uninsured adolescents in America, many have no regular source for health care. Even insured adolescents underutilize care. In one large study in New York state, upper middle-class adolescents who could identify a private physician stated that they would be unwilling to utilize that physician for many sensitive concerns, such as sexuality or drug problems, for fear that their parents would find out.

18. Should adolescents receive health care without parental involvement?

Although parental involvement is generally beneficial and should be strongly encouraged, the ability to provide confidential care to adolescents, with the minor's own consent, is essential to ensure access to health care. Consent and confidentiality are separate legal issues. Consent is a basic legal requirement for the provision of health care to patients of all ages. In general, minors under the age of 18 require parental consent for medical treatment. However, because of the compelling interest of the state in encouraging adolescents to seek early health care for pregnancy, sexually transmitted diseases, and substance abuse, courts and legislatures have created numerous exceptions to parental consent that enable adolescents to obtain care independently for these health concerns. Numerous studies have shown that adolescents 14 and older are as competent as adults to make informed choices about health care.

Confidentiality refers to maintaining privacy of medical information. Many adolescents are reluctant or completely unwilling to seek care without the assurance of confidentiality. Some require privacy as part of the normal process of developing autonomy; others may face hostile or abusive reactions from alienated or dysfunctional families if sensitive information is disclosed. Medical record information is usually not released without the patient's permission in accordance with the adolescent's legal right to privacy. Every state has specific statutes related to a minor's access to health care. Careful analysis of state legislation requiring parental notification shows no beneficial effect on family communication. Adolescents unwilling to share private information with parents tend to delay care, avoid care, seek clandestine care, or utilize judicial bypass mechanisms to access medical care under their own consent. The major documented effects of such legislation are delay in timely diagnosis and treatment and increased medical risk. Other studies demonstrate that many adolescents willingly involve their families (even if there is no legal requirement) if they believe that their families will be supportive and nonjudgmental. The most effective means for parents to ensure involvement in their adolescent's health care decisions is to establish open, trusting communication from early childhood forward.

19. How can adolescent access to health care be improved?

1. **School-based and school-linked clinics.** At local, state, and national levels, implementation of school-based and school-linked health services is seen as one means to overcome barriers to care. Services range from professional telephone consultations with school-based personnel to comprehensive on-site health clinics that provide primary care, mental health services, social services, and other support. Advantages of school-based clinics include accessibility and affordability as well as greater access to preventive care and intervention.

2. **Increased caregiver training in adolescent medicine.** Training programs in pediatrics, family practice, internal medicine, and obstetrics and gynecology have recognized the need to provide specific training in adolescent medicine. Nurse practitioner and physician assistant training programs have likewise added adolescent medicine to curriculum components. Specialty board certification in adolescent medicine became available in 1994. Such efforts should increase the adolescent medicine skills of the next generation of health care providers.

3. **Expanded health care insurance through new health care delivery systems.** A cornerstone for improving the health of adolescents will be mechanisms to reimburse a wide range of providers and service settings for the time-consuming care that adolescents require. Inclusion in capitated health insurance programs and health maintenance organizations may improve access. "Safety-net" features for homeless, emancipated, out-of-school, unemployed, and other disenfranchised youth are essential.

20. When do adolescents become sexually active?

Middle-to-late adolescence has always been the average age for initiation of sexual intercourse. Since the late 1960s ("the sexual revolution"), greater numbers of younger adolescents have become sexually active. The 1995 National Youth Risk Behavior Survey of students in grades 6–12 confirmed little change from the 1992 report that 54% of all high school students had begun sexual intercourse, with 39% having sex in the 3 months prior to the survey. Rates increase rapidly during high school, with 25% of 8th graders, 40% of 9th graders, and 72% of 12th graders reporting sexual intercourse. The median age of first intercourse reported by students is 16.1 years for males and 16.9 years for females. Intercourse is only one aspect of sexual activity. A recent study found that of adolescents who are virgins, one-third reported that they had engaged in genital touching of a partner and one-tenth had participated in oral-genital sex.

21. Why is there so much concern about adolescent sexuality?

The medical consequences of adolescent sexual activity are a national health concern, particularly unintended pregnancy, sexually transmitted diseases (STDs), and HIV infection. One million adolescents still become pregnant each year, although only 400,000 are school-aged minors (17 years and younger). Over 3,000,000 cases of STDs occur in adolescents annually. It is estimated that the number of adolescents with HIV infection doubles every 14 months; AIDS is now the seventh leading cause of death in the 15–24 year-old age group.

22. Should the primary care provider support contraceptive use?

Yes. Health promotion goals for adolescents include postponement of sexual activity until psychosocial maturity and consistent use of condoms and contraceptives by those who engage in sexual intercourse. Abstinence is highly effective in preventing pregnancies and STDs if used consistently and correctly; in actual practice, however, abstinence has a failure rate of 24% in teenaged couples attempting to use it for 1 year. The level of condom use by adolescents has tripled since 1979; nearly 70% report use of condoms with their last coitus. The actual pregnancy rate in sexually active adolescents has decreased 17% since 1976, reflecting an increased use of contraception. New methods of contraception highly appropriate for adolescents include Norplant (5-year subcutaneous implant), Depo-Provera (intramuscular injection every 12 weeks), and improved birth control pill formulations with fewer side effects. If the social environment is supportive, adolescents can be highly effective contraceptive users, as has been well demonstrated in other Western countries. Caregivers should ensure that all adolescents receive anticipatory guidance about safer sex practices and have access to condoms and contraceptives when needed. Despite the perception of crisis, responsible sexual behavior by adolescents has increased.

CONTROVERSY

23. Should "abstinence-only" be the sexuality education message for adolescents?

Adolescent sexuality remains a highly controversial issue, as families, schools, and primary caregivers seek the most effective strategies to promote responsible health behaviors and reduce health risks. During the past decade the vast majority of professional health and educational organizations achieved consensus about the need for comprehensive sexuality education. Recently, there has been a surge in political advocacy by proponents of abstinence-only education, and in 1997 over $88 million dollars in federal and matching state funds were awarded to educational programs teaching abstinence only. By definition, these programs must teach that abstinence from sexual activity outside marriage is the expected standard for all school-aged adolescents, that a mutually faithful monogamous relationship in the context of marriage is the expected standard for human sexual activity, and that sexual activity outside the context of marriage is likely have harmful psychological and physical effects. The funded programs may not discuss contraception or condom use. Proponents of abstinence-only education argue that discussion of contraception and condoms sends an inappropriate mixed message to youth. They propose that if you firmly tell young people to abstain from sexual intercourse, they will. Propopents of abstinence-only programs often state that their own (unpublished) evaluations show that "just-say-no" programs are effective. At present no published studies in the professional literature indicate that abstinence-only programs will result in delay of intercourse.

Proponents of comprehensive sexuality education ("abstinence-plus") also support educational programs emphasizing that sexual abstinence is a desirable objective and the most effective method for prevented unintended pregnancy and STD/HIV infections. In addition, however, they advise young people who engage in intercourse to use contraception and condoms. Effective comprehensive sexual education programs also help to develop cognitive decision-making abilities and to teach young people communication and conflict resolution skills to resist peer pressure. Multiple reviews conclude that programs most effective in changing young people's behavior are those that address abstinence-plus contraception and STD prevention.

Young people need support for abstaining from premature sexual activity, but they also need affordable, sensitive, and confidential reproductive health services and life opportunities that offer them reasons not to become teenaged parents. Rather than being confused about mixed messages, health professionals may offer one very clear message: protect your health and your future—either by abstaining from sexual intercourse or by using effective contraception and condoms.

BIBLIOGRAPHY

1. Blum RW, Beuhring T, Wunderlich M, Resnick MD: Don't ask, they won't tell: The quality of adolescent health screening in five practice settings. Am J Public Health 86:1767–1772, 1996.
2. Centers for Disease Control: Youth risk behavior surveillance. MMWR 45:53–54, 1996.
3. Costa FM, Jessor R, Fortenberry JD, Donovan JE: Psychosocial conventionality, health orientation, and contraceptive use in adolescence. J Adolesc Health 18:404–416, 1996.
4. Coupey SM, Kierman LV (eds): Adolescent sexuality: Preventing unhealthy consequences. Adolesc Med State Art Rev 3:1, 1992 [entire issue].
5. Elster AB: Confronting the crisis in adolescent health: Visions for change. J Adolesc Health 14:505–508, 1993.
6. Elster A, Kuznets N: AMA Guidelines for Adolescent Preventive Services (GAPS). Baltimore, Williams & Wilkins, 1994.
7. Ford CA, Millstein SG: Delivery of confidentiality assurances to adolescents by primary care physicians. Arch Pediatr Adolesc Med 151:505–509, 1997.
8. Friedman HL: Promoting the health of adolescents in the United States of America: A global perspective. J Adolesc Health 14:509–519, 1993.
9. Friedman SB, Fisher M, Schonberg SK (eds): Comprehensive Adolescent Health Care, 2nd ed. St. Louis, Mosby, 1997.
10. Ginsburg KR, Slap GB, Cnaan A, et al: Adolescents' perceptions of factors affecting their decisions to seek health care. JAMA 273:1913–1918, 1995.
11. Haffner DW: What's wrong with abstinence-only sexuality education programs. Seicus Rep 25(4):9–13, 1997.
12. Hofmann AD, Greydanus DE: Adolescent Medicine, 3rd ed. Norwalk, CT, Appleton & Lange, 1997.
13. Knight JR: Adolescent substance use: Screening, assessment, and intervention. Contemp Pediatr 14:45–72, 1997.
14. McAnarney ER, Kreipe RE, Orr DP, Comerci GD (eds): Textbook of Adolescent Medicine. Philadelphia, W.B. Saunders, 1992.
15. Millstein SG, Gans J: Delivery of S.D./HIV preventive services to adolescents by primary care physicians. J Adolesc Health 19:249–257, 1996.

16. Purcell JS, Hergenroeder AC, Kozinetz C, et al: Interviewing techniques with adolescents in primary care. J Adolesc Health 20:300–305, 1997.
17. Schuster MA, Bell RM, Kanouse DE: The sexual practices of adolescent virgins: Genital sexual activities of high school students who have never had vaginal intercourse. Am J Public Health 86:1570–1576, 1996.
18. Slawkowski DJ: Adolescent medicine and law. Adolesc Med State Art Rev 4:204–218, 1993.
19. Stout JW, Kirby D: The effects of sexuality education on adolescent sexual activity. Pediatr Ann 22:120–126, 1993.
20. Styne DM: New aspects in the diagnosis and treatment of pubertal disorders. Pediatr Clin North Am 44:505–529, 1997.
21. Tafelski T, Boehm KE: Contraception in the adolescent patient. Prim Care 22:145–159, 1995.
22. Woods ER, Lin YG, Middleman A, et al: The associations of suicide attempts in adolescents. Pediatrics 99:791–796, 1997.

103. THE ELDERLY PATIENT

Evelyn Hutt, M.D.

1. What is functional assessment? Why is it important?

Functional assessment is a formalized way of paying attention to how a patient manages the details of daily life. We assume that most young patients are cognitively intact, can get around in their homes, get into and out of the bathroom and bath tub safely, and do their own cooking, shopping, and eating. However, because the prevalence of disabilities in performing activities of daily living (ADLs) is so high among elders (10% of community-dwelling elders have at least one deficit in ADL performance) and because neither patients nor careproviders are accustomed to thinking of such matters as part of medical care, we need a more formal way of including such information in our review of systems. Several brief questionnaires are available for use in clinical practice. Consistent use of any one will provide insight into how the patient functions in daily life.

As the physician manages more incurable or chronic disease, it becomes increasingly important to improve the quality and independence of a patient's life. If we have not asked how well a patient is managing (by performing a functional assessment) when he or she presents, we (1) miss significant treatable problems and (2) do not know whether we have affected the patient's day-to-day function positively or negatively.

2. Which special aspects of the physical exam need evaluation during assessment of an elder?

Perceptual function, cognitive and emotional function, and gait.

3. When a patient presents to the clinic with a new change in mental status, how do you know whether the patient is delirious, depressed, or demented?

The difference between delirium and dementia can be recognized clinically. Delirious patients have an altered level of consciousness (either depressed or agitated), whereas simply demented patients are awake, alert, and calm. Ascertaining the patient's baseline status from a reliable source is crucial. A patient who presents with abnormal mental status should be presumed to be delirious rather than demented. Delirium is a serious but often treatable manifestation of disease. Patients known to be demented by reliable history or chart documentation often present with acute worsening of mental status as the only sign of infection, myocardial infarction, or central lesion from a fall.

Distinguishing between depression and dementia can be difficult. Paradoxically, patients who present with complaints of memory problems are more likely to be depressed than demented. Other clues to depression include difficulty with concentration out of proportion to other deficits in the mental status exam; recent major losses (family members, friends, health, independence); sleep disturbance; and weight loss. Even after brief formal screening for both depression and cognitive deficits (for example, with the Geriatric Depression Scale and Mini-Mental Status Exam), the diagnosis may not be clear. Referral for neuropsychiatric testing or a trial of antidepressants may be helpful.

4. What major derangements should be considered in the etiology of delirium?

The mnemonic **DELIRIUM** is a helpful reminder of the many treatable causes of delirium.

D = **D**rugs. Unfortunately, the list of potential offenders is extensive. Most important are anticholinergics, which are very common in over-the-counter medications and often impair cognitive function. Other side effects particularly bothersome to older people include dry mouth, constipation, and urinary retention. All psychoactive medications may induce delirium. A thorough drug history is therefore the first step in sorting out the cause of delirium. Elimination of as many agents as possible and reduction of the remainder to the lowest possible dose are helpful.

E = **E**lectrolytes. Electrolyte imbalance and other metabolic disturbances may impair cognitive function. Examples include hypo- and hypernatremia, hypo- and hyperkalemia, hypo- and hypercalcemia, hypo- and hypermagnesemia, hypo- and hyperglycemia, hypoxia, and hypercarbia.

L = **L**ow temperature (hypothermia) and **L**unacy. High temperature, of course, also may induce delirium. Acute psychosis is uncommon in elders without a prior history.

I = **I**ntoxication and **I**ntracranial processes. Alcoholism is no less prevalent among elders than among younger populations. The diagnosis of alcoholism is particularly easy to overlook in elderly women. Intracranial processes include subdural hematomas, neoplasms, and infection. If no other cause of delirium is apparent, the elder presenting with an acute or subacute change in cognitive function should have a brain imaging study.

R = **R**etention, either urinary or fecal. Prevalence of retention as a true cause of delirium is difficult to ascertain, but the problem is easy to relieve. It should be considered causal only if the patient improves and other, more serious causes have been considered.

I = **I**nfection. Infection is the most important treatable cause of delirium. The *only* presenting sign of infection in an older person may be a change in mental status. Because immune function declines with age, elders may have pneumonia, urosepsis, or an abdominal catastrophe without pain, fever, or an elevated white blood cell count.

U = **U**nfamiliar surroundings with decreased sensory input. In this disorder, often described as the sundowning phenomenon, patients with subclinical dementia function well until a strange environment combines with impaired vision and hearing to induce confusion. Simple expedients may ameliorate the problem: well-lit room, undisturbed sleep, clock, calendar, familiar pictures and visitors, and easy access to food, water, and toilet.

M = **M**yocardial infarction and other causes of decreased central perfusion. Like infection, acute cardiovascular events may present without localizing signs.

5. Which tests should be used to evaluate a patient with dementia? Why?

About 10% of dementia cases are at least partially reversible, including those caused by hypothyroidism, B_{12} deficiency, syphilis, and depression. Thus, evaluation should be directed at reversible etiologies. Although normal pressure hydrocephalus can be treated, the associated dementia generally does not reverse. Subdural hematomas may cause a subtle and subclinical decline in mental status without localizing neurologic findings and should be investigated in anyone with a history of both associated symptoms and a recent fall.

A reasonable laboratory work-up for dementia, once delirium has been excluded, includes levels of thyroid-stimulating hormone (TSH) and B_{12}, Venereal Disease Research Laboratory test, liver function tests, and a complete blood count. Whether a computed tomographic (CT) or magnetic resonance imaging (MRI) scan of the head is necessary remains controversial and depends on the unique presentation of the patient (e.g., possibility of subdural hematoma).

6. Discuss the major options for the treatment of depression in an older patient.

Three major modalities are available for the treatment of depression: psychotherapy, medication, and electroconvulsion.

Psychotherapy has the clear advantage of fewer side effects, but it may be difficult to persuade older people to begin such treatment because of their cultural bias against expression of affect and "complaining." The cognitive behavioral model offers a more acceptable and less embarrassing style of therapy. The primary care provider should be aware of who in the psychotherapeutic community offers this approach and is comfortable treating older patients.

Medications are readily available for treatment and may be divided into roughly four groups: tricyclics, serotonergics, psychostimulants, and others (see table). Use of tricyclics entails the risks of anticholinergic side effects, which may be decreased by choosing the metabolite compounds, nortriptyline or desipramine. Nortriptyline is somewhat more sedating than desipramine. If respiratory depression is a concern, protriptyline can be used. An electrocardiogram should be obtained for underlying conduction delay, and dosing should begin at 25 mg. It is useful to measure drug levels at this dose, particularly in the presence of renal insufficiency. A 4–6-week trial at adequate levels is needed to produce benefit.

There are no controlled studies of the use of the newer serotonergic agents (fluoxetine, sertraline, and paroxetine) in an older population. Fluoxetine commonly causes gastrointestinal distress and anorexia. It has a long half-life and should be used cautiously if a major symptom of the depression has been weight loss. Psychostimulants, chiefly methylphenidate, are useful when a more rapid response is needed to gauge whether the patient is likely to respond to medication. The beginning dose is 5 mg 2 or 3 times/day. Other agents include trazodone and bupropion. Trazodone may be particularly useful in patients with underlying lung disease. Bupropion is newer, more expensive, and not well studied in older populations.

Antidepressants in the Elderly

	ADVANTAGES	DISADVANTAGES
Tricyclics	Short-acting Inexpensive	Anticholinergic side effects Overdose Cardiac conduction delays Monitoring
Serotonergics	Fewer side effects of drowsiness, dry mouth, constipation	Long half-life (days) Expensive
Psychostimulants	Rapid response	Tremor Sleeplessness
Other: trazodone	Little respiratory depression Few cardiac effects	Orthostatic hypotension Sedating

Electroconvulsive therapy (ECT) is a highly effective treatment for older depressed patients. It probably is safer and has fewer side effects than tricyclic antidepressants. Because of the fear and horror that it engenders in many people, it is an underused modality. Primary care providers should known which psychiatrists in their area are comfortable using ECT in older patients.

7. Why do elderly patients fall?
A combination of extrinsic (environmental) and intrinsic (to the patient) factors increase the risk of falling. Extrinsic factors such as clutter in the home, poor lighting, throw rugs, and slippery bathtubs are probably the most easily correctable. Intrinsic precipitants include (in decreasing order of importance) drugs, cognitive impairment, disability of the lower extremities, abnormal balance and gait, and foot problems. The risk of falling increases linearly with the number of risk factors.

8. Which particular type of drug is associated with morbidity from falls?
All classes of sedatives (anxiolytics, antidepressants, and neuroleptics) are associated with falls and hip fractures. Both dosage and half-life of the medication are related to incidence of falls.

9. What are the consequences of falls for the elderly?
Only 5% of falls result in a fracture. Serious soft-tissue injury occurs in another 10%. Such injuries account for 9,500 deaths/year. Falls that do not result in injury may have the serious

consequence of fear, leading to reduced activity. Of patients who decide to enter nursing homes, 40% say that falls and instability contributed to that decision.

10. What are the most important causes of visual impairment in the elderly?

The majority of visual impairment in older patients is due to three conditions:

Cataracts affect 13% of people 65–74 years of age and over 40% of those over 75. Early in the course, decline in distant visual acuity and difficulty in tolerating glare may be the presenting complaints. In most patients cataract removal and lens implantation can be done on an outpatient basis. A common late complication is delayed opacification of the posterior capsule, which occurs in up to 50% of patients. It can be managed in 90% of patients with yttrium-aluminum-garnet (YAG) laser treatment.

Macular degeneration affects 6.4% of people 65–74 years of age and about 20% of those over 70. Two types are identified clinically: nonexudative, which is managed expectantly, and exudative, which is managed with argon laser photocoagulation. Ninety percent of patients have the nonexudative type.

Glaucoma affects 3% of people over 65 years of age. Prevalence rates are higher among African-Americans.

11. How common is hearing impairment among the elderly?

About one-third of people over the age of 65 years are hearing-impaired. Close to one-half of those over age 80 are affected. Men are more commonly affected than women. Given this prevalence, when you interview an older patient, be sure that he or she can see your face. Speak clearly, reduce background noise, use gestures, and check often for comprehension. Inexpensive amplifiers ($40) are available for office use. Drugs that are ototoxic should be used sparingly: aminoglycosides, erythromycin, vancomycin, loop diuretics, and nonsteroidal antiinflammatories.

12. How are pharmacokinetics altered by the usual aging process?

As people age, the proportion of body water to fat shifts toward fat. This shift changes the volume of distribution as well as the half-life for all drugs. Lipophilic agents, which affect the central nervous system, tend to have much longer half-lives in older people. In general, drug absorption is not affected by age, nor is liver metabolism if the liver is healthy. Whether renal function necessarily declines with age is controversial, but practically speaking, it usually does. A simple formula for calculating creatinine clearance—$(140 - age) (\times 0.85$ for women$)$ divided by the serum creatinine—can be used to adjust dosing intervals in renally excreted drugs.

13. What is an advance care directive?

An advance care directive is a written and witnessed document specifying treatment preferences in the event that a patient becomes incompetent. Two forms exist: living wills, which generally become effective when the patient is both terminally ill and incompetent, and durable powers of attorney for health care, which appoint a surrogate decision maker and express treatment preferences, whether or not a terminal condition exists. Laws about the formulation and enactment of both directives vary from state to state, but all older patients, as well as patients with serious chronic illness, should be provided the opportunity to discuss end-of-life options.

14. When should elder abuse be suspected?

Although hard data are lacking, abuse is thought to affect at least 3% of the elderly population (1–2 million elders/year). As with the problem of child abuse, neglect is probably much more common. In general, the physician should screen for abuse when the patient fits the "typical victim" profile, when the caregiver fits an "abuser profile," and when certain symptom complexes are found.

The **typical victim profile** includes patients with multiple frailties and behavioral problems, such as dementia, incontinence, nocturnal shouting, wandering, and paranoia.

The **abuser profile** includes overburdened caregivers who live with the elder, are sleep-deprived, and/or have marital and work-related stresses of their own. Abusers also may be socially isolated and have a history of substance abuse, psychopathology, or other domestic violence.

Symptom complexes that should arouse suspicion include unexplained weight loss, signs of trauma (multiple fractures, falls, dislocations, bruises of varying ages, burns in unusual places, genital pain, or bleeding), and decubitus ulcers. Psychosocial manifestations include excessive fear, depression, infantile behavior, confusion over or ignorance of the patient's own financial situation, and the caregiver's refusal to let the patient see the doctor alone. The physician should persist in repeated screening, even in the face of denial. Fear may keep the victim from reporting abuse.

15. Which vaccines should be routine?

All people over 65 years of age should have yearly influenza vaccines, pneumococcal vaccine polyvalent (Pneumovax) at least once, and tetanus booster every 10 years. Whether Pneumovax should be repeated every 10 years is controversial; there is no clear evidence in either direction. Because vaccination rates are so low, from a public health point of view efforts should focus on one Pneumovax per elder.

Changes in Preventive Care for the Elderly

Vaccines	Yearly influenza
	1 Pneumovax
	Tetanus booster every 10 years
Lipid profiles	In the absence of cardiovascular disease, discontinue at age 70–75 years
Papanicoloau smears	If routinely negative, discontinue at age 70 years

16. When can you stop checking cholesterol?

The answer depends on whether the patient has known cardiovascular disease. For patients with known disease, no upper age limit applies, and treatment guidelines are no different for elders than for middle-aged patients. In the absence of cardiovascular disease, screening probably may end at age 70 or 75 years. This guideline takes into account the 10 years needed to show an effect of cholesterol reduction on the incidence of myocardial infarction and life expectancy. Virtually no data are available about the utility of lowering cholesterol in women. Consideration should be given to treating people with LDL levels greater than 100 plus age; the approach needs to be individualized.

17. Should elders continue to be screened for breast, cervical, and colon cancer?

The incidence of breast and colon cancer rises continuously with age, whereas the incidence of cervical cancer reaches a plateau. Therefore, it makes sense to set no upper limit on screening for breast and colon cancer, but Papanicoloau smears may be stopped in the early 70s if the patient has had several negative exams.

18. How and why should you skin-test for tuberculosis in the elderly?

Tuberculosis (TB) screening should be performed. TB is more common among the elderly, who are at greater risk of reactivation as they age and become less immunocompetent. Skin testing is an important part of baseline data so that TB may be appropriately considered when the patient becomes ill. A control skin test should be placed simultaneously to distinguish anergy from a negative response. The purified protein derivative (PPD) test should be repeated in 2–4 weeks if it is negative to allow for anamnestic response. This practice prevents the false diagnosis of recent conversion, if the patient undergoes TB testing in the future.

19. What vitamin supplements should elderly people take?

People over 65 whose nutritional intake is adequate need no supplementary vitamins. However, because most people consume inadequate amounts of calcium (< 1000 mg/day), calcium supplementation is both prudent and low risk. Because homebound and nursing home residents are especially likely (38–54%) to be vitamin D-deficient, vitamin D supplementation is beneficial.

20. How common is protein-calorie malnutrition in the elderly?
About 11–22% of elderly outpatients are malnourished. Indicators of nutritional risk include one or fewer meals per day, absence of fruits and vegetables in diet, depression, loneliness, low income, and difficulty with shopping.

21. What medications have potential utility in the prevention and treatment of dementia?
Although clinical trials are not available, epidemiologic and animal studies suggest that estrogen replacement therapy may slow cognitive decline. Possible mechanisms include direct and indirect neurotransmitter effects, mood improvement, and slower progression of atherosclerosis. Because of strong evidence that estrogen is useful in preventing osteoporosis and retarding atherosclerosis, consideration should be given to broadening its use among elderly women, with the caveat that prolonged use may increase the risk for breast cancer. Less strong epidemiologic evidence from the EPESE study suggests that NSAIDs may protect against cognitive decline. However, because NSAID use is associated with a four-fold increased risk of hospitalization for peptic ulcer disease, its routine use cannot be suggested.

Two classes of drug are available for treatment: acetylcholinesterase inhibitors and antioxidants. The cholinesterase inhibitors, donepezil and tacrine, produce modest improvement in some measures of cognition but not function. Tacrine has a high incidence of hepatotoxicity. Both medications may cause nausea, vomiting, and insomnia and are expensive. Selegiline and vitamin E have recently been shown to improve function but not cognition in moderate Alzheimer's disease. The study needs to be replicated before use of either drug can be recommended.

BIBLIOGRAPHY

1. American Geriatric Society: Hearing and visual impairment. In Geriatric Review Syllabus. New York, American Geriatric Society, 1989.
2. Anentzberger GJ, Lachs MS, O'Brien JG, et al: Elder mistreatment: A call for help. Patient Care June 15:93–130, 1993.
3. Birge SJ: Is there role for estrogen replacement therapy in the prevention and treatment of dementia? J Am Geriatr Soc 44:865–870, 1996.
4. Council on Scientific Affairs: Elder abuse and neglect. JAMA 257:966–971, 1987.
5. Donepezil (Aricept) for Alzheimer's disease. Med Lett 39:53–54, 1997.
6. Francis J, Kapoor WN: Delirium in the hospitalized elderly. J Gen Intern Med 5:65–79, 1990.
7. Gloth FM III, Gundberg CM, Hollis BW, et al: Vitamin D deficiency in homebound elderly persons. JAMA 254:1683–1686, 1995.
8. Kane RL, Ouslander JG, Abrass IB: Essentials of Clinical Geriatrics, 3rd ed. New York, McGraw-Hill, 1994.
9. Lachs MS, Feinstein AR, Cooney LM, et al: A simple procedure for general screening for functional disability in elderly patients. Ann Intern Med 112:699–706, 1990.
10. Lipowski ZJ: Delirium in the elderly patient. N Engl J Med 320:578–582, 1989.
11. McGreevy JF, Franco K: Depression in the elderly. J Gen Intern Med 3:498–507, 1988.
12. Ray WA, Griffin MR, Schaffner W, et al: Psychotropic drug use and the risk of hip fracture. N Engl J Med 318:363–369, 1987.
13. Roose SP, Glassman AH: Cardiovascular effects of tricyclic anti-depressants in depressed patients with and without heart disease. J Clin Psychiatry 7:1–18, 1989.
14. Sano M, Ernesto C, Thomas RG, et al: A controlled trial of selegeline, alpha-tocopherol, or both as treatment for Alzheimer's disease. N Engl J Med 336:1216–1222, 1997.
15. Satel SL, Nelson JC: Stimulants in the treatment of depression: A critical review. J Clin Psychiatry 50:241–249, 1989.
16. Thompson LW, Gallagher D, Breckenridge JS: Comparative effectiveness of psychotherapies for depressed elders. J Consult Clin Psychol 55:385–390, 1987.
17. Tinetti ME, Speechley M: Prevention of falls among the elderly. N Engl J Med 320:1055–1060, 1989.
18. Tinetti ME, Speechley M, Ginter SF: Risk factors for falls among elderly persons living in the community. N Engl J Med: 219:1701–1708, 1988.
19. United States Public Health Service: Prevention and control of tuberculosis in facilities providing long-term care to the elderly. MMWR 39:7–20, 1990.
20. Woolf SH, Kamerow DR, Lawrence RS, et al: The periodic health examination of older adults: The recommendations of the U.S. Preventive Services Task Force. J Am Geriatr Soc 38:933–942, 1990.

104. THE OBESE PATIENT

Daniel H. Bessesen, M.D., and Laura M. Lasater, M.D.

1. What is obesity?

Obesity is a degree of overweight that is associated with increases in morbidity and mortality. The concept of "ideal body weight" originated with the Metropolitan Life Insurance studies, which demonstrated a J-shaped relationship between body weight and morbidity. People who weighed less than or more than a certain amount experienced excessive rates of mortality. More recently the concept of an "ideal" body weight has been questioned. Recent studies suggest that the increase in mortality observed with being underweight was related to smoking-associated mortality (smokers weigh less than nonsmokers) and preexisting cancer, which were not controlled in earlier studies. Modern studies demonstrate that the relationship between body weight and mortality is essentially linear when corrected for preexisting illness and smoking. This relationship was seen for women in the large Nurses Health Study cohort, the Harvard Alumni Study, and the recently published Cancer Prevention Study I.

2. How is obesity diagnosed?

Most clinicians now use the body mass index (BMI) to diagnose obesity. The BMI is calculated by dividing weight in kg by height in meters squared. A BMI of 25 or less is normal. A BMI from 25–26.9 indicates overweight; 27–29.9, obesity; 30–34.9, moderate obesity; 35–39.9, severe obesity; and > 40, morbid obesity.

Body Weights in Pounds According to Height and Body Mass Index*

HEIGHT (IN)	BODY MASS INDEX, kg/m²													
	19	20	21	22	23	24	25	26	27	28	29	30	35	40
	◄─────────────────── BODY WEIGHT, lb ───────────────────►													
58	91	96	100	105	110	115	119	124	129	134	138	143	167	191
59	94	99	104	109	114	119	124	128	133	138	143	148	173	198
60	97	102	107	112	118	123	128	133	138	143	148	153	179	204
61	100	106	111	116	122	127	132	137	143	148	153	158	185	211
62	104	109	115	120	126	131	136	142	147	153	158	164	191	218
63	107	113	118	124	130	135	141	146	152	158	163	169	197	225
64	110	116	122	128	134	140	145	151	157	163	169	174	204	232
65	114	120	126	132	138	144	150	156	162	168	174	180	210	240
66	118	124	130	136	142	148	155	161	167	173	179	186	216	247
67	121	127	134	140	146	153	159	166	172	178	185	191	223	255
68	125	131	138	144	151	158	164	171	177	184	190	197	230	262
69	128	135	142	149	155	162	169	176	182	189	196	203	236	270
70	132	139	146	153	160	167	174	181	188	195	202	207	243	278
71	136	143	150	157	165	172	179	186	193	200	208	215	250	286
72	140	147	154	162	169	177	184	191	199	206	213	221	258	294
73	144	151	159	166	174	182	189	197	204	212	219	227	265	302
74	148	155	163	171	179	186	194	202	210	218	223	233	272	311
75	152	160	168	176	184	192	200	208	216	224	232	240	279	319
76	156	164	172	180	189	197	205	213	221	230	238	246	287	328

* Each entry gives body weight in pounds (lb) for a person of a given height and body mass index. Pounds have been rounded off. To use the table, find the appropriate height in the left hand column. Move across the row to a given weight. The number at the top of the column is the body mass index for the height and weight. (From NIH Technology Assessment Conference Panel: Methods for voluntary weight loss and control. Ann Intern Med 116:942–949, 1992.)

The BMI serves as a surrogate measure of fat mass, which can be measured more directly by underwater weighing, dual energy x-ray absorptiometry, electrical impedance, or skin fold measurements. However, these measures are not generally available to most clinicians, and for most people BMI provides a reasonable estimate of fat mass. The health risks of obesity are also related to the distribution of fat. A growing number of studies have demonstrated that excessive adipose tissue that accumulates in a central or upper body distribution (android or male pattern) is associated with more adverse health consequences than lower body obesity (gynoid or female pattern). Central obesity can be diagnosed by calculating a ratio of the waist circumference divided by the maximal circumference of the hips. This so-called waist:hip ratio defines central obesity if it is greater than 0.85 in women or 1.0 in men.

3. What are the health consequences of obesity?

Obesity is clearly associated with some of the most common illnesses, including diabetes, hypertension, hyperlipidemia, coronary artery disease, degenerative arthritis, gallbladder disease, and cancer of the endometrium, breast, prostate, and colon. The incidence of these conditions rises steadily as body weight increases. In general, the more one weighs, the greater the health risks. It is surprising how risks increase with even modest gains in weight. Health risks are magnified in people with a positive family history of obesity-associated diseases. The absolute risk of adverse health consequences increases as the person ages, but the relative risk declines. This decline in the relative risk of obesity-associated mortality was demonstrated in data from the Cancer Prevention Study I.

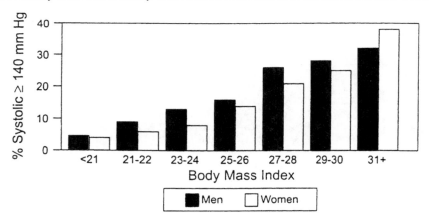

BMI and the risk of hypertension. (From Canadian Guidelines for Healthy Weights. Cat. No. H39-134 1989E: 1988:69.)

BMI and the risk of coronary artery disease. (From Colditz GA, Meir SJ, et al: A prospective study of obesity and risk of CHD in women. N Engl J Med 322: 882–890, 1990, with permission.)

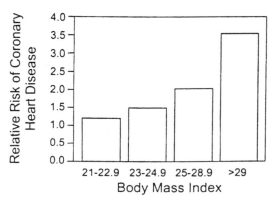

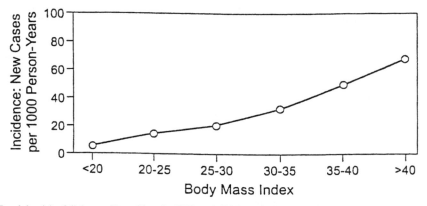

BMI and the risk of diabetes. (From Knowler WC, et al: Diabetes incidence in Pima Indians: Contributions of obesity and parental diabetes. Am J Epidemiol 113:144–156, 1981, with permission.)

BMI and Body Weight Associated with 20% and 50% Increases in Mortality from All Causes and Mortality from Cardiovascular Disease (CVD)

	20% INCREASE				50% INCREASE			
	MORTALITY FROM ALL CAUSES		MORTALITY FROM CVD		MORTALITY FROM ALL CAUSES		MORTALITY FROM CVD	
GROUP	BMI*	WEIGHT (lb)[†]	BMI	WEIGHT (lb)[†]	BMI	WEIGHT (lb)[†]	BMI	WEIGHT (lb)[†]
70 in. men								
30–44 yr	23.8	166	22.9	160	27.2	189	25.3	177
45–54 yr	24.2	169	23.2	162	28.1	196	26.0	181
55–64 yr	24.7	172	23.9	167	29.1	203	27.5	192
65–74 yr	28.2	197	26.5	185	37.0	258	33.2	232
75–84 yr	30.5	213	28.1	196	42.1	294	36.7	256
64 in. women								
30–44 yr	26.0	152	23.5	137	32.1	187	26.5	155
45–54 yr	24.8	145	23.2	135	29.4	171	25.8	151
55–64 yr	25.9	151	25.2	147	32.0	187	30.3	177
65–74 yr	29.9	174	29.0	169	40.8	238	38.7	226

* A body mass index of 21.0 was used as the reference value.
† For men, a height of 70 in. (178 cm) and weight of 146.5 lb (67 kg) were used as reference values. For women, a height of 64 in. (163 cm) and weight of 122.5 lb (56 kg) were used as reference values.
From Rosenbaum M, Leibel RL, Hirsch J: Obesity. N Engl J Med 337:396–407, 1997, with permission.

4. What are the economic consequences of obesity?

In 1980, 34 million Americans were obese. The overall costs of obesity in 1986 dollars was estimated to be $39.9 billion or 5.5% of national health care costs in 1986. Included were $22.2 billion for cardiovascular disease, $11.3 billion for diabetes, $1.5 billion for hypertension, and $1.9 billion for breast and colon cancer. This estimate does not include costs of musculoskeletal disorders, which may almost double the total figure. In addition, the loss in wages and productivity attributed to obesity approaches $20 billion per year. Finally, people attempting to lose weight spend 30–60 billion dollars annually on weight loss products, most of which have no proven benefit.

5. What are the psychological complications of obesity?

Situational depression and anxiety related to obesity are common. The obese person may suffer from discrimination that further contributes to difficulty with poor self-image and social isolation. In one study, obese adolescents were compared with adolescents who had other chronic health problems. Both groups were followed for 7 years. At the end of this period, obese women were 20% less likely to be married, made $6,700/yr less in income, and had 10% more poverty than controls. This effect was independent of baseline aptitude test scores and socioeconomic status. The concern shown by patients over how weight affects their lives is profound. It may be difficult or impossible for a care provider who has never experienced discrimination based on obesity to understand completely the experience of the obese person. It is important for care providers to examine closely their own feelings about obesity and to consider how their feelings affect the care that they provide to obese patients.

6. How common is obesity?

Obesity has reached epidemic proportions in the United States. The most recent study of the prevalence of obesity (The National Health and Nutrition Examination Survey [NHANES III]) conducted by the federal government demonstrates that one-third of all adult Americans are overweight (defined as 20% above ideal body weight). The NHANES studies have demonstrated that, despite a perception that consumption of low-calorie, low-fat foods and participation in regular exercise have increased, the prevalence of obesity has risen steadily over the past 30 years.

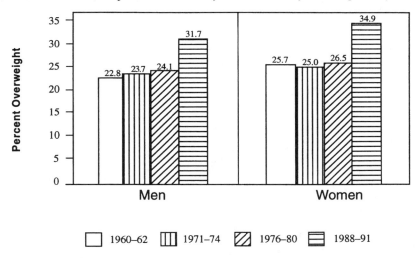

Percent of adult Americans who were overweight, 1960–1990. (From Kuczmarski RJ, et al: Increasing prevalence of overweight among U.S. adults. The National Health and Nutrition Examination Surveys, 1960–1991. JAMA 272:205–211, 1994, with permission.)

7. What causes obesity?

The regulation of body weight is complex. Multiple interrelated symptoms control caloric intake, macronutrient content of the diet, energy expenditure, and fuel metabolism. Models of obesity in mice have provided new and fundamental insights into the mechanisms involved in body weight regulation. Recent scientific developments have helped to foster a change in the way that people think about obesity. Professionals and lay people are increasingly viewing obesity as a chronic metabolic disorder much like diabetes or hypertension. This view requires a conceptual shift from the previous widely held belief that obesity is simply or cosmetic or behavioral problem. For obesity to develop, there must be a period of positive energy balance—that is, energy intake must exceed energy expenditure. The complex system regulating body weight and composition must be altered, ultimately achieving a new steady state at a higher weight. Maintaining energy balance is one of the most important jobs of any organism. From age 20–60 years the average human eats over 32 tons of food. A sustained negative imbalance between energy intake and expenditure is potentially life-threatening within a relatively short time. To maintain energy balance, the organism must assess energy stores within the body and the nutrient content of the diet, determine whether the body is in negative energy or nutrient balance, and adjust hormone levels, energy expenditure, nutrient movement, and consumatory behavior in response. These tremendously complex events involve thousands of gene products.

8. Do abnormal genes cause obesity?

The prevalence of obesity has dramatically increased in the past 60 years with minimal change in the human gene pool. The problem of human obesity is a classic gene-environment interaction. The genes that regulate body weight evolved somewhere between 200,000 and 1 million years ago, when the environmental forces controlling nutrient acquisition and habitual physical activity were dramatically different. A number of molecular-genetic approaches have been used to try to identify relevant genes. These efforts not only hold the promise of identifying physiologic mechanisms underlying the development of obesity but also may reveal novel targets for therapies.

9. Does a decrease in energy expenditure play a role in the development of obesity?

For obesity to develop, there must be an imbalance between caloric intake and caloric expenditure. For fat mass to increase, there must be an imbalance between the amount of fat consumed compared with the amount of fat oxidized. One possibility is that people become obese because of a reduction in energy expenditure. There are three components to energy expenditure:

1. **Basal metabolic rate (BMR)** is the amount of energy needed to keep sodium and potassium where they belong, to keep the body warm, to pump blood, to breathe, and to perform other basic functions.

2. **Energy expended in activity (EA)** is the most variable and may account for as little as 10–20% of total energy expenditure in people who are bedridden or as much as 60–80% in training athletes.

3. **Thermic effect of food (TEF)** is a relatively small component of energy expenditure and represents the increase in energy expenditure that follows the consumption of a meal.

Increasing evidence indicates that obesity is associated with a relative reduction in energy expended with activity. Evidence in favor of this hypothesis comes from the Pima Indians as well as obese Caucasians and previously obese people placed on weight-reducing diets. The role that reductions in BMR play in weight gain is more controversial. Regardless of the absolute level of energy expenditure, obesity results when the person fails to adjust accurately energy intake to changes in energy expenditure.

10. What approaches are available for the treatment of obese patients?

Treatment options include diet, exercise, drugs, surgery, and combinations of these modalities.

11. What is an appropriate goal for a weight-reducing program?

This important question has no simple answer. Increasing evidence indicates that many obese people have unrealistic expectations about the amount of weight that they may lose through a weight loss program. Most obese people would like to reach "ideal body weight." They accept a 20–30% weight loss as adequate but are disappointed if they lose only 5–10% of their initial weight. These desires stand in stark contrast to the magnitude of weight loss that has been seen with all treatment modalities short of surgery. The most effective diet, exercise, or drug treatment programs give roughly a 10% weight loss in most people. This degree of weight reduction has been associated with improvements in health-associated measures such as lower blood pressure, reductions in LDL cholesterol levels, improved functional capacity, and improved insulin sensitivity. However, this degree of weight reduction is disappointing to most patients unless the goal of the weight reduction program is clearly discussed before embarking on any plan. For many obese people, television and magazines define ideal body weight, and body weight is closely tied to self-esteem. Failure to lose weight may pose a serious threat to self-esteem. One of the most important roles that a health care provider can play for obese patients is to encourage them to separate body weight from self-worth. Secondarily it is important to help the patient adopt more realistic goals for a diet and exercise program. Most experts now believe that a sustained 5–10% weight loss (e.g., a 22-lb weight loss for someone who initially weighted 220 lb) is a realistic goal with probable medical benefits. The patient's goal may be to lose a lot of weight in a short period: "40 lb in 40 days." More realistic goals may be a gradual but sustained mild weight reduction. Alternatively, prevention of further weight gain may be an attainable goal, or the health care provider may encourage the patient to focus on eating and activity habits and not on a weight goal. In this manner, patients can be succeed independently of weight loss, and if they go off the behavioral program, they have relapsed independently of what the scale says.

12. What is the role of diet in the treatment of obese patients?

The mainstays of dietary modification in weight loss therapy have been a diet low in fat and calories. Whatever intervention is made must be lifelong to be beneficial. Therefore, it must be tolerable to the patient. The initial evaluation should include an assessment of whether the patient wants to change his or her diet; stages of change include precontemplative, contemplative, planning, action, and maintenance. In addition, the primary care provider should assess the current diet with a good nutritional history. This assessment can be done in a few minutes with a 24-hour dietary recall and a discussion of the composition of frequently eaten meals, including fast foods. Then slow, gradual dietary change should be encouraged. Simple dietary suggestions include (1) eating 3 meals per day, (2) eating only at meal times, and (3) eating only 1 serving. These suggestions help patients to focus on what they are eating. Most people know what they should eat. The problem is that they either do not pay attention to what they eat or do not find a "good diet" palatable. A nutritionist can help to tailor a diet to the individual patients' needs. A nutritional consultation, however, does not take the place of ongoing discussion and encouragement from the primary care provider. Many settings do not allow sophisticated behavioral modification techniques to be taught. The use of commercial programs such as Weight Watchers can provide reasonable nutritional counseling and social support. Many patients are surprised at the cost of these programs, which may be a deterrent to continued use. However, such programs involve no risk and may be cheaper in the long run than pharmacologic treatment. Unfortunately, many patients have already tried and failed at these approaches before they seek medical attention. The scientific literature supports the notion that for many people dietary approaches alone are not associated with a high level of success at achieving long-term weight loss.

13. What is the role of exercise in a weight loss program?

Exercise does not provide much weight loss in the short run. This observation may be frustrating for many patients, but the explanation is simple: the absolute caloric deficit produced by a moderate exercise program is insufficient to cause over a period of days or weeks the degree of negative energy balance necessary for marked weight reduction. Another problem is that the patient may preserve or even increase lean body mass at a time when fat mass is decreasing; thus the absolute amount of weight loss is reduced. However, over the long term the success of a weight loss program is substantially greater if exercise is included. A recent study of people who had successfully lost weight and kept it off for more than 1 year found that the unifying feature was that all of them exercise regularly. Although most patients and physicians think of an exercise program as at least 30 minutes of high-intensity exercise at least 3 times/week, it is important to remember that the expenditure side of the energy balance equation is equal to the intensity of the activity times the time. Many Americans watch television for 3–4 hours/day (21–28 hours/week). The energy expended while watching television is roughly equal to a sleeping metabolic rate. If such people simply reduce the time spent watching television and work around the house, the net effect on total energy expenditure may be larger than a program of higher-intensity exercise for only brief periods 1–3 times/week.

CONTROVERSIES

14. What are phen/fen and Redux?

Phen/fen is the combination of phentermine and fenfluramine. Redux is the trade name of dexfenfluramine. The two drugs were prescribed to over 8 million people in an effort to help them lose weight. They were removed from the market because of serious side effects (see question 16).

15. Can herbal medicines aid in weight loss?

The Food and Drug Administration became aware of the use of herbal medications purported to have the same mechanism of action as fen/phen without the side effects. These combinations usually include the herbal ingredient ephedra, commonly known as Ma Huang, and the herb *Hypericum perforatum*, also known as St. John's wort. The FDA does not approve their use in obese patients, considers them "drugs" in a weight loss program, and is taking regulatory action to remove them from the market because of the potential for serious side effects.

16. What side effects were observed with the use of phentermine/fenfluramine and dexfenfluramine?

Two serious, somewhat unexpected side effects were associated with the use of fenfluramine and dexfenfluramine: primary pulmonary hypertension (PPH) and valvular heart disease. Although it is not clear how commonly PPH occurred, the best data suggest that of 1 million people who took these medicines, between 28 and 50 will develop PPH, one-half of whom will die from the condition even if the medications are stopped. The frequency of valvular heart disease as a complication is not clear. Echocardiography has demonstrated a prevalence of valvular disease ranging from 30–38%. Such studies suggest that valvulopathy may be more common in people exposed to the drug for > 6 months. Aortic insufficiency was the most common lesion; only 18% of affected people had an audible murmur by auscultation. Based on these findings, the drugs were voluntarily withdrawn from the market in 1997.

17. How should a patient who was treated with fenfluramine or dexfenfluramine be followed?

There is no clear answer to this question. Because a high prevalence of valvular abnormalities was found in asymptomatic people exposed to these drugs, many of whom do not have a murmur by auscultation, some experts advocate that all exposed patients should have an echocardiogram. The rationale is that it is important for patients to know whether they have experienced a side effect. In addition, it has been advised that people with cardiac valvulopathy related to fenfluramine or dexfenfluramine should receive antibiotic prophylaxis if they undergo dental procedures. There are, however, some concerns with this approach. The first is that transthoracic echocardiography is more difficult in obese people, making the reliability of the study lower. Second, the natural history of this valvulopathy is unclear. Does it progress or regress once medication is stopped? There are no published data on which to base an answer, but unpublished observations suggest that at least in some people the disorder regresses with drug withdrawal. If this is the case, what does the care provider recommend to an asymptomatic patient with an abnormal valve? Experts recommend that echocardiography be repeated every 6 months.

18. What medications may become available in the next few years for treatment of obesity?

Orlistat, a pancreatic lipase inhibitor, reduces the absorption of fat by roughly 30%. It is given as 120 mg 3 times/day. Because it is not systemically absorbed, it probably will not be associated with PPH, although no firm data support this point. Orlistat should be available late in 1998 under the trade name Xenical. There were initial concerns of an increased risk of breast cancer in patients receiving the drug in premarketing trials. This concern is currently under study and is holding up final approval of the drug.

Sibutramine is a combination norepinephrine and serotonin reuptake blocker. Unlike fenfluramine and dexfenfluramine, it has no serotonin-releasing action and therefore is more like the serotonin-specific reuptake inhibitors currently used for treatment of depression. It is taken at doses ranging from 10–40 mg/day and produces weight loss in the range of 8–10% at doses of 20 mg and higher, somewhat less than the weight losses generally seen with the combination of fenfluramine and phentermine. In humans the drug works primarily by reducing appetite with minimal effects on energy expenditure. Sibutramine has been associated with an increase in blood pressure in some people, particularly at higher doses. The FDA required the manufacturer to examine the possibility that sibutramine may cause valvulopathy similar to that seen with fenfluramine and dexfenflu-ramine. Although this study has not yet been published, patients who were treated with sibutramine had no more cardiac valvular abnormalities identified by echocardiography than a control group. Sibutramine, which goes by the trade name Meridia, should be available in mid 1998.

Others. New developments in the basic sciences suggest that a number of regulatory systems may be potential targets for pharmacologic therapies. Recombinant leptin is currently in phase I trials. Like insulin, this peptide hormone must be administered parenterally. There is no published information about its efficacy, and it may interact with cytokine receptors at the site of infection to induce a local inflammatory response, which may limit its usefulness. Other drug companies are looking at compounds that interact with the downstream portions of the leptin-signaling pathway, in-cluding drugs that interact with the neuropeptide Y receptor subtype responsible for feeding effects. Cholecytokinin (CCK) is a gut hormone that inhibits feeding. A number of long-acting CCK ago-nists have been synthesized and are in the early stages of clinical trials. Stimulation of the beta$_3$-adrenergic receptor subtype causes increases in thermogenesis and energy expenditure in rodents. With the recent identification of uncoupling protein 3 in human skeletal muscle, it is hoped that a beta$_3$ agonist will increase energy expenditure in humans and aid in weight reduction. A number of these compounds have been synthesized and are in phase I clinical trials; however, bioavailability has been a major problem. This partial list gives some sense of the broad range of targets currently being examined as well as the unforeseen difficulties that may limit the usefulness of such compounds.

19. How long will a patient need to take a weight loss medicine?

In the past the FDA would allow only short-term use of weight loss medicines. However, experts now believe that obesity is a chronic illness like diabetes or high blood pressure and that a medicine used to help lose weight will work only as long as it is taken. Patients who take a weight loss medicine, lose weight, and then stop the medicine are likely to regain the lost weight. The same effect is observed when someone goes on a diet for a certain period, then stops the diet. this so-called "yo-yo" effect is probably not good for health. Unfortunately, we do not have good data about the safety or effectiveness of weight loss medicines used for 10–20 years. In general, if a primary care provider and a patient decide to use a weight loss medication, it should be used for a minimum of 3 months to determine whether the patient will lose at least 10% of body weight. Then consideration should be given to some form of chronic use in view of the available informa-tion about the risks and potential benefits of the medications, which is quite limited at this time.

20. Does the weight loss provided by medications improve health?

We do not know the answer to this question. One reasonable approach is to wait until more research is done to answer this important question clearly. Other medicines developed for other conditions, such as ventricular arrhythmias, have turned out to hurt more than to help. We know that in some people the weight loss accompanying the use of medicines is associated with de-creases in blood pressure, improved glucose control in patients with diabetes, reduced symptoms of degenerative arthritis, and reduced blood levels of cholesterol. Some people find that weight loss medicines reduce the occurrence of obsessive thoughts about eating, which may be their most important therapeutic effect. Although it makes intuitive sense that losing weight would im-prove health, it is not yet clear that losing weight *with medications* improves health. On the other hand, it is clear that increased weight is associated with health risks if nothing is done. The deci-sion whether the health benefits outweigh the risk and cost of weight loss medicines is an indi-vidual one that needs to be made on a case-by-case basis, based on less than adequate data, between the primary care provider and the patient.

21. So what is the role of pharmacologic therapy in the treatment of obesity?

Before the removal of fenfluramine and dexfenfluramine from the market, many primary care providers had the opportunity to experience firsthand the difficult issues raised by this ques-tion. Since the medications were removed, many who prescribed them have reevaluated the role of drugs in the treatment of obesity. A number of pharmaceutical companies, however, see a large potential market in this class of medications and are currently investing in drug development. This investment occurs at a time of dramatic new insights into the pathophysiology of obesity.

Probably there will always be a great demand for pharmacologic treatments from patients. Although it is easy to say that drugs should never be used or that it is up to the patient to assess the risk:benefit ratio, a more reasonable approach is probably somewhere between. It is clear that increasing body weight is associated with increased rates of morbidity and mortality. It is also clear that many patients lose more weight with drug treatment than with diet and exercise alone. Moreover, people fail to lose weight at all with standard diet and exercise counseling. The absolute health risks associated with obesity increase as BMI and age increase; it is also increases in patients with a positive family history of metabolic diseases. Therefore, the risk:benefit ratio for the use of a weight loss medication probably becomes favorable at some level of obesity if the medication does not have common severe side effects. Medications may be considered in patients with a BMI > 30 if comorbid conditions such as diabetes, hypertension, and degenerative arthritis are present or BMI > 33 in the absence of comorbid conditions. These criteria are conservative. The FDA has granted preliminary approval for the use of sibutramine in patients with a BMI > 30 in the absence of comorbid conditions and in patients with a BMI > 27 in the presence of comorbid conditions.

22. Should liposuction be advocated for obese patients?

In the only controlled trial, weight lost by liposuction was regained. In some patients the adipose tissue reaccumulated in the same site; in others, it reaccumulated elsewhere. Liposuction cannot be advocated as a weight loss strategy for patients with medically significant obesity.

23. What mechanical methods are available for the treatment of morbidly obese patients?

Morbid obesity has been variably defined as weight that is 100% or 100 lb above ideal. Another definition is BMI > 40. Such patients are at high risk for adverse health consequences. Surgical therapy may offer the best long-term chance for reducing body weight. The success rate for gastroplasty or gastric bypass is 60–70%, and the average weight loss is 30%. Many patients experience a marked improvement in preoperative morbidities, including resolution of diabetes, hypertension, and hyperlipidemia and improved rates of employment. In addition to operative morbidities, cholelithiasis is a relatively common complication. Recently laparoscopy has been used to do a procedure similar to banded gastroplasty. Initial results suggest that it has a lower rate of success than more traditional surgical treatments. The gastric balloon, popular a few years ago, has proved to be an unsafe mechanical treatment.

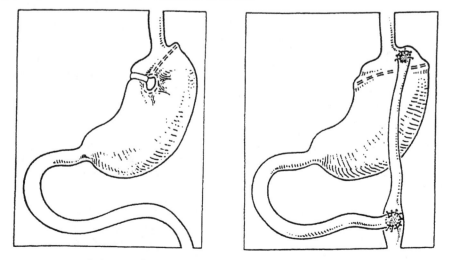

Gastroplasty *(left)* and gastric bypass *(right)* operations for the treatment of morbid obesity.

24. What is a very-low-calorie diet (VLCD)? When should its use be considered?

A VLCD is a nutritionally complete diet of 800 kcal/day that produces weight loss. Experienced teams in supervised settings should administer such diets. When VLCDs are used in this manner, complications are rare. The long-term results with VLCDs are no better than with other dietary programs. For this reason, VLCDs have limited usefulness. They may be helpful in patients who need a short-term weight loss to reduce the risk of a diagnostic or surgical procedure.

BIBLIOGRAPHY

1. Abenhaim L, et al: Appetite-suppressant drugs and the risk of primary pulmonary hypertension. N Engl J Med 335:609–616, 1996.
2. Bray GA: Drug treatment of obesity: Don't throw the baby out with the bath water. Am J Clin Nutr 67:1–2, 1998.
3. Bray GA: Obesity. Endocrinol Metab Clin North Am 25:781–1048, 1996.
4. Brownell KD: The LEARN Program for Weight Control, 7th ed. Philadelphia, American Health, 1997.
5. Cardiac valvuloplasty associated with exposure to fenfluramine or dexfenfluramine: U.S. Department of Health and Human Services interim public health recommendations. MMWR 46:1061–1066, 1997.
6. Conolly HM, Crary JL, McGoon MD, et al: Valvular heart disease associated with fenfluramine-phentermine. N Engl J Med 337:581–588, 1997.
7. Hirsch J: The treatment of obesity with drugs. Am J Clin Nutr 67:2–3, 1998.
8. Kushner J: The treatment of obesity with drugs: A call for prudence and professionalism. Arch Intern Med 157:602–604, 1997.
9. Leibel RL, Rosenbaum M, Hirsch J: Changes in energy expenditure resulting from altered body weight. N Engl J Med 332:621–628, 1995.
10. Long term pharmacotherapy in the management of obesity. JAMA 276:1907–1915, 1996.
11. Losing weight: What works and what doesn't. Consumer Rep June:347–357, 1993.
12. Manson JE, Faich GA: Pharmacotherapy of obesity—do the benefits outweigh the risks? N Engl J Med 335:659–660, 1996.
13. Methods for voluntary weight loss and control. Ann Intern Med 119:641–764, 1993.
14. Rosenbaum M, Leibel RL, Hirsch J: Obesity. N Engl J Med 337:396–407, 1997.
15. Stevens J, Cai J, Pamuk ER, et al: The effect of age on the association between body mass index and mortality. N Engl J Med 338:1–7, 1998.
16. Wolf AM, Colditz GA: Social and economic effects of body weight in the United States. Am J Clin Nutr 63:466S–469S, 1996.

105. THE CIGARETTE SMOKER

Thomas D. MacKenzie, M.D., M.S.P.H.

1. What is the current prevalence of cigarette smoking in the United States?

Cigarette smoking became the most popular form of tobacco consumption in the 1920s. Per capita cigarette consumption rose sharply during World War II and continued to rise until the 1950s. The first reports linking cigarette use with cancer emerged in the 1950s and were subsequently confirmed with other studies, leading to the famous Surgeon General's Report on Smoking and Health in 1964. Consumption eventually peaked in the late 1960s at over 4000 cigarettes per capita per year and has declined annually since. The prevalence of cigarette smoking (percentage of the adult population who smoke regularly) peaked at 41% and declined annually until 1990. Of great concern to public health officials is that the prevalence has remained static since 1990 at approximately 25% of the adult population. Moreover, recent data suggest that the prevalence of current cigarette smoking among teenagers has increased by 30% between 1991 and 1997.

2. At what age do people start to smoke?

The average age of initiation of regular cigarette smoking has been declining since the 1920s. For persons born between 1910 and 1920 the average age of initiation was approximately 20 years. Today the average age is 14.5 years. In 1992, 1 in 5 eighth graders reported smoking their first cigarette in fifth grade.

3. How do you quantify a person's smoking history?

Multiply the average number of packs smoked per day by the number of years of smoking to get the number of pack-years of smoking. For example, a 55-year-old woman who began smoking at age 15 and thinks that she smoked an average of $1\frac{1}{2}$ packs (30 cigarettes) per day has a 60 pack-year smoking history (1.5 packs $\times$ 40 years).

4. How is nicotine dependence defined?

According to the Diagnostic and Statistical Manual of Mental Disorders (DSM IV), a person meets criteria for nicotine dependence if any three of the following occur within a 12-month period:

1. The person smokes more cigarettes or smokes for a longer period than originally intended.

2. The person continuously desires or has made 1 or more unsuccessful attempts at cessation.

3. The person spends much time and energy getting cigarettes, smoking cigarettes, or recovering from their effects.

4. The person frequently smokes or suffers from withdrawal symptoms when expected to fulfill obligations at work, school, or home.

5. The person gives up important social, occupational, or recreational activities because of cigarette smoking.

6. The person continues to smoke despite the knowledge of having persistent or recurring social, psychological, or physical problems caused or exacerbated by the use of cigarettes.

7. The person needs increasing amounts of nicotine to achieve the desired effect or the person has diminished effect with continuing use of the same amount.

8. The person experiences characteristic nicotine withdrawal symptoms or uses nicotine to prevent withdrawal symptoms.

5. What are the four A's of smoking cessation counseling?

The National Cancer Institute's (NCI) manual "How to Help Your Patients Stop Smoking" and the 1996 Clinical Practice Guideline on Smoking Cessation from the Agency for Health Care Policy and Research (AHCPR) list four A's for office-based interventions:

1. **Ask** about smoking at every opportunity. Many experts have advocated that tobacco exposure should be assessed at every office visit as a fifth vital sign. It raises the awareness of smokers, nonsmokers, and office staff to the importance of cessation.

2. **Advise** all smokers to stop. Physician advice is a powerful and inexpensive tool for smoking cessation, especially when given in a "teachable moment" such as an office visit for bronchitis or a tobacco-related hospitalization.

3. **Assist** patients in the cessation effort. Any health care provider can assist the patient in setting a quit date. The date should be set as soon after the initial counseling session as possible. Nicotine replacement therapy should be offered to all patients except in special circumstances.

4. **Arrange** follow-up. A follow-up visit on or shortly after the quit date can improve success rates. The vast majority of relapses occur within the first 2 weeks after cessation.

For children and adolescents, the NCI recommends a fifth A: **Anticipatory guidance.**

6. The 1996 AHCPR Clinical Practice Guideline states that for primary care clinicians, all four A's are not appropriate for all smokers. How do you decide which patients should receive all four A's?

The **ask** step applies to all patients who visit a health care setting. The **advise** step is for all current smokers. After the advise step, the new guidelines strongly emphasize the importance of determining the willingness of the patient to attempt to quit. If he or she is willing to set a quit date, the clinician follows the **assist** and **arrange** steps. If the patient is not willing to attempt to quit, the guidelines recommend that the clinician make a "motivational intervention" to enhance the patient's motivation to stop (see next question).

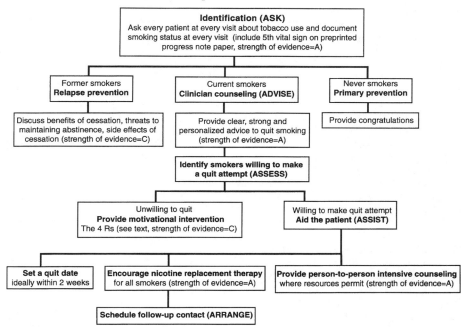

Clinical approach to smoking cessation counseling for adults.

7. What are the 4 R's of motivational interventions?

The 1996 AHCPR guideline lists the following components of clinical interventions designed to enhance motivation to quit smoking in patients who are not ready to make an attempt to quit:

1. **Relevance.** Information should be provided that is relevant to the patient's sociodemographic characteristics, disease status, health concerns, and social situation.

2. **Risks.** Acute, long-term, and environmental risks should be discussed with the patient.

3. **Rewards.** The clinician should highlight potential rewards of stopping that seem relevant to the patient.

4. **Repetition.** The motivational intervention should be repeated every time an unmotivated smoker visits the clinic.

8. What are typical nicotine withdrawal symptoms?

Craving for nicotine, irritability, frustration, anger, anxiety, difficulty in concentrating, restlessness, increased appetite, and decreased heart rate.

9. What happens to pulmonary function tests with smoking cessation?

The forced expiratory volume in 1 second (FEV_1) has been used as the marker of pulmonary function in several studies. Among all men over the age of 45 years, the FEV_1 typically declines at a rate of 20 ml/year as a natural consequence of aging. Smoking accelerates this age-related decline. For example, in the Honolulu Heart Program, men who continued to smoke showed a steeper rate of decline in FEV_1 of about 33 ml/year. Men who were able to quit in the first 2 years of the study rapidly reduced the rate of decline in FEV_1 to that of nonsmokers. Another study also showed that smoking intervention can significantly reduce the age-related decline in FEV_1 in middle-aged smokers with evidence of early chronic obstructive pulmonary disease.

10. How many times does a smoker attempt to quit before permanently giving up cigarettes?

Many times. Patients who have successfully given up smoking have often made several previous attempts to quit. Therefore, if a patient relapses after a period of abstinence, the physician should not consider him or her a "treatment failure." Support, understanding, and consideration of reenrollment in smoking cessation programs should be given.

11. What are the major short-term health benefits of smoking cessation?

1. The excessive risk of premature coronary heart disease falls by one-half within 1 year of abstinence.

2. Some of the toxic effects of cigarettes smoking that may lead to cardiac events, such as increased platelet activation, elevated carbon monoxide levels, and coronary artery spasm, are immediately reversible with cessation.

3. Pregnant women who stop during the first 3–4 months of pregnancy eliminate the risk of having a low-birth-weight baby.

12. Is inpatient smoking cessation treatment effective?

Five well-designed studies conducted with hospitalized smokers were reviewed for the AHCPR guideline. Inpatient counseling of varying intensity increased cessation rates by approximately 40%. The efficacy of the nicotine patch in hospitalized patients has not been well studied.

13. What are the major long-term benefits of smoking cessation?

1. Smoking cessation before age 35 eliminates the excessive mortality associated with smoking and translates into 7 more years of life compared with continuing smokers.

2. People who stop smoking between the ages of 45 and 55 years can extend their lives by approximately 4 years and can cut the excessive risk of death in half over the next 15 years compared with continuing smokers.

3. Even for smokers who can quite after age 65, there is significant improvement in overall survival compared with continuing smokers.

14. How much weight do people gain after they quit smoking?

In one large study of over 2500 smokers, the mean weight gain attributable to smoking cessation was 2.8 kg (6.2 lb) in men and 3.8 kg (8.4 lb) in women. Major weight gain (> 13 kg or 28.6 lb) occurred in 10% of men and 13% of women.

15. What are the 1996 U.S. Preventive Service Task Force (USPSTF) recommendations for smoking cessation counseling?

The USPSTF ranks its recommendations by the strength of the supporting evidence. The strongest favorable recommendation is an **A**, which implies that strong scientific evidence supports specific consideration of the recommendation in a periodic health examination. A **C** recommendation implies insufficient evidence to argue for or against its inclusion in a periodic health examination. The following recommendations received an A rating:

1. Tobacco cessation counseling is recommended on a regular basis for all patients who use tobacco products.

2. Pregnant women and parents with children living at home should be counseled about the potentially harmful effects of smoking on fetal and child health.

3. Prescription of nicotine patches or gum is recommended as an adjunct for selected patients.

The use of clonidine as an adjunct to smoking cessation counseling received a C rating. Clinical counseling of children, adolescents, and young adults to prevent smoking initiation also received a C rating based on the lack of evidence supporting its effectiveness.

16. How effective is nicotine replacement therapy?

Two recent metaanalyses of randomized, placebo-controlled trials of nicotine replacement therapy demonstrate that both nicotine gum and transdermal nicotine are highly effective aids for smoking cessation. Both agents approximately double the smoking cessation rates at 1 year compared with placebo. Success rates are also influenced by the degree of nicotine dependence and the intensity of counseling (see question 22).

17. How can a clinician assess the degree of tobacco dependency in an individual patient?
The Fagerström Test for Nicotine Dependence (FTND) is used to determine the degree of nicotine dependence for an individual patient. Studies have shown that highly dependent smokers benefit more from use of nicotine gum than less dependent smokers. However, the data for nicotine patches are mixed. Some recent studies suggest that the benefit of the patch may be more pronounced in smokers who are less dependent on nicotine.

Fagerström Test for Nicotine Dependence

QUESTIONS	ANSWERS	POINTS
1. How soon after you wake up do you smoke your first cigarette?	Within 5 minutes	3
	6–30 minutes	2
	31–60 minutes	1
	After 60 minutes	0
2. Do you find it difficult to refrain from smoking in places where it is forbidden (e.g., in church, at the library, in the cinema)?	Yes	1
	No	0
3. Which cigarette would you hate most to give up?	The first one in the morning	1
	All others	0
4. How many cigarettes/day do you smoke?	10 or less	0
	11–20	1
	21–30	2
	31 or more	3
5. Do you smoke more frequently during the first hours after waking than during the rest of the day?	Yes	1
	No	0
6. Do you smoke if you are so ill that you are in bed most of the day?	Yes	1
	No	0

From Heatherton TF, Kozlowski LT, Frecker RC, Fagerström KO: The Fagerström test for nicotine dependence: A revision of the Fagerström tolerance questioinnaire. Br J Addict 86:1119–1127, 1991.

18. What are the indications for nicotine polacrilex gum?
• The patient is motivated to quit (ready to set a quit date)
• The patient is able to follow a complex regimen.
• The patient has medium-to-high dependence on nicotine.
• The patient is able to abstain from smoking while using gum.

19. What is the mechanism of action of nicotine gum?
The gum contains nicotine bound to an ion-exchange resin in a gum base, which allows the nicotine to be released slowly. A low pH impairs the release of the nicotine. Once the nicotine is released, it is absorbed through the buccal mucosa. The systemic nicotine alleviates withdrawal symptoms normally associated with smoking cessation.

20. How is nicotine gum prescribed?
1. Use the FTND to determine the degree of dependence. Highly dependent ($\geq$ 5) smokers are given 4-mg nicotine gum for 6 weeks and then 2-mg nicotine gum until completion of therapy. Smokers with moderate-to-low dependence are prescribed 2-mg nicotine gum. The mean nicotine content of a cigarette is 1.8 ± 0.4 mg.
2. Prescribe one piece of gum every hour while the patient is awake. The patient should be instructed to chew the gum until he or she senses that the nicotine has been released and then to park the gum to allow absorption through the buccal mucosa. An acid environment from drinking juice, soda, or coffee greatly impairs absorption of nicotine.

3. Remove gum after 20 minutes.
4. Recommend tapering frequency of gum use after 3 months.

21. Discuss the length of treatment and dosing for nicotine patches.

Many randomized, controlled trials evaluating nicotine patches as an aid to smoking cessation suggest that the maximal benefit can be gained by using a 6–8-week course of daily patches. Although some patch manufacturers initially recommended nicotine patch use for up to 3 months, more recent studies have shown that end-of-treatment quit rates for 3 months of patch use are essentially the same as quit rates at the end of 4 weeks and worse than quit rates after 6 weeks of patch use. Studies suggest that 6–8 weeks is enough time for nicotine withdrawal symptoms to decrease and allows the patient to develop the new skills necessary to maintain abstinence. Many clinicians use high-dose patches uniformly in the initial 2–4 weeks and taper the dose at 2-week intervals thereafter. There is probably no significant difference in the efficacy of 24-hour vs. 16-hour patches.

22. What type of counseling is an effective adjunct to the use of nicotine patches?

Although the patch appears to be effective for some patients without counseling, counseling along with the patch uniformly increases quit rates. A meta-analysis of 17 nicotine patch studies rated counseling intensity levels according to four criteria: (1) the goal of the meeting was smoking cessation; (2) one or more weekly weekly meetings were held during the first 4 weeks of treatment; (3) the total number of meetings was greater than 7 in the first 12 weeks; and (4) counseling lasted more than 40 minutes. High-intensity counseling was shown to be more effective than low-intensity counseling. Furthermore, group counseling was more effective than individual counseling.

Abstinence Rates at 6 Months in a Meta-analysis of the Efficacy of Transdermal Nicotine by Format and Intensity of Counseling

	PLACEBO PATCH (%)	ACTIVE NICOTINE PATCH (%)
Counseling format		
Individual	7.7	20.0
Group	12.6	26.3
Counseling intensity		
Low	7.1	19.5
High	13.2	26.5

Adapted from Fiore MC, Smith SS, Jorenby DE, Baker TB: The effectiveness of the nicotine patch for smoking cessation: A meta-analysis. JAMA 271:1940–1947, 1994.

23. Can nicotine patches be used in patients with known coronary artery disease?

It is generally believed that the patch can be used in patients with stable angina if the patient understands that the patch is a *substitute* for cigarettes and is motivated to abstain totally. In one study of 156 patients with stable coronary artery disease, 14-mg patches were compared with placebo for 5 weeks. Quit rates were 36% for active patch users vs. 22% for placebo patch users. There was no increase in cardiac symptoms or complications in the active patch group. Patches are contraindicated in patients who have had a recent myocardial infarction or who have poorly controlled hypertension.

24. What strategies can be used to promote smoking cessation in a clinical setting?

A meta-analysis of 39 controlled trials of smoking cessation strategies showed that smoking cessation programs using several modes of *repeated* counseling and intervention are most effective for initial and long-term cessation. Interventions included physician and nonphysician individualized counseling, setting a quit date, nurse telephone follow-up, group counseling and classes, and use of written materials, cassettes, and videos. Carbon monoxide monitors are often used to verify abstinence and may be useful in the initial counseling stages by demonstrating the "poison" that builds up in the blood of the smoker. The use of nicotine patches or nicotine gum should be considered in all patients.

25. What is the cost-effectiveness of smoking interventions?

The cost-effectiveness of a therapy can be measured in dollars spent per quality-adjusted life year saved (QALY). Smoking cessation interventions are among the most cost-effective interventions in medicine. For comparison, hypertension screening costs $14,000–40,000 per QALY; annual mammography for women aged 50–69 years costs $46,000 per QALY. The table below shows that the cost per QALY for smoking cessation counseling is $1100–4000, depending on the intensity of counseling. When you use the nicotine patch as adjunctive therapy, the cost-effectiveness improves.

Costs and Cost-Effectiveness Ratios for Smoking Cessation Counseling Interventions With and Without Transdermal Nicotine*

| | COST/PARTICIPANT | | | |
INTERVENTION	SUCCESSFUL	FAILED	COST/QUITTER	COST/QALY[†]
Counseling alone				
Minimal	14.51	14.51	7922	4015
Full	75.55	75.55	2989	1515
Group intensive	53.14	53.14	2186	1108
Counseling with transdermal nicotine				
Minimal	246.25	141.40	4745	2405
Full	300.69	195.84	2715	1376
Group intensive	272.37	167.52	2310	1171

* Data from Cromwell J, Bartosch WJ, Fiore MC et al: Cost-effectiveness of the clinical practice recommendations in the AHCPR guideline for smoking cessation. JAMA 278:1759–1766, 1997.
[†] QALY = quality-adjusted life-year. Costs are discounted by 3% per year.

BIBLIOGRAPHY

1. Agency for Health Care Policy and Research Smoking Cessation Clinical Practice Guideline. JAMA 275:1270–1280, 1996.
2. Bartecchi CE, MacKenzie TD, Schrier RW: The global tobacco epidemic. Sci Am May:26–33, 1995.
3. Bartecchi CE, MacKenzie TD, Schrier RW: The human costs of tobacco use. Part I. N Engl J Med 330:907–912, 1994.
4. Burchfiel CM, et al: Effects of smoking and smoking cessation on longitudinal decline in pulmonary function. Am J Respir Crit Care Med 151:1778–1785, 1995.
5. Centers for Disease Control and Prevention: Cigarette smoking—attributable mortality and years of potential life lost—United States, 1990. MMWR 42:230–233, 1993.
6. Centers for Disease Control and Prevention: Cigarette smoking among adults—United States, 1992, and changes in the definition of current cigarette smoking. MMWR 43:342–346, 1994.
7. Centers for Disease Control and Prevention: Tobacco use among high school students—United States, 1997. MMWR 47:229–233, 1998.
8. Cromwell J, Bartosch WJ, Fiore MC, et al: Cost-effectiveness of the clinical practice recommendations in the AHCPR guideline for smoking cessation. Agency for Health Care Policy and Research. JAMA 278:1759–1766, 1997.
9. Doll R, Peto R, Wheatley K, et al: Mortality in relation to smoking: 40 years' observations in male British doctors. BMJ 309:901–911, 1994.
10. Fiore MC, Kenford SL, Jorenby DE, et al: Two studies of the clinical effectiveness of the nicotine patch with different counseling treatments. Chest 105:524–533, 1994.
11. Fiore MC, Smith SS, Jorenby DE, Baker TB: The effectiveness of the nicotine patch for smoking cessation: A meta-analysis. JAMA 271:1940–1947, 1994.
12. Heatherton TF, Kozlowski LT, Frecker RC, Fagerström KO: The Fagerström test for nicotine dependence: A revision of the Fagerström tolerance questionnaire. Br J Addict 86:1119–1127, 1991.
13. MacKenzie TD, Bartecchi CE, Schrier RW: The human costs of tobacco use. Part II. N Engl J Med 330:975–980, 1994.
14. Surgeon General: Reducing the Health Consequences of Smoking: 25 Years of Progress: A Report of the Surgeon General: Executive Summary. Rockville, MD, Department of Health and Human Services, 1989 [DHHS Publ. No. (CDC) 89-8411].
15. Surgeon General: The Health Benefits of Smoking Cessation. Washington, DC, Department of Health and Human Services, 1990, pp 473–515 [DHHS Publ. No. (CDC)90-8416].

16. Tang JL, Law M, Wald N: How effective is nicotine replacement therapy in helping people to stop smoking? BMJ 308:21–26, 1994.
17. U.S. Preventive Services Task Force: Guide to Clinical Preventive Services, 2nd ed. Baltimore, Williams & Wilkins, 1996.
18. Williamson DF, Madans J, Anda RF, et al: Smoking cessation and severity of weight gain in a national cohort. N Engl J Med 324:739–745, 1991.

106. THE PATIENT WITH ACQUIRED IMMUNODEFICIENCY SYNDROME

David W. Lehman, M.D., Ph.D.

1. When does a patient have acquired immunodeficiency syndrome (AIDS)?

AIDS is a clinical syndrome of acquired immunodeficiency resulting from infection with the human immunodeficiency virus (HIV). When a patient who is HIV-positive develops an opportunistic infection, a specific neoplasm, or other specified condition, the patient has AIDS. The most common opportunistic infections are *Pneumocystis carinii* pneumonia (PCP), *Mycobacterium avium* complex (MAC), cytomegalovirus (CMV), *Mycobacterium tuberculosis* infection, candidal esophagitis, coccidioidomycosis, and other fungal infections. The most common neoplasms are Kaposi's sarcoma and non-Hodgkin's lymphomas, but invasive cervical carcinoma is also AIDS-defining. Other AIDS-defining conditions include a CD4 < 200, pulmonary tuberculosis, recurrent pneumonia, HIV encephalopathy, and AIDS wasting syndrome.

Relative Risk of AIDS-defining Conditions as a Function of CD4 Count

May occur with higher CD4 counts (increased risk with lower counts)	
Tuberculosis	Kaposi's sarcoma
Herpes simplex or zoster	Systemic fungal infection
Rare, unless CD4 count < 200	
Pneumocystis carinii pneumonia	Progressive multifocal leukoencephalopathy
Non-Hodgkin's lymphoma	Wasting syndrome
AIDS dementia complex	Toxoplasmosis
Rare, unless CD4 < 50	
Mycobacterium avium complex	Cytomegalovirus disease

2. What risk factors for HIV disease should be assessed in primary care practice?

A complete history includes an assessment of HIV risk: male homosexual behavior, IV drug use (specifically needle sharing), sex with IV drug users, prostitution, sex with prostitutes, history of blood transfusion between 1978 and 1985, history of sexually transmitted diseases, and history of multiple sexual partners. Potential risk may be clarified by determining the frequency of safe/unsafe sex practices. The risk assessment process also may be used to educate patients about risk reduction, including safer sex and safer drug use.

3. When should the physician encourage the patient to be tested for HIV?

HIV testing should be recommended if a history of more than minimal risk is obtained. Because of the benefits of decreasing maternal-infant transmission with antiretroviral therapy, it is recommended that pregnant women be tested. Patients should be counseled about confidentiality issues and consent to testing. Some patients choose to be tested anonymously at an alternate test site.

4. How can the physician judge the patient's risk of transmission?

Parenteral blood products have the highest rate of transmission, although the rate has not been quantified. Although condom failures have been reported, the consistent, correct use of condoms with nonoxynol-9 is nearly 100% effective in preventing HIV transmission. Among specific sexual behaviors, unprotected receptive anal intercourse with ejaculation is the highest risk, estimated at 3% (3 of 100) for each act of anal sex. The risk for insertive partners in rectal sex is somewhat lower. The risk of male-to-female transmission has been studied by evaluating the proportion of infected women among the steady partners of infected men. The estimated rate of infection in women for each act of unprotected vaginal sex varies widely but may be 1 in 500. Female-to-male transmission is probably lower, although the low prevalence in women has limited collection of suitable data. The risk of transmission of HIV by unprotected oral sex for performing and receiving partners is unquantified.

5. How accurate is HIV testing?

The joint false-positive rate of sequential enzyme-linked immunosorbent assay (ELISA) and Western blot testing is about 0.1%, depending on the experience of the laboratory. In a population with a low prevalence of HIV infection, this false-positive rate may correspond to positive predictive values of less than 50%. False-negative tests in low prevalence populations are rare and result mainly from the window of time between infection and development of antibodies (usually < 3 months but rarely up to 6 months).

6. What are the natural history and prognosis of HIV infection?

On average, about 50% of untreated HIV-infected patients progress to AIDS in 10 years. Patients often gain a more positive outlook in learning that one-half of patients will *not* progress to AIDS after 10 years. Even in the asymptomatic stage viral synthesis is very active with as many as 10^{10} virions produced each day. The natural history of progression to AIDS has been studied in several populations:

- The San Francisco City Clinic Cohort: 54% progression after 11 years
- Transfusion recipients: 49% progression after 7 years
- Hemophiliacs: 25% progression after 9 years

Mathematical models predict that > 95% of untreated HIV-infected patients will eventually progress to AIDS, but the data do not allow us to conclude that every HIV-positive person will inevitably develop AIDS. The HIV RNA viral load is the single best predictor of survival. CD4 cell count and the viral syncytium-inducing phenotype predict outcome independently of viral load. A combination of these three markers predicts outcome more accurately. The median survival after developing of an AIDS-defining condition has increased about 48 months with current therapy.

7. How should the newly diagnosed HIV-positive patient be evaluated?

The complete history and physical exam for HIV-positive patients includes special emphasis on risk factors (timing of seroconversion if possible), psychosocial issues, systemic issues (fever and weight loss), and targeted organs: skin, oropharynx, lungs, gastrointestinal (GI) tract, and lymph nodes. Routine laboratory evaluation includes chest radiograph, complete blood count with differential and platelet count, levels of aspartate aminotransferase (AST), alanine aminotransferase (ALT), lactate dehydrogenase (LDH), bilirubin, alkaline phosphatase (AP), albumin, total protein, and creatinine; serologic test for syphilis, toxoplasmosis, and hepatitis B surface antigen (HBsAg); and assessment of HIV RNA viral load and T cells with subsets. Vaccinations (including diphtheria-tetanus, Pneumovax, and influenza) are updated, and purified protein derivative (PPD) skin testing is done. Hepatitis B vaccine is recommended for HBsAg-negative patients with ongoing risk behavior. Risk reduction behavior (tobacco cessation, alcohol moderation, IV drug cessation) should be encouraged. A nutritional evaluation and plan help patients to maintain a healthy weight.

8. How can a patient's clinical status, risk of disease progression, and response to therapy be determined?

The single best marker of clinical status is the viral load because it is the best predictor of progression to AIDS and death. The viral load is a measure of the number of copies of virus in a milliliter of blood. The combination of viral load and CD4 count gives a more accurate prediction of clinical status. For example, a patient with CD4 count > 750 and viral load < 500 has only a 3.6% risk of progressing to AIDS in 9 years; a patient with CD4 count of 201–350 and viral load of 10–30,000 has an 85% risk of progressing in 9 years and a 56% risk of progressing in only 3 years. Patients should be routinely monitored every 3–4 months. Because of intraassay and biologic variability, the viral load should be repeated within 2–4 weeks after baseline measurement or after a change in therapy, or after a significant change in viral load, which would lead to an adjustment in therapy. A 0.5-log (3-fold) decrease in viral load is the minimal change necessary for a positive response to therapy. Several drug regimens have been shown to decrease viral load by 1–2 logs (10- to 100-fold) or more. Treatment with antiretroviral drugs often leads to increases in CD4 count, but these higher counts do not restore the complete immune repertoire. Initiation of prophylaxis (for PCP and MAC) should be based on the lowest CD4 count and continued indefinitely if tolerated. A 1-log (10-fold) decrease in viral load on drug therapy (by week 8) is associated with a 65% decrease in risk of progression to AIDS. A 0.5-log increase or a return to within 0.5 log of baseline is an indication of treatment failure.

9. What are the goals of antiviral therapy?

Multiple goals have been proposed, ranging from eradication of infection (currently theoretical) to keeping the viral load undetectable or as low as possible (with CD4 count as high as possible) and the longer-term maintenance goal of keeping the patient healthy, functional, and free of side effects as long as possible. It would be preferable to restore immune function rather than only to stop further deterioration, even if eradication becomes possible.

10. What antiretroviral drugs are available?

Current antiretroviral (ARV) drugs represent three ways to prevent the synthesis of new HIV: nucleoside reverse transcriptase inhibitors (NRTIs), nonnucleoside reverse transcriptase inhibitors (NNRTIs), and protease inhibitors (PIs). The NRTIs are zidovudine, didanosine, zalcitabine, stavudine, and lamivudine. The available NNRTIs are nevirapine and delavirdine. The PIs are ritonavir, nelfinavir, indinavir, and saquinavir. Because of the high likelihood of the development of resistance to ARVs by HIV, monotherapy should not be used. Patients who choose to take drugs should take a combination of at least two drugs, and in most cases three drugs would be better. A combination of two NRTIs and one PI reduced viral load below detectable levels in 90% of one small series of patients at 24 weeks. Prior patient experience with one or more ARVs may alter the likelihood that the patient already has drug-resistant virus and should be a factor in choosing an appropriate drug regimen. Cross-resistance between drugs is a major problem, increases with partial/suboptimal treatment, and may decrease the effectiveness of future drug regimens. Research is ongoing, and most likely better drugs (more effective, improved dosing schedule, fewer side effects) will be available in the next 1–5 years.

No single drug regimen is best for all patients. A combination of two NRTIs with one PI or one NNRTI is frequently used. Because of the ongoing rapid flow of new clinical outcomes data and subsequent changing recommendations for therapy, physicians should consult recent expert recommendations for assistance in choosing the best drug regimen for a particular patient.

11. When should ARV treatment be started?

The timing and choice of ARVs are areas with rapidly evolving data about which physicians disagree. Well-informed patients often state their own preferences, which should be a major factor in the therapeutic decision process. Several groups and individuals have proposed algorithms for starting ARV treatment. These recommendations are extrapolations from limited clinical data about treatment of certain HIV clinical status categories. Data are not available for all HIV clinical status categories. The data are limited because outcomes were usually evaluated at 1–2 years at most and patients need to be treated for much longer periods.

Because the drug regimens can be difficult to follow and because the likelihood of drug-resistant mutants is high and increases when suboptimal drug regimens are followed, the decision to start drugs should follow careful patient education about the risks (all drugs have side effects, some of which are dangerous and some of which are annoying) and benefits of ARVs and the commitment of the patient to adhere to the drug regimen for at least 3 years and potentially for life. Present or past use of alcohol and/or other drugs should raise concerns about the patient's ability to make a long-term commitment to a complex drug regimen. Illicit drug use may counteract the benefits of ARVs and increase the likelihood of not following completely a drug regimen.

The usual indications for treatment include viral load > 3–10,000 copies/ml, CD4 count < 500 cells/μl, symptoms suggesting progression, and symptoms of primary infection. A falling CD4 count (> 100 decrease in CD4/year) or a rising viral load are also appropriate indications to start treatment. Many patients and their physicians choose to start ARVs even though the viral load is low and the CD4 count is high. Because such patients have a good prognosis even without drugs, they need to take drugs for many years to realize benefit and risk feeling worse in the interim because of drug side effects. Over such a long time, the likelihood of noncompliance and subsequent development of drug resistance increases.

12. Describe the common skin problems in HIV infection.

Up to 90% of HIV-positive patients have a skin disease. Kaposi's sarcoma is discussed in question 22 with other malignancies. The prevalence of skin infections is high. Among bacterial etiologies, *Staphylococcus aureus* is the most common, usually presenting as folliculitis or, less frequently, bullous impetigo, ecthyma, abscesses, or cellulitis. Among viral etiologies, herpes viruses (zoster and simplex) are the most common. The suggestion to assess HIV risk factors in all adults aged 18–50 years is especially applicable if such a patient (even up to 65 yr) presents with zoster. *Molluscum contagiosum* is common and especially difficult to eradicate in HIV-positive patients.

By virtue of taking more drugs, HIV-positive patients and patients with AIDS are at increased risk of drug reactions. The most common is due to trimethoprim/sulfamethoxazole (TMP/SMX) and presents as a diffuse maculopapular eruption. Other antibiotics, notably penicillins, are also common offenders. Among ARVs, nevirapine most often causes a rash.

13. What mouth problems are common in HIV infection?

Common oral lesions in HIV-positive patients have fungal, bacterial, viral, or neoplastic etiologies. The two most common types are hairy leukoplakia (white thickening of mucosal surfaces, often with vertical corrugations) and thrush (pseudomembranous candidiasis). Both have been shown to predict progression to AIDS independently of CD4 counts. Candidal infection also may present as angular cheilitis, candidal leukoplakia, or the erythematous form. Gingivitis and periodontitis are common bacterial complications of HIV disease. Kaposi's sarcoma may produce oral lesions.

14. What entities should be considered when an HIV-positive patient complains of dysphagia?

Candidal esophagitis is the most common cause of dysphagia; odynophagia and retrosternal chest pain are other frequent symptoms. Less common causes are CMV, herpes virus, and Kaposi's sarcoma. Response to empiric treatment for candidal infection with ketoconazole sometimes provides a presumptive diagnosis. Endoscopy with biopsies is needed for a definitive diagnosis.

15. Describe the neuropsychiatric complications of HIV infection.

The common neurologic manifestations may be due directly to HIV (e.g., AIDS dementia complex and peripheral neuropathy) or secondary to drugs or opportunistic disease, including fungal (*Cryptococcus* sp.), protozoan (toxoplasmosis), myocbacterial, and viral infections. Peripheral neuropathy presents as a painful sensation with limited sensory or motor deficits. *Cryptococcus neoformans* meningitis is the most common fungal infection of the central nervous system in HIV-positive patients. Other fungal pathogens are histoplasmosis and coccidioidomycosis. *Toxoplasma gondii* causes encephalitis and focal intracerebral lesions, which are ring-enhancing on computed tomographic (CT) scan. Progressive multifocal leukoencephalopathy (PML), caused by the human polyomavirus (JC), commonly presents insidiously over weeks with focal neurologic deficits. AIDS dementia complex is an organic mental disorder with cognitive deficits (confusion, memory loss, impaired concentration or mental slowing), behavioral manifestations (depressed affect or agitation), and motor symptoms (weakness, unsteady gait, or decreased coordination). The common psychiatric manifestations include adjustment, affective, and anxiety disorders. An increased prevalence of substance abuse is self-evident among intravenous drug users but also has been described empirically in the male homosexual population.

16. When should the primary care physician seek hematologic consultations for HIV disease?
    Anemia, leukopenia, and thrombocytopenia may occur singly or in combination either as a direct manifestation of HIV disease or as a result of opportunistic infections or neoplasms, drug effects, or nutritional deficiencies. In many instances, the primary care physician may diagnose and manage the penias of HIV infection. Anemia is the most common abnormality, occurring in up to 85% of patients with AIDS. Isolated anemia is associated with *Mycobacterium avium* or parvovirus infection. Hemolytic anemia may occur in patients who are deficient in glucose 6-phosphate-dehydrogenase and treated with dapsone. Zidovudine may cause anemia that requires transfusions, neutropenia, and thrombocytopenia. Ganciclovir, pentamidine, trimethoprim, and cancer chemotherapeutic agents commonly cause neutropenia. Isolated immune thrombocytopenia may occur as a manifestation of HIV infection or AIDS. Diagnosis and treatment of immune thrombocytopenia may require bone marrow biopsy and hematologic consultation. In some instances, treatment of appropriate patients (CD4 counts < 500) with AZT has led to marked improvement of thrombocytopenia. In addition, the administration of growth factors (erythropoietin and granulocyte colony-stimulating factor [G-CSF]) may be helpful in some instances.

17. Contrast the clinical presentations and management of the various forms of pneumonia in HIV-positive patients.
    Pneuomocystis carinii pneumonia (PCP) is the most common AIDS-defining condition and usually occurs only in severely immuncompromised patients (CD4 < 200). Prophylaxis against PCP has been shown to prolong life for HIV-infected patients. Several agents are available for PCP prophylaxis: TMP/SMX (first-line), dapsone, and aerosolized pentamidine. Patients should be monitored for the occurrence of side effects that require a change to a different agent. Clinical presentation includes fever, nonproductive cough, and progressive shortness of breath; pleuritic chest pain is uncommon. Supportive evidence includes an elevated LDH, hypoxia or at least an increased alveoloarterial oxygen gradient, and a diffuse interstitial infiltrate on chest radiograph. Diagnosis is made by fluorescent antibody stain of induced sputum (64% sensitive) or, if necessary, bronchoalveolar lavage specimens (97% sensitive). Treatment options include TMP/SMX, pentamidine, TMP/dapsone, clindamycin/primaquine, and atovaquone with the addition of steroids for acute disease.
    Bacterial pneumonia, which is AIDS-defining if recurrent, occurs with increased frequency in HIV-positive patients. The most common pathogens include *Streptococcus pneumoniae, Haemophilus influenzae,* and *Moraxella catarrhalis.* The presenting symptoms—fever, productive cough, and dyspnea—are often acute and of short duration. The chest radiograph more often shows lobar or segmental infiltrates. Blood cultures are positive in 40–80% of cases. The sputum Gram stain sometimes gives an immediate diagnosis. Empiric treatment with TMP/SMX provides excellent coverage of the common bacterial agents as well as PCP, pending definitive diagnosis.
    Mycobacterial infection, which occurs with pulmonary as well as systemic manifestations, is discussed in question 19. The herpes family causes pneumonia as well as infects other organs or occurs as a systemic disease (see question 20). Fungal agents include *Cryptococcus* sp., *Histoplasma* sp., and coccidioidomycosis.

18. Should HIV-positive patients be screened regularly for tuberculosis?
    Yes. *Mycobacterium tuberculosis* has been found in 3.8% of patients with AIDS, with a disproportionate increase in extrapulmonary sites. Intravenous drug users and ethnic minorities are at especially increased risk. The 1993 revised case definition added pulmonary tuberculosis as an AIDS-defining condition. Annual screening with PPD (a > 5-mm reaction is positive) is recommended for all HIV-positive patients who are not already known to be anergic. Because of frequent anergy, some physicians also recommend a screening chest radiograph, depending on local prevalence of tuberculosis. PPD-positive patients of whatever age should take prophylactic

isoniazid. Initial empiric treatment for active tuberculosis includes isoniazid, rifampin, and pyrazinamide; further adjustment depends on the presence of extrapulmonary tuberculosis and the local prevalence of multidrug-resistant strains.

19. Which patients are susceptible to MAC?

Disseminated MAC is a frequent late complication of HIV infection (up to 53% in one autopsy series). It occurs only in patients with < 100 CD4 cells (75% of patients in one series had < 19 CD4 cells). Antimicrobial prophylaxis against *M. avium* for patients with CD4 < 75 with prior opportunistic infections decreases the incidence of mycobacteremia and improves survival. Lifetime prophylaxis with clarithromycin, azithromycin, or rifabutin is recommended, although physicians must weigh the risks of drug toxicity, drug interactions, and detrimental effects on compliance of adding another drug to often complex medical regimens. The common clinical manifestations of MAC are fever, malaise, weight loss, anemia, neutropenia, chronic diarrhea, abdominal pain, and malabsorption. Diagnosis is by special blood culture techniques. Because of their low sensitivity and low positive predictive value, stool cultures are not recommended. MAC bacteremia is associated with increased risk of death. Various multidrug regimens have been recommended; the combination of clarithromycin, ethambutol, and rifabutin has been shown to improve clearance of *M. avium* bacteremia and to increase survival rates.

20. List the three most common viral infections in HIV-positive patients.

Herpes simplex infection has a high prevalence (95% seropositivity in homosexual men with AIDS) and sometimes has severe manifestations in HIV-positive patients, including esophagitis, pneumonia, and encephalitis. Some patients require chronic acyclovir suppression. **Herpes zoster** (recurrent varicella zoster infection) occurs frequently in HIV-infected patients, and the new diagnosis of zoster in any patient younger than 65 years should prompt a risk assessment and consideration of testing for HIV. Patients may experience multiple recurrences and systemic dissemination. **Active CMV** is a frequent late complication of AIDS (in one series the median CD4 count was 19, and 75% of patients had < 46 CD4 cells). Clinical manifestations include retinitis, pneumonia, encephalitis, and severe diarrhea.

21. How should an HIV-positive patient with diarrhea be evaluated and treated?

First, a diagnosis should be sought to identify treatable etiologies of diarrhea. Stool should be cultured for bacteria and examined microscopically for parasites. *Mycobacterium avium intracellulare* (MAI) is best identified by blood cultures (see question 19). Common bacterial etiologies include *Salmonella, Shigella,* and *Campylobacter* spp., *Giardia lamblia, Entamoeba histolytica,* and, less commonly, *Cryptosporidium* sp. and *Isospora belli* (parasitic agents). A toxin from *Clostridium difficile* should be considered when the patient has been taking antibiotics. In one series CMV colitis was the most common cause of diarrhea; diagnosis requires identification of CMV and biopsy of mucosal ulcers. If no specific cause is identified, symptomatic treatment with nonspecific antidiarrheal drugs may provide significant benefit to patients.

22. Which malignancies are associated with HIV infection?

The AIDS-defining opportunistic malignancies are Kaposi's sarcoma (most common), non-Hodgkin's lymphoma, and invasive cervical carcinoma. Kaposi's sarcoma (KS) usually presents as violaceous, palpable nodules of the skin or oral mucosa; it also may involve the GI tract, lungs, and lymph nodes. About 70% of non-Hodgkin's lymphoma is B-cell lymphoma and usually presents as advanced extranodal disease. Three-fourths of patients with non-Hodgkin's lymphoma have CD4 counts < 80; the disease may present as a primary lymphoma of the central nervous system but usually not until patients are severely immunocompromised (CD4 < 50). Invasive cervical carcinoma was added as an AIDS-defining condition in the revised case definition of 1993.

23. Describe the special issues associated with HIV in women.

The rising frequency, epidemiology, and severity of HIV infection in women present special issues. The fastest growing AIDS group is women. Intravenous drug use is responsible for 59%

of AIDS cases in women, either directly (39%) or indirectly (20%) through sex with an injection drug user. Minorities are disproportionately represented; 74% of women with AIDS are African-American or Hispanic. AIDS is now the most common cause of death among women of color ages 25–44 years in the United States and the third most common cause of death among all U.S. women in that age group. Women tend to present in more advanced stages of disease, in part because up to 50% with heterosexual sex as a risk factor were unaware of their risk. As in men, PCP is the most frequent AIDS-defining diagnosis. Some opportunistic infections, including PCP, *Streptococcus pneumoniae*, esophageal thrush, and CMV colitis, are more common in women than in men. Candidal vaginitis is the most frequent symptom of early immunodeficiency and may occur in the presence of CD4 counts > 500. HIV-infected women also appear to have vaginal warts and cervical dysplasia (associated with human papilloma virus) both more frequently and more severely than noninfected women. Treatment with AZT during pregnancy and delivery plus 6 weeks of AZT for the newborn reduces the risk of maternal-infant transmission from 33% to 8%.

24. When and how should advance care directives be discussed with HIV-infected patients?
    The 100% mortality rate associated with an AIDS diagnosis impels a discussion of advance care directives so that the extent and type of endstage care complies with the patient's wishes. This discussion is best initiated by a caring primary care provider within a long-term provider/patient relationship. Postponing the discussion until emergent hospital admission and expecting the admitting house officer (unfamiliar to the patient and subject to frequent distractions) to help the patient understand the issues needed to make an appropriate decision is a disservice to the patient. Physicians must accept the responsibility to anticipate situations in which a clear advance directive will improve patient care and initiate discussion of this issue in a timely manner. There is increasing discussion of physician-assisted suicide. More than 80% of patients who request physician assistance to end their lives do not commit suicide. The request is often a call for help in dealing with a range of issues related to endstage disease and needs to be evaluated for its broader implications.

BIBLIOGRAPHY

 1. British Guidelines Co-ordinating Committee: British HIV Association guidelines for antiretroviral treatment of HIV seropositive individuals. Lancet 349:1086–1092, 1997.
 2. Burman WJ, et al: The case for conservative management of early HIV disease. JAMA 280:93–95, 1998.
 3. CAESAR Coordinating Committee: Randomised trial of addition of lamivudine or lamivudine plus loviride to zidovudine-containing regimens for patients with HIV-1 infection: The CAESAR trial. Lancet 349:1413–1421, 1997.
 4. Carpenter CCJ, et al: Antiretroviral therapy for HIV infection in 1998: Updated recommendations of the International AIDS Society—USA panel. JAMA 280:78–86, 1998.
 5. Centers for Disease Control and Prevention: Update: Mortality attributable to HIV infection among persons aged 25–44 years—United States, 1994. MMWR 45:121–125, 1996.
 6. Deeks SG: Practical issues regarding the use of antiretroviral therapy for HIV infection. West J Med 168:133–139, 1998.
 7. Deeks SG, Smith M, Holodny M, Kahn JO: HIV-1 protease inhibitors. JAMA 277:145–153, 1997.
 8. Haas JS, et al: Discussion of preferences for life-sustaining care by persons with AIDS. Arch Intern Med 153:1241–1248, 1993.
 9. Horsburgh CR: Advances in the prevention and treatment of *Mycobacterium avium* disease. N Engl J Med 335:428–430, 1996.
10. Kobayashi JS: The evolution of adjustment issues in HIV/AIDS. Bull Menninger Clin 61:146–188, 1997.
11. Mellors JW, et al: Plasma viral load and CD4+ lymphocytes as prognostic markers of HIV-1 infection. Ann Intern Med 126:946–954, 1997.
12. Moore RD, Chaisson RE: Natural history of opportunistic disease in an HIV-infected urban clinical cohort. Ann Intern Med 124:633–642, 1996.
13. Price RW: Neurological complications of HIV infection. Lancet 348:445–452, 1996.
14. Saag MS: Use of HIV viral load in clinical practice: Back to the future. Ann Intern Med 126:983–985, 1997.
15. Sande MA, Volberding PA (eds): The Medical Management of AIDS, 5th ed. Philadelphia, W.B. Saunders, 1997.
16. Sharpstone D, Bazzard B: Gastrointestinal manifestations of HIV infection. Lancet 348:379–383, 1996.
17. Sperling RS, et al: Maternal viral load, zidovudine treatment, and the risk of transmission of human immunodeficiency virus type 1 from mother to infant. N Engl J Med 335:1621–1629, 1996.
18. Tschachler E, Bergstresser PR, Stingl G: HIV-related skin diseases. Lancet 348:659–663, 1996.

107. THE PATIENT WITH ANOREXIA AND/OR WEIGHT LOSS

Lawrence G. Smith, M.D.

1. What is medically important weight loss?

Any degree of weight loss can be significant, but most experts define loss of 5% of body weight over 6 months as medically important if the patient was not on a reduced calorie diet or undergoing diuretic therapy. Greater amounts of weight loss are more often associated with serious disease.

2. When does anorexia need to be evaluated?

Anorexia without weight loss is rarely the result of serious disease. Side effects of medication, changes in taste, gastrointestinal (GI) and liver disease, or psychiatric conditions need to be considered. However, the basic evaluation of serious anorexia parallels that of unintentional weight loss.

3. Is it important to verify weight loss?

Weight loss is a common complaint to primary care physicians. Over one-half of such patients have been found not to have sustained significant weight loss and need no evaluation. Verifying weight loss is essential; methods include comparison with earlier weights, demonstration of change in clothing size, clear confirmation from friends or relatives, or visible signs of cachexia.

4. What are the major causes of weight loss?

The data in the table below combine several studies. Of note is that studies of inpatients showed a higher percentage of serious organic disease, whereas studies of outpatients showed a higher percentage of psychiatric disease.

*Causes of Weight Loss**

CAUSE	RELATIVE FREQUENCY (%)	CAUSE	RELATIVE FREQUENCY (%)
Psychiatric disease	4	Hyperthyroid disease	2
Malignancy	22	Other severe physical disease	10
Gastrointestinal disease	11	Medication effects	3
Food intake disorders	4	No cause found	24

* Estimates compiled from four studies with a total of 407 patients.

5. Do serious illnesses often present only as weight loss?

Although most serious illnesses, such as cancer, endstage heart disease, chronic obstructive pulmonary disease, arthritis, or renal failure, are associated with significant involuntary weight loss, this loss usually occurs long after the disease is diagnosed. It is rare for someone to have weight loss from a serious organic illness that is not obvious at the time of evaluation.

6. Does occult malignancy present as weight loss?

Most studies have shown that malignancy is an uncommon cause of weight loss, and occult malignancy is very rare. In all series, most malignancies were obvious at initial visits, and all were diagnosed by 6 months after the first evaluation. Extensive evaluations searching for occult malignancy are not appropriate in patients with weight loss.

7. What causes weight loss and increased appetite?

Few conditions truly produce the combination of weight loss and increased appetite. Possibilities include hyperthyroidism, diabetes mellitus, and perhaps malabsorption syndromes. Psychiatric disorders such as schizophrenia or a primary eating disorder also need to be considered.

8. Why do patients not maintain adequate food intake?

Anorexia is not the only reason for inadequate food intake. Pain associated with eating, as in esophageal and gastric diseases, may lead to aversion of food. Dental problems, taste disorders, neurologic difficulties, social conditions, financial problems, and many other factors may contribute to poor nutrition. In evaluating poor food intake, an open-minded approach is important.

9. How extensive should the initial evaluation be?

Serious organic disease is usually obvious at the time of presentation. All studies emphasize the high sensitivity of a good history and physical examination. The table below shows a typical initial screening panel of laboratory studies.

Initial Screen for Weight Loss

Complete history
Complete physical examination, including mental status and functional assessment
Complete blood count
Sequential multiple analysis—12 tests
Urinalysis
Chest radiograph
Stool—occult blood
Upper GI series if abdominal symptoms are present
Thyroid tests if symptoms are suggestive or patient is elderly

10. When should the physician look extensively for occult disease?

The answer is probably never. Occult serious disease is rare and usually becomes evident quickly on follow-up. Specifically, CT scans to discover unsuspected problems have not proved useful in the setting of weight loss. The exception may be the patient with a high level of alkaline phosphatase and low level of serum albumin; in one study, the incidence of positive findings was high in such patients.

11. Approximately 25% of patients with weight loss have no specific diagnosis. How long does follow-up need to be continued?

If no illness is obvious at 6 months, it is highly unlikely that the weight loss is due to undiagnosed organic disease. Serious social or psychiatric problems, however, may have been missed.

12. What pyschiatric disorders are associated with weight loss?

Most studies show depression as the most common psychiatric disorder in all patients with weight loss and the most common diagnosis overall in outpatients with weight loss. In addition, schizophrenia, conversion disorder, and the primary eating disorders of anorexia nervosa and bulimia are seen occasionally. Addiction to drugs and alcohol also may present with profound weight loss.

13. How are primary eating disorders recognized?

Patients with eating disorders are typically young adult white women of middle-to-upper socioeconomic class. Bulimic patients present at an older age than patients with anorexia nervosa. Symptoms are vague and usually result from weight loss (e.g., amenorrhea, fatigue, weakness) or vomiting (e.g., electrolyte abnormalities). Patients rarely seek help on their own and, despite being thin, perceive themselves as overweight. They are at risk for life-threatening problems from weight loss and vomiting. Bulimics frequently also abuse laxatives and diuretics. A team approach with psychiatric evaluation and nutritional support is essential.

14. What social conditions may present as weight loss?

Poverty, isolation, lack of transportation, and inability to cook or shop for food are only some of the social problems associated with significant weight loss. If suspicion is high, a social service referral and a home visit may be valuable.

15. Are elderly patients of special concern?

Decreasing functional states, dementia, stroke, and decreasing taste for and interest in food are some of the geriatric problems accounting for weight loss. A careful neurologic exam, Mini-Mental Status evaluation, functional assessment, and screening for depression are particularly useful in the elderly. Because hypothyroidism may present in its apathetic form in elderly patients, routine thyroid function studies are probably in order. The elderly are also particularly susceptible to the anorectic side effects of medication.

16. Is weight loss a normal occurrence of aging?

It is true that most community-dwelling elderly patients show a gradual loss of weight at the extremes of age. However, studies have shown that the typical change in body weight is 0.5% per year. Weight loss of greater than 5% is almost always indicative of a serious problem. Weight loss has been described as one of the earliest findings of dementia in community-dwelling adults along with other neurologic and psychological problems.

CONTROVERSIES

17. Does forced feeding benefit the patient when weight loss is due to serious organic illness?

Despite many clinical trials, especially among patients with terminal cancer, attempting to reverse cachexia with forced feeding, including total parenteral nutrition, has shown little evidence of overall benefit. Transient weight gain has been reported but without consistent benefit to functional status or survival.

18. Are medications effective in the weight loss associated with serious systemic illness?

Several interventions have failed to pass scientific scrutiny, including introgastric and parenteral nutrition as well as drug treatment with cyproheptadine and anabolic steroids. However, several drugs have been evaluated in placebo-controlled trials and shown to be effective in improving appetite, sense of well-being, and body mass in patients with cancer and AIDS. Examples include metoclopramide, megestrol acetate, corticosteroids (especially dexamethasone), and delta-9-tetrahydrocannabinol (THC).

BIBLIOGRAPHY

1. Barrett-Connor E, Edelstein S, Corey-Bloom J, et al: Weight loss precedes dementia in community-dwelling older adults. J Am Geriatr Soc 44:1147–1152, 1996.
2. Coodley G, Loveless M, Merrill T: The HIV wasting syndrome: A review. J Acquir Immune Defic Syndr 7:681–694, 1994.
3. Garfinkel P, Garner D, Kaplan A, et al: Differential diagnosis of emotional disorders that cause weight loss. Can Med Assoc J 129:939–945, 1983.
4. Marton K, Sox H, Krupp J: Involuntary weight loss: Diagnostic and prognostic significance. Ann Intern Med 95:568–574, 1981.
5. McKinley M, Goodman-Black J, Lesser M, et al: Improved body weight status as a result of nutrition intervention in adult, HIV-positive outpatients. J Am Diet Assoc 94:1014–1017, 1994.
6. Nelson K, Walsh D, Sheehan F: The cancer anorexia-cachexia syndrome. J Clin Oncol 12:213–225, 1994.
7. Rabinovitz M, Pitlik S, Leifer M, et al: Unintentional weight loss. Arch Intern Med 146:186–187, 1986.
8. Reife C: Involuntary weight loss. Med Clin North Am 79:299–313, 1995.
9. Sullivan D, Martin W, Flaxman N, Hagen J: Oral health problems and involuntary weight loss in a population of frail elderly. J Am Geriatr Soc 41:725–731, 1983.
10. Thompson M, Morris L: Unexplained weight loss in the ambulatory elderly. J Am Geriatr Soc 39:498–500, 1991.
11. Von Roenn J: Management of HIV-related body weight loss. Drugs 47:774–783, 1994.
12. Wallace J, Schwartz R, LaCroix A, et al: Involuntary weight loss in older outpatients: Incidence and clinical significance. J Am Geriatr Soc 43:329–337, 1995.
13. Wise G, Craig D: Evaluation of involuntary weight loss. Where do you start? Postgrad Med 95(4):143–146, 149–150, 1994.

108. THE PATIENT WITH CANCER

Kathleen Ogle, M.D.

1. What pitfalls should be avoided in telling a patient that he or she has cancer?

The clinician who makes a diagnosis of cancer bears the brunt of the patient's initial emotional reaction. Thus, in most instances, a certain diagnosis must be made before informing the patient or consulting the oncologist. A presumed surprise or error in diagnosis only adds additional suffering for the patient and disrupts the trust of the physician/patient relationship. Compassionate communication of the diagnosis and reassurance that all appropriate measures will be taken are important. It is crucial to avoid the pitfall of attempting to estimate the duration of remaining life; such estimates are frequently proved wrong or, worse yet, become self-fulfilling prophecy.

The patient's cultural background, socioeconomic status, education level, and personal experience influence psychological response to a diagnosis of cancer. A large difference between the provider's cultural beliefs and those of the patient and family may lead to difficulties. An example is the taboo, common in Asian cultures, that forbids telling the patient of the diagnosis. A compromise between biases of the provider and the patient must be sought.

Patients with testicular cancer or Hodgkin's disease frequently recall with bitter resentment having been told soon after diagnosis that they are "lucky" to have such a curable neoplasm. In fact, considering the strenuous treatment that they face, such a comment, however well-meaning, is quite cruel and obviously should be avoided.

2. Should an attempt at antineoplastic treatment be made at the time of diagnosis of all cancers?

No. Some cancers are so indolent that in essence they "coexist" with the patient and may never require treatment. In other circumstances, the general health of the patient precludes attempts at treatment of the malignancy. Numerous randomized trials of anticancer treatment demonstrate that patients confined to bed for ≥ 50% of an average day (i.e., poor performance status) are unlikely to benefit from treatment. This seems to be true whether or not the poor performance status is due to malignancy.

3. Which cancers can be cured with current therapy?

Around 50% of new cancer diagnoses can be successfully treated, and early diagnosis improves the chance of cure by surgery or local irradiation. Advanced cancers frequently curable with chemotherapy include some leukemias, Hodgkin's disease, some lymphomas, testicular and germ-cell cancer in adults, and many childhood malignancies. Chemotherapy or hormone therapy adds years of life often without signs of active malignancy in patients with certain other cancers, such as small-cell lung cancer, breast cancer, prostate cancer, colorectal cancer, and ovarian cancer. When other malignancies spread beyond the local site, treatment is palliative.

4. When a patient presents with a metastatic cancer of unknown primary site, what are the appropriate diagnostic tests to consider?

For the majority of patients who present with widespread carcinoma for which no obvious primary site is apparent, a complete history and physical examination (including pelvic and rectal exams) should be followed by a chest radiograph, a mammogram in women, and laboratory tests and radiographs designed to investigate symptoms or abnormal signs. Meticulous screening for intraabdominal cancers or occult bronchogenic tumors does not affect outcome and is unnecessary in most cases. Following this evaluation, the patient should be referred to an oncologist for further therapy.

5. What are the most common symptoms of advanced cancer?

Pain is a major symptom in cancer; up to 70% of patients with advanced cancer experience significant pain. Most studies indicate that undertreatment of cancer-related pain is a pervasive problem in the United States. Other common symptoms of advanced malignancy are fatigue, loss of appetite, weight loss, dyspnea, and excessive somnolence.

6. What are the greatest fears expressed by patients with cancer?

When questioned about beliefs and fears surrounding dying and death, persons of all ages identify several areas of concern. Loss of autonomy and dignity, disfigurement, and loss of body control and mental awareness are cited frequently. Fear of abandonment by family and friends as well as by health care providers is often high on the list. However, fear of a painful death is paramount; cancer and pain are inextricably linked in the minds of patients. Acknowledgment of common fears and concerns by the physician accomplishes a great deal in alleviating them. Patients are rarely confident or self-aware enough to verbalize their anxieties about death, and the health care professional should raise the topic. In particular, reassurance that the patient will not be abandoned in the dying process is crucial and should take place early in the discussion of terminal illness.

7. What is the best approach to the management of pain in a patient with cancer?

Pain in the terminally ill should be managed as if it were a separate problem from the underlying disease. Physical pain in a patient with cancer may be related to the malignancy, to debility resulting from cancer, or to treatment; it also may be unrelated to cancer. An effort should be made to diagnose and treat more readily reversible causes of pain (such as constipation, stomatitis, headache from brain edema, infection in locally advanced tumors). If a focal site of cancer metastasis is found to cause pain, local radiation is used to alleviate the symptom. When it is determined that the cause of pain is not reversible or is unknown, analgesic therapy should be appropriate to the level of pain, as perceived by the patient.

8. What pain syndromes occur in patients with cancer? How do they affect therapy?

Three types of pain can be recognized as separate syndromes requiring somewhat different management strategies:

Somatic or musculoskeletal pain results from pressure on peripheral nerves by masses and organ infiltration. This type of pain is generally more localized and intense; it may be intermittent and tends to be the most responsive to narcotic analgesics. When somatic pain originates from bone metastases, the frequently associated inflammation may respond well to antiinflammatory drugs.

Visceral pain may result from compression of autonomic nervous pathways, as in deep-seated tumors of the abdomen, or from obstruction of bowel or other visceral organs. This pain is less localized by the patient and often associated with other unpleasant sensations, such as nausea; in addition, it often has a component that is constant and a component that is intermittent but much more severe. Visceral pain may be associated with hyperesthetic areas on overlying skin. It usually responds to narcotic analgesics, but higher doses may be required.

Neuropathic pain results from destruction of nerves and causes associated burning and hyperesthesia in the affected region. Episodes of associated lancinating pains may be excruciating but very brief. Neuropathic pain is the least responsive to opioids. Adjunctive medications such as tricyclic antidepressants or anticonvulsants are often needed. Corticosteroids as an adjunct to analgesics may be useful in both somatic and neuropathic pain syndromes.

9. How should analgesics be used in terminally ill patients?

The most important tenets of pain control in terminally ill patients are the following five rules:

1. **Use scheduled doses** of analgesics in addition to "as needed."
2. **Adjust the dose frequently.** The goal is to control the pain to a tolerable level within a few hours, if possible.
3. **Allow the patient to control dosing** and dose adjustment as much as possible.
4. The **oral route** for analgesics is preferred.
5. **Use a sufficient dose** to control the pain. It is better to "overshoot" and titrate downward.

An occasional patient with pain due to cancer may require only acetaminophen, aspirin, or some other nonsteroidal antiinflammatory agent. However, the majority of patients with cancer who experience pain require more potent analgesics at some point.

10. When does the physician switch to a narcotic for pain control? How are narcotics safely used?

For moderate pain or pain that is not controlled with nonnarcotic analgesics, it is appropriate to use mild opioids such as codeine or oxycodone. As soon as the mild opioids fail to control pain, or if a patient presents with severe pain, it is appropriate to begin a potent opioid such as morphine sulfate. The tables below present the oral and parenteral dose equivalencies to morphine sulfate of common narcotic analgesics and compare three common potent opioids.

Narcotic Dose Equivalents for Chronic Pain Control

ORAL DOSE (mg)	ANALGESIC	PARENTERAL DOSE (mg)
15	Morphine	5
150	Meperidine	50
100	Codeine	60
10	Oxycodone*	10
10	Methadone	5
4	Hydromorphone	2
2	Levorphanol	1
NA	Fentanyl patch	25 μg/hr†

NA = not applicable.

* Oxycodone is available primarily in combination with acetaminophen or aspirin; recently immediate-release and slow-release products became available as oxycodone alone.

† Fentanyl patch dose equivalent to 10–20 mg/day of parenteral morphine or 30–60 mg/day of oral morphine.

Potent Narcotic Analgesics

Morphine sulfate (MS)	**Methadone**
Available routes of administration	Available only orally
Oral, buccal, sublingual	Variable duration of analgesia
Slow-release oral pill	Duration of analgesia not equivalent to duration of sedating effects because of accumulation of metabolites
Rectal	Cheap
IV, IM subcutaneous	Not cross-reactive in morphine-allergic patients
Intrathecal	**Fentanyl**
Intraventricular	Routes: topical (dermal absorption) or IV
Slow-release pills	New product (Duragesic): fentanyl transdermal patch
8-, 12-, or 24-hour duration of analgesia	Excellent alternative to MS infusion in patient unable to swallow
Ease of administration, dosing	Very expensive (but not as much as IV morphine)
Can be given rectally	Slow onset of action, depot effect in subcutaneous tissue, and variable rate of absorption
Expensive	

IV = Intravenous, IM = intramuscular.

Morphine sulfate has several advantages over other potent opioids: (1) it is available by any route of administration; (2) it is well absorbed orally; (3) the potency ratio of oral to parenteral dosage is predictable; and (4) it is relatively less expensive than many potent opioids. It is also available in three slow-release formulations that allow dosing every 8, 12, or 24 hours. Rapid-onset morphine for oral dosing is available in low- or high-concentration liquids as well as in far less expensive pills. Rapid-onset morphine can be used for breakthrough pain in a patient on slow-release tablets or as a means to achieve rapid pain control in a patient with severe pain.

Anticipatory management of the side effects of opiates is required for effective pain control. All patients taking narcotic analgesics have some decrease in gut motility, which results in constipation in the majority and nausea in a significant proportion. Stool softeners and a mild antiemetic should be prescribed along with the first prescription for a narcotic, even codeine. A bowel program to prevent constipation should be taught to patients and caregivers. Other less frequent but sometimes distressing narcotic side effects include urinary retention, pruritus, excessive sweating, and myoclonic jerking. Reassurance may be all that is necessary for the last three; urinary retention occasionally requires use of an indwelling catheter.

11. What is the maximal dose of narcotics?

The dose required to achieve analgesia in an individual patient is *whatever dose is necessary. No evidence suggests that a maximal dose of narcotic analgesic exists.* Physiologic tolerance is an expected outcome of chronic opiate use and should be anticipated. Patients may require hundreds, even thousands, of milligrams of morphine per day, yet remain awake, even ambulatory. Respiratory depression and somnolence are rarely significant problems because of the rapid development of tolerance in the vast majority of patients. However, even if respiratory depression does occur, it may be viewed as a secondary effect and should not lead to hesitation on the part of the provider to use whatever dose is needed to control terminal pain or discomfort. Naloxone should be avoided in patients taking chronic narcotics, because it precipitates immediate narcotic withdrawal symptoms and causes extreme pain and suffering.

12. What special problems relate to treatment of cancer pain in infants and children?

One needs a high index of suspicion for pain when dealing with children, along with observational techniques and parental reporting for infants and facial scales or other visual aids in young children. Children express chronic pain through rapid (within days) behavioral changes, such as apathy, depression, and withdrawal, rather than by overt crying. Initial doses of opioids need to be adjusted downward for infants under 6 months of age but are otherwise used in doses proportional to weight. Infants and children develop narcotic tolerance the same as adults and may require high doses for pain control.

13. How are pharmacologic adjuncts to analgesics used to improve pain control in patients with malignancy?

1. Nonsteroidal antiinflammatory agents may be used at standard doses as part of the treatment of bone pain due to malignancy.

2. Nortriptyline, desipramine, amitriptyline, imipramine, and doxepin at one-tenth to one-half the doses used for antidepressant effects may be prescribed for neuropathic pain, sleep, and depression associated with a diagnosis of cancer.

3. Lancinating pains and neuropathic pain may be treated with carbamazepine at 100–200 mg orally 2 or 3 times daily. Other anticonvulsants also have been used successfully.

4. Corticosteroids have been used at high doses (e.g., dexamethasone, 8–40 mg/day) for control of brain edema and resultant headaches or for nerve root or spinal cord compression symptoms. At low doses (e.g., dexamethasone, 0.75 mg/day, or prednisone, 10–20 mg/day) corticosteroids are sometimes helpful in treating pain from diffuse bone metastases or visceral pain from deep-seated intraabdominal tumors.

5. Antihistamines, cannabinoids, and amphetamines have been reported anecdotally to help alleviate pain.

6. Topical drugs, such as local anesthetics applied to ulcers or capsaicin cream to painful or dysesthetic intact skin, may be helpful.

7. Pamidronate, an intravenous biphosphonate that directly inhibits osteoclast activity, has been shown in randomized trials to improve bone pain significantly and to reduce skeletal fractures in patients with multiple myeloma and breast cancer metastatic to bone with lytic lesions.

14. Should any drugs be avoided in the management of cancer pain?

Mixed narcotic agonist/antagonist drugs, such as pentazocine (Talwin), should be avoided. Meperidine given orally has poor bioavailability. Parenteral meperidine is somewhat useful for acute pain, but the duration of action is too short for chronic pain; long-acting metabolites may cause confusion and, on rare occasions, precipitate seizures. Methadone has long-acting metabolites that can accumulate and cause sedation even after the analgesic effect has worn off, making it less useful for chronic pain management. Given its cheaper price, however, methadone may offer an attractive alternative to long-acting morphine compounds with careful titration in selected patients. Benzodiazepines as an adjunct to cancer pain may paradoxically sedate the patient enough to prevent the expression of pain but do little to abate the sensations. Heroin has no role in the management of cancer pain. Heroin is hydrolyzed to morphine in the body, and its analgesic effects are identical; however, the metabolites of heroin have neurostimulatory effects that may lead to extreme abuse.

15. What nonpharmacologic adjuncts are useful in the management of cancer pain?

Unquestionably, the emotional state of a patient with cancer vastly affects perception of pain. Anxiety about approaching death, uncertainty, anger, loss of control, and fear of abandonment exacerbate perception of pain. Recognition of fears and sometimes simply naming them may dissipate anxiety. Treatment of overt depression by pharmacologic means should be considered.

Relaxation and self-hypnosis techniques can be taught to patients. Distraction plays an important role in lessening perception of pain. Humor, music, pets, travel, fulfilling long-desired wishes—even a return to work or a long-neglected hobby—may help individual patients to be less aware of pain. Sometimes merely suggesting such an alternative allows patients to find their own options. Spiritual support provides others with a powerful alleviating factor.

Acupuncture, chiropractic treatments, and therapeutic massage may be beneficial to individual patients. The practitioner of such treatments must be given sufficient information about the patient's malignancy so that injury is avoided.

16. How should the cancer patient with back pain be assessed?

Rapidly. A frequent complication of cancer is spinal cord or cauda equina compression from metastases. Such compression is a medical emergency, because any delay in diagnosis and therapy may result in permanent loss of neurologic function. The patient's neurologic function at the time of discovery of spinal cord compression is the most important factor in predicting outcome. Patients who develop neurologic compromise without appropriate evaluation after initial reports of back pain or, worse yet, progress neurologically under direct observation of health care workers are grossly mismanaged. It is extremely important to make every effort to diagnose and treat spinal cord compression before abnormal neurologic findings appear.

In 90% of patients with spinal cord or cauda equina compression, pain in the back is the primary symptom. The pain may be exacerbated by movement, coughing, straining, or lying down. The pain also may have a radicular component, sometimes only with the exacerbating maneuver. Radicular pain allows fairly precise localization of the lesion. Pain usually proceeds neurologic symptoms by weeks to months. Weakness and sensory loss are next, followed rapidly first by urinary retention and constipation, then by paraplegia and loss of bowel and bladder continence. Once neurologic symptoms begin, progression to complete and permanent paraplegia may take only a few hours.

17. Which malignancies most commonly metastasize to the spine?

The malignancies that most commonly metastasize to the spine are cancers of the lung, breast, and prostate, myeloma, lymphoma, and renal-cell carcinoma. Most often spinal cord compression occurs in a patient with a known cancer, but it is not uncommonly the presenting symptom of malignancy. The location of cord compression is most often the thoracic spine (70%), followed by the lumbar (20%) and cervical (10%) spines. More than one area of spine may be involved, and several locations may threaten the cord. Compression most often results from a mass that begins in the vertebral body or neural arch and extends into the spinal canal, compressing the epidural space. More rarely a tumor may form in the epidural or intradural spaces without bone involvement.

18. What should you do if a patient with cancer develops signs of cord compression?

Any patients with cancer and signs of cord compression requires immediate treatment, followed by imaging of the suspected area of involved spine and spinal cord. Intravenous dexamethasone should be given (10–20 mg) with a 4-mg dose repeated every 4–6 hours while immediate neurologic, neurosurgical, and oncologic consultations are arranged and before imaging studies are done.

19. What should be considered in a patient with cancer and change in mental status?

The patient with cancer who presents with a mental status change, either directly or by corroborative history from the caregiver, should undergo a careful neurologic examination. In the presence of focal abnormalities or complaints of headache, a structural cause should be assumed; however, many patients with structural central nervous system lesions have no focal findings on exam. Evaluation consists of metabolic screening laboratory tests, review of drug therapy, and an imaging study of the central nervous system (lumbar puncture, if indicated).

Causes of Changes of Mental Status in Patients with Cancer

Structural	Metastasis, carcinomatosis, hemorrhage, or stroke
Infectious	Meningitis
Metabolic	Hypercalcemia, hyponatremia, hyperglycemia, or hypoglycemia
Drugs	Sedatives, antiemetics, anxiolytics, antineoplastics: ifosfamide, high-dose cytosine arabinoside, 5-fluorouracil (rare), interferons, and interleukin-2
Miscellaneous	Pain, constipation, depression, psychosis

20. What is the most common metabolic paraneoplastic syndrome? How is it treated?

Hypercalcemia is the most frequent metabolic abnormality due to paraneoplastic syndrome. It is commonly associated with lung tumors, breast cancer, multiple myeloma, and renal-cell cancer. It may be due to production by the tumor of a parathyroid hormone-like molecule, to direct lysis of bone by metastases, or to both. Symptoms of a high level of serum calcium include confusion, nausea, constipation, polydipsia, and polyuria.

Urgent treatment is required for calcium > 12 mg/dl or if the patient is symptomatic. Normal saline and diuresis should be used when calcium is extremely high (e.g., > 14 mg/dl), followed by the institution of the appropriate drug treatment. Pamidronate is the treatment of choice for most patients and may be safely given on an outpatient basis over 3–5 hours at a dose of 60–90 mg by vein. Its effects begin within 24–48 hours and last 3–6 weeks. Other less successful or more toxic options include gallium nitrate, plicamycin, calcitonin, or oral diphosphonates. Corticosteroids work only in hypercalcemia due to hematologic malignancy—and then often only transiently. Nonsteroid antiinflammatory agents are ineffective except in a few very mild cases.

21. What are the common causes of dyspnea in a patient with cancer?

Patients with cancer are at risk for **pulmonary embolism**. A hypercoagulable state accompanies adenocarcinomas, particularly carcinoma of the prostate, pancreas, and breast. Patients with breast cancer who undergo chemotherapy are at especially high risk for thromboembolic events. Other patients at extremely high risk are adults with primary brain tumors, probably because of an association with hemiparesis, but even in the absence of paralysis, pulmonary emboli are seen with high frequency in patients with glioma.

The **superior vena cava (SVC) syndrome** usually presents with dyspnea as well as facial and arm swelling, conjunctival edema, venous engorgement on the chest wall or in the neck, and, on rare occasions, somnolence. The SVC may be blocked by extrinsic pressure, intravascular invasion, or thrombosis from an indwelling catheter, usually in association with lung carcinoma, mediastinal lymphomas, germ-cell cancer, and occasionally breast cancer. SVC syndrome is a diagnosis easily made by physical examination and chest radiograph; invasive studies are rarely necessary, and it is rarely a true emergency. Maintaining the patient in an upright posture is the most important initial step in management; some patients temporarily feel better with corticosteroids or mild diuresis. Depending on the underlying tumor type, treatment may be radiation or chemotherapy; anticoagulation is recommended only in catheter-induced thrombosis.

Pleural and pericardial effusions caused by malignant studding of the serosal surface or by mediastinal lymphatic obstruction are also common causes of dyspnea. Lung, breast, and ovarian cancers are common causes of effusions, but lymphomas, leukemias, and many other tumors may involve the pleura or pericardium. A pleural effusion large enough to cause dyspnea is usually quite apparent on exam and chest radiograph. A pericardial effusion requires a higher index of suspicion. Patients with dyspnea and tachycardia with no other explanation should be carefully evaluated for both pericardial effusion and the equally insidious pulmonary embolus.

22. How may the patient with cancer be potentially immunocompromised?

1. Altered cellular immunity may develop, as in patients receiving corticosteroids and patients with lymphoid malignancies.

2. Cancer patients may be anatomically or functionally asplenic and thus at risk of early death from bacterial infections.

3. Many hematologic cancers cause decreased or absent production of normal immunoglobulins.

4. Insufficient numbers of granulocytes may result from treatment or from the disease process.

5. Macroscopic host defenses may be impaired as a result of breaks in the skin or mucous membranes, visceral or bronchial obstruction, or indwelling catheters.

23. What information is necessary to evaluate the urgency of fever in the patient with cancer?

Several important questions should be asked about every febrile patient with cancer:

1. What is the patient's leukocyte and granulocyte count?

2. What is the relationship of the fever to the patient's last session of chemotherapy and most recent blood product transfusion?

3. Is the patient receiving antibiotics? What type? For how long?

4. What is the fever pattern? Is this the first fever, or has the patient been febrile for some time?

The patient who is granulocytopenic may not have sufficient white blood cells to produce pus and therefore may have no localizing findings at all. Similarly, patients receiving corticosteroids may not show fever or other symptoms, even in the presence of active infection.

24. When are empirical antibiotics used in patients with cancer? What is the rationale for their use?

The febrile granulocytopenic patient, who is both at greatest risk for and least likely to present with obvious evidence of serious infections, requires immediate empirical coverage. Granulocytopenia is defined as less than 500 granulocytes per cubic microliter of blood. The absolute granulocyte count (AGC) is calculated by multiplying the total leukocyte count by the added percentage of neutrophils plus bands; it is also often referred to as the absolute neutrophil count (ANC). Granulocytopenic patients are at particular risk for spontaneous bacteremia, especially from gram-negative organisms. Because of observations in patients and animal studies of granulocytopenia and infection, empirical antibiotics are now considered standard treatment for the febrile granulocytopenic patient.

25. Which empirical antibiotics are appropriate?

Antibiotic combinations designed to provide the broadest spectrum of bacterial coverage for staphylococci and gram-negative organisms (including *Pseudomonas* sp.) are appropriate if the patient has no localizing symptoms or signs. Additional coverage should be considered in unique clinical situations. Acceptable combinations include:

1. Aminoglycoside plus antipseudomonal penicillin (APsP) or APsP plus clavulanic acid or

2. Antipseudomonal cephalosporin with or without aminoglycoside

Other broad-spectrum antibiotics that may prove useful include the quinolones, the new erythromycin derivatives, and the carbopenems and monobactams. The first two are good choices in persons with both penicillin and cephalosporin allergies.

26. What is the practical approach to the outpatient who is undergoing treatment for cancer and whose white blood cell counts are dropping?

The vast majority of cancer therapy is safely given in an outpatient setting. One result is that many patients experience iatrogenic myelosuppression at home. Most chemotherapy regimens have a predictable peak time of cell death, which usually starts 7–10 days after drug administration and lasts for a few days. If a patient develops absolute granulocytopenia (< 500) but feels well and remains afebrile, no intervention is needed. Patients should be instructed to check their temperature twice a day and to report fevers or symptoms of infection. The counts should be repeated daily or every other day until the AGC rises above 1000. Patients with moderate fever and moderately low granulocyte counts (i.e., 500–1000) or patients who are "on the rise" probably can be safely placed on a broad-spectrum oral antibiotic but should be checked frequently. Hematopoietic growth factors are unnecessary for management of uncomplicated neutropenia following chemotherapy.

27. When should patients with cancer be transfused?

Anemia caused by chemotherapy is likely to be slow in onset and slow to reverse. Packed red blood cell transfusions should be cautiously considered. There is no absolute hemoglobin level at which all patients require blood transfusions. A young person may tolerate a hemoglobin of 7 gm/dl or lower with only mild fatigue, whereas a patient with angina or congestive heart failure may require a hemoglobin of 9 or 10 gm/dl to avoid severe symptoms. Erythropoietin injections, now approved for cancer-related anemia, improve the hematocrit, but their expense and slow onset of action must be balanced against the benefits of decreasing transfusions.

Thrombocytopenia caused by chemotherapy in an outpatient is rarely severe enough to require transfusions. For several decades the standard cut-off that indicated a need for prophylactic platelet transfusions to prevent spontaneous bleeding has been 20,000 platelets/μ^3. Recently this time-honored criterion has been seriously questioned. It may be safe and reasonable to wait until the level is 10,000 or less. This controversy awaits further study.

28. What is the role of nutritional support in the management of patients with cancer?

For the most part studies of nutritional support in patients with cancer do not show any benefit. Both total parenteral nutrition (TPN) and oral or enteral concentrated feedings fail to achieve increases in lean body mass. Indeed, in two randomized trials of TPN vs. supportive care, patients with metastatic cancer who were treated with nutritional supplementation actually had a shortened survival. When a specific mechanical problem prevents normal eating or when severe treatment-associated mucositis prevents eating because of pain, TPN may be of value for a limited time. Under such circumstances the goal is specific: temporary support until relief of mechanical obstruction by surgery or healing of mucosa and return to a normal diet.

Food and water have great symbolic significance to patients and especially to family members, representing a life-prolonging basic function. It is a source of tremendous emotional distress for family members to be asked to sit by and watch their loved one apparently starve. In a survey of hospice workers, however, death associated with malnutrition and dehydration was observed to be peaceful and not accompanied by pain. Denial on the part of family members also may influence their inability to accept the patient's lack of nutritional support. A commonly expressed concern is that "if only he could gain some weight, he'd be strong enough to fight the cancer." Yet for the patient with profound anorexia due to advanced cancer, being forced to eat is often burdensome and intrusive. This common end-of-life symptom may be an adaptive mechanism. Education of patients and family members as well as health care workers is crucial. Families must be helped to understand the lack of benefit and the potential harm of forced nutrition in a terminally ill patient. No effective appetite stimulant has yet been identified for cancer-associated anorexia.

29. What is hospice care?

Hospice care is intended simply to control symptoms of terminal conditions, to alleviate pain, and to allow a peaceful death. The first hospice was opened in 1967 by Dr. Cicely Saunders in London. A hospice may be in the home or in a specially designed facility. After death, bereavement counseling is an important part of a hospice program.

30. How should the primary care physician follow a patient with cancer after treatment is successfully completed?

The intention of follow-up after antineoplastic treatment is to detect problems that can be treated successfully, whether complications or recurrences of cancer. Only a handful of cancers can be cured or adequately treated after a relapse: testicular cancer, Hodgkin's disease, certain lymphomas, some leukemias, and occasionally breast cancer recurrence. Such patients should be aggressively followed, according to instructions from the treating oncologist. No other cancers in adults can be successfully eradicated a second time, except in rare circumstances. Thus there is no real justification for routine radiographic and laboratory screening in the posttreatment phase; yet this is precisely what many patients have undergone and have been "taught" to expect. Certainly screening with costly imaging studies such as computerized scans or nuclear medicine scans has been shown to have virtually no impact on patient survival or even on palliation; indeed, the anxiety surrounding the testing may be antipalliative. Great controversy exists over the value of routine serum tumor markers (except in testicular cancer) during follow-up.

31. What are the major types of problems to expect in long-term survivors of successful cancer treatment?

1. **Social adjustments** are frequent in survivors of cancer. Many report problems with obtaining employment and with eligibility for health or life insurance. Many patients experience long-term anxiety about the possibility of relapse, especially at the time of visits to the doctor.

2. **Persistent physical problems** include sexual dysfunction manifesting as ejaculatory disturbances in men and vaginal dryness that leads to dyspareunia in women; infertility in both men and women; fibrosis or inflammation in irradiated areas or surgical scars; growth retardation and learning problems in children; cataracts in recipients of head or whole-body radiation; cardiomyopathy in persons treated with cardiotoxic drugs or chest radiation; accelerated atherosclerosis in radiation fields; and hypertension, Raynaud's phenomenon, and hypercholesterolemia in survivors of testicular cancer.

3. **Higher risk for the development of another cancer** or for second malignancies that are treatment-induced. Early after chemotherapy (< 5 years) for various cancers (best described after Hodgkin's disease), about 5% of patients develop chemotherapy-induced acute myelogenous leukemia or a myelodysplastic disorder. Patients treated with radiation, particularly in childhood or young adulthood, are at risk for second radiation-induced cancers in the treated areas. These second cancers may not begin to appear until the second or third decade after treatment.

32. What is the role of genetic testing for familial cancer syndrome?

There has been an explosion of basic science discoveries about inherited syndromes that place affected persons at markedly increased risk for cancer. Overall, however, only 5–10% of all cancers in the U.S. annually are due to an inherited cancer syndrome. For each type of malignancy, several different gene mutations may have been inherited and may lead to an increase in the development of malignancy. Some common cancers, such as breast cancer, have been found in very-high-risk families to be associated with three or more different genetic defects. At this time, testing for so-called "cancer genes" cannot be recommended as a routine test. The complexities of determining the cancer family pedigree, deciding which test (if any) is appropriate, interpreting test results with the knowledge of false-positive and false-negative rates, and individual and family counseling required before and after testing are highly problematic. Hallmarks of a family with a possible inherited cancer syndrome are early onset, three or more first-degree relatives with the same cancer, bilateral cancers in paired organs, and a pattern consistent with autosomal dominant inheritance. Families with a suspected familial cancer syndrome are best served by referral to a specialized center with oncology and genetic expertise.

CONTROVERSY

33. Is physician-assisted suicide an issue for those who care for patients with cancer?

Recent legal decisions about physician-assisted suicide have received widespread coverage in lay and professional press. Patients with cancer may ask about the physician's opinion on this subject or may request such a service. Ideally, this matter should never require implementation. If proper care of terminally ill patients' needs, including treatment of suicidal depression and relief of all terminal symptoms, were the norm, there would be no need for physician-assisted suicide. This controversial area remains for the present a decision for each physician and patient to address individually.

BIBLIOGRAPHY

1. American Pain Society Quality of Care Committee: Quality improvement guidelines for the treatment of acute pain and cancer pain. JAMA 274:1874–1880, 1995.
2. Angell M: The Supreme Court and physician-assisted suicide—The ultimate right. N Engl J Med 336:50–53, 1997.
3. Berenson JR, Lichtenstein A, Porter L, et al: Efficacy of pamidronate in reducing skeletal events in patients with advanced multiple myeloma. Myeloma Aredia Study Group. N Engl J Med 334:488–493, 1996.
4. Bilezikian JP: Management of acute hypercalcemia. N Engl J Med 326:1196–1203, 1992.
5. Blatt J, Olshan A, Gula MJ, et al: Second malignancies in very-long-term survivors of childhood cancer. Am J Med 93:57–60, 1992.
6. Boring CC, Squires TS, Tong T: Cancer statistics, 1993. Cancer 43:7–26, 1993.
7. Burke W, Petersen G, Lynch P, et al: Recommendations for follow-up care of individuals with an inherited predisposition to cancer. I: Hereditary nonpolyposis colon cancer. Cancer Genetics Studies Consortium. JAMA 277:915–919, 1997.
8. Burke W, Daly M, Garber J, et al: Recommendations for follow-up care of individuals with an inherited predisposition to cancer. II: BRCA1 and BRCA2. Cancer Genetics Studies Consortium. JAMA 277:977–1003, 1997.
9. Byrne TN: Spinal cord compression from epidural metastases. N Engl J Med 327:614–619, 1992.
10. Dahl JL: Effective pain management in terminal care. Clin Geriatr Med 12:279–300, 1996.
11. Emanuel EJ: Pain and symptom control: Patient rights and physician responsibilities. Hematol Oncol Clin North Am 10:42–56, 1996.
12. Foley KM: Competent care for the dying instead of physician-assisted suicide. N Engl J Med 336:54–58, 1997.
13. Foley KM: The treatment of pain in cancer. N Engl J Med 313:84–95, 1985.
14. Hainsworth JD, Greco FA: The treatment of patients with cancer of an unknown primary site. N Engl J Med 329:257–263, 1993.
15. Hortobagyi GN, Theriault RL, Porter L, et al: Efficacy of pamidronate in reducing skeletal complications in patients with breast cancer and lytic bone metastases. Protocol 19 Aredia Breast Cancer Study Group. N Engl J Med 335:1785–1791, 1996.
16. Jadad AR, Bowman GP: The WHO analgesic ladder for cancer pain management: Stepping up the quality of its evaluation. JAMA 274:1870–1873, 1995.
17. Kanner R: Recent advances in cancer pain management. Cancer Invest 11:80–87, 1993.
18. Loescher JL, Welch-McCarthy D, Leigh SA, et al: Surviving adult cancers. I. Physiologic effects. Ann Intern Med 111:411–432, 1989.
19. Miller RJ, Albright PC: What is the role of nutritional support and hydration in terminal cancer patients? Am J Hospice Care Nov/Dec:33–38, 1989.
20. Pizzo PA: Management of fever in patients with cancer and treatment-induced neutropenia. N Engl J Med 328:1323–1332, 1993.
21. Raghavan D, Cox K, Childs A, et al: Hypercholesterolemia after chemotherapy for testis cancer. J Clin Oncol 10:1386–1389, 1992.
22. Rhymes JA: Clinical management of the terminally ill. Geriatrics 46(2):57–67, 1991.
23. Welch-McCaffrey D, Hoffman B, Leigh SA, et al: Surviving adult cancers: Psychological and social effects. Ann Intern Med 111:517–524, 1989.
24. Yellen SB, Cella DF, Bonomi A: Quality of life in people with Hodgkin's disease. Oncology 7(8):41–45, 1993.

109. THE PREOPERATIVE PATIENT

Jeffrey Pickard, M.D.

1. What test(s) must be done before surgery?

The simple answer is that no test is considered essential for preoperative evaluation. In general, tests should be based on the type of surgery (e.g., urinalysis before urologic surgery) and the patient's current and past medical history (e.g., chest radiograph for patients with chronic obstructive pulmonary disease [COPD]). Practically speaking, however, certain tests are ordered almost routinely, because they can be obtained relatively easily and cheaply (e.g., complete blood count, urinalysis, electrocardiogram [EKG], and chest radiograph in the elderly).

2. How does age affect the outcome of surgery?

The answer is somewhat controversial. Some studies consider age over 70 years to be an independent risk factor. Recent studies, however, have challenged this notion, suggesting that the patient's underlying physiology is much more important than age alone. Age may be a risk factor only in that the elderly are more likely to have underlying disease.

3. What type of anesthesia is the safest?

There is a fairly common misconception that spinal anesthesia is safer and better tolerated than general anesthesia. However, both confer equal risks of postoperative fatal and nonfatal myocardial infarctions. Regional or local anesthesia may be less risky than general or spinal anesthesia. The type of anesthesia should be determined by the anesthesiologist.

4. Which types of surgery are inherently riskier than others?

Vascular surgery appears to carry the greatest risk, both because the procedures are physiologically stressful and because patients who require such procedures have a high incidence of coronary artery disease. Intrathoracic, intraperitoneal, and emergency procedures are also high risk.

5. What is meant by a patient's preoperative cardiac risk index?

The preoperative cardiac risk index refers to a quantitative assessment of a patient's risk of adverse cardiac outcome intra- or postoperatively; it is based on various preoperative clinical, historical, and laboratory variables. The first, and probably most widely used, of these indices was published by Goldman et al. in 1977.

Computation of the Cardiac Risk Index

CRITERIA	MULTIVARIATE DISCRIMINANT-FUNCTION COEFFICIENT	POINTS
1. History		
Age > 70 yr	0.191	5
MI in previous 6 mo	0.384	10
2. Physical examination		
S_3 gallop or JVD	0.451	11
Important VAS	0.119	3
3. Electrocardiogram		
Rhythm other than sinus or PACs on last preoperative EKG	0.283	7
> 5 PVCs/min documented at any time before operation	0.278	7
4. General status		
$Po_2 < 60$ or $Pco_2 > 50$ mmHg	0.132	3
K < 3.0 or $HCO_3 < 20$ mEq/L		
BUN > 0.50 or Cr > 3.0 mg/dl,		
abnormal SGOT, signs of chronic liver disease		
or patient bedridden from noncardiac causes		
5. Operation		
Intraperitoneal, intrathoracic, or aortic operation	0.123	3
Emergency operation	0.167	4
Total possible points		53

MI = myocardial infarction, JVD = jugular vein distention, VAS = valvular aortic stenosis, PACs = premature atrial contractions, PVCs = premature ventricular contractions, Po_2 = partial pressure of oxygen, Pco_2 = partial pressure of carbon dioxide, K = potassium, HCO_3 = bicarbonate, BUN = blood urea nitrogen, Cr = creatinine, SGOT = serum glutamic oxaloacetic transaminase.

Cardiac Risk Index

CLASS	POINT TOTAL	NO OR ONLY MINOR COMPLICATION (N = 943)	LIFE-THREATENING COMPLICATION* (N = 39)	CARDIAC DEATHS (N = 19)
I (N = 537)	0–5	542 (99%)	4 (0.7%)	1 (0.2%)
II (N = 316)	6–12	295 (93%)	16 (5%)	5 (2%)
III (N = 130)	13–25	112 (86%)	15 (11%)	3 (2%)
IV (N = 18)	> 26	4 (22%)	4 (22%)	10 (56%)

* Documented intraoperative or postoperative myocardial infarction, pulmonary edema, or ventricular tachycardia without progression to cardiac death.
From Goldman L, Caldera DL, Nussbaum SR, et al: Multifactorial index of cardiac risk in noncardiac surgical procedures. N Engl J Med 297:845–850, 1977, with permission.

6. How does a history of myocardial infarction affect a patient's perioperative risk?

Most investigators and clinicians believe that within the first 3–6 months after myocardial infarction, perioperative cardiac morbidity and mortality are significantly increased. Therefore, nonemergent surgery should be delayed, if possible, until after this period. After 6 months, perioperative risk remains relatively stable, assuming the absence of sequelae (e.g., congestive heart failure, rhythm disturbances). Some authors believe that the level of risk returns to preinfarct levels (< 1% in the general population), whereas others believe that the risk remains somewhat elevated (2–8%).

7. Which patients should be evaluated for coronary artery disease (CAD) before surgery?

Patients who undergo high-risk procedures such as those listed above (especially vascular procedures that require cross-clamping of the aorta) may require additional evaluation for CAD, such as an exercise treadmill test (ETT). Patients with unstable angina, new EKG changes (especially ischemic), or high cardiac risk indices also should be considered for further cardiac evaluation. Patients who are unable to exercise (e.g., patients with peripheral vascular disease) or who have baseline EKG abnormalities may require a dipyridamole-thallium scan or dobutamine stress echocardiogram to detect ischemia. Patients with evidence of ischemic disease on noninvasive testing may require coronary angiography with an eye toward angioplasty or coronary artery bypass grafting (CABG) before high-risk surgery. These procedures, of course, have their own operative risks, but patients who have had successful revascularization may reduce their perioperative cardiac risk to approximately that of the normal population.

8. How does the presence of hypertension affect perioperative risk?

Hypertension as an independent risk factor is notably absent from both Goldman's and Detsky's scoring systems. Mild-to-moderate hypertension appears to be generally well-tolerated during and after surgery. However, patients with diastolic blood pressure > 110 mmHg or systolic blood pressure > 170 mmHg are at increased risk of perioperative morbidity and should have their blood pressure controlled before going to surgery, if possible.

9. How should antihypertensive medications be adjusted in patients who are undergoing elective surgery?

Assuming adequate control of blood pressure, most antihypertensive medications should be continued until surgery and restarted posoperatively when the patient resumes oral intake. Guanethidine and monoamine oxidase (MAO) inhibitors are rarely used and probably should be avoided perioperatively. Earlier case reports suggested that abrupt withdrawal of both clonidine and beta blockers was associated with rebound hypertension and ischemia and recommended that both agents should be tapered before surgery. According to current recommendations, however, these medications are continued during the perioperative period. If necessary, transdermal clonidine and intravenous beta blockers may be used while oral intake is prohibited.

10. Describe the perioperative management of patients taking medication for diabetes.

Ideally, patients should be euglycemic perioperatively, but this goal is often not practical, because the risks of hypoglycemia may be substantial. Therefore, patients generally are allowed to be somewhat hyperglycemic. Patients taking insulin should be given approximately one-half of the usual morning dose of neutral protamine Hagedorn (NPH) or Lente insulin on the morning of surgery and should be maintained on a continuous infusion of dextrose until oral intake is resumed. Fingerstick glucoses should be obtained at regular intervals during prolonged procedures. Levels of blood sugar should be checked, either by fingerstick or phlebotomy, every 4–6 hours postoperatively until the patient is able to resume normal oral intake. Small doses of subcutaneous regular insulin may be used to maintain blood glucose levels ≤ 250 mg/dl, if possible. Patients with type I diabetes or patients who are difficult to control may require insulin drips. Patients taking oral hypoglycemic agents usually do not require significant adjustment of medications. Some authors recommend discontinuing chlorpropamide 2–3 days before surgery because of its prolonged half-life and risk of hypoglycemia. However, this is an issue only in the rare patient with type II diabetes who is euglycemic on oral medications.

11. What is the value of preoperative pulmonary function tests (PFTs)?

In patients with no history of pulmonary problems, PFTs are of little or no value and should not be routinely ordered. Although some authors believe that severely obese patients are at risk for postoperative pulmonary complications, few data support the use of PFTs as part of the preoperative evaluation. Patients with a history of lung disease (COPD, asthma, smokers with productive cough) or signs and symptoms of pulmonary dysfunction (wheezing, dyspnea) may be at risk for postoperative pulmonary complications. In such patients, PFTs may be helpful in identifying patients with severe disease (FEV ≤ 0.5 L; hypercapnia) but otherwise are of little help in quantifying the risk of postoperative pulmonary complications.

12. How should patients with potential pulmonary problems be evaluated before surgery?

As stated above, patients with pulmonary disease are at increased risk for postoperative pulmonary complications, and their respiratory status should be optimized before surgery. Chest radiographs are usually obtained for baseline values but rarely change management. Other risk factors may include length of surgery (> 3.5 hours), surgical factors (intrathoracic surgery and intraabdominal procedures, especially those close to the diaphragm), and smoking (> 20 years or > 1 pack/day actively). There is no difference in risk between general and spinal anesthesia, although procedures done under regional or local anesthesia may have lower risk.

13. How should you manage a patient with asthma perioperatively?

Assess the patient for signs and symptoms of airflow obstruction, such as awakening at night, increased use of bronchodilators, and recent steroid use (inhaled or systemic). Steroids should be considered for use both before (2–3 days) and after (taper over 1 week) surgery because perioperative asthma exacerbations increase the risk of pulmonary complications. Wound infections, pneumonia, and adrenal insufficiency are not increased in patients with asthma who are treated with steroids perioperatively.

14. How should cigarette smokers be counseled before surgery?

Although only a small percentage of smokers will quit when advised to do so by their physicians, all smokers should be advised to quit before elective surgery. Abstinence for at least 2 months is necessary to decrease postoperative pulmonary complications significantly.

15. What are the important preoperative predictors of postoperative renal failure?

Patients with elevated serum creatinine (> 1.2 mg/dl) have a 3–4-fold increase in postoperative renal insufficiency compared with patients whose creatinine is normal. A rising serum creatinine perioperatively and left ventricular dysfunction are also significant risk factors for postoperative renal failure.

16. Which patients should be placed on prophylactic antibiotics perioperatively?

The goal of prophylactic antibiotics is to decrease the potential morbidity of postoperative infections when the procedure is likely to contaminate normally sterile areas or when the potential for infection of a prosthetic device exists (e.g., heart valve, artificial joint, vascular graft).

Most surgical procedures (75%) are **clean** and normally require no antibiotic prophylaxis, although some experts recommend antibiotic prophylaxis in all surgeries. Approximately 15% are **clean-contaminated** procedures, in which gastrointestinal, genitourinary, or respiratory mucosa are invaded. Likelihood of infection in such cases is about 10%. The remaining procedures are either **contaminated** (e.g., fresh trauma) or **dirty** (e.g., trauma more than 4 hours old); rates of infection in these cases are 20% and ≥ 40%, respectively.

17. What regimens are recommended for perioperative antibiotic prophylaxis?

Although there are about as many antibiotic regimens as there are surgical procedures, general recommendations are provided in the table below.

Recommended Regimens for Perioperative Antibiotic Prophylaxis

PROCEDURE	POSSIBLE INDICATIONS	ANTIBIOTIC REGIMEN
Cardiovascular (e.g., CABG, valve replacement, pacemaker)	Transthoracic wires	Cefazolin, 1 gm IV preoperatively; alternative: vancomycin
Upper GI tract	Age, local infection	Cefazolin, 1 gm IV preoperatively; alternatives: clindamycin, metronidazole
GU tract (e.g., TURP)		Cefazolin, 1 gm IV preoperatively; alternatives: clindamycin, ciprofloxacin
GU (e.g., hysterectomy)	Prolonged procedure	Cefazolin, 1 gm IV preoperatively
Orthopedics (e.g., joint arthroplasty)		Cefazolin, 1 gm IV preoperatively with q 6 hr × 24 hr; alternative: vancomycin
Peripheral vascular (e.g., AAA repair)		Cefazolin, 1 gm IV preoperatively and q 6 hr × 24 hr
Thoracic surgery		Same as above

CABG = coronary artery bypass graft, IV = intravenously, GI = gastrointestinal, GU = genitourinary, TURP = transurethral prostatectomy, AAA = abdominal aortic aneurysm.

CONTROVERSY

18. How should patients on chronic anticoagulation be managed perioperatively?

There is no standard regimen to prepare patients on chronic warfarin therapy for surgery. Patients with prothrombin time (PT) < 20 and international normalized ratio (INR) < 2.9 rarely have significant postoperative bleeding problems. However, most patients on warfarin therapy can safely be taken off their medications 3–4 days before surgery and restarted postoperatively when oral intake is resumed. Patients at high risk for thromboembolic disease (e.g., patients with mechanical valves or mitral stenosis or patients who have had recurrent thromboembolism in the past) may be switched to full-dose heparin (preferably by continuous intravenous infusion) 3–4 days before surgery. The heparin may be stopped approximately 6 hours before the procedure and restarted as soon as adequate postoperative hemostasis has been attained (usually the evening after surgery or 12 hours after the procedure). Patients requiring dental surgery rarely bleed while on warfarin therapy; thus discontinuance is usually unnecessary. Likewise, routine cataract surgery is avascular and does not necessitate reversal of anticoagulation. Accumulating data indicate that subcutaneous low-molecular-weight heparin may be superior to warfarin in preventing postoperative thromboembolism.

BIBLIOGRAPHY

1. Anderson DR, O'Brien BJ, Levine MN, et al: Efficacy and cost of low-molecular-weight heparin with standard heparin for the prevention of deep vein thrombosis after total hip arthroplasty. Ann Intern Med 119:1105–1112, 1993.
2. Cygan R, Waitzin H: Stopping and restarting medications in the perioperative period. J Gen Intern Med 2:270–283, 1987.
3. Eagle KA, Brundage BH, Chaitman BR, et al: Guidelines for perioperative cardiovascular evaluation for noncardiac surgery: An abridged version of the report of the American College of Cardiology/American Heart Association task force on practice guidelines. Mayo Clin Proc 72:524–531, 1997.
4. Hayden SP, Mayer ME, Stoller JK: Postoperative pulmonary complications: Risk assessment, prevention and treatment. Cleve Clin J Med 62:401–407, 1995.
5. Hull R, Raskob G, Pineo G, et al: A comparison of subcutaneous low-molecular-weight heparin with warfarin sodium for prophylaxis against deep-vein thrombosis after hip or knee implantation. N Engl J Med 329:1370–1376, 1993.
6. Kroenke K: Preoperative evaluation: The assessment and management of surgical risk. J Gen Intern Med 2:257–269, 1987.
7. Lawrence VA, Page CP, Harris GD: Preoperative spirometry before abdominal operations: A critical appraisal of its predictive value. Arch Intern Med 149:280–285, 1989.
8. Lewis RT, Weigand FM, Mamazza J, et al: Should antibiotic prophylaxis be used routinely in clean surgical procedures: A tentative yes. Surgery 118:742–747, 1995.
9. Mohr DH, Jett JR: Preoperative evaluation of pulmonary risk factors. J Gen Intern Med 3:277–287, 1988.
10. Narr BJ, Warner ME, Schroeder DR, Warner MA: Outcomes of patients with no laboratory assessment before anesthesia and a surgical procedure. Mayo Clin Proc 72:505–509, 1997.
11. Schade DS: Surgery and diabetes. Med Clin North Am 72:1531–1543, 1988.
12. Thomas DR, Ritchie CS: Preoperative assessment of older adults. J Am Geriatr Soc 43:811–821, 1995.
13. Velanovich V: Preoperative laboratory evaluation. J Am Coll Surg 183:79–87, 1996.
14. Wolf H: Low-molecular-weight heparin. Med Clin North Am 78:733–743, 1994.

110. THE PREGNANT PATIENT

Jeffrey Pickard, M.D.

1. At 37 weeks' gestation, a 20-year-old primigravida who has received optimal prenatal care is noted to have proteinuria, edema of both upper and lower extremities, and a 5-pound weight gain over the preceding week. Her blood pressure, which has been normal for pregnancy, now measures 136/92. What is the diagnosis?

The triad of hypertension, edema, and proteinuria occurring late in pregnancy is a classic presentation of preeclampsia. Preeclampsia occurs 6–8 times more commonly in primigravidas than in multigravidas. It is almost never seen before 20 weeks' gestation (except with trophoblastic diseases) and usually occurs near term.

2. How is preeclampsia managed?

The only definitive treatment of preeclampsia is delivery. Hypertension is only a sign of preeclampsia, and treatment of the blood pressure does little to alter the course of the disease. Diuresis for edema likewise does not alter the underlying pathophysiology and in fact may be counterproductive and adversely affect fetal outcome, because intravascular volume is already depleted in women with preeclampsia.

The triad of proteinuria, edema, and hypertension is not specific for preeclampsia. Edema may be seen during normal pregnancy, as may low levels of proteinuria. Hypertension late in pregnancy may be previously unrecognized chronic hypertension, or it may be transient hypertension of pregnancy. If the fetus is not yet mature, it may be appropriate to monitor the pregnancy closely in hope of delaying delivery.

3. What laboratory evaluations should be done in a woman who presents with hypertension during the second half of pregnancy?

A complete blood count should be obtained. Hemoglobin and hematocrit may be elevated, because hemoconcentration may occur in preeclampsia. Thrombocytopenia and evidence of hemolysis on the smear may suggest severe preeclampsia. Liver function tests (transaminase, lactate dehydrogenase), uric acid, and creatinine also may be elevated in cases of severe preeclampsia.

4. Describe the evaluation of a woman who presents with hypertension before week 20 of gestation.

In addition to obtaining the laboratory data mentioned above, a careful history should be obtained with emphasis on duration of elevated blood pressure, blood pressure in previous pregnancies, previous diagnostic evaluation, and symptoms associated with secondary causes of hypertension. Pregnant women, especially young pregnant women, with chronic hypertension or hypertension during the first half of pregnancy are more likely than other patients to have secondary causes of hypertension. Pheochromocytoma, although rare, is associated with high maternal mortality, and appropriate screening should be done with even minimal suspicion.

5. What is HELLP?

    H = Hemolysis
    E = Elevated
    L = Liver enzymes
    L = Low
    P = Platelets

This syndrome, associated with severe preeclampsia, is rapidly progressive and life-threatening to both mother and baby. Regardless of the stage in pregnancy at which it occurs, the HELLP syndrome is an emergency and requires immediate termination of pregnancy.

6. How does the nonpharmacologic management of hypertension differ in pregnant and nonpregnant patients?

As in nonpregnant patients, mild-to-moderate hypertension should be treated with nonpharmacologic modalities first, especially when the diastolic blood pressure is between 90 and 99 mmHg. However, nonpharmacologic strategies for blood pressure control during pregnancy differ from those used in nonpregnancy.

Weight reduction is frequently recommended for blood pressure control in nonpregnant patients but should not be recommended during pregnancy. Salt (sodium) restriction should not be recommended during pregnancy unless the patient has been on a sodium-restricted diet before becoming pregnant. Volume status may be important for maintaining uteroplacental perfusion in the pregnant hypertensive patient, whose intravascular volume is usually lower than that in normotensive patients.

Because of its unknown effect on uteroplacental blood flow, exercise should be discouraged in pregnant women with hypertension. Whereas its effectiveness has not been well studied in chronic hypertension, bed rest during pregnancy enhances uteroplacental blood flow, reduces premature labor, lowers blood pressure, and promotes diuresis in women with hypertension.

7. How should drugs be used to treat hypertension during pregnancy?

The goal of treating hypertension during pregnancy is to minimize short-term risks of elevated blood pressure to the mother without compromising fetal well-being. Pharmacologic therapy may be necessary if nonpharmacologic maneuvers are unsuccessful in lowering blood pressure or if diastolic blood pressure exceeds 99 mmHg.

First-line therapy for hypertensive pregnant women not already on medication is methyldopa, the only drug that is both efficacious for lowering maternal blood pressure and unquestionably safe for the fetus. Second-line therapy is usually hydralazine, because other than methyldopa, it is the drug with most frequent use during pregnancy and generally is considered safe for the fetus. However, it is not highly effective as a single agent because of the reflex tachycardia and increased cardiac output that it causes. Other agents used to treat hypertension during pregnancy are beta blockers, labetolol, and nifedipine. Because of their theoretical effect on uteroplacental perfusion, thiazides are usually not begun during pregnancy but may be continued when already in use by a hypertensive woman who becomes pregnant. Angiotensin-converting enzyme inhibitors are relatively contraindicated during pregnancy because of their association with high rates of fetal loss in animals and because of several case reports of anoxic renal failure, sometimes fatal, in neonates exposed in utero. Other agents used to treat hypertension during pregnancy are beta blockers, labetalol, and nifedipine. Nifedipine has not been associated with adverse fetal effects in humans, but studies in pregnant sheep have demonstrated fetal acidosis and hypoxia.

Antihypertensive Medications in Pregnancy

MEDICATION	DAILY DOSE	COMMENTS
Methyldopa	500 mg–2 gm	Drug of choice during pregnancy
Hydralazine	40–200 mg	Second-line therapy; associated with reflex tachycardia
Hydrochlorothiazide	25–50 mg	Potentially decreases uteroplacental perfusion, may be continued during pregnancy if patient already taking it
Beta blockers (e.g., propranolol)	40–240 mg	Case reports of neonatal hypoglycemia, bradycardia, ? mild intrauterine growth retardation
Calcium channel blockers (e.g., nifedipine)	30–120 mg	Limited data in humans; fetal acidosis and hypoxia in sheep
Labetalol	200–1000 mg	Probably safe; limited data in humans
Angiotensin-converting enzyme inhibitors	—	Contraindicated; teratogenic in animals; anoxic renal failure in human neonates

8. What is the long-term prognosis of women who have hypertension during pregnancy?

Women with transient hypertension during one pregnancy have recurrent hypertension in up to 90% of subsequent pregnancies as well as a high likelihood of developing chronic hypertension in the future. In contrast, women who do not have hypertension during pregnancy, especially after age 25 years, have a low likelihood of developing chronic hypertension.

Women who develop preeclampsia-eclampsia during their first pregnancy have about a 10% chance of having preeclampsia in subsequent pregnancies. Their risk of developing chronic hypertension is no different from that of the general population. Women with chronic hypertension have an increased risk of developing preeclampsia when they become pregnant.

9. Describe normal maternal carbohydrate metabolism during pregnancy.

Early in pregnancy, usually at about 10 weeks' gestation, fasting glucose levels fall to as low as 60 mg/dl and either remain at this level or continue to decrease slightly throughout gestation. This early drop in maternal glucose levels occurs before the conceptus is large enough to have an effect and probably is due to an enhancement (increased sensitivity) of insulin-mediated glucose assimilation related primarily to the large rise in placental hormones (especially estrogen).

Basal insulin levels, normal during the first half of pregnancy, rise sharply (50–100%) during the second half of pregnancy. Throughout most of pregnancy, the stimulation of insulin in response to glucose load increases. Overall, insulin sensitivity in pregnancy is about 20% of that in the nonpregnant state. The mechanism for the decreased tissue responsiveness to insulin is not completely understood but probably relates to hormonal changes of pregnancy, such as elevated levels of prolactin, cortisol, and other counterregulatory hormones. The human placenta produces placental lactogen, an insulin antagonist, in increasingly larger amounts after 20 weeks. In addition to a decrease in insulin-receptor binding, postreceptor response to insulin at the tissue level also may be diminished.

10. How do the metabolic changes in a diabetic pregnancy affect the fetus?

Glucose crosses the placenta by facilitated diffusion so that fetal glucose levels are only slightly lower than the mother's. Maternal insulin does not cross the placenta. Maternal hyperglycemia, therefore, leads to fetal hyperglycemia. The fetal pancreas, which starts producing insulin between weeks 9 and 11, secretes large amounts of insulin to control glucose levels. Studies of fetal and infant pancreases exposed to diabetes in utero have documented beta-cell hypertrophy and hyperplasia. Amino acids are actively transported across the placenta and also stimulate fetal secretion of insulin. These and other substrates are stored in adipose and other insulin-responsive tissues and lead to macrosomia as well as organomegaly of heart, lung, spleen, liver, and adrenal glands. Hyperinsulinemia at birth leads to neonatal hypoglycemia in as many as 75% of infants of diabetic mothers. Other consequences of poor metabolic control include neonatal hypercalcemia, polycythemia, hyperbilirubinemia, and respiratory distress syndrome (RDS).

11. What is the White classification?

This classification schema was devised by Priscilla White to categorize women with progestational diabetes on the basis of duration of disease, age at onset, mode of therapy, and presence of vascular complications. Current modifications now include gestational diabetes, either as a separate category or as defined by treatment (diet vs. insulin). Classes A–D correlate with slight increases in fetal mortality, whereas classes F and higher are also associated with increased maternal risk.

White Classification

CLASS	AGE AT ONSET*	DURATION*	INSULIN
A_1	Any	Any	–
A_2	Any	Gestational[†]	+
B	≥ 20 years	< 10 years	+
C	10–19 years	10–19 years	+
D	< 10 years	≥ 20 years	+
R	Proliferative retinopathy or vitreous hemorrhage		+
F	Nephropathy		+
RF	Retinopathy and nephropathy		+
H	Heart disease, usually coronary artery disease		+
T	Renal transplant recipient		+

* Either age at onset or duration determines class.
[†] Gestational diabetes mellitus (GDM) is often classified separately. In the original White classification, class A was diabetes of any age or duration that did not require insulin.

12. Discuss the other possible adverse outcomes of pregnancy in a woman with diabetes.

The incidence of major congenital anomalies associated with type I diabetes is as high as 10% in some studies, an overall risk of 2–4 times that of control populations. Patients in poor metabolic control and patients with vascular disease are at higher risk. Most likely, metabolic disturbances (hyperglycemia, hypoglycemia) during the period of organogenesis (weeks 3–8) are responsible for the malformations (mostly sacral agenesis and complex cardiac defects). Women who are in good metabolic control at the time of conception and through the first trimester appear to be at much lower risk of having either infants with congenital anomalies or first-trimester spontaneous abortions. Women in class F, R, or RF of the White classification are more likely to have infants with intrauterine growth retardation as well as premature infants.

Maternal morbidity is increased in diabetic pregnant women with retinopathy or nephropathy. Nephropathy (defined by proteinuria) may worsen during pregnancy, but the worsening is rarely permanent. Retinopathy (especially proliferative changes) worsens in a substantial number of women during pregnancy and may not completely regress after delivery.

13. What is gestational diabetes mellitus (GDM)? How is it diagnosed?

GDM is diabetes that is first diagnosed during pregnancy (although it may have existed before pregnancy). Every woman should be screened for GDM, usually between 24 and 28 weeks of gestation, with a randomly administered 50-gram glucose load. Plasma $\geq$ 140 mg/dl; 1 hour after ingestion indicates the need for further diagnostic testing, which consists of administering a 100-gram glucose load to a fasting woman and then measuring hourly glucose levels for 3 hours (see criteria below). If any two values are abnormal or if the fasting glucose is elevated, the patient has GDM and is followed accordingly.

Three-hour Glucose Tolerance Test

TIME	PLASMA GLUCOSE LEVEL (mg/dl)
Fasting	$\geq$ 105
1 hour	$\geq$ 190
2 hours	$\geq$ 165
3 hours	$\geq$ 145

14. What are the criteria for beginning insulin therapy in women with GDM?

Some authors advise starting prophylactic insulin in all women diagnosed with GDM. Most clinicians, however, assess control of diabetes by regularly checking fasting and 2-hour postprandial levels of serum glucose. Adequate control is indicated by a fasting level < 105 and a 2-hour postprandial level < 120. If either value is exceeded twice within 1 week, insulin is usually begun.

15. Describe the changes in respiratory physiology during pregnancy.

Normal pregnancy is a state of mild, compensated respiratory alkalosis. During the first trimester, the pregnant woman hyperventilates by increasing tidal volume by up to 50%. Respiratory rate stays fairly constant. Arterial pH is normal (7.40–7.45) because of renal compensation so that levels of serum bicarbonate fall. Such changes probably occur because of progesterone effects and remain constant throughout pregnancy. Both expiratory reserve volume (ERV) and residual volume (RV), which together make up the functional residual capacity (FRC), fall by a total of 20%, mostly during the third trimester. Vital capacity (VC) is essentially unchanged.

16. How should asthma be managed during pregnancy?

Pregnancy changes the management of asthma very little. Medications used to treat asthma in the nonpregnant patient also may be used during pregnancy. The one possible exception is saturated solution of potassium iodide (SSKI), which occasionally has been used as a mucolytic. The iodine crosses the placenta easily and theoretically may cause fetal thyroid abnormalities.

17. Describe the hemodynamic changes of pregnancy.

By early in the third trimester, cardiac output is increased by up to 500% over prepregnancy levels because of a marked increase in plasma volume (40–50%) and a lesser increase (20–30%) in red cell mass. This increased output causes a physiologic anemia of pregnancy. Despite the marked increase in cardiac output, however, blood pressure falls during pregnancy because of arteriolar vasodilation and a marked decrease in systemic vascular resistance. Pulmonary pressures are largely unchanged. Organs with the largest increase in perfusion are the kidneys, breasts, skin, and uterus.

18. How does pregnancy affect thyroid function?

Despite earlier reports to the contrary, the size of the normal thyroid gland usually does not change significantly during pregnancy when iodine intake is adequate. Because of the effects of estrogen, thyroid-binding globulin level rises 2–3 times above normal, and levels of total thyroxine (T_4) and total triiodothyronine (T_3) rise concomitantly. Levels of free T_4 and free T_3 stay within the normal to low-normal range. Levels of thyroid-stimulating hormone (TSH) may fall slightly during early pregnancy because of the weak thyroid-stimulating activity of beta human chorionic gonadotropin (hCG) but return to normal during the second and third trimesters.

19. How does renal disease affect pregnancy?

Renal disease, especially moderate-to-severe renal disease (serum creatinine > 1.4 mg/dl) increases the risks of preterm delivery, cesarean section, fetal growth restriction, maternal hypertension, and preeclampsia. Fetal survival is moderately reduced (~93%).

Maternal renal function may be markedly affected by pregnancy in women whose initial serum creatinine is > 1.4 mg/dl. Only 60% of women have stable renal function 6 months after delivery. Thirty-five percent of women whose initial serum creatinine is ≥ 2.0 mg/dl are at risk for endstage renal failure as a result of pregnancy.

20. How does pregnancy affect the diagnosis of hyperthyroidism?

Diagnosis of hyperthyroidism during pregnancy may be difficult because signs and symptoms such as tachycardia, palpitations, heat intolerance, emotional lability, and diaphoresis may be seen with normal pregnancy. Poor weight gain and persistent tachycardia along with a goiter suggest the diagnosis. Laboratory evaluation is made by demonstrating elevated values of free T_3, free T_4, and suppressed TSH. Transient hyperthyroidism also may be seen with hyperemesis gravidarum (persistent vomiting, tachycardia, and weight loss during pregnancy). Hyperthyroidism in this setting is transient and does not require treatment.

21. How should a woman with seizures be treated during pregnancy?

A patient whose seizures are controlled by medication generally should continue medication during pregnancy. Although no antiepileptic agent is safe during pregnancy, uncontrolled seizures are harmful to both mother and fetus. If a woman has been seizure-free for 2 years, she may attempt to discontinue medication before becoming pregnant. If withdrawal is successful, she may be followed expectantly during gestation.

If possible, women taking valproic acid should change to another medication before becoming pregnant. Although published data in humans are not completely clear, valproic acid has been implicated in a number of congenital anomalies, but the major concern is neural tube defects. Trimethadione is clearly associated with a constellation of congenital anomalies and should be avoided during pregnancy.

22. How does infection with the human immunodeficiency virus (HIV) affect pregnancy?

The incidence of perinatal transmission is 20–30% without treatment. However, treatment of HIV-infected women with zidovudine during pregnancy and delivery has been shown to decrease the incidence of vertical transmission by about two-thirds. Zidovudine also should be given to the newborn, and breast-feeding should be discouraged because of the risk of transmission via colostrum and breast milk. Zidovudine is well tolerated by the fetus and the newborn but should not be given during the first trimester of pregnancy. Anemia and growth retardation have been observed in newborns of women treated with zidovudine during gestation.

23. What is the significance of asymptomatic bacteriuria during pregnancy?

Asymptomatic bacteriuria may occur in up to 5–10% of pregnant women. Unlike their non-pregnant counterparts, up to 40% of these women may develop infections. Such infections may have a deleterious effect on pregnancy, especially if pyelonephritis ensues. Therefore, all pregnant women with asymptomatic bacteriuria should be treated with antibiotics. In women with recurrences, daily suppressive doses of antibiotics may be indicated until after delivery.

24. How should a pregnant woman with deep venous thrombosis be treated?

In general, warfarin should be avoided during pregnancy, because it crosses the placenta and has been associated with fetal malformations as well as neurologic dysfunction. In a pregnant women with a documented blood clot, acute therapy should be given with intravenous heparin followed by intermittent (2 or 3 times/day) subcutaneous heparin for several weeks in doses adequate to keep the midinterval partial thromboplastin time at 1.5–2 times control. Thereafter, she should be maintained on low-dose subcutaneous heparin (5,000–10,000 U twice daily) until delivery.

Warfarin is then generally substituted until 4–6 weeks after delivery. A woman taking warfarin may breastfeed her baby.

Women who have had thrombosis in a prior pregnancy are generally considered to be at risk if they again become pregnant. They are treated with low-dose subcutaneous heparin throughout gestation. Although opinions differ as to the proper dose, heparin levels apparently fall as pregnancy proceeds, if the amount is not increased accordingly. We therefore recommend 5,000 U subcutaneously twice daily in the first trimester; 7,500 U twice daily in the second trimester; and 10,000 U twice daily in the third trimester. Because the risk of thromboembolic events may persist in the early postpartum period, warfarin is used as above.

Low-molecular-weight heparin may have some advantages during pregnancy because of its longer half-life, which may allow once daily dosing with fewer bleeding complications. Low-molecular-weight heparin does not cross the placenta and has been used safely during pregnancy.

BIBLIOGRAPHY

1. Barbour LA, Pickard J: Controversies in thromboembolic disease during pregnancy: A critical review. Obstet Gynecol 86:621–633, 1995.
2. Bares VA: Diabetes and pregnancy. Med Clin North Am 73:685–700, 1989.
3. Connor EM, Sperling RS, Gelber R, et al: Reduction of maternal-infant transmission of human immunodeficiency virus type I with zidovudine treatment. N Engl J Med 331:1173–1180, 1994.
4. Gianopoulos JG: Cardiac disease in pregnancy. Med Clin North Am 73:639–651, 1989.
5. Glinoer D, de Nayer P, Bourdoux P, et al: Regulation of maternal thyroid during pregnancy. J Clin Endocrinol Metab 71:276–287, 1990.
6. Greenberger PA, Patterson R: Management of asthma during pregnancy. N Engl J Med 312:897–902, 1985.
7. Jones DC, Hayslett JP: Outcome of pregnancy in women with moderate or severe renal insufficiency. N Engl J Med 335:257–265, 1996.
8. Jovanonic-Peterson C, Petersen CM: Pregnancy in the diabetic woman: Guidelines for a successful outcome. Endocrinol Metab Clin North Am 21:433–455, 1992.
9. Mestman JH, Goodwin TM, Montoro MM: Thyroid disorders of pregnancy. Endocrinol Metab Clin North Am 24:41–71, 1995.
10. Nelson-Piercy C, Letsky EA, de Swiet M; Low-molecular-weight heparin for obstetric thromboprophylaxis: Experience of sixty-nine pregnancies in sixty-one women at high risk. Am J Obstet Gynecol 176: 1062–1068, 1997.
11. Shuster EA: Seizures in pregnancy. Emerg Med Clin North Am 12:1013–1025, 1994.
12. Sibai BM: Drug therapy: Treatment of hypertension in pregnant women. N Engl J Med 335:257–265, 1996.
13. Sperling RS, Shapiro DE, Coombs RW, et al: Maternal viral load, zidovudine treatment, and the risk of transmission of human immunodeficiency virus type I from mother to infant. N Engl J Med 335: 1621–1629, 1996.

XV. Drug Interactions

111. COMMON DRUG INTERACTIONS AND TOXICITY

Donald B. Hansen, B.S. Pharm, Pharm D., Julie Rifkin, M.D., and Robert Valuck, Ph.D., R.Ph.

1. List five levels at which drug interactions may occur.

1. Gastrointestinal absorption interactions
2. Plasma protein-binding interactions
3. Metabolic enzyme interactions
4. Renal excretion interactions
5. Pharmacodynamic interactions

2. If a pair of drugs is stated to interact, must one be stopped?

Not necessarily. Interactions range from effects that are detectable only with laboratory testing to effects that are clinically significant—and predictably so. If an interaction is known to produce clinically significant effects, it can be tracked as it occurs, and dosages can be adjusted to compensate. If other agents are available and the potential for adverse outcome is great, alternative therapy should be offered.

3. Does all drug interaction result in an adverse drug reaction (ADR)?

A drug interaction does not necessarily result in an ADR, even with documentable changes in drug level or physiologic parameters. The specific definition of an ADR varies but usually addresses the following issues: severity of outcome; whether the drug met therapeutic indications; and whether the adverse reaction occurred after an overdose, on withdrawal, or as a failure of the expected pharmacologic action.

4. What is a reportable ADR?

A reportable ADR is defined as a reaction that is (1) suspected to be secondary to drug therapy, (2) uncommon or not described in the package insert, or (3) severe in nature, requiring treatment or prolonging hospitalization. All ADRs should be recorded in the progress notes of the patient's medical record, along with outcome and treatment. ADRs that fit the above criteria should be reported to the institution through the mechanism approved by the local Pharmacy and Therapeutics Committee. If the institution does not have a mechanism for forwarding the information to the Food and Drug Administration (FDA), the physician may call the FDA directly at 1-800-FDA-1088. Such reports contribute to postmarketing surveillance of the drug.

5. How can I determine the likelihood that a drug caused an adverse event?

Perhaps the most important problem in assessing ADRs is determining whether there is a causal relationship between consumption of the drug and occurrence of an adverse event. Various algorithms are available to assist the clinician in determining the causal probability of a suspected ADR. The algorithms range from simple to complex; some have been automated and put into computer software format. Each clinician may find a different algorithm most useful in his or her practice setting. One time-tested, well-validated example of an ADR probability assessment scale is that of Naranjo et al., who suggested a list of 10 questions to assess ADR causality. The questions, answer choices, and score values are as follow:

QUESTIONS	ANSWERS AND VALUES		
	YES	NO	DON'T KNOW
1. Are there previous *conclusive* reports of this reaction?	+1	0	0
2. Did the adverse event appear after the suspected drug was administered?	+2	−1	0
3. Did the adverse reaction improve when the drug was discontinued or a *specific* antagonist was administered?	+1	0	0
4. Did the adverse reaction reappear when the drug was readministered?	+2	−1	0
5. Are there alternative factors (other than the drug) that could have caused the reaction?	−1	+2	0
6. Did the reaction appear when a placebo was given?	−1	+1	0
7. Was the drug detected in the blood (or other fluids) in concentrations known to be toxic?	+1	0	0
8. Was the reaction more severe when the dose was increased or less severe when the dose was decreased?	+1	0	0
9. Did the patient have a similar reaction to the same or similar drugs in any previous exposure?	+1	0	0
10. Was the adverse event confirmed by any objective evidence?	+1	0	0

To calculate a causal probability for an ADR, sum the scores for the 10 questions, and refer the total score to the following ranges;

Score	ADR causal probability
9–13	Definite
5–8	Probable
1–4	Possible
(−)4–0	Doubtful

The resulting causal probability category for the suspected ADR gives the clinician a crude but fairly reliable method for determining whether in fact a drug has caused an adverse event. Several adverse event reporting systems in the United States use similar questions (if not the entire Naranjo algorithm) for determination and classification of ADRs.

6. Do drug interactions occur with alcohol and caffeine?

Yes. Alcohol abuse in patients taking warfarin prolongs the prothrombin time and predisposes to gastric microbleeding. Alcohol also disturbs glycemic control, adding to the hypoglycemia produced by drugs such as sulfonylureas. Metronidazole inhibits the metabolic oxidation of alcohol and may produce the disulfiram reaction of nausea, vomiting, and malaise in the presence of alcohol. The effect varies highly among the population.

Caffeine blocks the antiarrhythmic effects of adenosine IV; like theophylline, it is a competitive agonist for the adenosine receptor. Because the antagonism is competitive, the effect varies and may be clinically important only in the heavy coffee drinker. Ciprofloxacin and enoxacin (but probably not ofloxacin) inhibit the metabolism of caffeine and theophylline, resulting in higher levels than anticipated and requiring dosage adjustment.

7. Define steady-state concentration.

Steady state is achieved when the dosage intake per unit of time equals the elimination rate and fluctuations between peak and trough plasma levels remain fairly constant. Most drugs are eliminated by first-order kinetics. The time required to achieve steady state for first-order kinetic medications can be determined by the half-life of the drug. Steady-state levels generally are achieved at the end of 3–4 half-lives.

8. When is a loading dose used?

A loading dose is used when it is necessary to provide a rigid therapeutic concentration of a drug, often in the presence of a long half-life. Classes of drugs for which loading doses are used include aminoglycosides, antiarrhythmics, and anticonvulsants.

9. What are the pitfalls in the interpretation of plasma drug concentrations?

Drug levels must be interpreted in light of the patient's clinical status. The major pitfall in interpreting drug assays probably relates to timing of the blood level. A rule of thumb is that 5.5 drug half-lives are needed before steady-state concentrations are achieved. Accurate peak and trough levels cannot be measured except at steady-state concentrations. Sample timing is critically important. Thus, the best time to draw drug levels is immediately before the next dose, during a steady-state infusion, or at least 8 hours after a dose when the drug is taken twice daily. Renal and hepatic alterations of half-life must be considered. The patient's age, height, and sex as well as possible alterations in drug absorption, binding, and active metabolites may have unpredictable effects on plasma drug levels.

10. Which drugs commonly require monitoring by serum levels? Why?

1. **Aminoglycosides** may cause nephrotoxicity and/or ototoxicity at high levels and are significantly affected by changes in creatinine clearance. Serum peak and trough levels are therefore useful for monitoring. Optimal sampling strategies for single daily dose aminoglycosides have yet to be determined.

2. **Tricyclic antidepressants** display great variations in blood level, depending on dosage. African-Americans usually have 50% greater blood levels than Caucasians for the same dose schedule. In geriatric patients conventional doses may lead to toxic levels. Furthermore, symptoms of overdose may mimic the symptoms for which the drug was prescribed. Steady-state plasma levels are achieved after about 2 weeks on a given dosage.

3. Serum levels of **anticonvulsant medications** are helpful in assessing compliance and during use of more than one anticonvulsant. Plasma concentrations of a given drug may increase or decrease when a second agent is added.

4. Serum levels of **digoxin** are useful to confirm or prevent toxicity. Advanced patient age, renal insufficiency, and/or concomitant use of quinidine elevate digoxin levels.

11. How does an anaphylactoid reaction differ from anaphylaxis?

Anaphylaxis and anaphylactoid reactions produce identical clinical signs and symptoms but differ in the mechanism and predictability of the reaction. Anaphylaxis is an immunoglobulin E (IgE)-mediated event that occurs after exposure in a previously sensitized person. The anaphylactoid reaction is not IgE-mediated and does not require previous exposure to the inciting substance. Both reactions may cause various symptoms, including flushing, urticaria, angioedema, tachycardia, hypotension, syncope, shock, laryngeal edema, wheezing, diaphoresis, abdominal pain, diarrhea, and vomiting. The symptoms are due to intact cell-derived and basophil-derived mediators. A classic example of an anaphylactoid reaction is the response to radiocontrast.

A person who has had one anaphylactoid reaction has a 60% chance of a second reaction when exposed to the same agent. No specific characteristics identify a patient who may be at risk for an anaphylactoid reaction initially or on a repeat exposure. Measures to decrease the repeat reactions include pharmacologic prophylaxis with diphenhydramine and corticosteroids.

12. Can orally administered drugs cause anaphylaxis?

Yes. Penicillin given orally or parenterally is the most common cause of anaphylaxis. The anaphylactic death rate is approximately 1–2/10,000 patients treated with penicillin. A personal or family history of allergies does not predict who will react to penicillin. A person with a history of any penicillin allergy is assumed to be allergic to all penicillins, unless a skin test to both major and minor determinants is negative. Cephalosporins cannot be considered a safe alternative because of cross-reactivity.

13. Which patients should not be given charcoal after an overdose? Which patients should not be induced to vomit?

Activated charcoal must not be given if ingestion of a corrosive substance is suspected (e.g., ammonia, bleach). In such patients it has no proved efficacy and obscures an endoscopic examination. The use of activated charcoal after acetaminophen overdose is generally not recommended because it binds to the antidote, N-acetyl-L-cysteine (NAC), in vitro. If ingestion of Tylenol and other agents is suspected, administration of activated charcoal within the first 4 hours may be useful.

Syrup of ipepac should not be used to induce emesis in patients who are comatose, experience seizures, or have an inadequate gag reflex. Suspected ingestion of corrosive substances is a contraindication to emesis, because exposure to the vomitus causes reinjury. Ingestion of poorly absorbed hydrocarbons (e.g., gasoline, kerosene) is not treated by emesis because the risk of aspiration outweighs the potential for central nervous system depression. Suspicion of coingestion of sharp, solid objects negates emesis therapy.

14. Name five drug overdoses that may cause arrhythmogenic death and thus require electrocardiographic (EKG) monitoring.

Drug toxicity may alter the intrinsic firing rate of pacemaker cells or conduction in one pathway, thus allowing the formation of a reentry circuit that triggers tachydysrhythmia. Dysrhythmias may result from both altered conduction and altered automaticity. Several drug overdoses may cause arrhythmogenic death, including (1) digoxin, (2) virtually all classes of antiarrhythmic drugs, (3) tricyclic antidepressants (overdoses prolong PR and QRS intervals and cause various other EKG abnormalities), (4) phenothiazine (overdoses cause dysrhythmia and hypotension), and (5) cocaine. Thus, cardiac monitoring is essential in cases of overdose or toxicity.

15. When should patients be treated for acetaminophen toxicity?

Patients should be treated for acetaminophen toxicity whenever it is suspected. Treatment is life-saving and nontoxic. If a patient presents within 4 hours of ingestion, gut decontamination may be used. NAC should be given within 8–10 hours of ingestion but may be effective up to 24 hours after ingestion. Therapy should be guided by levels corresponding to the Rumack-Matthew homogram but initiated promptly if toxicity is suspected. **Do not delay** therapy with NAC past 8–12 hours to await drug levels.

16. What is a toxicology screen? When is it cost-effective?

No single, inexpensive method detects all toxins. A toxicology screen does not provide blood levels of specific substances or drugs. Blood toxic screens generally detect the presence of benzodiazepines, barbiturates, cocaine, methadone, nicotine, caffeine, salicylates, and tricyclics. Qualitative evidence of metabolites of therapeutic agents and drugs of abuse is found in the urine rather than the serum.

A specific request for a blood level aids in management of toxicity due to acetaminophen, salicylates, carboxyhemoglobin, methemoglobin, methanol, ethylene glycol, lithium, iron, digoxin, theophylline, organophosphates, ethanol, phenytoin, lead, and arsenic.

Patients with an altered sensorium for whom the physical examination and available history fail to provide a cause should be suspected of having a toxic-metabolic disorder. Unexplained hypo- or hyperthermia, distinctive odors, miotic or mydriatic pupils, abdominal pain, nausea, vomiting, tremors, seizures, and coma are clues to poisoning syndromes. Various laboratory abnormalities may be due to drug toxicity, including unusual coloration of urine, hemolysis, coagulopathy, elevated levels of creatine phosphokinase (CPK), rhabdomyolysis, electrolyte abnormalities, and anion and/or osmolar gap.

17. What are the principles of treating drug overdoses?

1. Support the patient. Airway protection, oxygenation, and treatment of circulatory collapse should be initiated immediately.

2. Reduce further drug absorption. When appropriate, induced emesis, gastric lavage, oral activated charcoal, and/or cathartics should be used.

3. Enhance drug elimination. Alkalinization, diuresis, hemodialysis, and hemoperfusion are possibilities.

4. Give an antagonist or antidote, if possible. Only 5% of poisons have specific antidotes.

5. Prevent recurrences. Education, psychiatric evaluation, and rehabilitation should be initiated to decrease recurrent ingestions.

18. What principles should be followed in prescribing drugs for elderly patients?

Factor that predispose older patients to adverse drug reactions include multisystem disease, greater severity of disease, female sex, small body size, hepatic or renal insufficiency, and previous drug reactions. The following principles are useful for prescribing mediations to people over 65 years of age:

1. Ask about use of over-the-counter medications.

2. Simplify a patient's drug regimen whenever possible (avoid polypharmacy).

3. Remember that creatinine clearance, gastrointestinal motility, total body water, lean body mass, cardiac output, hepatic mass, and hepatic blood flow are decreased in the elderly.

4. In general, use smaller doses of medications (50% or less).

19. Which common drugs are likely to cause side effects in elderly patients and thus should be avoided?

Several medications place elderly patients at risk for adverse side effects. Any medication that may cause sedation, syncope, or confusion places the patient at risk for a fall. Other side effects to be avoided include urinary retention, anorexia, urinary incontinence, constipation, and dry mouth. Drugs to be avoided in the elderly patient include amitriptyline, propoxyphene, dipyridamole, chlorpropamide, chlordiazepoxide, diazepam, indomethacin, methyldopa, propranolol, and muscle relaxants.

20. Which disease states lead to alteration in drug pharmacokinetics?

1. **Renal insufficiency** is associated with toxic levels of drugs that are cleared by urinary excretion. Commonly used antibiotics that require dosage adjustment in patients with renal insufficiency include aminoglycosides, penicillins and cephalosporins, and vancomycin. Reduced doses may be administered at normal intervals, or the usual dose may be administered less frequently.

2. **Liver disease** leads to altered pharmacokinetics in an unpredictable manner. Biotransformation of drugs metabolized primarily by the liver may be accelerated or impaired. Overall, hepatic drug clearance is often only mildly to moderately altered by liver dysfunction, and liver function tests do not predict the degree of alteration in drug clearance. However, patients with portocaval shunts do have first-pass hepatic metabolism or high blood flow to the liver. Concentrations of propranolol, lidocaine, meperidine, and phenytoin are notably increased in patients with liver failure.

3. **Hypotension and circulatory insufficiency** alter pharmacokinetics, because the body preserves blood flow to the heart and brain at the expense of other organs. The effective volume of distribution is smaller, and the central nervous system and heart are exposed to higher drug concentrations than found in the plasma. There are no useful methods to determine the exact alteration in drug dose in this setting. In patients with heart failure, lower doses of lidocaine, procainamide, and theophylline are used. Loading doses should be conservative, and the patient must be followed closely for indications of drug toxicity.

BIBLIOGRAPHY

1. Bochner BS, Lichtenstein LM: Anaphylaxis. N Engl J Med 324:1785–1790, 1991.
2. Ellenhan MJ, Barcelaux D: Medical Toxicology: Diagnosis and Treatment of Human Poisoning. New York, Elsevier, 1988.
3. Gentry CA, Paloucek EP, Rodvold KA: Prediction of acetaminophen concentrations in overdose patients using a Bayesian pharmacokinetic model. J Toxicol 32:17–30, 1994.
4. Hoffman RS, Smilkstein MJ, Howland MA, Goldfrank MR: Osmol groups revisited: Normal values and limitations. J Toxicol 31:81–93, 1994.
5. Jacobs DS, Kaston BL, et al: Laboratory Test Handbook, 2nd ed. Baltimore, Williams & Wilkins, 1990.
6. Montamat SC, Cuoack BJ, Vestal RE: Management of drug therapy in the elderly. N Engl J Med 321:303–309, 1991.
7. Naranjo CA, Busto U, Sellers EM, et al: A method for estimating the probability of adverse drug reactions. Clin Pharmacol Ther 30:239–245, 1981.
8. Talbert RL: Drug dosing in renal insufficiency. J Clin Pharmacol 34(2):99–110, 1994.
9. Wilcox SM, Himmelstein DU, Woodhandler S: Inappropriate drug prescribing for the community-dwelling elderly. JAMA 272:292–296, 1994.

INDEX

Page numbers in **boldface type** indicate complete chapters.